Lucas's Pathology of Tumors of the Oral Tissues

Lucas's Pathology of Tumors of the Oral Tissues

Roderick A. Cawson MD FDSRCS (England) FDSRCPS (Glasgow) FRCPath
Emeritus Professor in Oral Medicine and Pathology, Eastman Dental Institute for Oral Health Care Sciences, University of London, London, UK, and Department of Surgery, Guy's Hospital, London, UK

William H. Binnie BDS DDS MSD FDSRCPS (Glasgow) FRCPath
Professor and Chairman of Diagnostic Sciences, Baylor College of Dentistry – A Member of the Texas A&M University Systems, Dallas, Texas, USA

Paul Speight BDS PhD FDSRCPS FRCPath
Professor of Oral Pathology, Eastman Dental Institute for Oral Health Care Sciences, London, UK, and Honorary Consultant in Oral Pathology, University College Hospitals NHS Trust, London, UK

Andrew W. Barrett BDS MSc PhD FDSRCS(Edin) DipRCPath
Lecturer and Honorary Senior Registrar in Oral Pathology, Eastman Dental Institute for Oral Health Care Sciences, University of London, London, UK

John M. Wright DDS MS
Professor and Director of Pathology, Baylor College of Dentistry – A Member of the Texas A&M University System, Dallas, Texas, USA

with a contribution by

Peter Thorogood BSc PhD
Professor and Head of the Department of Developmental Biology, Institute of Child Health, University of London, London, UK

FIFTH EDITION

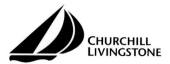

CHURCHILL LIVINGSTONE

LONDON • EDINBURGH • NEW YORK • PHILADELPHIA • SYDNEY AND TORONTO 1998

CHURCHILL LIVINGSTONE
A division of Harcourt Brace & Co Limited

© Harcourt Brace & Co Ltd 1998

◢▱ is a registered trade mark of Harcourt Brace and Company
Limited 1998

First edition 1964
Second edition 1972
Third edition 1976
Fourth edition 1984
Fifth edition 1998

ISBN 0 443 03990 9

British Library Cataloguing in Publication Data
A catalogue record for this book is available from the British
Library.

Library of Congress Cataloging in Publication Data
A catalog record for this book is available from the Library of
Congress.

Medical knowledge is constantly changing. As new information
becomes available, changes in treatment, procedures, equipment
and the use of drugs become necessary. The editors/authors/
contributors and the publishers have, as far as it is possible, taken
care to ensure that the information given in the text is accurate
and up to date. However, readers are strongly advised to confirm
that the information, especially with regard to drug usage,
complies with latest legislation and standards of practice.

The
publisher's
policy is to use
**paper manufactured
from sustainable forests**

Produced by Addison Wesley Longman China Limited, Hong Kong
C&C/01

Contents

Preface

'Lucas's Pathology of Tumors of the Oral Tissues' has been justifiably esteemed for its textual content as well as the superb quality and setting of the black and white illustrations. We feel honoured therefore to have been asked to rewrite this new edition.

This fifth edition largely follows the approach used by Professor Lucas but with the passage of fourteen years since the last edition several changes have inevitably had to be made. First and most obviously, advances in technology have made it possible to have the illustrations in color.

Second, new entities have become recognized in the intervening years and have been included. Knowledge about well recognized tumors has also accumulated and has been included.

Third, the arrangement of the text has been changed slightly. Emphasis has therefore been placed on odontogenic tumors and cysts which have been brought together in the early part of the book. This is partly because some of these tumors are cystic and some of the cysts, notably odontogenic keratocysts, behave in tumor-like fashion. To take an extreme example also, the differential diagnosis between glandular odontogenic cyst and intraosseous mucoepidermoid carcinoma has been seriously discussed. The general pathologist will also be less familiar with these lesions than tumors which only incidentally affect the oral soft tissues and jaws and it was obviously appropriate to bring them together.

Fourth, non odontogenic tumors have been dealt with in greater detail, as oral pathologists accredited or in training, will be less familiar with them. Furthermore, the standards for accreditation have risen so considerably in recent years that it gave another reason for treating these diseases more extensively.

Fifth, considerably more emphasis has been placed on behavior and management, particularly because the response to treatment is an important guide as to a tumor's potential. Moreover, it is by no means certain that some tumors in the oral regions behave in the same way as their counterparts in other regions. Certainly, the operative constraints on surgery in the head and neck area also affect the outcome. Some tumors are however so uncommon in the oral and perioral regions that reports of the response of small numbers of them are conflicting, but need to be considered.

Finally, a few particularly rare diseases, such as mastocytosis of the jaws, have been included with the aim of drawing attention to them in the hope that awareness will lead to enhancement of knowledge by encouraging the reporting of more cases.

Our aim therefore has been to help general pathologists who will see relatively little material from the orofacial region as well as oral pathologists in position or in training.

Acknowledgements

We would like to express our appreciation of the fact that we have had the privilege of access to Professor Ivor Kramer's extensive collection of histopathological material. We must also thank the clinicians – unfortunately too numerous to mention by name – who have kindly submitted material to us over the years.

Embryology and histology of the oral tissues

Introduction to the diagnosis of oral tumors

1

Most processes in the histopathological investigation of tumors of the oral cavity are the same as those followed at any other site, but there are factors attributable to the anatomical locality which may need to be considered. There are also tumors which are seen only in the jaws.

JAW LESIONS

RADIOLOGY

Other than the special stains discussed below, radiology is the most frequent diagnostic aid requested by oral histopathologists, most of whom will issue no more than a differential diagnosis without the aid of appropriate films. All osteolytic and osteosynthetic tumors can affect the maxilla and mandible, albeit rarely. However, the jaws are distinguished by the presence of teeth and, as a consequence, are the commonest skeletal site for cysts which, though benign in all but exceptional cases, have variable radiographic appearances. These will be discussed in more detail with the individual lesions. Anomalies in the odontogenic apparatus also give rise to a group of tumors seen at no other anatomical site. Several of these have similar histological features, and the information available in radiographs may be essential for accurate diagnosis. For many lesions, 'conventional' views such as panoramic tomographs, periapical, and occlusal radiographs or, for lesions extending into the maxillary sinuses, occipitomental films are all that are required. Sialography may be useful for neoplasms of the major salivary glands. However, computed tomography and magnetic resonance imaging have provided better visualization of tumors affecting the complex three-dimensional structure of the facial skeleton and base of skull. Because of the rarity of many jaw tumors, radiologists may be unfamiliar with their appearances and clinical behavior, and the diagnostic histopathologist should have no hesitation in requesting films for inspection.

Other techniques, for example ultrasonography and technetium scanning, provide little extra information that cannot be gleaned by using one or other of the above means.

PREPARATION OF HARD-TISSUE SPECIMENS

As with any other bony resection, partially or totally excised jaw specimens need to be radiographed before demineralization, ideally in at least two planes. After blocks of the attached soft tissues have been selected, the entire resection can be slowly demineralized with organic acids. Immersion in strong mineral acids such as nitric acid should be avoided in order to retain the architecture of the specimen as much as possible. This is especially important in maxillectomies, where the bony skeleton is fragile and easily disrupted. By contrast, the density of mandibular bone means that decalcification time may be protracted for longer than is desirable, in which case transverse sections, usually in a buccolingual plane, can be removed with a band saw and decalcified separately from the remainder, which is left in formalin. Even then, specimens containing dental tissues can take several weeks to decalcify adequately before processing is possible.

Occasionally it is necessary to prepare ground sections of teeth, the usual indication for this being the need to identify developmental dental abnormalities, for example amelogenesis or dentinogenesis imperfecta. In such situations it is customary to take the necessary ground sections before decalcifying the remainder of the tooth for processing and wax embedding.

ORAL MUCOSA

The request form must include the site of the biopsy, since normal oral mucosa shows regional variations in structure. Epithelium lining the cheeks, vestibules, ventral surface of the tongue, floor of mouth, and soft palate is normally nonkeratinized. By contrast, the stratified squamous epithelium covering the hard palate and gingivae is orthokeratinized. Keratinized filiform and fungiform papillae and, posteriorly, lymphoid follicles, circumvallate papillae, and taste buds may be seen on the surface of the mucosa of the dorsal surface of the tongue. Parakeratinization, mild epithelial hyperplasia, and chronic inflammatory cell infiltration are frequent and unremarkable findings at any oral site and reflect day-to-day trauma to the mucosa. In older patients, degenerative or inflammatory changes are common findings in salivary tissue. Minor salivary gland tumors affect the upper lip more frequently than the lower lip. Malignant salivary disease relatively more frequently affects the minor and sublingual glands than the submandibular and parotid glands. The presence of striated muscle or minor salivary gland on the deep aspect provides evidence as to the adequacy of the depth of the biopsy.

SPECIAL STAINS

The structures peculiar to the oral and perioral region call for frequent use of some special stains. Mucin stains in particular may be necessary to establish the glandular nature of a poorly differentiated carcinoma; periodic acid/Schiff (PAS) stains should be used with and without diastase digestion. Alcian blue or mucicarmine are valuable adjunctive stains. Many oral pathology laboratories routinely stain all mucosal biopsies with PAS to determine the presence of *Candida* in order to recommend antifungal treatment if necessary, particularly in dysplastic hyperkeratoses where candidal infection possibly has a role in progression towards frank malignancy.

PAS staining can also confirm the presence of mucous metaplasia in the epithelial lining of odontogenic cysts, but there are no stains uniquely used for odontogenic tissues. Immunohistochemistry has shown that coexpression of cytokeratins 5 and 19, whilst by no means specific, is characteristic of odontogenic epithelium[1] and may therefore be of use in determining the origin of ectopic epithelial tissue. Immunohistochemistry has so far proved unhelpful in the identification of salivary tumors. Despite claims that S100 expression identifies some salivary adenocarcinomas, few specialists in this field would regard this as having any diagnostic specificity. Otherwise, immunohistochemistry is used at orofacial sites as it is elsewhere; the antibodies most often used are those to intermediate filaments and CD45 RA or RB (leucocyte common antigen) in anaplastic tumors; those to S100 protein if a neural or melanocytic lesion is suspected (supported by HMB45, MELAN-A, or NKI/C3 to confirm melanoma); those to CD3 or CD45RO (T cells), CD19 or CD20 (B cells), or CD21 (follicular dendritic cells) to determine ontogeny in lymphomas; and those to κ and λ light chains to determine monotypic expression in B cell or plasmacytic tumors.

A marker for invasive potential of dysplastic oral mucosal lesions has yet to be identified and, despite early promise, changes in cytokeratin profiles are unhelpful. Recent work using molecular biologic techniques such as the polymerase chain reaction and in situ hybridization have shown, however, that progression to mucosa-associated lymphoid tissue (MALT) lymphoma may be predicted from analysis of the lymphoid infiltrate in the salivary glands of patients with Sjögren's syndrome.[2] When this happens, the site of the tumor may be at any MALT site.

CYTOPATHOLOGY

EXFOLIATIVE CYTOLOGY

Cytopathology is not used as an investigation of oral disease as it has been in the cervix. The easy access for biopsy means that exfoliative cytology has minimal advantages, especially as it provides less information than conventional histopathology. Nevertheless, Ogden et al[3] showed that quantitative oral exfoliative cytology could determine changes in the nuclear/cytoplasmic ratio in neoplastic keratinocytes and so might have a role in identifying subjects with field change who might be at risk of a second oral malignancy. Furthermore, smears from malignant and normal oral mucosa show differences in expression of cytokeratins[4] and p53.[5] Despite these findings, the technique still awaits general recognition as a diagnostic tool. One possible indication for this method is where biopsy is inadvisable because of avascularity, for example in areas exposed to therapeutic irradiation.

FINE-NEEDLE ASPIRATION CYTOLOGY

Despite the frequently bland cytology and often focal distribution of salivary neoplasms, cytopathology of fine-needle aspirates can produce a definitive diagnosis in over 85% of salivary tumors, with high sensitivity (89%) and specificity (94%) but low false-positive and false-negative values (4%).[6] The attainment of such accuracy demands extensive experience and a high standard of vigilance. Schelkun & Grundy,[7] analyzing fine-needle aspirates from 213 head and neck lesions found a false-positive rate of 0.5% and a false-negative rate of 2.3%. Sensitivity was 81% and specificity 99% for malignant tumors. A more traditional, but gradually disappearing, application of aspiration has been in cysts, aspirates from which are stained with hematoxylin and eosin (H&E), PAS and Papanicolaou, with an unfixed, unstained smear in an aqueous mountant also analyzed. Shimmering cholesterol crystals may be observed under polarized light in radicular and dentigerous cysts, although they are not pathognomonic.

REFERENCES

1. Gao Z, Williams DM, Cruchley AT 1989 Cytokeratin expression of the odontogenic epithelia in dental follicles and developmental cysts. J Oral Pathol Med 18: 63–67
2. Jordan RC, Pringle JH, Speight PM 1985 High frequency of light chain restriction in labial gland biopsies of Sjögren's syndrome detected by in situ hybridization. J Pathol 177: 35–40
3. Ogden GR, Cowpe JG, Green MW 1991 Detection of field change in oral cancer using oral exfoliative cytologic study. Cancer 68: 1611–1615
4. Ogden GR, McQueen S, Chisholm DM, Lane EB 1993 Keratin profiles of normal and malignant oral mucosa using exfoliative cytology. J Clin Pathol 46: 352–356
5. Ogden GR, Cowpe JG, Chisholm DM, Lane DP 1994 p53 immunostaining as a marker for oral cancer in diagnostic cytopathology – preliminary report. Cytopathology 5: 47–53
6. Kocjan G, Nayagam M, Harris M 1990 Fine needle aspiration cytology of salivary gland lesions: advantages and pitfalls. Cytopathology 1: 269–275
7. Schelkun PM, Grundy WG 1991 Fine needle aspiration biopsy of head and neck lesions. J Oral Maxillofac Surg 49: 262–267

The embryology and histology of the oral tissues

P. Thorogood

In order to understand many of the pathologic processes that affect the face and mouth, knowledge of how the orofacial complex is formed in the embryo, together with an appreciation of the developmental history of its component tissues, is a prerequisite. In this sense, the orofacial complex can be regarded as a modular structure, with contributions from diverse cell lineages. Its embryonic development comprises a sequence of highly coordinated patterns of growth and morphogenetic events such as cell migration, fusion of epithelia, tissue invaginations and evaginations, cell polarization, tissue interactions/cell signaling, and directed extracellular matrix secretion. These developmental events are precisely coordinated in a spatiotemporal sense, thereby generating a structure in which all the modular contributions are anatomically 'in register,' thus ensuring functional integration. Therefore, position and timing become critically important at the cell level during orofacial development. The morphogenetic complexity means that the orofacial region is particularly sensitive to perturbation by genetic mutation or environmental teratogens, and this is reflected in the fact that one-third of all major birth defects involve the head and face.[1]

CELL LINEAGE AND THE EVOLUTION OF THE HEAD

The diversity of cell lineages within the embryonic head is fundamentally important. In this respect the dual source of mesenchyme, from the 'ectomesenchyme' of the neural crest *and* from mesoderm is pivotal. Indeed, much of the connective tissue and the peripheral nervous system in the head, face, and neck is derived from the cephalic neural crest,[2,3] with the ectodermal placodes making a significant contribution to the cranial sensory ganglia.[4] Thus, the greater part of the skeletal tissue and the cranial ganglia, the odontoblasts of the teeth, the corneal stromal fibroblasts, the fascia of the facial muscles, the smooth muscle associated with major blood vessels, dermis, the stroma of the salivary glands, and melanocytes have a common embryonic origin. They are all derived from that transient population of cells, the neural crest, which emerges by a localized de-epithelialization at the margin of the neural plate during neurulation and which proceeds to migrate throughout the body of the embryo

(Fig. 2.1). The question of what generates the enormous diversity of crest-derived tissues remains unsettled. Evidence from different experimental strategies supports either intrinsic multipotency within neural crest cells, or interactions between crest cells and their environment, or both. In contrast to the crest derivatives, mesodermal mesenchyme (i.e. mesenchyme derived from the internalization of cells during gastrulation) makes a proportionately much smaller contribution, providing a source of angiogenic tissue, a limited amount of connective tissue, the bones of the occipital region of the skull, part of the otic capsule, all the striated muscle, and the tongue musculature.

In a functional sense the mouth and buccal cavity should not be regarded as a single organ system but as a complex of interdependent organs and tissue systems. Orofacial morphogenesis is topographically complex. Here it will be dealt with in a general sense, with emphasis on the mouth and embryonic oropharynx, and referring to other organ systems within the head whenever

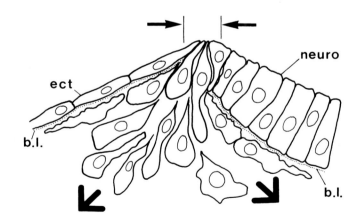

Fig. 2.1 Diagram of cranial neural crest origin. The interface is shown between the neuroectoderm (neuro) and the ectoderm (ect) during early neurulation and depicted in a transverse plane (the midline is off to the right). At this interface, within the region defined by the small arrows, the cells lose their epithelial organization, concomitant with changes in adhesive relationships between neighboring cells and the dissolution of the basal lamina (b.l.). The cells 'liberated' at this point constitute the neural crest and proceed to migrate throughout the forming head of the embryo. This is in contrast to events in the head, where the crest arises before neurulation has been completed, and the more posterior 'trunk' neural crest originates *after* neurulation has been completed. (From Thorogood P, Ferretti P 1992 Br Dent J 173: 301–306.)

necessary. For fuller accounts of craniofacial developmental anatomy, see Larsen;[5] for craniofacial fetal pathology, see Ferguson;[6] and for the molecular biology of craniofacial morphogenesis and dysmorphogenesis, see Thorogood.[7]

EMBRYONIC DEVELOPMENT AND MORPHOGENESIS OF THE OROFACIAL COMPLEX

MORPHOGENESIS OF THE HUMAN FACE

The first outward indication of morphogenesis is a lifting of the anterior end of the axis from the surrounding extraembryonic tissues, the so-called 'head fold,' at the beginning of the fourth week of embryonic life and, by the end of that week, the gradual emergence of a series of bulges and intervening grooves on the ventrolateral aspects of the early head. The most rostral of these (in a virtually terminal location) is a midline process, termed the frontonasal mass. Flanking this, and first distinguishable during the fifth week, are the paired olfactory placodes and areas of thickened ectoderm, which will subsequently invaginate to give rise to much of the olfactory organs, including the chemosensory neurons. The medial and lateral edges of these placodes will grow into the paired, bilateral, medial, and lateral nasal processes (Fig. 2.2), followed by the paired and bilateral maxillary processes. Collectively, these processes or primordia will give rise to the upper and mid-face (Fig. 2.2). Moving caudally back along the embryonic axis there are a series of paired ventrolateral processes called the branchial arches, each separated from its neighbors fore and aft by a groove in the surface ectoderm, termed the pharyngeal groove, and matched by an outpocketing from the foregut internally, called the branchial or pharyngeal

pouch. At these points between adjacent arches, the surface ectoderm and the endoderm lining the foregut are in close approximation.

The arches are remnants of the gill arches of a vertebrate ancestor and, although fewer in number, retain some of their primitive characteristics. Likewise, the grooves and pouches together represent the embryonic gill clefts of that ancestor. Thus, each arch and associated pouch originally formed a set of structures (skeletal, vascular, muscular, neural, and glandular) comprising a single functional unit in a repeating metameric series. However, one characteristic of arch evolution has been the specialization of each arch, with its developmental potential being deployed in unique and axial-level-specific ways (see later). The maxillary process, which gives rise to the tissues of the upper jaw, is regarded as an anterior protrusion from the first or 'mandibular' arch, which itself gives rise to most of the lower jaw (Fig. 2.3). Thus, the embryonic mouth or stomodaeum is largely surrounded by first arch-derived tissues. Branchial arches are generally numbered 1, 2, 3, 4, and 6, the fifth arch being assumed to have been lost during the course of evolution. It is also assumed that the ancestral chordates possessed an arch anterior, or rostral, to what we currently regard as the first arch. This 'premandibular' arch is thought to have swung forward during the course of evolution to give rise to the anterior part of the skull base, the trabeculae cranii, providing support for the new anterior additions to the ancestral brain, structures that we now regard as the fore- and midbrain or prosencephalon and mesencephalon, respectively. The progressive shift forward of the ancestral second arch, which we now regard as arch 1 or the mandibular arch, permitted the development of a biting and masticatory function. At a later stage, proximal elements from this arch and from the second or 'hyoid' arch became secondarily modified as the

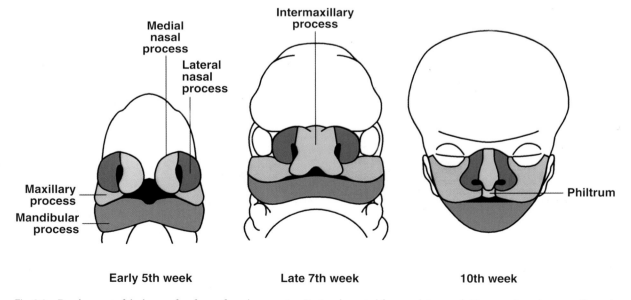

Fig. 2.2   Development of the human face from a frontal perspective. During the period from week 5 to week 10, a coordinated process of growth brings the facial primordia into contact at precise locations and at precise times. Fusion, continued growth, and epithelial remodeling ensues and generates the recognizable features of the face by the end of week 10 (after Larsen 1993).[5]

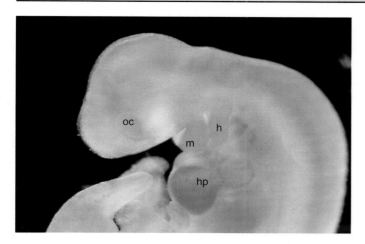

Fig. 2.3 Left lateral view of a human embryo, 4½ weeks after conception. The key features of the early face can be seen including the optic cup (oc), the mandibular (m), and hyoid (h) processes; at this stage the heart primordium (hp) has not yet descended into the thoracic region.

conductive elements of the middle ear. It can thus be seen that the changing morphology and pattern of these arch elements, generated by mutational changes to the mechanisms controlling their development, provided the foundation for the explosive evolution of the vertebrates from a primitive chordate ancestor and, ultimately, for the development of the human face.

During the sixth week, as the olfactory placodes thicken and invaginate to form the nasal pits, the frontonasal mass, comprising largely neural crest derived from the anterior mesencephalon (and possibly prosencephalon), grows forward and downward. The lateral and medial margins of the invaginating placodes grow and, as the lateral and medial nasal processes, contact the maxillary primordia on each side during the seventh week (see Fig. 2.2). The three-branched contact seam so formed is the site at which adhesion and fusion occur. Remodeling of the ectoderm

at the points of contact eliminates the seams and generates epithelial continuity across the forming upper face. The ectoderm along the interface between the lateral nasal process and the adjacent maxillary process, the nasolacrimal groove, separates and sinks into the subjacent mesenchyme, where it goes on to form the nasolacrimal duct draining from the conjunctiva into the nasal cavity.

The contribution of these three processes on each side of the forming face will provide the cheeks and the wings or alae of the nostrils (see Fig. 2.2). Failure of fusion at these points, for any reason, will result in unilateral or bilateral facial clefting (Fig. 2.4). Coincident with the formation of the maxillary region, the frontonasal mass grows to provide a body of tissue between the medial nasal processes, the so-called intermaxillary process, which will provide the midfacial tissue, including much of the nose and the philtrum. Again, a failure to attain a critical mass for any of the processes or primordia involved will result in facial clefting, in this case midline clefting. The two sides of the face continue to develop in a semi-autonomous fashion, but the lack of midline union causes an often wide midfacial cleft.

The mandibular process, which will give rise to the lower jaw, is rarely affected by clefting since fusion is not a feature of its development. Nevertheless, a pattern of growth coordinated with that of the upper and midface is essential to provide a balanced physiognomy and functional integration. For example, both hypo- and hyperplastic mandibles will be dysfunctional with regard to dental occlusion. In rare instances, lateral clefting back from the angle of the mouth to the external meatus of the ear is seen, but the etiology is not always clear and may reflect some vascular crisis earlier in development.

The first branchial cleft, between the first and second branchial arches, deepens and sinks inwards to develop into the external auditory canal or meatus; internally the corresponding first branchial pouch grows into the tubotympanic recess, which will subsequently become the tympanic cavity of the middle ear and

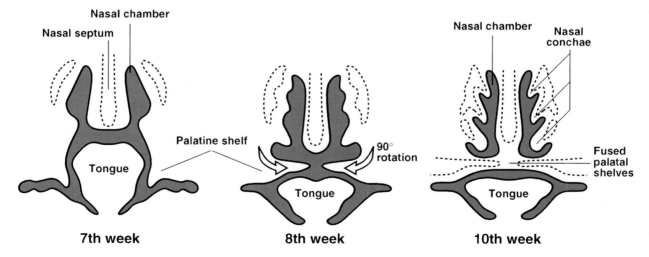

Fig. 2.4 Morphogenesis of the palatal shelves during development of the oropharynx, seen in a transverse plane. The palatal shelves initially point ventrally, but around the eighth week of development they rotate 90° to point medially after which continued growth brings them into midline contact and fusion ensues to create the secondary palate (after Larsen 1993).[5]

the Eustachian tube, which maintains continuity to the oropharynx. Intimately linked with this is the derivation of the auditory ossicles of the middle ear from the proximal mesenchyme of the first arch. Ths latter provides the incus and malleus, while the second arch provides the stapes. Concomitantly, during the fourth to seventh weeks of development, the otic placode invaginates, sinks inwards, and starts to form the vestibular system of the inner ear. The ossicles themselves form within loose mesenchyme, which becomes engulfed by the expanding tympanic cavity and, whilst the stapes comes to lie adjacent to the oval window of the inner ear, the endodermal lining of the tympanic cavity and the ectoderm of the meatus, with a small fibrous layer sandwiched between them, develop into the tympanic membrane or eardrum.[5] The external auricle of the ear is formed from condensations of tissue from both the first and the second arches, which surround the proximal part of the first branchial groove or cleft. As the cleft itself sinks inwards to form the meatus, these auricular hillocks grow, fuse, and undergo a morphogenesis to produce the complex topography of the auricle. From their initially low position on the embryonic neck the auricles migrate progressively dorsally to coordinate with the morphogenesis of the meatus. Given the developmental complexity of forming the inner, middle, and external parts of the ear, this organ is, predictably, susceptible to disruption. Thus, dysmorphic first arch syndromes can affect ossicle development, as well as components of the jaw, and may result in conductive deafness. Even relatively mild disturbances to this sensitive event may result in misshapen, small, or absent auricles. Growth of the auricular hillocks and their morphogenesis into an auricle takes place largely during the fetal stages, even though the hillocks are themselves first distinguishable at the sixth week of embryogenesis.

Caudal to the first arch, the branchial arch series becomes progressively obscured by the caudalward extension of the second arch. During the sixth week, it grows backwards, as a sheet-like structure, over the third, fourth, and sixth arches to fuse with the body wall at a point adjacent to the position of the descending heart primordium. The transient space enclosed by this second-arch-derived process is normally lost in subsequent tissue re-modeling, but may persist as a lateral cervical (branchial) cyst, sometimes with fistulae draining externally, internally (into the oropharynx), or both.

By early fetal stages the landmarks of the human face have been established; during the second and third trimesters, allomeric growth will transform it into the more familiar face of the neonate. However, the dramatic events producing the external topography are paralleled by an equally complex internal morphogenesis involving the oropharynx and the branchial pouches.

MORPHOGENESIS OF THE STOMODAEUM AND OROPHARYNX

In the initial stages of first-arch development, the primitive mouth, or stomodaeum, is separated from the foregut by a layer of apposed ectoderm externally and endoderm internally. This buccopharyngeal membrane breaks down late during the fourth week of development, thereby creating continuity with the primitive foregut. The through cavity so formed is the oropharynx. The tongue forms on the floor of the oropharynx with contributions from arches 1,2, and 4 and from the occipital somites. During the fifth week, a small endodermal invagination from the dorsal surface of the tongue grows and migrates downwards into the developing neck, where the cells will form the thyroid gland at a site anterior to the future larynx. Physical continuity with the dorsum of the tongue is briefly maintained as the thyroglossal duct, but this connection is lost as development proceeds; small foci of ectopic thyroid tissue occasionally result from fragmentation of the thyroid primordium as it descends into the neck.

During the early fourth week of embryonic life, a placodal structure on the roof of the stomodaeum invaginates dorsally towards the underside of the overlying forebrain. This structure, known as Rathke's pouch, becomes associated with a ventral downgrowth from the forebrain, the infundibulum, and together they will form the pituitary gland. Initially, the site of invagination of Rathke's pouch can be seen on the roof of the stomodaeum, but this continuity is soon lost as pituitary development proceeds. Rathke's pouch itself gives rise to the adenohypophysis and pars intermedia, while the neurohypophysis forms from the infundibulum.

Initially the nasal cavity and oropharynx are only separated by a posterior extension of intermaxillary-process-derived tissue, the primary (soft) palate, separating them rostrally. Full anatomical separation of the two is achieved by the formation of the secondary (hard) palate from the bilateral palatal shelves, which grow ventromedially into the oropharynx from the medial surface of the maxillary processes (see Fig. 2.4). Initially the shelves project almost ventrally and lie lateral to the tongue primordium. However, starting at the eighth week they rotate through 90° to point medially, and then grow to fuse in the midline. The nasal cavity thereby becomes separated from the oropharynx, except at the posterior extreme, and the nasal cavity becomes divided into two bilateral passages by the downward growth of the nasal septum.

Like many other phenomena that occur during craniofacial development, morphogenesis of the palate is highly sensitive to perturbation from a variety of causes. For example, reduced growth of the mesenchyme within the shelves, or an oversized tongue primordium impeding their rotation will both cause palatal clefting. Given the interrelationship with maxillary development and the development of the soft palate from the intermaxillary process, it is not surprising that cleft palate often accompanies facial clefting.

The developmental fate of the tissues lining the pharyngeal pouches is complex. The morphogenesis and growth of the first pouch to form the tubotympanic recess (and subsequently the tympanic cavity and the Eustachian tube) has already been dealt with, but even from that brief account it is evident that allomeric growth and tissue relocations are an integral feature. With the development of the remaining pouches these phenomena are

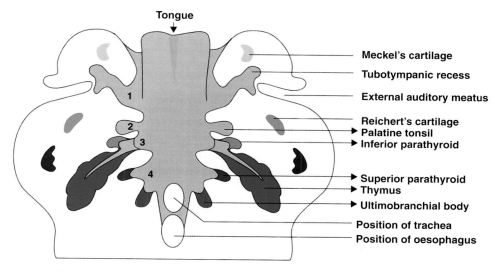

Fig. 2.5 Diagram of the oropharynx depicted in a coronal plane and illustrating the developmental fate of branchial-pouch-derived tissues. Rostral is uppermost and the pouches are numbered 1–4; the angular midline object at the top of the figure is the dorsum of the tongue (after Larsen 1993).[5]

even more dramatic, with some cell populations being relocated to sites in the lower neck and even the chest (Fig. 2.5). The endoderm and associated mesenchyme of the second pouch gives rise to the palatine tonsils, differentiating from the end of the third trimester onwards. During weeks 5–7, endodermal cells from the third and fourth pouches descend through the forming neck to give rise to the inferior and superior parathyroids, respectively (the third-pouch-derived cells descend further than their more caudal counterparts to an inferior location). Starting at 6 weeks, a similar route of descent is traced by the cells of what is variously interpreted as a pocket of the fourth pouch or, more controversially, as a vestigial fifth pouch, to give rise to parafollicular or calcitonin-producing cells of the thyroid. The precise derivation of these cells, from pouch endoderm, associated mesenchyme, or groove ectoderm, is still to be determined. The most dramatic of all of these descents is that displayed by the cells that will form the stroma of the thymus. These originate from tissue proliferations at the distal tip of each third pouch during weeks 4–5 and subsequently relocate in the anterior chest wall where full morphogenesis of the thymus gland ensues.

During the fourth week, the respiratory diverticulum grows out as an evagination from the underside of the foregut. During the following week it branches for the first time. The left and right branches will go on to form the right and left bronchial buds, which branch progressively to form the respiratory tree, and the stem itself develops into the trachea and larynx. The epithelial lining of the respiratory tract is thus endodermal in origin, although the surrounding stroma is mesodermal. Rostral to the opening of the respiratory diverticulum, at the approximate level of the fourth arch, the epiglottis develops from about 6 weeks onwards from the paired bilateral arytenoid swellings, but the tissue derivation of the epiglottis and its supporting cartilages is not entirely clear.

MORPHOGENESIS OF THE MUSCULOSKELETAL SYSTEM

The major part of the skull is produced by ectomesenchymal cells of neural crest origin. In fact, the mesodermal contribution, which was originally thought to include the bones of the cranial vault, has recently been reassessed. The first five somites, the occipital somites, together with the nonsegmented cephalic mesoderm, become incorporated into the skull to form the occipital bones and a major part of the otic capsule. All the remaining parts of the skull, including the rostral part of the cranial base, the facial skeleton and jaws, a minor part of the otic capsule, the bones of the cranial vault, and the cells of the sutures, are derived from the neural crest.[8] A combination of epigenetic tissue interactions (in the neurocranium) and genetic specification (in the viscerocranium, see later) seems to be involved in determining the intricate patterns of skeletogenic differentiation that subsequently take place.[9,10]

However, it is the viscerocranium, the skeleton of the jaws and of the throat, that primarily concerns us here. This is, predictably, derived in large part from the branchial arch mesenchyme and reflects, in a highly modified fashion, the original metameric series of ancestral arch cartilages (see earlier). The elements are embryonically derived largely from the hindbrain neural crest (see later), with a contribution from the midbrain crest to the mandibular arch. The independent upper jaw articulation of lower vertebrates has been lost in mammals, including humans (see earlier), and the skeletal elements of both upper and lower jaws form from a variety of (dermal) membranous and endochondral bones (Fig. 2.6). Thus, the ectomesenchyme of the maxillary process gives rise not only to the cartilaginous alisphenoid, which undergoes endochondral ossification, but also to the maxillary bone of the upper jaw and the zygomatic bone of the

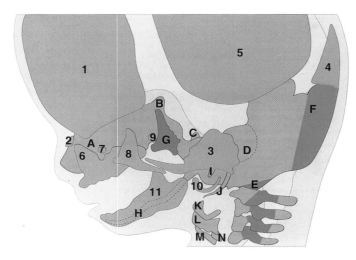

Fig. 2.6   The facial skeleton at approximately 12 weeks. Membrane bone is shown in orange, cartilage in blue, and areas of endochondral ossification within the cartilage in green (after Williams 1995)[15]. Cartilage elements: A, nasal capsule; B, orbitosphenoid; C, postsphenoid; D, otic capsule; E, exoccipital; F, supraoccipital; G, alisphenoid; H, Meckel's cartilage (buried within 11); I, malleus; J, styloid cartilage; K, hyoid cartilage; L, thyroid cartilage; M, cricoid cartilage; N, arytenoid cartilage. Membrane bone elements: 1, frontal bone; 2, nasal bone; 3, squama of temporal bone; 4, squama of occipital bone; 5, parietal bone; 6, maxilla; 7, lacrimal bone; 8, zygomatic bone; 9, medial pterygoid plate; 10, tympanic ring; 11, mandible.

cheek, both of which, as membrane bones, form directly from it. In a comparable fashion, the mandibular bone of the lower jaw is a composite structure derived partly from endochondral ossification of Meckel's cartilage (the original arch cartilage) and partly from the membrane bones, which closely invest Meckel's cartilage. In a sense, therefore, the rod-like Meckel's cartilage acts as a structural template, determining the pattern of ossification in and around it. More proximally, first-arch ectomesenchyme gives rise to the squamous portion of the membranous temporal bone and to the cartilaginous primordia of the incus and the malleus (see earlier). Both maxillary and mandibular bones provide the foundation for the dentition, even though the mesenchymal component of the tooth germ, including the actual bone of attachment, may have a different origin along the rostrocaudal axis of the neural crest.

More caudally, the second-arch cartilage or Reichert's cartilage, develops into structures supporting not only the lower jaw (reflecting its primitive function) but also the tongue and larynx, as well as making a contribution to the middle ear (see Fig. 2.6). Thus, part of Reichert's cartilage undergoes endochondral ossification to produce the stapes. Other parts give rise to the styloid process of the temporal bone, the stylohyoid ligament, and the lesser cornua and upper rim of the hyoid bone. Within the third arch, the cartilage gives rise to the greater and remaining part of the hyoid bone. Finally, ectomesenchyme from the fourth arch, perhaps with a contribution from the sixth arch, provides skeletal support for the larynx, in the form of the thyroid, cuneiform, corniculate, arytenoid, and cricoid cartilages. All these structures are well formed by 10 weeks of development, with the most rostral

having commenced development as skeletogenic condensations from about 5 weeks onwards.

Paraxial mesoderm, including the occipital somites, is the sole source of myogenic cells in the head.[11,12] Like myogenic cells elsewhere in the body, these cells have no intrinsic pattern specification of their own and when heterotopically grafted develop according to the site of grafting.[13] Facial musculature appears to be patterned entirely by the crest-derived connective tissue cells,[14] but the molecular and cellular mechanisms by which this patterning is specified is unknown.

Individual populations of myogenic cells, whether derived from paraxial mesoderm, somitomeres, or occipital somites, display relocation during craniofacial morphogenesis, as a result of cell migration, displacement, and/or allomeric growth. However, the origin of each muscle primordium is indicated by its innervation since, during this relocation, a branch of the cranial nerve specific to the branchial arch at the axial level of origin is carried with the myogenic condensation. As a result, the origin of the facial musculature can be mapped as shown in Figure 2.7, revealing dramatic relocation. Although a precise account of the origin of facial musculature is outside the scope of this chapter (see Williams[15]), a useful working summary can be made. The extrinsic ocular muscles derive from mesoderm in the periocular region. First-arch-associated mesoderm gives rise to the muscles of mastication (temporalis, masseter, and anterior belly of the digastric). Second-arch-associated mesoderm undergoes a very extensive relocation into a frontal location to produce the muscles of facial expression (frontalis, orbicularis oculi, orbicularis oris, buccinator, posterior belly of the digastric, and stylohyoid). Mesoderm from arches three, four, and six gives rise to the stylopharyngeus, cricothyroid, and intrinsic laryngeal muscles,

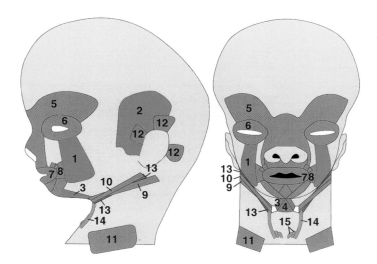

Fig. 2.7   Facial musculature at approximately 12 weeks: (left) left lateral view; (right) frontal view. The derivation of muscles from the mesoderm of individual branchial arches is indicated by colour coding: first arch, green; second arch, orange; third arch, purple; fourth arch, blue. 1, Masseter; 2, temporalis; 3, anterior belly of the digastric; 4, mylohyoid; 5, frontalis; 6, orbicularis oculi; 7, orbicularis oris; 8, buccinator; 9, posterior belly of the digastric; 10, stylohyoid; 11, platysma; 12, auricularis; 13, stylopharyngeus; 14, inferior constrictor of pharynx; 15, cricothyroid.

respectively. Meanwhile, the myogenic cells derived from the occipital somites differentiate into the extrinsic and intrinsic lingual muscles (except the palatoglossus).

For accounts of the morphogenesis of a wide range of tissue systems during craniofacial development generally, see Le Douarin et al[16] and Noden.[17] *Gray's Anatomy*[15] provides a comprehensive overview of the developmental anatomy.

MOLECULAR MECHANISMS UNDERLYING THE MORPHOGENETIC SPECIFICATION OF OROFACIAL TISSUES

Our understanding of the developmental mechanisms involved in the building of the head and face has grown enormously over recent years. The application of new technologies in novel experimental strategies using traditional animal-model systems (chiefly avian and murine) has generated fresh paradigms. Analysis of craniofacial development is no longer the rather intractable problem that it was once thought to be. Thus, the creation of heterospecific chimeras and the advent of new lipophilic fluorochromes such as DiI have transformed our understanding of cell fate, lineage, and neural crest migration. Refinement of older immunocytochemical techniques coupled with confocal microscopy has created higher levels of resolution of distribution of specific proteins. Molecular techniques, including in situ hybridization and reverse transcriptase polymerase chain reaction (RT-PCR), have enabled not only the definition of precise spatiotemporal patterns of gene expression, but also genetic engineering to create transgenic models to elucidate the functional role of specific genes.[7]

Here we will deal solely with the lower face, which is largely derived from the branchial region of the embryonic axis. This comprises those axial levels approximating to the hindbrain or rhombencephalon, within which the branchial arches develop. Tissue recombination experiments, in which the ectodermal and mesenchymal components of facial primordia were interchanged, have demonstrated that the specification of growth and morphogenetic fate in the arches resides in the mesenchymal component.[18] The focus of our attention therefore becomes the rhombencephalic crest, which gives rise to most of the branchial-arch mesenchyme (with the exception of the myogenic lineage, discussed earlier). Given that much of the mid- and lower face and the jaw skeleton is arch derived, hindbrain crest is clearly profoundly important in the formation of the face. Furthermore, as will become apparent, it is the mode of rhombencephalic crest migration, imposed by the organization of the hindbrain, that ensures anatomical registration between axial structures and the metameric array of branchial arches.

The rhombencephalon is itself a segmented structure with eight neuromeres known as rhombomeres (R1–R8). Each of these is now known to constitute a unit of lineage restriction, which has early commitment to a particular developmental fate.[19] Migration of neural crest from the rhombencephalon is not random, but has been shown to be orderly and discrete insofar as

crest cells from particular rhombomeres migrate into particular branchial arches.[20] Thus, from work using animal-model systems we find an evolutionarily conserved pattern of R1 and R2 crest migrating into the first arch, R4 crest into the second arch, and crest from R6 into the third arch (R3 and R5 produce either no or negligible amounts of crest due to programmed cell death, which eliminates crest precursors within the neural primordium).[21]

Almost concomitant with this finding was the observation that some conserved regulatory genes, the homologs in *Drosophila* of which are involved in specifying parts of the body plan, display expression domains that coincide with rhombomere boundaries. In particular, the more-3′ genes of the *Hox* gene family are expressed in domains which, whilst extending forward from the caudal region, have anterior limits of expression, or 'anterior cut-offs', which are arranged in a staggered array at successive rhombomere boundaries. Given that the rhombomeres represent units of lineage restriction and that the homologs of the genes concerned have an ancestral role in specifying morphogenetic fate, then the possibility arises that these *Hox* genes have a role in specifying position within the hindbrain.[22]

There are 38 *Hox* genes in all vertebrates studied to date, including humans, and within the genome they are organized into four clusters on different chromosomes. From work on animal-model systems it has emerged that the rostrocaudal sequence of the anterior cut-offs within the hindbrain maps with the sequential position of each *Hox* gene within its respective cluster, along the 3′ to 5′ polarity of the chromosome. Thus, the more 3′ the gene, then the more rostral its cut-off (Fig. 2.8) and it is the more 3′ *Hox* genes that concern us when considering the head. This relationship has been termed the 'rule of structural colinearity', which also has a temporal dimension in that the more 3′ genes are expressed before the more 5′ genes with their more caudal cut-offs.[23]

The four clusters of these *Hox* genes (typically identified as a, b, c, and d; and as A, B, C, and D in humans) reflect a common origin from a single ancestral cluster far back in our evolutionary past. As a result, there is a relationship between equivalent genes existing within different clusters but reflecting their common origin from an ancestral gene. This relationship is seen in their high sequence homology and equivalent 3′ to 5′ positions within their respective clusters. Such genes sharing a common ancestor are termed paralogs, and the groups so defined as paralogous groups. Thus, in the mouse *Hoxa-3* is paralogous to *Hoxb-3* and *Hoxd-3*. Significantly, paralogous *Hox* genes share the same expression domains (see Fig. 2.8) and there is believed to be a certain degree of functional redundancy between the members of any one paralogous group; that is to say, they may share functions totally or in part. Human *Hox* genes are organized in an identical way to those in the animal-model systems, that is to say with four clusters A, B, C, and D present, in this case, on chromosomes 7, 17, 12, and 2, respectively (Fig. 2.9).

The relevance of this to development of the orofacial region arises from the fact that, as neural crest cells emigrate from the rhombencephalon, they continue to express the particular combination of *Hox* genes that characterized the axial or rhomb-

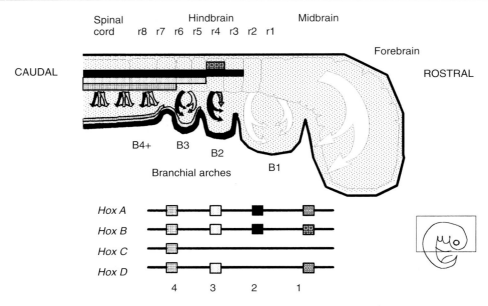

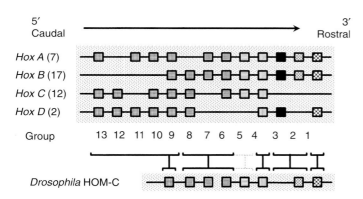

Fig. 2.8 The branchial *Hox* code as elucidated in the mouse embryo, illustrating the relationship between expression domains of the 3′-most *Hox* genes in the rhombomeres (r1–r8) in the developing hindbrain and branchial arches (B1–B4+), and their position within their respective clusters (A–D) on individual chromosomes. Paralogous groups are defined vertically across the clusters and these 3′-most paralogous groups are numbered 1–4. Note the correspondence (as indicated by hatching) between an individual gene in its cluster, its paralogs in other clusters, and their spatial expression domain in the rhombomere, in streams of migrating crest cells (arrows) and in the ectodermal covering of each arch (migration of crest cells from particular axial levels is indicated by arrows). Spatial colinearity is seen in the rostral-to-caudal sequence of anterior cut-offs of expression (from right to left) and the location of the individual genes 3′ to 5′ along each chromosome (also from right to left). Note that no *Hox* genes are expressed in those crest cells migrating from the first two rhombomeres into the first arch (which is thought to reflect a 'default' branchial arch specification) or in those migrating rostrally from the mid- and forebrain. The location of the diagram vis à vis the rest of the embryo is indicated in the inset. (Diagram kindly supplied by Dr Paul Hunt.)

Fig. 2.9 Schematic representation of the human *Hox* gene clusters (A–D) and their chromosomal locations (in parentheses). Clusters are aligned so that paralogous genes belonging to the same group correspond vertically. The *Drosophila* HOM-C complex, which is thought to resemble the single ancestral complex, and the known homologies with vertebrate genes are shown below. The direction of transcription is indicated by the arrow. Genes situated at the 3′ end of the clusters are expressed more rostrally and earlier than genes at the 5′ end. It is the genes of paralogous groups 1–4 that have anterior cut-offs within the branchial region and which are thought to have a critical role in morphogenetic specification during orofacial development (see also Fig. 2.8) (after Vieille-Grosjean et al 1997).[25]

encephalic level from which they arose. Given the likely function of these regulatory genes in specifying morphogenetic fate, and that streams of crest cells each expressing different combinations of *Hox* genes migrate to colonize different branchial arches, one model that has emerged is that the crest cells thereby determine the identity (i.e. morphogenetic fate) of each arch by virtue of the arch-specific combination of *Hox* genes expressed. This has led to the concept of a branchial arch 'hox code' underlying the morphogenetic specification of the arches and, therefore, of the lower face and orofacial region.[24] It is also relevant that the other tissues in each arch (ectoderm, endoderm, and mesoderm) are all initially naive with regard to *Hox* gene expression and an arch-specific pattern of expression is imposed upon them secondarily by the incoming crest cells. This accords with the classic tissue recombination experiments (see earlier) and means that the fate of each arch and its contribution to the orofacial region is the consequence of a specification event taking place within the neural primordium at a much earlier stage of development. Although it is outside the scope of this brief account, this putative role of *Hox* genes has been tested using transgenic strategies whereby individual *Hox* genes can be knocked out or expressed

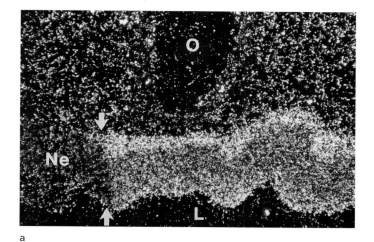

a

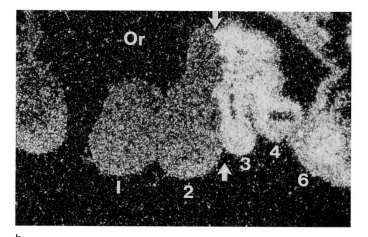

b

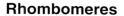
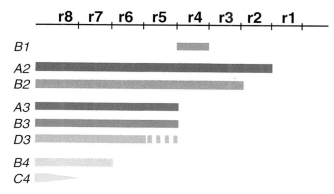

Rhombomeres

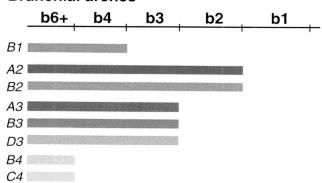

Branchial arches

Fig. 2.10 Autoradiographic in situ hybridization revealing expression of *HOXA-3* in the branchial region of a 4-week post-conception human embryo (dark-field microscopy). **a** Coronal section through the hindbrain showing the neuroepithelial wall (Ne) of one side of the rhombencephalon, the lumen of the rhombencephalon (L), and the otocyst lateral to the hindbrain (O). Rostral is to the left. Note the sharp anterior cut-off of expression at the junction between rhombomeres 4 and 5 (arrows). **b** Similar plane of section showing expression in the branchial arches on the opposite side of the same embryo. Rostral is to the left. The branchial arches, seen here on one side of the oropharynx (Or), are labeled 1, 2, 3, 4, and 6. Note the dramatic anterior cut-off (arrows) at the interface between arches 2 and 3 (Vieille-Grosjean et al 1997).[25]

Fig. 2.11 The *Hox* code for the human branchial region, summarizing expression data for eight genes that are coexpressed in this region at 4 weeks of embryonic development. The nested nature of the expression domains, and the common domains shared by members of any individual paralogous group (2, 3, or 4), are clearly evident (Vieille-Grosjean et al 1997).[25]

ectopically and, broadly speaking, the results to date support such an interpretation.[7]

Does any of this have relevance to the development of the human orofacial region? Recently, *Hox* gene expression has been studied in the early embryonic human head, at four and five weeks post-conception (Fig. 2.10), and the human branchial *Hox* code has been elucidated (Fig. 2.11). The human code was found to be identical to that defined for all other vertebrate species to date.[25] Although gene expression alone provides limited information on gene function, given the correspondence between the datasets from different species, it is very probable that the branchial *Hox* code in humans operates in a fashion equivalent to that

in, say, the mouse. In fact, this correspondence between expression data from the mouse and human provides a degree of vindication for the use of the former as an experimental model from which to extrapolate to human craniofacial development and dysmorphogenesis (including the transgenic manipulation of individual *Hox* genes to define their function). Moreover, it can be concluded that the branchial hox code is a part of the evolutionarily ancient process of building a head, but has not necessarily been deployed to specify morphology that is uniquely human. The upstream control of *Hox* genes (i.e. what it is that sets up the nested pattern of expression domains initially in the neural primordium) and the identity of their downstream targets (i.e. which genes are the targets for regulation by *Hox* genes) remain the focus of much research activity.

MORPHOGENESIS OF THE TEETH

DEVELOPMENT OF THE ENAMEL ORGAN

The sites of tooth development first become apparent during the

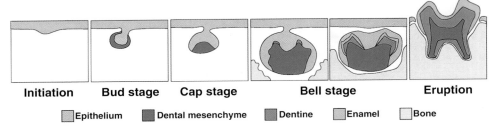

Fig. 2.12   Stages in the development and eruption of the teeth. (Diagram kindly supplied Dr Irma Thesleff (Thesleff 1997)[26])

sixth week of embryonic life with the formation of the primary epithelial band. This is a ridge of thickened epithelium running the whole length of the jaws along the crest of the alveolar ridges. The epithelium proliferates down into an area of condensed mesenchymal tissue. The primary epithelial band divides to form an outer process or vestibular lamina, which will separate the lips and cheeks from the jaws, and an inner process, which forms the dental lamina from which the teeth develop. By the eighth week a series of bud-like swellings develop in the dental lamina, one for each deciduous tooth to be formed. These will form the enamel organs of the teeth, and initially consist of simple aggregates of epithelial cells, but these soon proliferate and undergo morphogenesis to produce the classically described stages of development of the enamel organ: the cap stage and bell stage (Fig. 2.12).[26] At the time when the enamel organs first appear, the underlying neural-crest-derived mesenchyme becomes condensed and richly cellular, forming an area called the dental papillae, which gives rise to dentine and ultimately forms the tooth pulp. As the enamel organ develops, the dental papilla gradually invaginates into the center of the cap-like structure. The condensed mesenchyme on the outer or convex surface of the organ will form the dental follicle. The combined structure of enamel organ, dental papilla, and dental follicle is the tooth germ.

The epithelial cells of the enamel organ differentiate into a peripheral layer of low columnar cells surrounding a central area of polyhedral or stellate cells, which are separated by a significant amount of glycosaminoglycans and form the stellate reticulum. By the eleventh week the cells on the deep surface invaginate into the bud to form the cap stage. This continues until, by the fourteenth week, the enamel organ resembles a bell. By the time this stage is reached, four distinct layers are apparent. The outermost layer or external enamel epithelium is composed of low cuboidal cells. The internal enamel epithelium lines the deep surface of the enamel organ on the concave or inward surface of the cap or bell. This layer is composed of tall columnar cells that differentiate progressively to form the ameloblasts. The internal and external enamel epithelia are separated by the stellate reticulum, but adjacent to the internal enamel epithelium the cells condense to form the fourth layer, the stratum intermedium. At this stage the bell shape of the enamel organ roughly maps out the shape of the tooth crown, and there may be folds in the

internal enamel epithelium corresponding to the occlusal pattern of the developing tooth (Fig. 2.13). The internal and external enamel epithelia are continuous at the open edge of the bell shape, and here form the cervical loop. This is a site of active cell proliferation, which results in a downgrowth of epithelium between the dental follicle and dental papilla. This subsequently forms the epithelial root sheath (sheath of Hertwig), which encloses the tooth pulp and delineates the root morphology (Fig. 2.14).

As the enamel organs of the deciduous teeth develop the dental lamina continues to proliferate to form branches from which develop the enamel organs of the permanent teeth. Later the dental lamina breaks down and small residual islands of odontogenic epithelial cells may remain in the overlying oral mucosa. These cell rests or 'epithelial pearls' (pearls of Serres) may give rise to odontogenic cysts. By the late bell stage the whole tooth germ lies free, and gradually becomes encased in the bone of the developing jaw.

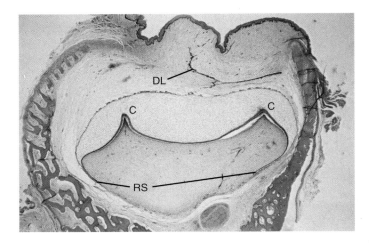

Fig. 2.13   Histologic section of a tooth germ enclosed within its bony crypt. The enamel organ is in the late bell stage and the internal enamel epithelium is folded in a pattern which will determine the shape of the tooth crown; in this case, two developing cusps (C) can be seen. Other structures to note are: the remnant of the dental lamina (DL) extending from the external enamel epithelium up towards the oral epithelium, and the developing root sheath (RS) extending downwards from the margins of the bell.

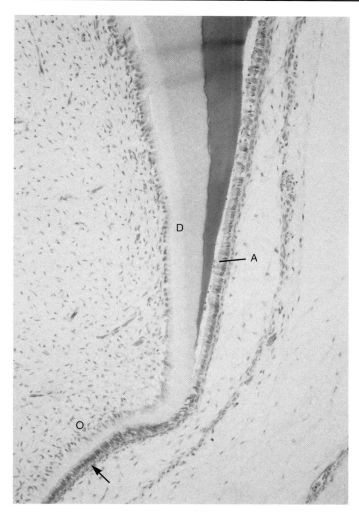

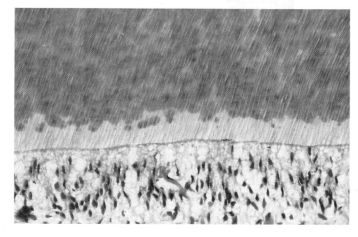

Fig. 2.15 High-power view of the odontoblast layer. The odontoblasts are long columnar cells, which form elongated processes that pass upwards through the dentine in the parallel dentinal tubules. Adjacent to the odontoblasts there is a pale layer of unmineralized predentine containing globules of mineralizing tissue (interglobular dentine).

Once the matrix is about 5 mm thick it begins to mineralize, but the dentine adjacent to the odontoblast, the predentine, never mineralizes. The basement membrane that existed between the ameloblasts and the odontoblasts is broken down, so that eventually enamel and dentine are in direct contact at the amelodentinal junction. Adjacent to the enamel, the superficial dentine, or mantle dentine, has branching tubules and is less regular than the later formed circumpulpal dentine.

Mineralization of dentine proceeds by the formation of crystallites within matrix vesicles, which are secreted by the odontoblast processes. Crystal growth then continues around each nidus to form spherical or globular masses called calcospherites, which coalesce to form a uniformly mineralized structure. In immature dentine, or in dental defects associated with poor mineralization, the separate globules of mineralized tissue can be seen within the uncalcified matrix. This is referred to as interglobular dentine (see Fig. 2.15).

The dentine of the tooth root is formed by odontoblasts that differentiate adjacent to the epithelial root sheath, which has proliferated down from the cervical loop (see Fig. 2.14). Much of the root dentine is laid down after crown formation, both during and after tooth eruption. No enamel is deposited in this region, and eventually the root surface becomes covered by cementum. After root dentine formation has started the epithelial root sheath disintegrates, but leaves odontogenic epithelial rests (rests of Malassez) that remain as a network of epithelial cells in the periodontal ligament throughout life. These cells contribute particularly to the formation of radicular cysts.

Mature dentine is composed of 70% inorganic material, 20% organic material, and 10% water. The principal inorganic component is hydroxyapatite and the organic element is composed mostly of fibres of type I collagen embedded in a proteoglycan matrix. Unlike bone or cementum, dentine does not contain cell bodies but only the elongated odontoblast processes, which pass

Fig. 2.14 High-power view of the root sheath of Hertwig (arrow) showing differentiation of odontoblasts (O) on the outer aspect of the pulpal tissue. Note that the ameloblasts (A) are already well differentiated but that the pale eosinophilic dentine (D) forms first, followed by the darker enamel, which is then laid down onto the dentine surface.

DEVELOPMENT AND STRUCTURE OF DENTINE

By the late bell stage, cells of the internal enamel epithelium have begun to differentiate towards ameloblasts and exert an inductive influence on the most superficial mesenchymal cells of the dental papillae, which as a result differentiate to become odontoblasts. These eventually produce dentine, which is the first dental hard tissue to be formed (Fig. 2.14). The odontoblasts, originally derived from the neural crest, are columnar cells with a large cell body and a secretory process. Dentine is deposited initially as an organic matrix composed of collagen in a proteoglycan ground substance. As the matrix is deposited the odontoblasts migrate centripetally towards the center of the dental papillae, and the secretory processes elongate so that the final mineralized dentine contains tubules through its full thickness, each containing a single odontoblast process (Fig. 2.15).

through the whole thickness of the dentine, from the pulp to the amelodentinal junction, within dentinal tubules that are 2–4 μm in diameter. In normal dentine the tubules follow a smooth, curved course and are evenly spaced, but in dysplastic dentine, secondary dentine, and dentine found in tumors the tubules may be wider, irregular, and frequently branched.

After tooth formation, dentine continues to be laid down slowly throughout life, mainly as regular secondary dentine, on the pulpal aspect, but also as peritubular dentine. Thus, with age, the pulp chamber diminishes in size and the dentinal tubules may become obliterated to form translucent or sclerotic dentine. Irregular secondary dentine or reactive dentine may also be deposited, more rapidly than regular secondary dentine, in response to noxious stimuli, particularly attrition and dental caries.

DEVELOPMENT AND STRUCTURE OF ENAMEL

Enamel formation begins in the late bell stage, but only after dentine has been deposited and initiates a signal for the final differentiation and secretory activity of ameloblasts. The differentiated ameloblast is a tall columnar cell showing reversal of polarity; that is, the nucleus moves to the pole of the cell furthest from the basement membrane or dentine (Fig. 2.16). Next to the dentine the ameloblast cytoplasm becomes granular, and from here the enamel is secreted. As the cell retreats and lays down enamel, a small pyramidal extension (the Tomes process) develops. Thenceforth enamel is secreted as a mineralized matrix in a well-organized orientation giving the enamel a prismatic structure. After the enamel has been formed it undergoes a period of maturation when the residual organic matrix is removed to produce a highly mineralized structure composed primarily of crystals of hydroxyapatite.

As the enamel is laid down the ameloblasts retreat, eventually obliterating the stellate reticulum and coming into contact with

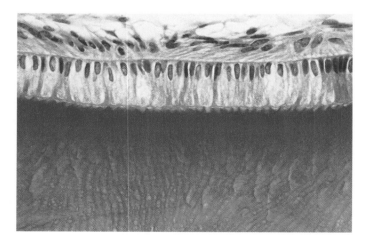

Fig. 2.16   High-power view of ameloblasts showing a regular monolayer of columnar cells with the nuclei polarized away from the enamel surface. In this decalcified section the matrix of the immature enamel can be clearly seen and the prism margins are visible as a fish-scale pattern.

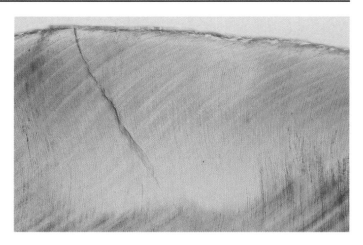

Fig. 2.17   A ground section of enamel shows the fine prisms passing upwards, perpendicular to the tooth surface (top). Regular incremental lines, the striae of Retzius, cross the enamel obliquely.

the external enamel epithelium. When enamel production is complete, the ameloblasts shrink, become cuboidal and, with the external enamel epithelium, form the reduced enamel epithelium, which invests the crown of the tooth until eruption.

Mature enamel is composed of 96% inorganic material and can only be demonstrated in ground sections. It is made up of long rods or prisms about 4 nm in diameter, which run the full thickness of the enamel and are mostly perpendicular to the tooth surface or, on the lateral tooth surfaces, run upwards from the amelodentinal junction (Fig. 2.17). In ground sections the prisms are crossed obliquely by regular incremental lines called the striae of Retzius. The prismatic structure may also be seen in decalcified sections of immature enamel when the residual organic matrix clearly delineates the prism boundaries (see Fig. 2.16). The shape varies with the plane of section, but a characteristic appearance is seen in transverse or oblique sections when the prisms are seen as interdigitating keyhole-shaped structures or may resolve as a fish-scale appearance. Immature enamel is seen in developing teeth, but is also a feature of some odontogenic tumors, particularly odontomas.

DEVELOPMENT AND STRUCTURE OF CEMENTUM

The details of cementum formation, particularly the internal cementum laid down on the dentine surface, are poorly understood. However, it is agreed that cementum is essentially a modified type of bone that is derived from the mesenchymal cells of the dental follicle. Cementum formation appears to be initiated by the breakdown of the epithelial root sheath, which allows dentine to come into contact with mesenchymal cells, which differentiate into cementoblasts. The first-formed cementum is acellular, or primary, cementum which covers the whole of the tooth root and provides an anchor for the collagen fibers of the

eloping tooth. Before eruption, but after formation of the tooth crown, the follicle contributes to the formation of the periodontal ligament, but residual follicle can be seen on a radiograph as a well-demarcated radiolucent area surrounding the crown. As well as the residual odontogenic mesenchyme, this structure contains the reduced enamel epithelium and residual epithelial rests derived from the dental lamina. These structures frequently give rise to odontogenic cysts and tumors, particularly follicular (dentigerous) cysts associated with unerupted teeth and probably also keratocysts and tumors, including ameloblastoma and ameloblastic fibroma.

TOOTH ERUPTION

'Tooth eruption' is the term given to tooth movement into the mouth. Eruption starts as soon as formation of the dentine and enamel of the crown is completed, and does not depend entirely on the formation of the root. The actual mechanism of tooth eruption is not known, but it is probably multifactorial. However, an important component of the mechanism is the presence of the dental follicle and its development into the periodontal ligament. As the tooth moves towards the mucosal surface the reduced enamel epithelium covering the crown fuses with the oral epithelium and then breaks down to provide a conduit for the tooth to move through. Although outside the scope of this chapter, knowledge of the chronology of tooth development and the order of eruption is important for an understanding of the pathology of the region, particularly for the differential diagnosis of odontogenic tumors and cysts in younger individuals.

STRUCTURE OF THE MATURE TOOTH AND PERIODONTIUM

The mature tooth is composed of a pulp enclosed in dentine, which is anchored, via the cementum, to the alveolar bone by the connective tissue fibers of the periodontal ligament. The oral component is covered by the enamel of the tooth crown. The tooth pulp is composed of loose fibrous connective tissue, which contains the blood, lymphatic, and nerve supplies that pass into it at the apex, often through multiple small foramina. In aging pulps, small irregular or spherical calcifications, referred to as pulp stones, are common. Sometimes these may be composed of tubular dentine.

The periodontal ligament develops from the dental follicle and is composed of dense collagen fibers that run in bundles from the cementum to the alveolar bone (see Fig. 2.18), except at the alveolar crest where some fibers join adjacent teeth or run into the gingivae. On either side of the periodontal ligament the fibers are inserted into the bone and cementum via collagenous bundles called Sharpey's fibers. The principal cell of the periodontium is the fibroblast, but osteoblasts, osteoclasts, and cementoblasts are also present. The lineage relationships between these cell types are unknown but, with the exception of the

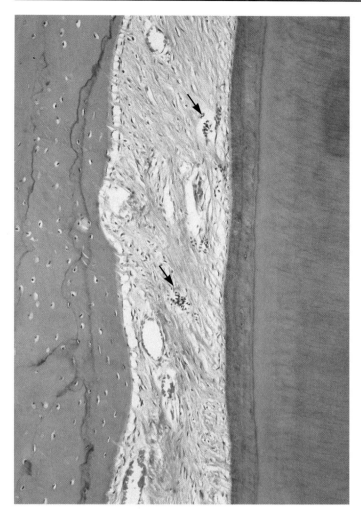

Fig. 2.18 The periodontal ligament is composed of dense bundles of collagen fibers which pass downwards from the bone (left) and insert into the cementum (right). Small islands of odontogenic epithelium (rests of Malassez) can be seen close to the tooth surface (arrows).

periodontal ligament (Fig. 2.18). Secondary, or cellular, cementum is laid down later and is mostly deposited over the apical third of the root. It is laid down more rapidly and, as a result, cementoblasts become incorporated into the structure. Unlike osteocytes, however, cementocytes are more widely distributed and have canaliculi orientated towards the periodontal ligament. Cementum is slowly deposited throughout life, but deposition may increase to compensate for excess tooth wear. Hypercementosis may also result from inflammation in the periapical region and from other causes.

THE DENTAL FOLLICLE

The dental follicle is the sac of condensed mesenchymal cells that surrounds the developing tooth germ. As the jaw ossifies, the bone surrounds the follicle to form a crypt enclosing the dev-

osteoclast, all are thought to be derived from the neural crest. Also, epithelial rest cells, derived from the epithelial root sheath, are arranged as a fine network throughout the periodontal ligament.

STRUCTURE OF THE ORAL MUCOSA

The oral cavity is lined by a moist mucous membrane that is continuous with the skin at the vermilion border of the lips. The mucosa of the mouth has a basic structure of stratified squamous epithelium overlying a vascular fibrous connective tissue called the lamina propria, but there are regional variations reflecting the different functional requirements at different sites.[27] In places there is also a submucosa composed of loose fatty connective tissue containing a variable number of minor salivary glands. In many areas, however, a submucosa is absent and the mucous membrane is attached directly to the underlying bone or muscle.

THE ORAL EPITHELIUM

The mucosa is covered by stratified squamous epithelium, which is composed of four cell layers (Fig. 2.19). The basal layer abuts directly onto the basement membrane and is the site of cell proliferation and renewal. As each basal cell divides it produces a new stem cell and a second cell, termed a transit amplifying cell, which may divide a few times before migrating towards the surface and undergoing terminal differentiation. In epidermis the basal layer is usually composed of a single layer of cells, but in oral epithelium a single layer is often not distinct and the basal layer may be two or three cells thick. The next most superficial layer is the prickle cell layer or stratum spinosum, which forms the bulk of the epithelium and may be very wide depending on the overall thickness of the epithelium. The cells of this layer are

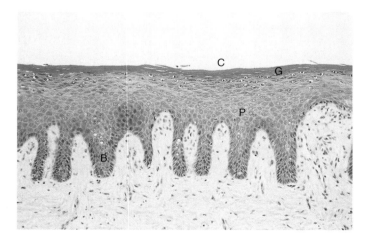

Fig. 2.19 Low-power view of palatal mucosa which is covered by stratified squamous epithelium. Cell layers: B, basal layer; P, prickle cell layer or stratum spinosum; G, granular cell layer or stratum granulosum; C, cornified layer. In palatal epithelium this layer is composed of orthokeratin.

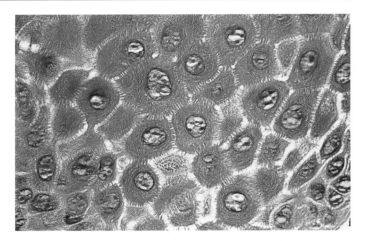

Fig. 2.20 High-power view of the cells of the prickle cell layer, showing prominent desmosomes between the cells.

larger and polygonal or rounded, with well-developed and prominent desmosomes that produce the prickled or spiny appearance on light microscopy (Fig. 2.20).

Superficial to the prickle cell layer is the granular cell layer (stratum granulosum), which is only 2–3 cells thick and is only present in epithelium that has undergone full orthokeratinization. The cells of the granular cell layer are flattened and contain dark-staining keratohyaline granules, which contain profiligrin, a precursor to the cornified envelope. The most superficial layer is the keratinized or cornified layer, which is composed of flattened cells that are devoid of organelles but packed with keratin tonafilaments. These cells are shed from the surface but are constantly renewed by cells migrating up from the basal layers. In fully keratinized epithelium the surface layer is composed of ortho-keratin, but at some sites in the mouth, including most of the lining mucosa, keratinization may be 'incomplete,' so that nuclei are retained in the cornified cells and the granular cell layer is missing. In this case the surface layer is referred to as 'parakeratinized.' In nonkeratinized oral epithelium the surface cells do not keratinize and retain their organelles, although they may be slightly flattened and desmosomes are less prominent. In this case the outermost layer is referred to as the surface or superficial layer (Fig. 2.21).

CELL TYPES IN THE ORAL EPITHELIUM

The above description only relates to epithelial cells and keratinocytes, which make up the bulk of the epithelium (see Fig. 2.20). However, other cells may be present within the epithelial layers. Melanocytes are dendritic cells that form a network in the basal layers and produce melanin. Langerhans cells are also dendritic cells, but are of the macrophage lineage and serve as intraepithelial antigen-presenting cells. They are found in the lower prickle cell layers above the basal layer (Fig. 2.22). Merkel cells are sensory receptor cells found in the basal layer adjacent to

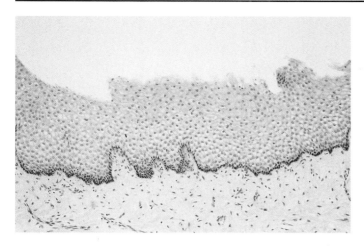

Fig. 2.21 Low-power view of lining mucosa. The epithelium is nonkeratinized and is nucleated throughout the surface layers. Unlike the epithelium of the palate, lining epithelium has a relatively flat basement membrane, with poorly developed rete ridges.

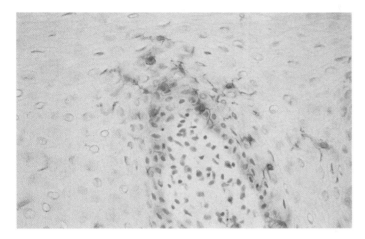

Fig. 2.22 High-power view of oral epithelium stained by the immunoperoxidase method to show Langerhans cells. These dendritic cells are distributed in the basal and lower prickle cell layers.

nerve fibers. Lymphocytes, usually T-cells, may also be found within the epithelium and are particularly prominent in inflammatory mucosal diseases. In routine light microscopy the nonkeratinocytes usually appear as small rounded cells surrounded by a clear halo. The dendritic nature of the Langerhans cells and melanocytes is not usually apparent, and special stains are needed for precise identification.

THE LAMINA PROPRIA

The oral epithelium is supported by a layer of vascular fibrous connective tissue called the lamina propria. This is divided into two layers: the papillary layer, which fills the connective tissue papillae between the epithelial rete ridges; and a deeper reticular layer, which contains dense collagen bundles. The main cell of the lamina propria is the fibroblast, which secretes the collagens and ground substance of the extracellular matrix, although mast cells, macrophages, and lymphocytes are also present.

The lamina propria provides structural support for the oral mucosa, and the density of the collagen bundles may vary from site to site depending upon the mechanical loads imposed.

REGIONAL VARIATIONS IN THE ORAL MUCOSA

Different parts of the mouth are subjected to different functional stresses and, as a consequence, the structure of the mucosa varies to accommodate them. It is important for a pathologist to appreciate the variations because a thickened epithelium which may be normal at one site may represent a pathological change at another adjacent site. The main variations involve the thickness or pattern of the keratin layers, the density of the fibrous connective tissue, or the presence or absence of a submucosa. There are three types of oral mucosa: lining mucosa, masticatory mucosa, and specialized mucosa.

LINING MUCOSA

This forms the largest proportion of the oral mucosa and covers the cheeks, lips, floor of the mouth, ventral surface of the tongue, the vestibules, and the soft palate. It has a nonkeratinized epithelium with a relatively poorly formed system of rete ridges (see Fig. 2.21). The lining mucosa must be distensible, and it therefore has a loose fibrous lamina propria and a thick fibrofatty submucosa. Minor salivary glands are abundant in the submucosa of the lips and soft palate but are also present elsewhere. The lining mucosa itself may vary in thickness. In the cheeks, where there may be considerable lateral shear forces, the epithelium is thick and may have quite well-developed, elongated, and branching connective tissue papillae. Here also, where the teeth often rub against the epithelium, there may be a degree of keratinization in the form of a layer of surface parakeratin. In the floor of the mouth where there are few forces, but where the movement of the tongue demands flexibility, the epithelium is very thin, with few papillae and a very loose and thick submucosa.

MASTICATORY MUCOSA

The mucosa of the hard palate and gingivae is composed of a thick keratinized epithelium overlying a dense fibrous lamina propria which is bound down directly to the periosteum without an intervening submucosa. The epithelial–connective tissue interface must resist the forces of mastication, and therefore has a large surface area in the form of long and well-developed rete ridges and connective tissue papillae (see Fig. 2.19).

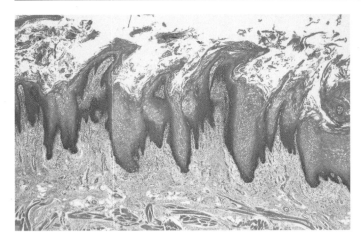

Fig. 2.23 A low-power view of the specialized mucosa of the dorsum of the tongue. There is a well-developed rete structure and filiform papillae project from the surface.

SPECIALIZED MUCOSA

The mucosa of the dorsal surface of the tongue is specialized for mastication and taste. It is heavily keratinized and is arranged into papillae, the most numerous of which are the filiform papillae which cover the surface of the tongue and give it a rough or velvety texture (Fig. 2.23). The filiform papillae are composed of cones of epithelium with a central connective tissue core and surmounted by a hair-like projection of keratin. Fungiform papillae are small dome-shaped structures with a nonkeratinized surface. They are randomly arranged towards the anterior aspect of the tongue and contain occasional taste buds on their surface. The circumvallate papillae are larger and are arranged in a V-shaped row between the anterior two-thirds and the posterior one-third of the tongue. They are flat-topped papillae surrounded by a trench. Serous saliva, from the glands of von Ebner, is secreted into the trench and taste buds are located on the lateral wall of the papillae. On the lateral aspects of the tongue in the posterior third there may be well-developed folds, often referred to as foliate papillae. These are not particularly well developed in humans, but when present may contain some taste buds or may overlie normal lymphoid tissue, sometimes referred to as lingual tonsil.

THE GINGIVAE

The gingivae are the cuff of oral mucosa, which surrounds and is attached to the teeth and periodontal structures (Fig. 2.24). The integrity of the lining of the mouth is maintained by the close attachment of the epithelium to the surface of the teeth via the junctional epithelium, which is continuous with the oral epithelium at the gingival margin. The lamina propria of the gingivae contains collagen bundles arranged into gingival fibers, which maintain the attachment of the mucosa to the alveolar bone and teeth.

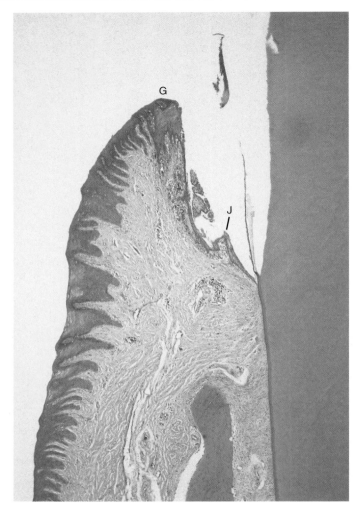

Fig. 2.24 A low-power view of the gingiva, the junctional epithelium (J) lines the gingival sulcus and is continuous with the oral epithelium at the gingival margin (G). The integrity of the lining of the mouth is maintained by the close attachment of the junctional epithelium to the enamel of the tooth, which cannot be seen in this decalcified section.

THE DEVELOPMENT AND STRUCTURE OF THE SALIVARY GLANDS

The salivary glands are usually divided into two groups according to size and location: the paired major glands and the intraoral minor salivary glands. The major glands comprise the parotid, submandibular, and sublingual glands, while the minor glands are mostly small mucous glands located beneath the epithelium in all parts of the mouth except the gingivae and anterior hard palate.

DEVELOPMENT OF THE SALIVARY GLANDS

The salivary glands begin to develop in the fourth week of intra-uterine life when the anlage of the parotid gland first appears.

carry the main blood vessels and nerves and the large interlobular ducts. These eventually drain into a single excretory duct that discharges saliva into the mouth. Within the lobules the epithelial component is arranged into many closely packed secretory units, each composed of a secretory endpiece that drains successively into intercalated and striated ducts (Fig. 2.26).

The endpieces actively secrete the saliva and consist of a group of cells arranged around a central lumen. There are two types of secretory cell in human salivary glands: serous cells and mucous cells. Serous cells form rounded compact endpieces, called acini, which contain numerous basophilic secretory granules on routine staining. Mucous cells are plump polygonal cells with a clear, mucus-filled cytoplasm. They usually form short tubular structures referred to as 'tubuloacini'. The parotid glands are wholly serous (Fig. 2.26), while the sublingual and intraoral glands are

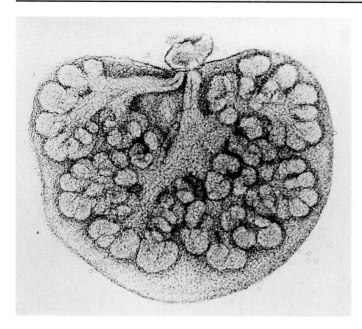

Fig. 2.25 Developing rat salivary gland in vitro shows the typical branching morphogenesis. The epithelium has repeatedly branched to form multiple ductal structures, each ending in a terminal bulb that will become a secretory endpiece. (Photograph kindly provided by Dr Patricia Hardman (Hardman & Spooner 1992).[28])

This is followed by the submandibular and sublingual glands at about 6 and 8 weeks, respectively. The minor salivary glands begin to form between 8 and 12 weeks. Development is similar for all the glands, and begins with a downgrowth of epithelium from the lining of the stomodeum. This forms a solid cord of cells that grows into the underlying mesenchyme and branches to form multiple epithelial strands with bulbous terminals, which will eventually form the secretory endpieces (Fig. 2.25). The centers of the solid strands are hollowed by degeneration of the cells, so that by 6 months an intact ductal system has formed. Secretion commences at around the time of birth.

Although it is the epithelial component that forms the characteristic structure of the salivary glands, in vitro studies have revealed that at the embryonic primordium stage the epithelium has absolute dependence upon the investing mesenchyme if it is to undergo the typical branching morphogenesis (see Fig. 2.25). This epithelial–mesenchymal interaction is mediated through the extracellular matrix of the basement membrane; the turnover of matrix and the sequential release and binding of growth factors at the tips of the growing epithelial buds appear to be crucial parts of this interaction.[28]

HISTOLOGY AND STRUCTURE OF THE SALIVARY GLANDS

The fully developed gland has an overall resemblance to a bunch of grapes divided into lobules by connective tissue septa, which

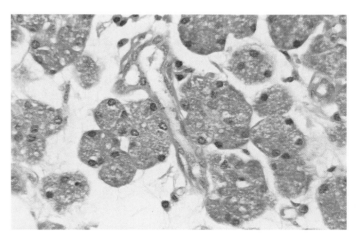

Fig. 2.26 High-power view of the parotid gland showing the acinar cells arranged into groups of secretory endpieces. Centrally three endpieces open into an intercalated duct.

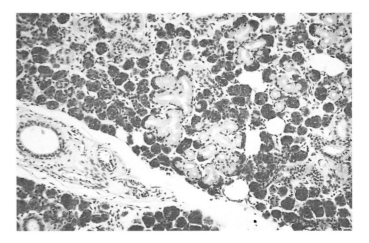

Fig. 2.27 Low-power view of the mixed submandibular gland stained with the periodic acid Schiff technique. Pale-staining mucous acini can be seen among the darker serous acini, and in places serous cells form caps or demilunes at the tips of the mucous tubules.

almost entirely mucous. The submandibular is a mixed gland that contains serous acini as well as mucous tubuloacini. Many of the mucous endpieces are surrounded by serous cells to form serous caps or demilunes, which drain into the same lumen (see Fig. 2.27).

The secretory endpieces are invested by myoepithelial cells that lie within the basement membrane and embrace the acini and intercalated ducts with long branching processes. Although of epithelial origin, the myoepithelial cells are contractile and have some features of smooth muscle, including parallel arrays of actin filaments. The myoepithelial cells function to support the secretory units and may also facilitate secretion by contracting and causing the ejection of preformed saliva. These cells are also an important component of some tumors, in particular pleomorphic adenoma and myoepithelioma, where the characteristic myxoid or mucoid stroma is of myoepithelial origin.

REFERENCES

1. Gorlin RJ, Cohen MM, Levine LS 1990 Syndromes of the head and neck, 3rd edn. Oxford University Press, New York
2. Le Douarin NM 1982 The neural crest. Cambridge University Press, Cambridge
3. Hall BK, Horstadius S 1988 The neural crest. Oxford University Press, Oxford
4. Webb JF, Noden DM 1993 Ectodermal placodes: contributions to the development of the vertebrate head. Am Zool 33: 434–447
5. Larsen WJ 1993 Human embryology. Churchill Livingstone, New York
6. Ferguson MWJ 1991 The orofacial region. In Wigglesworth JS, Singer DB (eds) Textbook of fetal and perinatal pathology. Blackwell, Oxford, vol 1, p 843–879
7. Thorogood P (ed) 1997 Embryos, genes and birth defects. Wiley, Chichester, p 197–229
8. Couly GF, Coltey PM, Le Douarin NM 1993 The triple origin of skull in higher vertebrates: a study in quail-chick chimeras. Development 117: 402–429
9. Thorogood P 1993 The differentiation and morphogenesis of cranial skeletal tissues. In Hanken J, Hall BK (eds) The vertebrate skull, University of Chicago Press, Chicago, vol 1, p 112–152
10. Hanken J, Thorogood P 1993 Evolution of the skull: a problem in pattern formation. Trends in Ecology and Evolution 8: 9–15
11. Noden DM 1983 The embryonic origins of avian cephalic and cervical muscles and associated connective tissues. Am J Anat 168: 257–276
12. Couly GF, Coltey PM, Le Douarin NM 1992 The developmental fate of the cephalic mesoderm in quail-chick chimeras. Development 114: 1–15
13. Trainor P, Tan S-S, Tam PPL 1994 Cranial paraxial mesoderm: regionalisation of cell fate and impact on craniofacial development in mouse embryos. Development 120: 2397–2408
14. Noden DM 1983 The role of neural crest in patterning of avian cranial skeletal, connective and muscle tissue. Dev Biol 96: 296–312
15. Williams LP 1995 Gray's anatomy, 38th edn. Churchill Livingstone, Edinburgh
16. Le Douarin NM 1993 Patterning of neural crest derivatives in the avian embryo: in vivo and in vitro studies. Dev Biol 159: 24–49
17. Noden DM 1991 Cell movements and control of patterned tissue assembly during craniofacial development. J Craniofac Genet Dev Biol 11: 192–213
18. Richman JM, Tickle C 1989 Epithelia are interchangeable between facial primordia of chick embryos and morphogenesis is controlled by the mesenchyme. Dev Biol 136: 201–210
19. Fraser S, Keynes R, Lumsden A 1990 Segmentation in the chick hindbrain is defined by cell lineage restrictions. Nature 344: 431–435
20. Lumsden A, Sprawson N, Graham A 1991 Segmental origin and migration of neural crest cells in the hindbrain region of the chick embryo. Development 113: 1281–1291
21. Graham A, Heyman I, Lumsden A 1993 Even-numbered rhombomeres control the apoptotic elimination of neural crest cells from odd-numbered rhombomeres in the chick hindbrain. Development 119: 233–245
22. Krumaluf R 1994 *Hox* genes in vertebrate development. Cell 78: 191–201
23. Duboule D, Dollé P 1989 The structural and functional organisation of the murine *Hox* gene family resembles that of *Drosophila* homeotic genes. EMBO J 8: 1497–1505
24. Hunt P, Gulisano M, Cook M et al 1991 A distinct Hox code for the branchial region of the vertebrate head. Nature 353: 861–864
25. Vieille-Grosjean I, Hunt P, Gulisano M, Boncinelli E, Thorogood P 1997 Branchial *Hox* gene expression and human craniofacial development. Dev Biol 183: 49–60
26. Thesleff I 1997 The teeth. In Thorogood P (ed) Embryos, genes and birth defects. Wiley, Chichester, p. 329–348
27. Squier CA, Johnson N, Hopps RM 1976 Human oral mucosa. Development, structure and function. Blackwell, Oxford
28. Hardman P, Spooner BS 1992 Salivary epithelium branching morphogenesis. In Fleming TP (ed.) Epithelium organization and development. Chapman & Hall, London, p 353–375

Odontogenic tumors

Ameloblastoma

3

Because of the limitations of early microscopy and dependence on drawings, there is uncertainty as to who provided the first accurate descriptions of an ameloblastoma. Gorlin[1] firmly identifies Cusack[2] in Dublin, as recognizing it as early as 1827. Falkson[3] gave a detailed description in 1879, and Baden[4] has discussed its early history. Bouquot & Lense[5] give credit to Wedl[6] for the first histopathological description in 1853, although his book on oral pathology was not published until 1870. Wedl called the tumor 'cystosarcoma or cystosarcoma adenoides,' but suggested that it could have arisen from a tooth bud or the dental lamina. Bouquot & Lense[5] also ascribe the first histological drawing of ameloblastoma to Wagstaffe[7] in 1871.

Gorlin[1] credits Malassez[8] with introducing the term *adamantine epithelioma* and Derjinsky with introducing the term *adamantinoma* in 1890. Ivy and Churchill[9] were the first to encourage adoption of the term *ameloblastoma*, although Gorlin[1] points out that Galippe[10] suggested the term appreciably earlier.

A few still cling to term 'adamantinoma,' but it should be avoided as obsolete and a possible source of confusion with the so-called adamantinoma of long bones.

INCIDENCE

Early large series examining the relative frequency of the different types of odontogenic tumors, such as that by Bhaskar[11] suffer from the fact that several other entities have been identified since that time. Regezi et al[12] in an analysis of 706 odontogenic tumors (12 types, but including periapical cemental dysplasia) found ameloblastomas to account for 11%. Daley et al[13] found that ameloblastomas comprised 13.5% of 392 odontogenic tumors of 20 currently recognized types. They also compared the relative incidence of ameloblastomas with cysts of the jaws. Thus there were only 79 ameloblastomas to 7287 jaw cysts of all types. The relative rarity of ameloblastomas as shown by their infrequency among this large body of material also makes clear the difficulties in acquiring valid data on the behavior and effect of treatment, particularly of tumor subtypes.

Race and gender distribution

Shear and Singh,[14] in South Africa, calculated the age-standardized

incidence of ameloblastomas as 2.09 per million for black African males and 1.55 for females. In white males, the age-standardized incidence was 0.42 and in white females 0.23 per million. In West Africa, Adekeye[15] found that 62.4% of 109 ameloblastomas were in males (1.7 : 1). Günhan et al[16] found that ameloblastomas accounted for no fewer than 36.5% of 403 benign odontogenic tumors in Turkey, while Wu & Chan,[17] from analysis of 204 583 surgical specimens found ameloblastomas to account for a remarkable 61% of 82 odontogenic jaw tumors in Hong Kong Chinese.

Age and gender distribution

Ameloblastomas are rare in children, and reviews of large series have confirmed an average age at presentation of between 33 and 44 years[18–20] in the USA and similar findings in the Far East.[21,22] However, in West Africa, Adekeye[15] found a mean age at presentation of 26.3 years with 80% of patients being less than 40 years old.

These findings have been confirmed by an analysis of reports in the major European languages as well as Korean and Japanese of 3677 ameloblastomas, by Reichart et al.[23] They found that, worldwide, the median age was 35 years with a range of 4–92 years. Males accounted for 53% of cases and females 47%. However, the mean age at presentation was 28.7 years in blacks, 39.9 years in Caucasians, and 41.2 years in Asians. The average age of patients from developing countries was 27.7 years, while that of patients from industrialized countries was 39.1 years.

These figures apply to ameloblastomas in general. Maxillary ameloblastomas may be seen at a later age. Tsaknis & Nelson[24] found the average age of 24 patients with maxillary ameloblastomas to be 45.6 years. The male/female ratio was 2.4 : 1, but the patients were members of the US military, before females were accepted in the armed services. Extraosseous ameloblastomas also appear to affect an older group of patients and also show a greater male preponderance than the intraosseous type.

In the case of unicystic ameloblastomas, as discussed below, there also appears to be a significant male preponderance, but presentation is earlier, being more frequent in the second and third decades. However, relatively few cases have been reported.

Site distribution

Small & Waldron[19] found 81% of ameloblastomas to have been in the mandible, and of these 70% were in the molar–ramus area. Forty-seven per cent of maxillary ameloblastomas were in the molar region, and 20% in the antrum and floor of the nose. In Waldron & El Mofty's breakdown of the sites of 110 ameloblastomas,[20] 83% were in the mandible, 61% were in the molar area, 12.5% in the premolar area, and 11% in the anterior area. Of 14 maxillary ameloblastomas, 50% were in the anterior area, 43% in the posterior area, and 7% in the premolar area.

Reichart et al[23] noted that the mandible was affected over five times as frequently as the maxilla. They also showed that in blacks the incisor region was relatively more frequently affected than in Caucasians and Asians.

Desmoplastic ameloblastomas appear to be unusual in that the relatively few reported cases have equally frequently involved the maxilla or mandible. This type of ameloblastoma is also unusual in that it frequently forms in the anterior part of the jaw, and many specimens have been detected before they exceeded 2 cm in diameter.

Unicystic ameloblastomas

Shteyer et al[25] found that these affected a younger age group, the average age being 10.8 years. Gardner & Corio[26] in their analysis of 46 plexiform, unicystic ameloblastomas also concluded that they were more frequent in patients less than 30 years old. The majority (82%) contained a tooth and appeared radiographically as dentigerous cysts. All were in the mandible, and males were affected twice as frequently as females.

Ackerman et al,[27] in a study of 57 unicystic ameloblastomas, concluded that the gender and site distribution corresponded with that of solid and multicystic ameloblastomas, but the mean age at diagnosis of 23.8 years was significantly younger.

Clinical features

Ameloblastomas grow slowly and typically cause no symptoms until a swelling becomes noticeable. Occasionally, small tumors may be first seen in a routine radiograph. As the tumor enlarges it forms a hard, rounded swelling, but later thinning of the bone allows eggshell cracking to be elicited. However, the slow growth of the tumor may allow reactive bone formation almost to keep pace with it. As a result, the jaw may become grossly enlarged and distorted, as shown in early illustrations. If neglected further, the tumor can perforate the bone and, ultimately, spread into the soft tissues, making subsequent excision difficult. Even large tumors rarely cause pain, although Ueno et al[21] reported pain in 25% of their patients. Other effects include: difficulties with managing a denture; displacement, mobility, and resorption of teeth; and paresthesia if the inferior dental canal is invaded. Rarely, an ameloblastoma can ulcerate through the mucosa, but such a complication or production of enormous tumors is likely only to be seen in the developing world or in illustrations to early texts.

RADIOGRAPHY

At least 85% of ameloblastomas form rounded, well-defined, multilocular, cyst-like radiolucent areas with well-defined margins. Variants include a honeycomb pattern of radiolucency, a soap-bubble appearance, or, rarely, a few large radiolucent areas with small daughter cysts nearby. The bony margins are typically scalloped (Fig. 3.1).

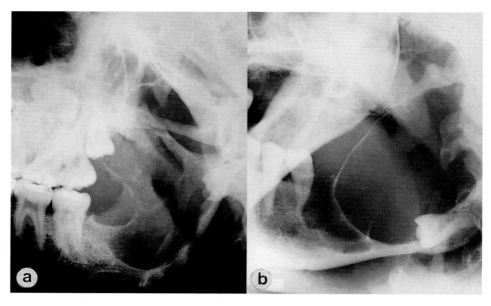

Fig. 3.1 Ameloblastoma. Radiographs showing **a** the typical multilocular appearance and **b** an appearance resembling a dentigerous cyst. This is more typical of plexiform unicystic ameloblastomas.

A monolocular well-defined cavity, which frequently contains a tooth, is the usual appearance of unicystic ameloblastomas.

Ameloblastomas preferentially infiltrate medullary bone, often without inducing resorption. The radiographic margins are not therefore accurate indicators of the extent of involvement. Compact, cortical bone mainly undergoes pressure resorption rather than invasion, but may eventually be perforated. Periosteum is rarely penetrated.

Buccal and lingual expansion of the cortical plates may be seen on an occlusal radiograph, but is not pathognomonic of ameloblastoma (Fig. 3.1). The roots of adjacent teeth are frequently displaced or resorbed.

Overall, therefore, the appearances can often strongly suggest an ameloblastoma, but differentiation from keratocysts, other tumors of the jaws, or hyperparathyroidism by radiography alone is not reliable.

The uncommon desmoplastic ameloblastoma is unusual in that it can resemble a fibro-osseous lesion radiographically, and of the cases reported by Waldron & El Mofty[20] most were no more than 1.0–2.0 cm in maximum diameter. None of the six cases where radiographs were available resembled conventional ameloblastomas. Radiographic appearances included irregular radiolucent areas containing fine irregular calcifications and having indistinct borders. Others had a mixed radiolucent/radiopaque appearance with indistinct borders. Kaffe et al[28] found that only 3 of 15 cases appeared multilocular, only 2 had well-defined margins, and all except one had a mixed radiolucent/radiopaque appearance. Tooth displacement was seen in 92%, but roots were resorbed in only 33% of these cases.

Waldron & El Mofty[20] describe 11% of their 116 ameloblastomas as unicystic. This variant particularly involves the posterior part of the body of the mandible, and the majority surround the crown of a displaced molar tooth. The radiolucent area is frequently well circumscribed with the result that the tumor may not be distinguishable radiographically from a radicular, dentigerous or other non-neoplastic cyst. Eversole et al[29] described the radiographic findings in 31 cases of unicystic ameloblastoma and noted that 52% were associated with unerupted third molars and usually appeared as unilocular pericoronal radiolucencies.

MICROSCOPY

Although distinct subtypes are described here, Reichart et al[23] found that 15.5% of 1593 ameloblastomas showed mixed histological appearances.

Follicular ameloblastomas. These are the most readily recognizable and most common type. From a total of 1593 cases from reports and reviews, Reichart et al[23] found that they accounted for 33.9% cases.

Follicular ameloblastomas consist of islands or trabeculae of epithelial cells in a connective tissue stroma (Fig. 3.2). These epithelial islands consist of a core of loosely arranged polygonal or angular cells, resembling stellate reticulum, surrounded by a well-organized single layer (palisade) of tall, columnar, ameloblast-

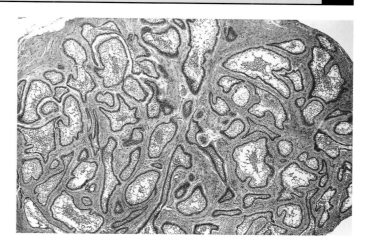

Fig. 3.2 Ameloblastoma. Low-power view showing typical islands of a follicular tumor in a fibrous stroma.

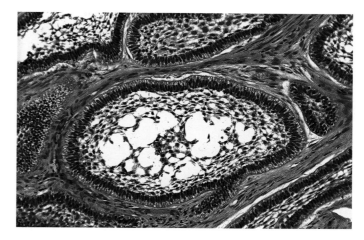

Fig. 3.3 Ameloblastoma, follicular type. Higher power view showing typical ameloblast-like cells with reversed nuclear polarity, surrounding stellate reticulum-like epithelial cells with incipient cyst formation.

like cells with nuclei at the opposite pole to the basement membrane (reversed nuclear polarity) (Fig. 3.3). This peripheral cell layer tends to show cytoplasmic vacuolization. In other specimens, or other parts of the same tumor, the peripheral cells may be cut obliquely or be more cuboidal and resemble basal cells.

Cyst formation is common and varies from microcysts within a predominantly solid tumor, to an almost completely cystic tumor. Cysts develop particularly within the epithelial islands as a result of degeneration of the stellate reticulum-like cells. Approximately 75% of ameloblastomas are at least partially cystic.

As with most other ameloblastomas the margins are ill-defined and infiltration of surrounding cancellous bone can be seen.

Plexiform ameloblastomas. These were found by Reichart et al[23] to account for 30.2% of 1593 cases. They consist largely of thin trabeculae of epithelium typically bordered by less-well-differentiated columnar cells than the ameloblast-like cells of the follicular type. The stroma consists of loose, vascular, sparsely

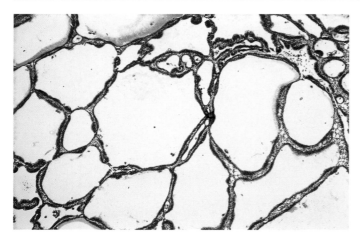

Fig. 3.4 Plexiform ameloblastoma. Strands of small darkly staining cells surround stellate reticulum-like cells. Extensive microcystic change is due to stromal degeneration.

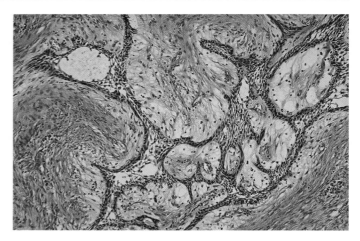

Fig. 3.6 Plexiform ameloblastoma. Higher power view of the nondescript-looking epithelium.

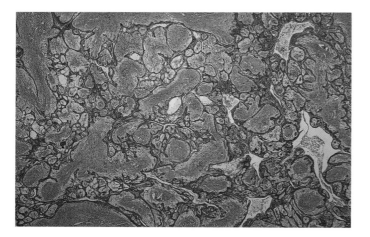

Fig. 3.5 Plexiform ameloblastoma showing strands of darkly staining cells in a dense fibrous stroma.

cells. They excluded from this study any unicystic ameloblastomas that showed histological patterns typical of other types of ameloblastoma. Solid masses of tumor cells may also extend into the lumen, or islands of tumor may infiltrate the fibrous wall. However, to be categorized as unicystic, the ameloblastoma tissue must be confined to the cyst and not extend into the wall (Figs 3.7 and 3.8a). It is important, therefore, to note that the diagnosis of unicystic ameloblastoma cannot be made on the basis of a unilocular radiographic appearance or a single incisional biopsy. Multiple areas need to be evaluated to confirm that the tumor does not extend beyond the cyst wall.

It must be emphasized that not all unicystic ameloblastomas are pure plexiform in type. Ackermann et al,[27] in their study of 57 unicystic ameloblastomas, defined three subgroups. Group 1 (42%) consisted of a unilocular cyst with a nondescript but variable epithelial lining, frequently with typical ameloblastoma cells in the basal layer in some parts. Inactive odontogenic cell rests might be present in the fibrous wall, but there was no

cellular connective tissue. Microcyst formation is common and typically due to stromal degeneration (Figs 3.4–3.6). Degeneration of the stroma rather than of the epithelium is difficult to understand, especially as the stromal blood vessels also disappear or may be seen as ghostly outlines surrounding erythrocytes.

Plexiform ameloblastomas are more frequent in the maxilla, and most maxillary ameloblastomas are plexiform in part at least.

Plexiform unicystic ameloblastomas. These were first described by Robinson & Martinez[30] and are now accepted as a distinct subtype with a lower recurrence rate after surgery. Shteyer et al,[25] in reviewing mural ameloblastomas, concluded that they formed 9.7% of 835 reported ameloblastomas: 83% of them contained a tooth and simulated dentigerous cysts.

Unicystic ameloblastoma is defined as a single cystic cavity that shows ameloblastomatous differentiation in the lining. As defined by Gardner & Corio,[26] these tumors show no ameloblast-like cells but do show a net-like pattern of trabeculae of squamous

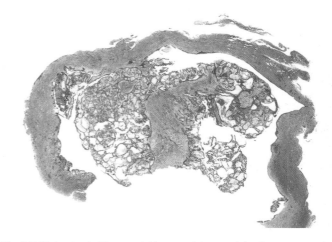

Fig. 3.7 Unicystic plexiform ameloblastoma. A large nodule of tumor protrudes into the cyst cavity.

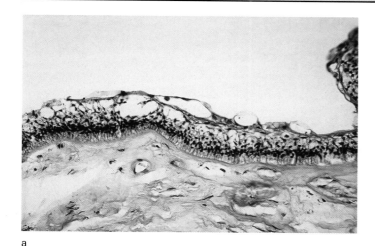

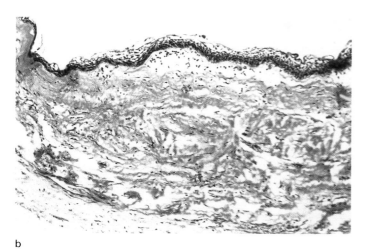

Fig. 3.8 a Unicystic ameloblastoma showing a flattened cyst lining that retains ameloblast-like cells in the basal layer. **b** Unicystic ameloblastoma showing a flattened cyst lining resembling that of a non-neoplastic cyst.

infiltration by neoplastic epithelium. Group 2 lesions (9%) featured intraluminal plexiform proliferation but no infiltration of the cyst wall. In Group 3 lesions (49%), plexiform- or follicular-type ameloblastoma, sometimes in continuity with the cyst lining, infiltrated the wall. The lining of the cystic area becomes flattened and can resemble that of a non-neoplastic cyst (Fig. 3.8b). Biopsy of part of the cyst wall, therefore, can led to a misdiagnosis of a non-neoplastic cyst, unless an area of ameloblast-like cells is seen.

Incidentally, this cystic overgrowth of ameloblastomas, with obliteration of the normal microscopic features of the tumor in the flattened cyst wall, is one reason for earlier beliefs that ameloblastomas can originate in non-neoplastic cysts. Thus, Leider et al,[31] in an analysis of 33 cystic ameloblastomas, confirmed that 'ordinary' (stratified squamous) epithelium could be identified the cyst lining in 88% of cases, and concluded that unicystic ameloblastomas were most likely to have arisen as a result of neoplastic change in an odontogenic cyst. However, Shear[32] firmly dismisses this idea (as discussed later). If there is any doubt, Saku

et al[33] report that cystic as well as solid ameloblastomas bind the lectins UEA-1 and BSA-1, enabling them to be differentiated from non-neoplastic odontogenic cysts, which do not. In this way it may be possible to identify with certainty the residuum of a non-neoplastic cyst from which an ameloblastoma may have arisen.

Acanthomatous ameloblastomas. These accounted for 11.3% of 1593 ameloblastomas reviewed by Reichart et al.[23] Acanthomatous ameloblastomas show squamous metaplasia of the central core of epithelium of the tumors, which otherwise resemble the more common follicular type. Keratin formation may be prominent and the tumor may be mistaken for a squamous cell carcinoma (Fig. 3.9). Ferreiro[34] found that four acanthomatous ameloblastomas reacted strongly with anti-CEA but that a single example of the follicular type failed to do so.

Papilliferous keratoameloblastomas. These may be a variant or a different entity. It was first described by Pindborg.[35] Further cases reported since then[36,37] have brought the total number of cases to three. Histologically, there are sheets of epithelial follicles, separated by bands of connective tissue. The follicles are mostly lined by papilliferous epithelium and filled with necrotic debris or, sometimes, desquamated keratin. The lining epithelium consists of large rounded cells with central, vesiculated nuclei and prominent nucleoli. These same cells clad the connective tissue core of the papilliferous projections. The remaining follicles are lined by parakeratinizing stratified squamous epithelium. No ameloblast-like cells are seen. This variant accounted for 0.1% of 1593 ameloblastomas reviewed by Reichart et al.[23]

Granular cell ameloblastomas. These are also rare; they accounted for 3.5% of the ameloblastomas reviewed by Reichart et al.[23] They usually resemble the more common follicular type, but the epithelium, particularly in the centers of the tumor islands, forms sheets of large eosinophilic granular cells resembling those of other granular cell tumors (Figs 3.10 and 3.11). This change may be so extensive that the peripheral columnar cells are replaced, making the tumor difficult to recognize in a small biopsy specimen. Granular-cell formation was thought to be an aging or degenerative change, but can be seen in ameloblastomas in young persons.

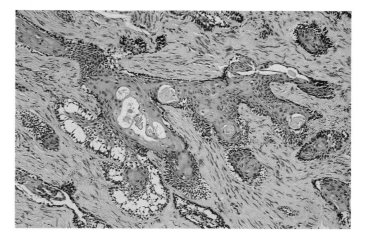

Fig. 3.9 Acanthomatous ameloblastoma with squamous metaplasia of the stellate reticulum-like cells.

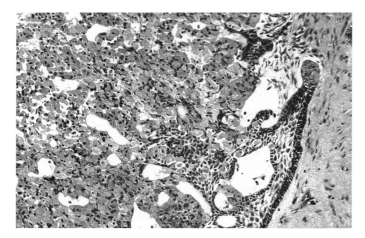

Fig. 3.10 Granular cell ameloblastoma. Low-power view.

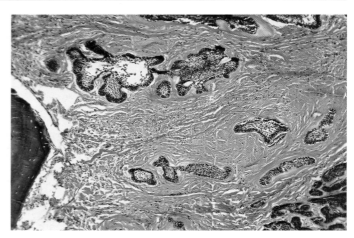

Fig. 3.12 Desmoplastic ameloblastoma. Only scattered islands of tumor lie in a dense fibrous stroma.

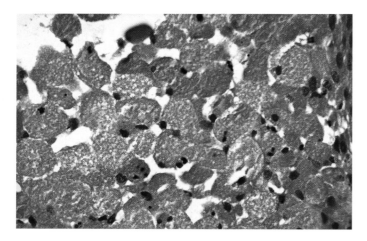

Fig. 3.11 Granular cell ameloblastoma. Higher power view of the eosinophilic granular cells.

Navarrete & Smith[38] investigated the ultrastructure of this variant, and found that the granules consisted mainly of pleomorphic, osmiophilic, lysosome-like organelles.

Desmoplastic ameloblastomas. According to Philipsen et al,[39] these were first described (in the Japanese literature) by Takigawa et al[40] and by Uji et al.[41] Eversole et al[29] were the first to describe the tumor in the English language, and reported three cases in detail. This variant accounted for 1.4% of 1593 ameloblastomas reviewed by Reichart et al.[23]

Desmoplastic ameloblastomas have been reviewed by Ashman et al,[42] and in more detail by Philipsen et al,[39] who analyzed the findings in 29 reported cases. These tumors consist predominantly of dense collagenous fibrous tissue in which there are small, irregular islands of neoplastic epithelium. These islands are rounded or angular, and may have slender straggling extensions. There is little or no cyst formation, and ameloblast-like cells are typically only present in small foci on the periphery of some islands of epithelium. Stellate reticulum-like tissue is also absent from the interior of the epithelial islands, which consist of densely packed

spindle-shaped or polygonal cells (Fig. 3.12). Squamous metaplasia or foci of keratinization may occasionally be seen centrally, and this variant may be difficult to recognize as an ameloblastoma. Calcification in the fibrous stroma and, occasionally, bone formation is seen.

Basal cell ameloblastomas. These formed only 1.4% of the 1593 ameloblastomas reviewed by Reichart et al.[23] They consist of darkly staining cells in a predominantly trabecular pattern with little evidence of palisading at the periphery. Rare examples of extraosseous basal cell ameloblastomas have been mistaken for basal cell carcinomas. However, the latter do not affect the oral cavity (Fig. 3.13).

Clear cell ameloblastoma. This was described by Müller & Slootweg[43] and by Waldron et al,[44] who termed it an odontogenic carcinoma. Ng & Siar[45] reported a peripheral ameloblastoma with clear cell differentiation. Apart from the fields of clear cells, these tumors were follicular or plexiform ameloblastomas, and thus differed from the clear cell odontogenic carcinoma, which shows no features of ameloblastoma (see Fig. 7.1).

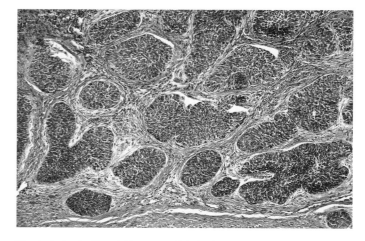

Fig. 3.13 Basal cell ameloblastoma. Solid islands of basaloid hyperchromatic cells are interspersed by fibrous stroma.

Ng & Siar[45] could find only the four reports already quoted of ameloblastomas with clear cell change. Only the maxillary ameloblastoma reported by Waldron et al[44] caused death from local spread of disease 14.5 years after maxillectomy and radiotherapy, while the patient reported by Müller & Slootweg[43] was free from disease 15 years after conservative marginal resection. None developed metastases.

Too few cases have been reported to determine whether these tumors are variants of clear cell odontogenic carcinoma. However, their failure to metastasize casts doubts on whether they should be regarded as truly malignant as Waldron et al[44] believed, or whether indeed they are significantly different from other ameloblastomas.

Rarely, mucous cells can be seen in ameloblastomas, but their presence does not seem to affect the tumor behavior.

BEHAVIOR AND MANAGEMENT

The diagnosis should be confirmed by biopsy, but occasionally may be made only after excision. This is particularly true of cystic ameloblastomas, when tumor tissue is found in only a limited area of mural thickening.

Ameloblastomas are, with rare exceptions, benign and slow growing, but relentlessly infiltrative. Death only results from involvement of vital tissues, by maxillary ameloblastomas in particular.

It is generally believed that histological variations in solid ameloblastoma do not affect tumor behavior. Hartman,[46] from a survey of the results of treatment of 15 granular cell ameloblastomas, concluded that they were more likely to recur than other types. However, 10 of those that recurred had been treated by methods now regarded as inadequate, namely, enucleation, curettage, and irradiation. Cranin et al[47] have reported a pulmonary metastasis, considered to have been haematogenous, from a massive granular cell ameloblastoma that was neglected for 45 years.

More recently, Reichart et al,[23] from their extensive review, have concluded that the histological subtype may affect the risk of recurrence. Thus, of a total of 144 ameloblastomas where information was available, the recurrence rates for plexiform, follicular, granular cell, and acanthomatous types were 16.7%, 29.5%, 33.3%, and 4.5%, respectively. While these differences were statistically significant, the numbers of individual subtypes of tumor were small. However, more important than histological subtype in terms of behavior, is whether the tumor is multi- or unicystic.

Treatment of solid ameloblastomas is by wide excision including up to 1.5 cm of clinically normal bone around the margin. Sehdev et al[48] reported a recurrence rate of almost 90% after mere curettage of mandibular ameloblastomas and 100% for maxillary tumors. Although recurrence may not be evident for several years, curettage is clearly inadequate, particularly for solid ameloblastomas. Reichart et al,[23] from their analysis of 327 reported cases, found recurrence rates of 17.7% after radical and 22.6% after conservative surgery. However, reviews of treatment have shown widely variable recurrence rates.

Excision can be curative, but large tumors may require resection of the jaw and bone grafting. However, ameloblastomas are slow growing, typically infiltrate cancellous bone, and, as shown by Kramer,[49] only later erode compact bone. If, therefore, the lower border of the mandible is tumor free, it should be possible to preserve it and, by continuing dissection subperiosteally, avoid complete resection and bone grafting. Bony repair follows, and much of the jaw regenerates. Any residual tumor may take many years to recur and should be detectable at an early stage by regular radiographic follow-up. The latter is therefore mandatory. A further limited operation can then be carried out if necessary. This approach is generally less unpleasant for the patient, who must be warned of the necessity of regular follow-up and of the possibility of further surgery.

The chief risk with mandibular ameloblastomas is extension into the soft tissues, when it becomes difficult to define the tumor margins and vital structures may be endangered.

The value of radiotherapy has been reviewed by Gardner.[50] He concluded that radiotherapy can reduce the size of a tumor, but is not appropriate treatment for operable tumors. Its main use, therefore, is for inoperable tumors, particularly those in the posterior maxilla.

Plexiform unicystic ameloblastomas, by contrast, appear to have a considerably better prognosis than the more common type. They are frequently enucleated as cysts before their neoplastic nature is appreciated, but even with this form of treatment recurrence rates are low. Of 28 cases where Gardner & Corio[26] had follow-up information, the recurrence rate after enucleation or curettage was only 10.7% after an average period of 8.5 years. As a consequence, they advised avoidance of resection. Reichart et al[23] found a recurrence rate of 13.7% (73 cases) for unicystic ameloblastoma, as compared with an overall recurrence rate for solid ameloblastomas of 22.7%.

Robinson & Martinez[30] were the first to show the low recurrence rate of unicystic ameloblastomas, irrespective of the histological configuration, in 20 patients for whom follow-up data was available. Ackermann et al,[27] by contrast, suggested that unicystic ameloblastomas in which tumor had infiltrated the cyst wall (their group 3) should be treated aggressively, but those where there was no such infiltration (groups 1 and 2) could be treated conservatively. Thompson et al[51] reported recurrence, 5 years after enucleation, of a plexiform unicystic ameloblastoma with infiltration of the capsule.

Li et al[52] have compared the expression of proliferating cell nuclear antigen (PCNA) and Ki-67 in 14 unicystic and in a similar number of solid ameloblastomas. Cystic tumor lining showed relatively few PCNA-positive cells and a labeling index significantly lower than that for invading islands or intraluminal nodules. The labeling indices of solid follicular ameloblastomas were significantly higher than those of cystic ameloblastoma lining or intraluminal nodules. However, invading islands in the walls of cystic ameloblastomas showed a similar labeling index to that of solid ameloblastomas. There thus appears to be a biological basis for more vigorous treatment of cystic ameloblastomas with tumor proliferation within the fibrous wall.

The fact that cystic ameloblastomas can so closely resemble non-neoplastic cysts both radiographically and, to some degree, histologically also makes it mandatory to enucleate all cystic lesions completely, and to examine the entire cyst wall, particularly any mural thickenings, by microscopy. If mural plexiform ameloblastoma without infiltration of the wall is found, no further treatment may be necessary, but prolonged radiographic follow-up should be maintained. Extension of tumor through the fibrous cyst wall suggests that recurrence is likely, but operation may be delayed until this appears. Local excision may then be adequate, but prolonged observation is essential.

The management of ameloblastomas, including the many variants, has been reviewed by Williams.[53]

Maxillary ameloblastomas are particularly dangerous, partly because the bones are considerably thinner than those of the mandible and present less effective barriers to spread. Maxillary ameloblastomas tend to form in the posterior segment and to grow upwards to invade the sinonasal passages, pterygomaxillary fossa, orbit, cranium, and brain. They are thus potentially lethal.

Bredenkamp et al[54] reported five such cases, of which only two patients were known to be alive and disease free after periods of 14 months to 5 years. Four earlier cases were also reviewed: all had died or were presumed dead from their disease.

Radical excision of maxillary ameloblastomas at the earliest possible stage is essential. Effective reoperation is unlikely to be possible. Maxillectomy is usually the first requirement. However, there is limited information about the most effective surgical approach to ameloblastomas extending towards the skull base. Hell et al[55] have described the extensive surgery, including exenteration of an orbit, and extensive prosthetic reconstruction required for the removal of a recurrent follicular ameloblastoma that had extended into the skull base.

Postoperative radiotherapy may slow the growth of recurrences, but is little more than palliative. Chemotherapy has not been shown to be of any value.

Primary extraosseous (peripheral) ameloblastoma

Five per cent of the 116 ameloblastomas surveyed by Waldron & El Mofty[20] were extraosseous and superficial to the alveolar ridge. In Japan, Ueno et al[21] found that only 2% of 104 ameloblastomas were extraosseous. Older persons are predominantly affected. Reichart et al[23] also found that only 2% of 3677 ameloblastomas had been classified as peripheral.

El-Mofty et al[56] confirmed the findings of Gardner[57] that extraosseous ameloblastomas typically affect middle-aged patients. Nauta et al[58] found, from 53 reported cases, 60% of the patients to be male and the mandibular gingiva to be the site in 65%. Reichart et al[23] found the mandible to be affected five times as frequently as the maxilla. The incisor to premolar region was involved in 65%. Nauta et al[58] and Reichart et al[23] found the average age of

patients to be 50–51 years. In the eight cases presented by Gurol & Burkes,[59] the average age of patients was 62 years.

CLINICAL FEATURES

Clinically, peripheral ameloblastomas resemble fibrous nodules, pyogenic granulomas, or other peripheral hyperplastic swellings superficial to the alveolar ridge, and can interfere with the fit of a denture. They sometimes appear as erythematous plaques or, rarely, are polypoid or papillary.

They are slow-growing and cause little or no bone erosion. Any saucerization of the underlying bone is due to pressure rather than invasion.

The prominence of peripheral ameloblastomas usually leads to a request for treatment before they grow beyond 2 cm in diameter. However, Nauta et al[58] noted that one example had been allowed to grow to 12 cm × 6 cm in size.

In contrast to findings in Western countries, Zhu et al[60] found no fewer than 43 well-documented reports of peripheral ameloblastoma in the Japanese literature for the period 1967–1992. Three were located in the palatal or buccal mucosa. The most common site was the mandibular premolar region, but in the upper jaw the anterior region was more frequently affected than in Western patients.

HISTOGENESIS

Histologically, continuity with the mucosal epithelium is a significant feature, but multiple sections may have to be examined. El Mofty et al[56] found that, among 11 peripheral ameloblastomas, only one was pure follicular, one was basal cell, three were plexiform, and the remainder were of mixed type. By contrast, Zhu et al[60] noted that, of 43 Japanese cases, 19 were acanthomatous, seven were plexiform, three were follicular, and four were mixed. In the eight cases described by Gerol & Burkes,[59] only two were follicular, while three each were plexiform or acanthomatous (Fig. 3.14).

BEHAVIOR AND MANAGEMENT

Peripheral ameloblastomas can be managed by local excision. Reichart et al[23] found an overall recurrence rate of 9% (33 cases). In the event of recurrence, a further and wider local excision should be curative. This, of course, is in sharp contrast to soft tissue extensions of central ameloblastomas, which require wide excision and are difficult to control because of the difficulties in defining their margins.

Malignant ameloblastoma and ameloblastic carcinoma

These tumors are so uncommon that many pathologists may not

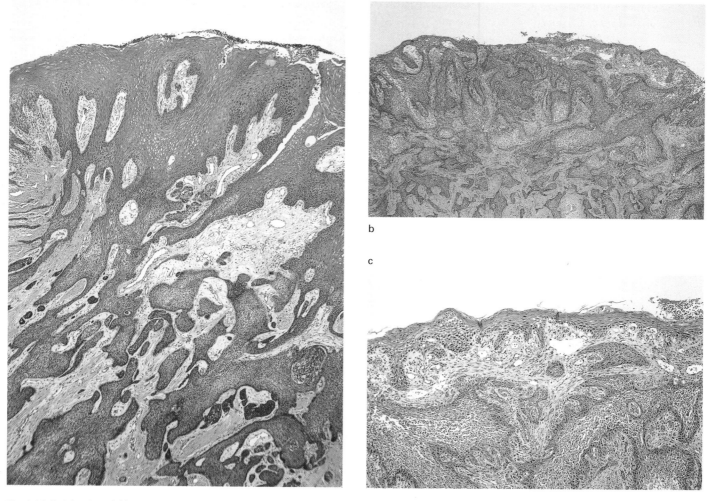

a

b

c

Fig. 3.14 Peripheral ameloblastoma. **a** Low-power view shows fusion with the mucosal epithelium, giving a pseudoepitheliomatous appearance. **b** Extension through the mucosal epithelium and a suggestion of early ulceration. **c** The mucosal epithelium shows reactive changes, and inflammation has permeated the islands of tumor.

see either type in a lifetime of practice. Moreover, the tumors are not recognized as separate entities in the 1992 WHO classification, although Slootweg & Müller[61] have made a strong case for their recognition. Hardly surprisingly, there has been some confusion about the terminology and the terms have sometimes been used indifferently.

In their analysis of 46 cases, Slootweg & Müller[61] categorized the tumors, with slight modifications, according to Elzay's classification.[62] These ameloblastomas thus fell into four groups: those where both the primary and metastatic growths consisted of well-differentiated ameloblastoma (20 reports); those where the metastasis was less well differentiated than the primary growth (two reports); those where both the primary and metastatic growth showed dedifferentiation (nine reports); and those where the jaw tumor was both locally aggressive and showed dedifferentiation, but lacked evidence of metastases (15 cases). Malignant ameloblastoma and ameloblastic carcinoma must also, of course, be distinguished from conventional ameloblastomas that have endangered life by extending towards vital structures.

MALIGNANT AMELOBLASTOMA

The term 'malignant ameloblastoma' has been given to an ameloblastoma that, despite typical histologic appearances, has given rise to pulmonary or nodal metastases. The metastases have retained the microscopic appearances of the primary growth. In addition to the 20 cases reviewed by Slootweg & Müller,[61] Kunze et al[63] reported another case and analyzed 25 others reported in the literature. They considered that in 80% of cases the metastases were of a pure or mixed plexiform type and, histologically, did not differ significantly from conventional, nonmetastasizing ameloblastomas. It was therefore not possible, they believed, to predict on the basis of morphology whether an ameloblastoma would metastasize. However, the chances of it so doing are exceedingly small.

Vorzimer & Perla[64] found tumor casts in the bronchi of a patient with pulmonary metastases. They argued that at least some of these deposits had resulted from aspiration implantation. This finding does not appear to have been confirmed but, if it were to be, the secondary tumor would be expected to grow as slowly as the primary and be associated with a moderately favorable prognosis. In the 20 cases analyzed by Slootweg & Müller,[61] the time between first manifestation of the primary tumor and the appearance of metastases ranged from 1 to 27 years. Survival, where known, ranged from 3 months to more than 9 years. Laughlin,[65] in an analysis of 42 published cases of metastasizing ameloblastomas and one of his own, found that the median duration of survival after treatment of the primary growth was 11 years, or 2 years after treatment of the metastasis. Nineteen of the 42 patients were known to have died from their disease. Also against the theory of implantation rather than true metastasis, was the fact that 75% of the secondary deposits were intrapleural or in hilar nodes and 15% were in cervical lymph nodes or spine. Other noteworthy findings were the wide age range (5–60 years, median 30.5 years) at the time of treatment and the high proportion of Japanese patients (25%). In some at least of these cases, such as the one reported by Ishikawa & Shimada,[66] it should be noted that the metastasis did not entirely replicate the primary tumor histologically, but showed areas of squamous carcinoma. In other reports the illustrations leave some doubt as to whether a case was truly a malignant ameloblastoma or should have been categorized as ameloblastic carcinoma. However, it is clear that the tumor reported by Houston et al[67] was a well-differentiated ameloblastoma that metastasized to a regional lymph node after 17 years, but retained the benign appearances of the parent tumor. As with a few other tumors, a benign cytological picture does not entirely exclude the potential for metastasis.

In summary, it appears that there have been a few well-authenticated cases where well-differentiated ameloblastomas have given rise to metastases that have replicated the histological appearances of the primary tumor.

BEHAVIOR AND MANAGEMENT

As already indicated, the diagnosis of malignant ameloblastoma can (by definition) only be made after it has metastasized. In one ameloblastic carcinoma and one recurrent ameloblastoma Kim & Yook[68] found remarkably high levels of PCNA activity, and this may also apply to malignant ameloblastomas. Otherwise, the possibility of metastasis from an ameloblastoma confirms the importance of careful prolonged follow-up. The treatment of choice for the primary tumor and recurrences is excision. Treatment of metastases to the lungs is by excision of a segment or lobe, or excision of other affected tissues. Radiotherapy may be used for metastatic disease not suitable for surgery, but its value is questionable. Ramadas et al[69] have claimed success with chemotherapy, but this has not been confirmed. Moreover, the toxic effects of combined chemotherapy have to be balanced against the unpredictable behavior of this tumor.

Overall, too few cases have been seen for a definitive treatment protocol to have evolved. Although the prognosis of reported cases has varied widely, a significant proportion of patients have died.

AMELOBLASTIC CARCINOMA

Corio et al[70] used the term 'ameloblastic carcinoma' for an ameloblastoma that shows cytological features of malignancy but is otherwise recognizable as an ameloblastoma and may later metastasize. In the later stages the microscopic appearances increasingly resemble those of a squamous cell carcinoma. Even more rarely, a tumor that initially has the microscopic features of a conventional ameloblastoma can behave in a more aggressive fashion, lose differentiation, particularly after multiple recurrences, and ultimately metastasize (Figs 3.15–3.18).

Slootweg & Müller[61] found reports of two such cases. Such a tumor in its histologically benign phase may simply represent an early stage of an ameloblastic carcinoma. However, absence of histologic features of malignancy in the first examination may be the result of incomplete inspection of the specimen. As mentioned

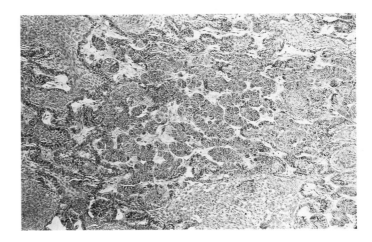

Fig. 3.15 Ameloblastic carcinoma. Low-power view shows a follicular configuration together with a suggestion of palisading and stellate reticulum-like epithelium.

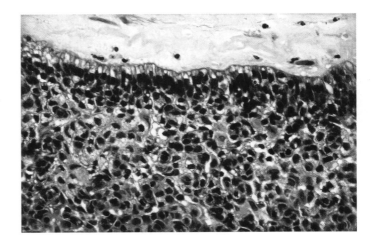

Fig. 3.16 Ameloblastic carcinoma. Higher power view shows peripheral ameloblast-like cells and prominent atypia of the deeper epithelium. This tumor gave rise to multiple metastases and caused the death of the patient.

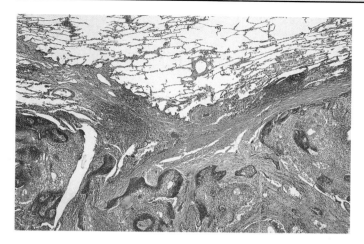

Fig. 3.17 Metastatic ameloblastoma in the lung. The tumor retains some resemblance to a follicular ameloblastoma.

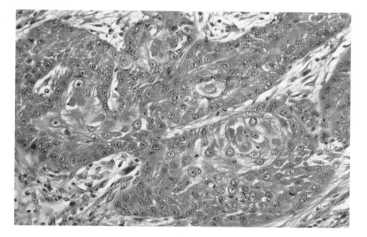

Fig. 3.18 Ameloblastic carcinoma. Another example showing a resemblance to a squamous cell carcinoma with mitotic figures.

earlier, Kim & Yook[68] found remarkably high levels of PCNA activity in one ameloblastic carcinoma and one recurrent ameloblastoma that they tested. Additionally, Müller et al[71] have shown that aneuploidy is significantly more frequent in ameloblastic carcinomas and is a strong predictor of malignant behavior. Müller et al,[71] in comparing the nuclear DNA content of 17 primary and five recurrent ameloblastomas, found the majority to be diploid, but there was no significant difference between them. By contrast 80% of ameloblastomas were aneuploid.

CLINICAL FEATURES

Clinically, ameloblastic carcinoma causes swelling of the jaw, but frequently it also causes pain and grows more rapidly than a conventional ameloblastoma. Like the latter, the mandible is most frequently involved. Radiographically, there is an ill-defined area of radiolucency in which Corio et al[70] noted focal radio-opacities.

Root resorption, perforation of the buccal and lingual plates of the jaw, and extension into the soft tissues illustrate the destructive potential.

Bruce & Jackson[72] summarized the features of ameloblastic carcinoma as a neoplasm showing histological evidence of malignant transformation of the ameloblastoma-like epithelium in the primary tumor, while metastases tended to resemble a less well-differentiated squamous cell carcinoma.

As to prognosis, three of the seven tumors reported by Corio et al,[70] for example, recurred within a year, while both of those reported by Slootweg & Müller[61] died within 2 years of the appearance of the metastasis.

Malignant change in peripheral ameloblastomas has been reported by Baden et al,[73] who found reports of only three previous cases.[74–76] The patient reported by Baden et al[73] was an 82-year-old male with a polypoid mass in the maxillary tuberosity region, and illustrates well how aggressive these tumors can become. Initially the tumor showed saucerization of the underlying bone and had the histologic features of an acanthomatous peripheral ameloblastoma. Excision was followed less than 3 months later by a recurrence that showed squamous cell carcinoma arising in a peripheral ameloblastoma. Aggressive surgery and radiotherapy were followed by further recurrences and extensive local spread. Histologically, the tumor had become an anaplastic carcinoma. Subtotal maxillectomy and several courses of radiotherapy failed to arrest its growth and the patient died with residual tumor less than 5 years after presentation.

BEHAVIOR AND MANAGEMENT

Recognition of ameloblastic carcinoma by the clinical and radiographic features is confirmed by the finding of malignant change in a tumor that otherwise resembles an ameloblastoma histologically. The problems of management are, therefore, those of an intraosseous carcinoma and, if the tumor has already metastasized, the prognosis is correspondingly poor.

MALIGNANT AMELOBLASTOMA WITH METASTASES TO THE LUNG AND HYPERCALCEMIA

Malignant ameloblastoma with metastases to the lung and hypercalcemia is distinctly unusual, but several cases have been reported.[77–80] Hypercalcemia in these cases appears to have resulted from the production of a parathyroid-hormone-like peptide, possibly prostaglandin E_2. The latter was detected in extracts from the tumor in the cases reported by Seward et al[77] and Inoue et al.[79] Bone destruction is the usual stimulus to tumor production of parathyroid-like hormone by, for example, carcinoma of the lung. However, this was not a feature of these ameloblastomas. In the case of most malignant tumors that cause hypercalcemia, survival is too short for renal calcinosis to develop, but this was seen in the malignant ameloblastoma reported by Seward et al.[77]

In contrast to these cases, Macpherson et al[81] have reported hypercalcemia by a benign ameloblastoma without metastases. Extracts from the tumor cells showed raised levels of interleukin-1 and a parathyroid-hormone-like substance: both of these can stimulate bone resorption and induce hypercalcemia. The latter resolved after surgical removal of the tumor.

PRIMARY INTRAOSSEOUS (SQUAMOUS CELL) CARCINOMA

Primary intra-alveolar carcinoma is a rare tumor that is presumed to arise from odontogenic rests, an odontogenic cyst, or an ameloblastoma. Müller & Waldron[82] considered that an origin in an odontogenic cyst accounted for the majority of cases, and traced 81 examples from 119 documented cases of intraosseous squamous cell carcinoma. Excluding central mucoepidermoid carcinomas, they defined three types, as proposed by Slootweg & Müller:[61]

1 Carcinoma originating in an odontogenic cyst
2A Malignant ameloblastoma;
2B Ameloblastic carcinoma arising de novo, ex ameloblastoma or ex odontogenic cyst
3 Keratinizing or nonkeratinizing intraosseous carcinoma arising de novo.

Kramer et al[83] use a somewhat similar classification in the current World Health Organization classification. However, it may not be possible always to assign a primary intraosseous carcinoma to one of these categories with certainty. Nor does it appear that these distinctions significantly affect the management or prognosis.

The peak incidence is in the sixth and seventh decades, and males are affected two to three times as frequently as females. Most cases appear to have originated in residual cysts in the posterior mandible. Primary intraosseous carcinomas with no evidence of origin in odontogenic cysts may originate from odontogenic rests, but it may be difficult to exclude the possibility that a carcinoma has entirely overgrown a cyst lining. To et al[84] reported three cases, but felt that several of 24 earlier cases were of dubious validity. They noted that in 50% of them diagnosis had been delayed by treatment of teeth thought to be causing the symptoms. Suei et al,[85] in reviewing 39 cases of primary intraosseous carcinoma reported between 1951 and 1991, found that only three had arisen in the anterior mandible and three in the anterior maxilla. Accelerated growth and pain are typical features, but neither may be obtrusive in the early stages. Spread to regional lymph nodes has been recorded in a minority.

Radiographically, neoplastic change may be suspected in a cyst-like lesion with ragged margins, but lesions can be well defined so that the diagnosis is not made until after enucleation.

Clinically and radiographically, therefore, primary intraosseous carcinomas cannot be reliably distinguished from infected cysts or other malignant tumors.

MICROSCOPY

The tumor is typically a well-differentiated squamous cell carcinoma that may or may not be keratinizing. According to the type, there may be microscopic evidence of an origin in a cyst or ameloblastoma. That it is a metastasis from a distant site should be excluded by clinical and radiographic investigation, particularly of the chest. Distinction from an intraosseous mucoepidermoid carcinoma may be made by the absence of mucous cells and mucicarmine staining. Squamous cell carcinoma of salivary glands is a recognized but uncommon entity, but examples arising from ectopic salivary gland tissue in the jaws do not appear to have been recorded.

The diagnosis of primary intra-alveolar carcinoma can only be made by excluding: bone invasion by a mucosal carcinoma, intraosseous salivary gland carcinoma (see Ch. 52), and a metastasis.

BEHAVIOR AND MANAGEMENT

From the viewpoint of management and prognosis, consideration of the precise origin or histogenesis of the carcinoma is likely to be considerably less significant than the extent of the tumor or the presence of metastases. However, metastases are slow to develop and are typically in the regional lymph nodes.

Treatment is preferably by radical excision, but many cases have been enucleated initially as cysts. If then carcinomatous change is found, radical excision should be carried out. The prognosis then appears to be relatively good, and the 5-year survival rate appears to be 30–40%. However, data are limited by the rarity of this disease and the brevity of follow-up in many cases.

AMELOBLASTOMAS ORIGINATING FROM ODONTOGENIC CYSTS

It was at one time believed that many, if not most, ameloblastomas originated from the epithelial lining of non-neoplastic odontogenic cysts. Indeed, since both ameloblastomas and odontogenic cysts originate from odontogenic epithelium, the possibility of neoplastic change in this epithelium cannot be excluded. However, it seems likely that in many cases of ameloblastomas thought to have arisen in cysts, there was confusion with unicystic ameloblastomas, as discussed earlier. In many of the reported cases it is impossible to determine from the illustrations whether the origin of an ameloblastoma from an odontogenic cyst had been adequately authenticated. Now that this diagnostic trap has become more widely appreciated, the number of reports of ameloblastomas originating in cysts has declined noticeably. Holmlund et al,[87] for example, reported three cases of solid ameloblastomas that developed at sites where cysts had been enucleated. Two of these cysts were radicular and the other was a dentigerous cyst; all were verified histologically.

The authors' caution in interpreting these findings seems justified in that cysts are usually enucleated entire, leaving no residual cyst epithelium for recurrence as either a cyst or neoplasm. It seems more likely, therefore, that, as these authors also suggest, the ameloblastomas originated from other embryonic epithelial rests in the region of the original cysts rather than from the cyst wall itself.

Shear & Singh[14] have also shown that black Africans have a high incidence of ameloblastomas but a low incidence of dentigerous cysts, while the reverse is true of whites. The high frequency of dentigerous cysts in the maxillary canine region also does not match the usual site distribution of ameloblastomas.

As discussed earlier, Saku et al[33] have reported that cystic as well as solid ameloblastomas bind the lectins UEA-1 and BSA-1, enabling them to be differentiated from non-neoplastic odontogenic cysts, which do not bind these lectins. It should therefore be possible to distinguish cystic ameloblastomas from ameloblastomas originating in non-neoplastic cyst epithelium with more certainty.

DIFFERENTIAL DIAGNOSIS

The diagnosis of typical ameloblastomas, particularly the follicular type with its well-defined ameloblast-like cells surrounding stellate reticulum-like tissue, should rarely be in doubt. However, inflammatory epithelial proliferation of a radicular cyst lining can produce arcaded and anastomosing configurations that might cause initial confusion with a plexiform ameloblastoma to the inexperienced eye. Conversely, cystic ameloblastomas can show proliferation of the epithelium of the wall that resembles that seen in an inflamed cyst, or be flattened and resemble the lining of a non-inflamed non-neoplastic cyst. Another possibility is that hydropic degeneration of the epithelial lining of an odontogenic keratocyst can occasionally produce an appearance with some resemblance to that of stellate reticulum. Other islets of epithelial proliferation in the walls of non-neoplastic cysts might conceivably be confused with ameloblastoma follicles, as shown in Figures 3.19 and 3.20. In the past also, squamous odontogenic tumors (see Ch. 5) have been mistaken for acanthomatous ameloblastomas.

In practice, the main risk is likely to be mistaking the flattened epithelium lining part of unicystic ameloblastoma for a nonneoplastic cyst. This problem is only likely to arise if the specimen is inadequate or examination is not thorough.

Rarely, ameloblastomas can resemble basal cell carcinomas, but the latter do not arise in the oral cavity. The problem should not therefore arise.

More difficult is the problem of distinguishing ameloblastomas from some salivary gland tumors, particularly adenoid cystic carcinomas, and particularly those arising from glands of the maxillary antral mucosa. Intraosseous salivary gland tumors of the mandible are mostly mucoepidermoid carcinomas, and it seems unlikely that the mucous cells could be confused with the ameloblast-like cells of ameloblastomas. In any case the configurations of these tumors is entirely different (see Ch. 52).

Occasionally, an ameloblastoma with extensive squamous metaplasia might resemble a squamous cell carcinoma, but the possibility of such a misinterpretation should be remote, particularly if account is taken of the clinical and radiographic findings.

The tumor that can show the closest histological resemblance to an ameloblastoma is the ameloblastic fibroma. Unlike ameloblastomas, the stroma of the latter consists of highly cellular mesenchyme resembling the immature dentine papilla. It also has a capsule and grows expansively.

Calcifying odontogenic cysts (ghost cell tumors), particularly the solid variant, frequently have a mantle of ameloblast-like cells. The different histologic configuration of calcifying odontogenic cyst and its characteristic ghost cells should usually allow it to be recognized readily (see Ch. 8).

Adenomatoid odontogenic tumors also feature ameloblast-like cells, and for this reason were formerly termed 'adenoameloblastomas.' However, the appearances of the latter are sufficiently distinctive, as discussed in Chapter 4, to prevent confusion.

Odontoameloblastoma

This rare neoplasm is essentially a tumor in which odontogenic cells have given rise to both an ameloblastoma and a composite odontoma. Thompson et al[87] listed synonyms that have been used. These include *ameloblastic odontoma*,[88] *soft and calcified odontoma*,[89] *adamanto-odontoma*,[90] and *calcified mixed odontogenic tumor*.[91]

Odontoameloblastomas formed 0.5% of 403 odontogenic tumors analyzed by Günhan et al,[16] but none were identified by Daley et al[13] among 445 odontogenic tumors, and it is not mentioned among the 706 odontogenic tumors analyzed by Regezi et al.[12]

Thompson et al[87] found that odontoameloblastomas affected persons aged between 6 months and 6 years, with the majority being children less than 16 years old. Males and females are equally frequently affected, although Hooker[88] and Gorlin & Goldman[92] reported a preponderance of males.

CLINICAL FEATURES

The site of predilection is the molar–premolar region of either the maxilla or mandible. Symptoms include slow expansion of the jaw, dull pain, and disturbance of occlusion.

Radiographically, odontoameloblastoma appears as a well-defined uni- or multilocular radiolucent area containing dense radioopacities either as solid masses or small particles.

MICROSCOPY

Odontoameloblastoma consists of ameloblastoma tissue juxtaposed with dentine and enamel of an odontoma. The example reported by Thompson et al[87] was unusual in that the ameloblastomatous component had infiltrated the odontoma tissue. In an

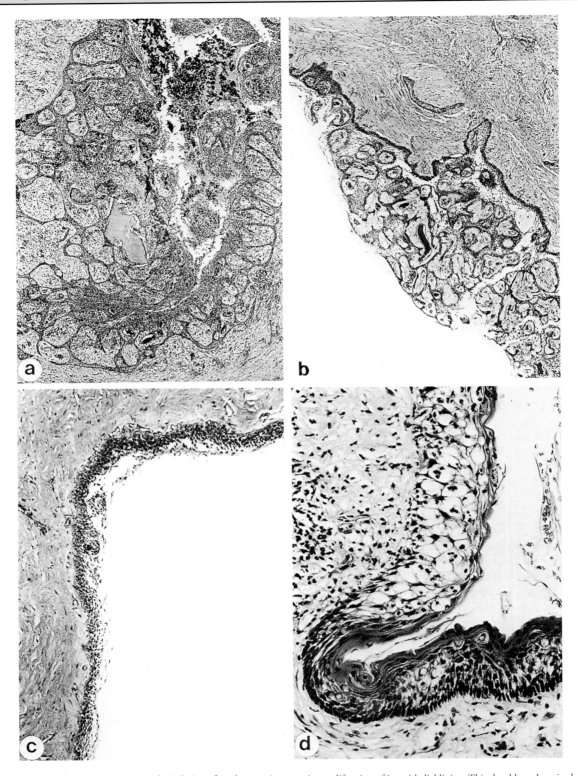

Fig. 3.19 a Radicular cyst. This common non-neoplastic lesion often shows quite extensive proliferation of its epithelial lining. This should not be mistaken for plexiform ameloblastoma. ×30. **b** A cystic area in an ameloblastoma that shows proliferation superficially similar to that in the wall of the cyst in **a**. ×30. **c** The cyst wall of a monocystic ameloblastoma. Note that the flattened tumor epithelium could be mistaken for non-neoplastic squamous epithelium. ×80. **d** A keratocyst of the mandible. Degenerative changes in the squamous epithelial lining, due to inflammation, produce a superficial resemblance to the stellate cells of ameloblastoma. ×22.

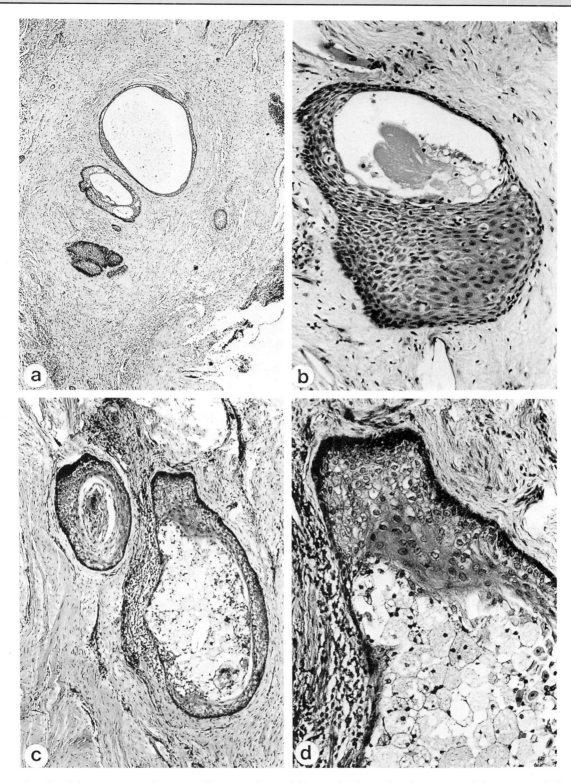

Fig. 3.20 Discrete islets of epithelium in non-neoplastic cyst walls may simulate ameloblastoma follicles. **a** Islets of squamous epithelium in the wall of a dentigerous cyst, showing central cyst formation. ×30. **b** Higher magnification of an islet similar to those shown in **a**. ×200. **c** Non-neoplastic islets showing cyst formation and degenerative changes in the cells, simulating ameloblastoma. ×80. **d** Higher magnification of a field from **c**. ×200.

odontoameloblastoma in an 11-year-old girl reported by Takeda et al,[93] dendritic cells containing melanin were widely distributed. Melanin of uncertain origin was also present in the epithelial cells. Slabbert et al[94] have reported a tumor in which infiltrating follicles of an ameloblastoma were associated with sheets of ovoid to spindle-shaped cells, abundant homogeneous eosinophilic extracellular material, and psammomatous dystrophic calcifications. They interpreted the eosinophilic material as dentinoid, and electron microscopy showed it to consist of interlacing collagen fibrils embedded in structureless ground substance. They concluded that this was an ameloblastoma showing induction of dentinoid production without concomitant enamel formation and termed it a *dentinoameloblastoma.*

DIFFERENTIAL DIAGNOSIS

LaBriola et al[95] reported a case but, when reviewing the literature, found that few of the 40 that they found met the clinical and pathological criteria of odontoameloblastoma. The chief cause of confusion is the ameloblastic fibro-odontoma, which is a variant of ameloblastic fibroma without the aggressiveness of the odontoameloblastoma. In ameloblastic fibro-odontoma the epithelial cells differentiate into functional ameloblasts before production of enamel matrix.

Odontoameloblastoma and ameloblastic fibro-odontoma both contain odontomatous tissue. The essential differences are that the ameloblastic fibro-odontoma lacks typical ameloblastoma epithelium and has an abundant stroma of immature dental papilla-like mesenchyme. Ameloblastic fibro-odontoma is usually seen at earlier ages than odontoameloblastoma, but there is an appreciable overlap.

HISTOGENESIS

Ameloblastomas clearly arise from odontogenic epithelium. The origin of these tumors from sites only where odontogenic epithelium is likely to persist, and the closeness of the resemblance of the ameloblastoma-like cells and stellate reticulum-like tissue, hardly permits any dispute.

The main source of contention is the stage of development of the odontogenic epithelium from which an ameloblastoma has arisen. The earlier belief that ameloblastomas arose from enamel organs is difficult to accept in view of the wide gap in years between the time of involution of enamel organs and the appearance of ameloblastomas.

A more probable origin for ameloblastomas is from odontogenic rests of the dental lamina. These are most common in the vicinity of the roots of the teeth, but may also be found in the overlying alveolar mucosa. They could therefore be the source of both intraosseous and the less common extraosseous ameloblastomas.

The observation that ameloblastomas may show a connection with the oral mucosa has led in the past to the theory that ameloblastomas arose from oral mucosa. Few now give credence to this idea, and it is generally accepted that growth of an ameloblastoma from within the jaw can extend until the alveolar mucosa is reached and the two different epithelia fuse together. That aside, ameloblastomas certainly do not arise from oral mucosa unrelated to the tooth-bearing areas. Confirmation of the origin of ameloblastomas from odontogenic epithelium has been provided by Snead et al,[97] who demonstrated that ameloblastoma epithelial cells express the amelogenin gene. This gene is otherwise only expressed by differentiated ameloblasts.

The possible origin of ameloblastomas from odontogenic cysts has already been discussed. Though such a possibility exists, and even if this process has been histologically authenticated, it can account for only a minute proportion of these tumors.

In summary, all the evidence points to the origin of ameloblastomas from derivatives or remnants of the dental lamina. In the case of odontoameloblastomas it is only possible to speculate that odontogenic epithelium undergoes divergent evolution, partly neoplastic to an ameloblastoma and partly to undergo hamartomatous change to an area of odontoma.

BEHAVIOR AND MANAGEMENT

The behavior of odontoameloblastoma is that of the ameloblastomatous component, namely progressive infiltration and local destruction of surrounding tissues. The treatment is also the same as for an ameloblastoma. Gunbay et al[97] have reported an odontoameloblastoma that had formed in an edentulous area of the anterior maxilla in an 11-year-old boy. This tumor showed no signs of recurrence 7 years after excision. However, too few cases have been reported to be certain about the ultimate prognosis, but it is likely to be similar to that of an ameloblastoma, and rigorous long-term follow-up is essential.

Extraoral tumors resembling ameloblastomas

CRANIOPHARYNGIOMA

The similarities between the ameloblastoma and craniopharyngioma have long been recognized. Both originate from oral ectoderm, but the craniopharyngioma arises from an outgrowth of the latter known as Rathke's pouch. Bernstein & Buchino[98] credit Onanoff with noticing the similarities between these tumors in 1892 and terming them *pituitary adamantinomas.* Bernstein & Buchino[98] have reappraised the similarities between these two types of tumor from a study of 27 craniopharyngiomas. They found that the main features distinguishing craniopharyngiomas from ameloblastomas are their copious ghost cell production, their predominantly cystic morphology, and the presence of osteoid or bone. The microscopic appearances of 20 of these craniopharyngiomas thus closely resembled calcifying odontogenic cysts. Only two resembled ameloblastomas and three were intermediate in configuration (Figs 3.21–3.25).

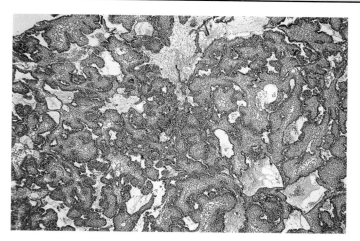

Fig. 3.21 Craniopharyngioma. Ameloblastoma-like type.

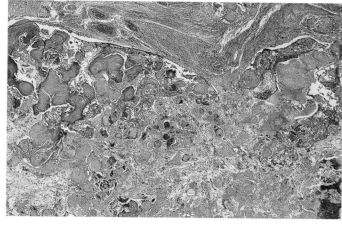

Fig. 3.23 Craniopharyngioma. Calcifying odontogenic cyst type.

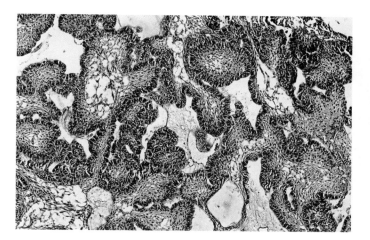

Fig. 3.22 Craniopharyngioma. Higher power view shows a resemblance to a follicular ameloblastoma.

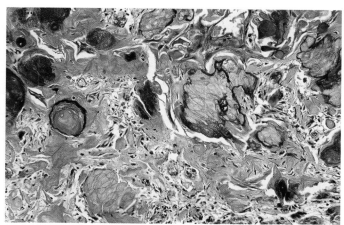

Fig. 3.24 Craniopharyngioma. Calcifying odontogenic cyst type. Higher power view than Figure 3.23 shows a striking picture of the abnormally keratinized (ghost) cells and calcifications.

ADAMANTINOMA OF LONG BONES

The so-called adamantinoma of long bones most frequently affects the tibia, but occasionally forms in soft tissue anterior to the bone. It is rare, and single case reports form the bulk of the literature.

Histologically there is wide variation in appearances. Rarely, there are follicles of loose edematous tissue resembling stellate reticulum surrounded by tall columnar cells. However, the latter lack the regular shape and reversed nuclear polarity of ameloblastoma cells. Other adamantinomas consist of small dark cells in strands or islets, resemble a Ewing's sarcoma, are angioblastic,[99] or show features of fibrous dysplasia. Czerniak et al[100] reviewed 25 cases and confirmed immunohistochemically that adamantinoma is epithelial and concluded that the osteofibrous dysplasia-like appearance is a reparative response that leads to spontaneous regression in some cases.

Hagendoorn[101] has shown widespread reactivity in all 34 specimens for keratins 14 and 19, and 74% showed reactivity for keratin 5. Focal reactivity for keratin 17 was seen in 50% of specimens. The keratin staining was independent of diverse histologic patterns, and the pattern was retained in recurrences and metastases. The different histologic types of adamantinoma appeared, therefore, to have a common histogenesis.

Some adamantinomas metastasize and are rapidly lethal, while others appear to regress spontaneously.

The histogenesis of the so-called adamantinoma remains speculative. Keratin staining indicates that it has epithelial characteristics, but there is nothing to suggest that there are epithelial rests within long bones from which it could originate.

There is in fact nothing to indicate that there is anything in common between ameloblastoma and so-called adamantinoma in terms of histogenesis and behavior. However, occasional adamantinomas of long bones show areas that have a superficial histological resemblance to an ameloblastoma.

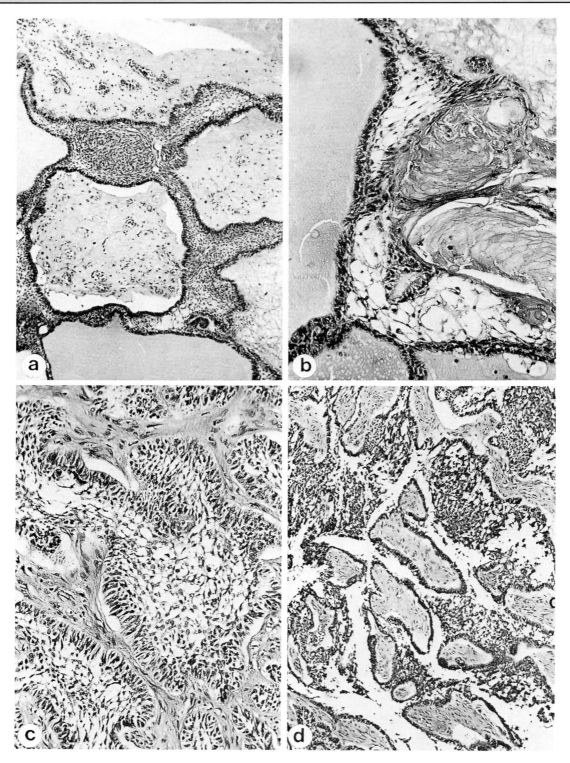

Fig. 3.25 a, b Craniopharyngioma. **a** The general pattern is similar to that of the plexiform type of ameloblastoma. ×80. **b** Higher magnification, showing how closely the histology resembles that of ameloblastoma, except for the presence of keratin, which is common in craniopharyngioma but rare in ameloblastoma. ×200.
c, d 'Adamantinoma' of the tibia. Two fields from the same tumor, showing in one field, **c** appearances very similar to ameloblastoma, while in the other, **d** the picture could be described as angioblastomatous. **c** ×22; **d** ×80.

REFERENCES

1. Gorlin RJ 1970 Odontogenic tumors. In Gorlin RJ, Goldman HM (eds) Thoma's oral pathology. CV Mosby, St Louis, p 481–515
2. Cusack JW 1827 Report of the amputations of the lower jaw. Dublin Hosp Rep 4: 1–38
3. Falkson R 1879 Zur Kenntnis der Kiefercysten. Virchows Arch 76: 504–509
4. Baden E 1965 Terminology of the ameloblastoma: history and current usage. J Oral Surg 23: 40–44
5. Bouquot HE, Lense EC 1994 The beginning of oral pathology. Part I: First dental journal reports of odontogenic tumors and cysts, 1839–1860. Oral Surg Oral Med Oral Pathol 78: 343–370
6. Wedl C 1870 Pathologie der Zahne mit besondere Rucksicht auf anatomie und Physiologie. A Felix, Leipzig
7. Wagstaffe WW 1871 Case of cystic sarcoma of lower jaw. Trans Pathol Soc London 22: 249–253
8. Malassez L 1885 Sur le rôle des debris épithéliaux paradentaires. Arch Physiol Norm Pathol 5: 309–340, 6: 379–449
9. Ivy RH, Churchill HR 1930 The need of a standardized surgical classification of the tumors and anomalies of dental tissues. Am Assoc Dent Sch Trans 7: 240–245
10. Galippe V 1910 Les débris épithéliaux paradentaires. Masson, Paris
11. Bhaskar SN 1968 Oral pathoolgy in the dental office: a survey of 20 575 biopsy specimens. J Am Dent Assoc 76: 761–766
12. Regezi JA, Kerr DA, Courtney RM 1978 Odontogenic tumors: analysis of 706 cases. J Oral Surg 36: 771–778
13. Daley TD, Wysocki GP, Pringle GA 1994 Relative incidence of odontogenic tumors and jaw cysts in a Canadian population. Oral Surg Oral Med Oral Pathol 77: 276–280
14. Shear M, Singh S 1978 Age-standardised incidence rates of ameloblastoma and dentigerous cyst on the Witwatersrand, South Africa. Commun Dent Oral Epidemiol 6: 195–199
15. Adekeye EO 1980 Ameloblastoma of the jaws: a survey of 109 Nigerian patients. J Oral Surg 38: 36–41
16. Günhan O, Erseven G, Ruacan S et al 1990 Odontogenic tumours: a series of 409 cases. Austr Dent J 35: 518–522
17. Wu PC, Chan KW 1985 A survey of tumours of the jawbones in Hong Kong Chinese: 1963–1982. Br J Oral Maxillofac Surg 23: 92–102
18. Gorlin RJ 1970 Odontogenic tumors. In Gorlin RJ, Goldman HM (ed) Thoma's oral pathology, 6th edn. Mosby, St Louis
19. Small IA, Waldron CA 1955 Ameloblastomas of the jaws. Oral Surg 8: 281–297
20. Waldron CA, El Mofty SK 1987 A histopathologic study of 116 ameloblastomas with special reference to the desmoplastic variant. Oral Surg Oral Med Oral Pathol 63: 441–451
21. Ueno S, Nakamura S, Mushimoto K, Shirasu R 1986 A clinicopathologic study of ameloblastoma. J Oral Maxillofac Surg 44: 361–365
22. Sirichitra V, Dhiravarangkura P 1984 Intrabony ameloblastoma of the jaws. An analysis of 147 patients. Int J Oral Surg 13: 187–193
23. Reichart PA, Philipsen HP, Sonner S 1995 Ameloblastoma: biological profile of 3677 cases. Eur J Cancer B, Oral Oncol 31: 86–99
24. Tsaknis PJ, Nelson JF 1980 The maxillary ameloblastoma: an analysis of 24 cases. J Oral Surg 38: 336–342
25. Shteyer A, Lustmann J, Lewin-Epstein J 1978 The mural ameloblastoma: a review of the literature. J Oral Surg 36: 866–872
26. Gardner DG, Corio RL 1984 Plexiform unicystic ameloblastoma. A variant of ameloblastoma with low-recurrence rate after enucleation. Cancer 53: 1730–1735
27. Ackermann GL, Altini M, Shear M 1988 The unicystic ameloblastoma: a clinicopathological study of 57 cases. J Oral Pathol 17: 541–546
28. Kaffe I, Buchner A, Taicher S 1993 Radiologic features of desmoplastic variant of ameloblastoma. Oral Surg Oral Med Oral Pathol 76: 525–529
29. Eversole LR, Leider AS, Hanson LS 1984 Ameloblastomas with pronounced desmoplasia. J Oral Maxillofac Surg 42: 735–740
30. Robinson L, Martinez MG 1977 Unicystic ameloblastoma. A prognostically distinct entity. Cancer 40: 2278–2285
31. Leider AS, Eversole LR, Barkin ME 1985 Cystic ameloblastoma. A clinicopathologic analysis. Oral Surg Oral Med Oral Pathol 60: 624–630
32. Shear M 1992 Cysts of the oral regions, 3rd edn. Wright, Bristol
33. Saku T, Shibata Y, Koyama Z, Cheng J 1991 Lectin histochemistry of cystic jaw lesions: an aid for differential diagnosis between cystic ameloblastoma and odontogenic cysts. J Oral Pathol Med 20: 108–113
34. Ferreiro JA 1994 Immunohistochemical analysis of salivary gland canalicular adenoma. Oral Surg Oral Med Oral Pathol 78: 761–765
35. Pindborg JJ 1970 Pathology of the dental hard tissues, 1st edn. Munksgard, Copenhagen, p 371–376
36. Lurie R, Altini M, Shear M 1976 A case report of keratoameloblastoma. Intl J Oral Surg 5: 245–249
37. Altini M, Slabbert H deV, Johnston T 1991 Papilliferous keratoameloblastoma. J Oral Pathol Med 20: 46–48
38. Navarrete AR, Smith M 1971 Ultrastructure of granular cell ameloblastoma. Cancer 27: 948–955
39. Philipsen HP, Ormiston IW, Reichart PA 1992 The desmo- and osteoplastic ameloblastoma. Histologic variant or clinicopathologic entity? Case reports. J Oral Maxillofac Surg 21: 352–357
40. Takigawa T, Matsumoto M, Sekini Y et al 1981 A case report of ameloblastoma proliferated like epulis of maxilla. Nihon Univ Dent J 55: 920–924 [in Japanese]
41. Uji Y, Kodama K, Sakamoto A, Taen A 1983 An ameloblastoma with interesting histological findings. Jpn J Oral Maxillofac Surg 29: 1512–1519 [in Japanese]
42. Ashman SG, Corio RL, Eisele DW, Murphy MT 1993 Desmoplastic ameloblastoma. A case report and literature review. Oral Surg Oral Med Oral Pathol 73: 479–482
43. Müller H, Slootweg P 1985 Clear cell differentiation in an ameloblastoma. J Max-fac Surg 14: 158–160
44. Waldron CA, Small IA, Silverman H 1985 Clear cell ameloblastoma – an odontogenic carcinoma. J Oral Maxillofac Surg 43: 707–717
45. Ng KH, Siar CH 1990 Peripheral ameloblastoma with clear cell differentiation. Oral Surg Oral Med Oral Pathol 70: 210–213
46. Hartman KS 1974 Granular cell ameloblastoma. A survey of twenty cases from the Armed Forces Institute of Pathology. Oral Surg Oral Med Oral Pathol 38: 241–244
47. Cranin AN, Bennet J, Solomon M, Quarco S 1987 Massive granular cell ameloblastoma with metastasis: report of a case. J Oral Maxillofac Surg 45: 800–804
48. Sehdev MK, Huvos AG, Strong EW, Gerold FP 1974 Ameloblastoma of the maxilla and mandible. Cancer 33: 324–333
49. Kramer IRH 1963 Ameloblastoma: a clinicopathological appraisal. Br J Oral Surg 1: 13–28
50. Gardner DG 1988 Radiotherapy in the treatment of ameloblastoma. Intl J Oral Maxillofac Surg 17: 201–205
51. Thompson IO, Ferreira R, van Wyk CW 1993 Recurrent unicystic ameloblastoma of the maxilla. Br J Oral Maxillofac Surg 31: 180–183
52. Li T-J, Browne RM, Matthews JB 1995 Expression of proliferating cell nuclear antigen (PCNA) and Ki-67 in unicystic ameloblastoma. Histopathology 26: 219–228
53. Williams TP 1993 Management of ameloblastoma: a changing perspective. J Oral Maxillofac Surg 51: 1064–1070
54. Bredenkamp JK, Zimmerman MC, Mickel RA 1989 Maxillary ameloblastoma. A potentially lethal neoplasm. Arch Otolaryngol Head Neck Surg 115: 99–104
55. Hell B, Heissler E, Gazounis G, Menneking H, Bier J 1994 Microsurgical and prosthetic reconstruction of patient with recurrent ameloblastoma extending into the skull case. Int J Oral Maxillofac Surg 23: 90–92
56. El-Mofty SK, Gerard NO, Farish SE, Rodu B 1991 Peripheral ameloblastoma: a clinical and histologic study of 11 cases. J Oral Maxillofac Surg 49: 970–974
57. Gardner DG 1970 Peripheral ameloblastoma. A study of 21 cases, including 5 reported as basal cell carcinoma of the gingiva. Cancer 39: 1625–1633
58. Nauta JM, Panders AK, Schoots CJF, Vermey A, Roodenburg JLN 1992 Peripheral ameloblastoma. A case report and review of the literature. Intl J Oral Maxillofac Surg 21: 40–44
59. Gerol M, Burkes EJ 1995 Peripheral ameloblastoma. J Periodontol 66: 1065–1068
60. Zhu EX, Okada N, Takagi M 1995 Peripheral ameloblastoma: case report and review of the literature. J Oral Maxillofac Surg 53: 590–594
61. Slootweg PJ, Müller H 1984 Malignant ameloblastoma or ameloblastic carcinoma. Oral Surg 57: 168–176
62. Elzay RP 1982 Primary intraosseous carcinoma of the jaws. Oral Surg 54: 299–303
63. Kunze E, Donath K, Luhr HG, Englehardt W, De Vivie R 1985 Biology of metastasizing ameloblastoma. Pathol Res Pract 180: 526–535
64. Vorzimer J, Perla D 1932 An instance of adamantinoma of the jaw with metastasis of the right lung. Am J Pathol 8: 445–453
65. Laughlin EH 1989 Metastasing ameloblastoma. Cancer 64: 776–780
66. Ishikawa T, Shimada Y 1954 A case of ameloblastoma with metastasis to the lower lip and lymph nodes. Gann 45: 311–313
67. Houston G, Davenport W, Keaton W, Harris S 1993 Malignant (metastatic) ameloblastoma: report of a case. J Oral Maxillofac Surg 51: 1152–1155
68. Kim J, Yook JI 1994 Immunohistochemical study on proliferating cell nuclear antigen expression in ameloblastomas. Eur J Cancer B, Oral Oncol 30: 126–131
69. Ramadas K, Jose C, Subhashani J, Chandi SM, Viswanathan FR 1990 Pulmonary metastasis from ameloblastoma treated with cisplatin, adriamycin and cyclophosphamide. Cancer 66: 1475–1479
70. Corio RL, Goldblatt LA, Edwards PA, Hartman KS 1987 Ameloblastic carcinoma: a clinicopathologic study and assessment of eight cases. Oral Surg 64: 570–576
71. Müller S, De Rose PB, Cohen C 1993 DNA ploidy of ameloblastoma and ameloblastic carcinoma of the jaws. Arch Pathol Lab Med 117: 1126–1131
72. Bruce RA, Jackson IT 1991 Ameloblastic carcinoma. Report of an aggressive case and review of the literature. J Cranio Max Fac Surg 19: 267–271
73. Baden E, Doyle JL, Petriella V 1993 Malignant transformation of peripheral ameloblastoma. Oral Surg Oral Med Oral Pathol 75: 214–219
74. Edmonson HD, Browne RM, Potts AJC 1982 Intraoral basal cell carcinoma. Br J Oral Surg 20: 239–247
75. Song-Chyr L, Chen Mei L, Lian-Jiuans H, Hsuch-Wan K 1987 Peripheral ameloblastoma with metastasis. Intl J Oral Maxillofac Surg 16: 202–204
76. McClatchey EC, Sullivan MJ, Paugh DR 1989 Peripheral ameloblastic carcinoma: a case report of a rare neoplasm. J Otolaryngol 18: 109–111
77. Seward GR, Beales SJ, Johnson NW, Sita Lumsden EG 1975 A metastasising ameloblastoma associated with renal calculi and hypercalcaemia. Cancer 36: 2277–2285
78. Madiedo G, Choi H, Kleinman JG 1981 Ameloblastoma of the maxilla with distant metastases and hypercalcemia. Am J Clin Pathol 75: 585–591
79. Inoue N, Shimojyo M, Iwai H et al 1988 Malignant ameloblastoma with pulmonary metastasis and hypercalcemia. Am J Clin Pathol 90: 474–481
80. Harada K, Suda S, Kayano T, Nagura H, Enomoto S 1989 Ameloblastoma with metastasis to the lung and hypercalcemia. J Oral Maxillofac Surg 47: 1083–1087

81. Macpherson DW, Hopper C, Meghji S 1991 Hypercalcaemia and the synthesis of interleukin-1 by an ameloblastoma. Br J Oral Maxillofac Surg 29: 29–33

82. Müller S, Waldron CA 1991 Primary intraosseous carcinoma. Intl J Oral Maxillofac Surg 20: 362–365

83. Kramer IRH, Pindborg JJ, Shear M, World Health Organization 1992 Histological typing of odontogenic tumours, 2nd edn. Springer-Verlag, Berlin

84. To EHW, Brown JS, Avery BS, Ward-Booth RP 1991 Primary intraosseous carcinoma of the jaws. Three new cases and a review of the literature. Br J Oral Maxillofac Surg 29: 19–25

85. Suei Y, Tanimoto K, Taguchi A, Wada T 1994 Primary intraosseous carcinoma: review of the literature and diagnostic criteria. J Oral Maxillofac Surg 52: 580–583

86. Holmlund A, Anneroth G, Lundquist G, Nordenram A 1991 Ameloblastomas originating from odontogenic cysts. J Oral Pathol Med 20: 318–321

87. Thompson IOC, Phillips VM, Ferriera R, Housego TG 1990 Odontoameloblastoma: a case report. Br J Oral Maxillofac Surg 28: 347–349

88. Hooker SP 1967 Ameloblastic odontoma: an analysis of 26 cases. Oral Surg Oral Med Oral Pathol 24: 375–379

89. Worley RD, McKee PE 1972 Ameloblastic odontoma: report of a case. J Oral Surg 30: 764–768

90. Shafer WG, Hine MK, Levy BM 1983 A textbook of oral pathology, 4th edn. CV Mosby, St Louis

91. Hoffman S, Hacoway JR, Krolls SO 1985 Intraosseous and parosteal tumors of the jaws. Armed Forces Institute of Pathology, Washington, DC, Fascicle 24, 2nd series

92. Gorlin RJ, Goldman HM 1970 Thoma's oral pathology, 6th edn. CV Mosby, St Louis

93. Takeda Y, Kuroda M, Suzuki A 1989 Melanocytes in odontoameloblastoma. A case report. Acta Pathol Japon 39: 465–468

94. Slabbert H, Altini M, Crooks J, Uys P 1992 Ameloblastoma with dentinoid: dentinoameloblastoma. J Oral Pathol Med 21: 46–48

95. LaBriola JD, Steiner M, Bernstein ML, Verdi GD, Stannard PF 1980 Odontoameloblastoma. J Oral Surg 38: 139–143

96. Snead ML, Luo W, Hsu RJ, Lau EC, Stenman G 1992 Human ameloblastoma tumors express the amelogenin gene. Oral Surg Oral Med Oral Pathol 74: 64–72

97. Gunbay T, Gunbay S, Oztop T 1993 Odontoameloblastoma: report of a case. J Clin Pediatr Dent 18: 17–20

98. Bernstein ML, Buchino JJ 1983 The histologic similarity between craniopharyngioma and odontogenic lesions: a reappraisal. Oral Surg 56: 502–511

99. Adler CP, Reichelt A 1985 Haemangiosarcoma of bone. Intl Orthopaed 8: 273–279

100. Czerniak R, Rojas-Corona RR, Dorfman HD 1989 Morphological diversity of long bone adamantinoma. The concept of differentiated (regressing) adamantinoma and its relationship to osteofibrous dysplasia. Cancer 64: 2319–2334

101. Hagendoorn PC 1993 Adamantinoma of long bones: keratin subclass reactivity with reference to its histogenesis. Am J Surg Pathol 17: 1225–1233

Adenomatoid odontogenic tumor 4

These uncommon lesions are completely benign, and may be hamartomas. Though formerly known as adenoameloblastomas, their behavior is quite different from that of ameloblastomas and they also have no glandular component.

INCIDENCE

Age and gender distribution

Daley et al,[1] in Canada, found that adenomatoid odontogenic tumors comprised 3.3% of 392 odontogenic tumors of 20 recognized types. Philipsen et al,[2] from their extensive analysis of 499 reported examples, found that these tumors were relatively more frequent in Africa, where they comprised up to 6.8% of odontogenic tumors compared with 3% to 4% in the USA, China, and several other countries. In 397 cases where data were available, 67% of the tumors were found between the ages of 10 and 19 years and 21% between the ages of 20 and 29 years. Four per cent arose before the age of 9 years and 8% at the age 30 years or older. Females were predominantly affected and accounted for 63%. As to site, the maxilla accounted for 64%, in the younger patients. By contrast, in patients over 30 years of age, the mandible was involved in 61%. In this age group also, 64.5% of the patients were males. However, the total number of patients aged 30 years or older was only 31.

CLINICAL FEATURES

Overall, adenomatoid odontogenic tumor most frequently appears in the anterior maxilla and forms a very slow-growing painless swelling or is noticed by chance on a radiograph.

Radiographically, adenomatoid odontogenic tumor appears as a rounded area of radiolucency with a well-defined outline, and in about 60% of cases contains faint radio-opaque foci. It commonly resembles a dentigerous cyst, since 75% are associated with an unerupted tooth. However, unlike a dentigerous cyst, the lesion may enclose part of the root, or forms on the lateral aspect of a tooth and resembles a lateral periodontal cyst. Nevertheless, its nature is frequently unsuspected until found (in most cases) to be solid at operation. Though microscopic calcifications are

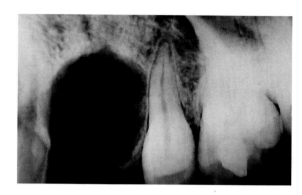

Fig. 4.1 Adenomatoid odontogenic tumor. The radiograph of this tumor in a 19-year-old girl shows the typical circumscribed, cyst-like appearance, but with minute flecks of calcification within the area of radiolucency.

typically present they are not normally visible in conventional radiographs (Fig. 4.1). However, in a particularly unusual example Nomura et al[3] reported a mandibular adenomatoid odontogenic tumor that appeared as a mixed radiopaque/radiolucent area with ill-defined boundaries. This lesion, in a 64-year-old male, had caused root resorption and tooth displacement, and having destroyed the buccal plate of bone had extended into the soft tissues. It had caused facial asymmetry and appeared clinically as a vascular, granulomatous mass extending over the alveolar ridge. Diagnoses such as osteosarcoma or an aggressive fibro-osseous lesion could not therefore be excluded from the clinical and radiographic findings. Despite these unusual features the tumor was, histologically, a conventional adenomatoid odontogenic tumor, apart from lack of a capsule and extensive osteodentine or cementum-like tissue at the periphery.

In their analysis of 499 examples, Philipsen et al[2] found that tumors containing a tooth (follicular variant) were three times as common as those that did not (extrafollicular variant), were recognized earlier (at a mean age of 17 years), and affected females twice as frequently as males. The extrafollicular variant was recognized at a mean age of 24 years and over 50% of all types were diagnosed between the ages of 13 and 19 years.

Teeth found in the follicular type of adenomatoid odontogenic tumor are almost invariably of the permanent series, and Philipsen et al[2] found only a single report of inclusion of a primary tooth.[4]

In the vast majority, the tumor-associated tooth is the permanent canine. Very occasionally, two or more teeth are embedded.

A rare extraosseous variant resembles a fibrous epulis clinically. It accounted for fewer than 3% of the cases analyzed by Philipsen et al.[2] Later, Philipsen et al[5] analyzed the findings in 14 peripheral adenomatoid odontogenic tumors and found that in the 12 where bony changes had been stated, bone loss was absent in five, slight in four, and a bone pocket had formed in three.

Philipsen et al[5] also described three rare variations of the adenomatoid odontogenic tumor in its relationship to teeth. One follicular tumor was associated with an impacted and displaced maxillary third molar, another mimicked a radicular cyst around the apex of a maxillary canine, and a peripheral (epulis-like) variant had produced a periodontal bone defect palatal to a maxillary incisor. They also reviewed and summarized the findings in the seven known follicular adenomatoid odontogenic tumors associated with impacted third molars, and showed that the mean age of patients (26.5 years) was approximately 10 years greater than that of patients with the more common types. However, calculation of this mean age was biased by a single case in a 53-year-old male.

MICROSCOPY

Adenomatoid odontogenic tumor is usually ovoid in shape, has a well-defined capsule, and is rarely more than few centimeters in diameter (Fig. 4.2). The most conspicuous feature is nodules or whorls of spindle-shaped or cuboidal epithelial cells. Around these highly cellular nodules, tumor cells form slender strands or cribriform patterns.

Within the cellular areas there are usually structures resembling ducts cut in cross-section; however, these are clearly spherical microcysts and, whatever the line of section, always appear circular in form. They are lined by columnar cells which resemble ameloblasts and usually have their nuclei polarized away from the lumen. These microcysts may contain homogeneous eosinophilic

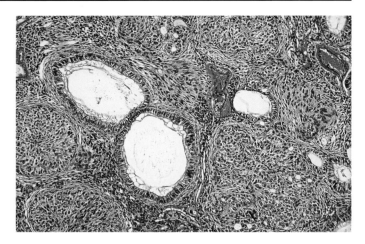

Fig. 4.3 Adenomatoid odontogenic tumor. Higher power view showing duct-like microcysts lined by ameloblast-like cells among whorls of more nondescript epithelium.

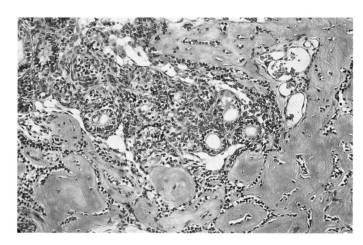

Fig. 4.4 Adenomatoid odontogenic tumor with calcifications and microcysts.

material (Fig. 4.3). Fragments of amorphous or crystalline calcification, which may be lamellated or sometimes resemble cementum, may be seen among the sheets of epithelial cells (Fig. 4.4). Occasionally, dentinoid or tubular dentine is formed.

The stroma is typically loose with scanty cellular elements, but contains thin-walled blood vessels, which are sometimes numerous. Degeneration of the vessel walls, endothelium, and perivascular connective tissue may be conspicuous.

Adenomatoid odontogenic tumors are usually solid as described, but are occasionally cystic, with tumor forming part of the cyst wall. Tajima et al[6] have reported an apparently unique example that was arising in the wall of a dentigerous cyst in a 15-year-old boy. Melanin pigmentation was seen in another rare variant.[7]

HISTOGENESIS

As Philipsen et al[5] have pointed out, there can be little doubt about the origin of adenomatoid odontogenic tumors from

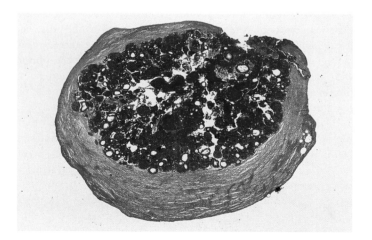

Fig. 4.2 Adenomatoid odontogenic tumor. Low-power view showing the dense circumscription of the epithelium.

epithelium of the dental lamina complex or its remnants. This is the only tissue the distribution of which conforms with the sites of formation of these tumors. As Philipsen et al[5] point out, dental lamina remnants are distributed only along the line of the gubernaculum dentis, a strand of fibrous connective tissue that runs in bony canals connecting the crypts of the developing tooth bud with the lamina propria of the gingiva. Thus proliferation of these epithelial remnants could lead to the formation of an extrafollicular tumor, or the tumor could envelop the underlying tooth. Moreover, in support of this concept, the tumor frequently encloses a considerable portion of the root of a tooth, as mentioned earlier. The permanent molars arise directly from the successional dental lamina that grows backward, beneath the oral epithelium from the dental lamina.

The stimulus to tumor production remains unknown. Further unanswered questions posed by Philipsen et al[5] are the reasons for the great excess of adenomatoid odontogenic tumors that arise from the parent rather than the successional dental lamina, for the preponderance of follicular over extrafollicular tumors, and for the strong predilection for involvement of the permanent canine tooth.

BEHAVIOR AND MANAGEMENT

Most adenomatoid odontogenic tumors have been recognized and treated when no more than a few centimeters in diameter. There has, therefore, been some doubt about their growth potential. Tsnaknis et al[8] reported an adenomatoid odontogenic tumor that had reached 12 cm in diameter in an 11-year-old girl. By contrast, Bedrick et al[9] reported one that had been present for 37 years and had reached only 2 cm × 1 cm × 1 cm, while Oehlers[10] reported two examples that had regressed spontaneously. Overall, therefore, there is scant information about growth potential. In practice, these lesions shell out readily and enucleation is almost invariably curative. However, Toida et al,[11] who surveyed 126 reported adenomatoid odontogenic tumours in Japan, found two that had recurred.[12,13] In the second of these there had been, uniquely, intracranial extension of one of the tumors.

Combined epithelial odontogenic tumors

Nodules of squamoid, polyhedral cells with eosinophilic cytoplasm, well-defined margins, and prominent intercellular bridges are sometimes seen in adenomatoid odontogenic tumor. The nuclei occasionally show mild pleomorphism due to degeneration, but true epithelial atypia has never been reported in these or any other areas of the epithelium. Also present may be deposits of amyloid-like material and globular calcifications, so that there is a resemblance to that of a calcifying epithelial odontogenic tumor.

This has led some workers[14,15] to propose the existence of a combined adenomatoid odontogenic and calcifying epithelial odontogenic tumor. Such tumors have also been reported by Takeda & Kudo,[16] Okada et al,[17] who carried out immunohistochemistry on one example, Siar & Ng,[18] and Montes et al,[19] who reviewed 10 previous reports.

However, Montes et al[19] concluded that calcifying epithelial odontogenic tumor-like areas in an adenomatoid odontogenic tumor were within the normal histopathological spectrum of the latter. Also, as Philipsen et al[2] point out, there is no evidence from the six reported cases that these histological appearances have any effect on the behavior of the tumor, and they strongly advise against the introduction of the concept of a hybrid tumor consisting of such biologically distinct lesions. Hicks et al[20] have analyzed the findings in nine reported cases, and confirmed that, as yet, unlike calcifying epithelial odontogenic tumors, none of the so-called combined tumors have recurred.

REFERENCES

1. Daley TD, Wysocki GP, Pringle GA 1994 Relative incidence of odontogenic tumors and jaw cysts in a Canadian population. Oral Surg Oral Med Oral Pathol 77: 276–280
2. Philipsen HP, Reichert PA, Zhang KJ, Nikai H, Yu QX 1991 Adenomatoid odontogenic tumor: biologic profile based on 499 cases. J Oral Pathol Med 20: 149–158
3. Nomura M, Tanimoto K, Takata T, Shimosato T 1992 Mandibular adenomatoid odontogenic tumor with unusual clinicopathologic features. J Oral Maxillofac Surg 50: 282–285
4. Mikukoshi A, Oshima I, Mizuno Y et al 1980 Adenomatoid odontogenic tumor in a 3-year-old boy. J Jpn Stomatol Soc 29: 605–606
5. Philipsen HP, Samman N, Ormiston IW, Wu PC, Reichert PA 1992 Variants of the adenomatoid odontogenic tumor with a note on tumor origin. J Oral Pathol Med 21: 348–352
6. Tajima Y, Skamoto E, Yamamoto Y 1992 Odontogenic cyst giving rise to an adenomatoid odontogenic tumor: report of a case with peculiar features. J Oral Maxillofac Surg 50: 190–193
7. Aldred MJ, Gray AR 1990 A pigmented adenomatoid odontogenic tumor. Oral Surg Oral Med Oral Pathol 70: 86–89
8. Tsnaknis PJ, Carpenter WM, Slade NL 1977 Odontogenic adenomatoid tumor: report of a case and review of the literature. Oral Surg 35: 146–150
9. Bedrick AE, Solomon MP, Ferber I 1979 The adenomatoid odontogenic tumour: an unusual clinical presentation. Oral Surg 48: 143–145
10. Oehlers FAC 1961 So-called adenoameloblastoma. Oral Surg 14: 712–725
11. Toida M, Hyodo I, Okuda T, Tatematsu N 1990 Adenomatoid odontogenic tumor: report of two cases and survey of 126 cases in Japan. J Oral Maxillofac Surg 48: 404–408
12. Fukaya M, Sato M, Umakoshi H et al 1971 A case report of adenoameloblastoma on the maxilla. Jpn J Oral Maxillofac Surg 17: 155–159
13. Takigami M, Ueda T, Imaizumi T et al 1988 A case of adenomatoid odontogenic tumour with intracranial extension. No Shinkei Geka 16: 775–779
14. Damm DD, White DK, Drummond JF et al 1983 Combined epithelial odontogenic tumor. Adenomatoid odontogenic tumor and calcifying epithelial odontogenic tumor. Oral Surg Oral Med Oral Pathol 55: 487–496
15. Bingham RA, Adrian JC 1986 Combined epithelial odontogenic tumor-adenomatoid odontogenic tumor and calcifying epithelial odontogenic tumor. J Oral Maxillofac Surg 44: 574–577
16. Takeda Y, Kudo K 1986 Adenomatoid odontogenic tumor associated with calcifying epithelial odontogenic tumor. Int J Oral Maxillofac Surg 15: 469–473
17. Okada Y, Mochizuki K, Sugimora K, Noda Y, Mori M 1987 Odontogenic tumor with combined characteristics of adenomatoid odontogenic tumor and calcifying epithelial odontogenic tumors. Pathol Res Pract 182: 647–657
18. Siar CH, Ng KH 1987 Combined calcifying epithelial odontogenic tumor and adenomatoid odontogenic tumor. Intl J Oral Maxillofac Surg 16: 214–216
19. Montes LC, Mosqueda TA, Romero del E, de la Piedra GM, Goldberg JP, Portilla RJ 1993 Adenomatoid odontogenic tumour with features of calcifying epithelial odontogenic tumour (the so-called combined epithelial odontogenic tumour). Clinico-pathological report of 12 cases. Eur J Cancer B, Oral Oncol 29: 221–224
20. Hicks MJ, Flaitz CM, Wong MEK, McDaniel RK, Cagle PT 1994 Clear cell variant of calcifying epithelial odontogenic tumour: case report and review of the literature. Head Neck 16: 272–277

Squamous odontogenic tumor

5

The squamous odontogenic tumor, first described by Pullon et al in 1975,[1] is a distinct entity but its appearances can be mimicked to varying degree by some other tumors.

INCIDENCE

Age and gender distribution

Daley et al[2] did not find a single example of the squamous type among 392 odontogenic tumors. In Turkey, Günhan et al[3] found five examples, representing 1% of 403 benign odontogenic tumors. This frequency seems unduly high, and Philipsen & Reichart[4] considered that the scarcity of reported cases was such that no conclusions could be drawn about the relative frequency of squamous odontogenic tumor compared with other odontogenic tumors. From analysis of the 36 acceptable cases reported at that time, they found that the female/male incidence was 1.8 : 1 and that the age distribution ranged from 8 to 74 years with a peak (36%) in the third decade. The median age of those affected was 31.5 years and the mean age was 38.2 years. The findings of Baden et al,[5] based on three new cases and 29 more acceptable examples reported at that time, are essentially similar.

Site distribution

Philipsen & Reichart[4] found that of 35 squamous odontogenic tumors where the location had been stated, seven were in the anterior mandible or maxilla, four were posterior to the maxillary canine, and seven were posterior to the mandibular canine. In addition, five were in multiple sites in both the upper and lower jaw, four were in both the anterior and posterior maxilla, and one was bilateral in the maxilla.

Thus the mandible, either anteriorly or posteriorly, is overall slightly more frequently affected, while maxillary tumors are more frequently located in an anterior segment.

CLINICAL FEATURES

Squamous odontogenic tumors mainly involve the alveolar process close to the roots of erupted teeth, which they may loosen. Mobility of teeth or painless swelling are the most common initial symptoms, and may be mistaken for periodontal disease. Pain is uncommon and some cases are found only by routine radiography.

Radiographically, squamous odontogenic tumors can mimic severe bone loss due to periodontal disease, or appear as a cyst-like area of radiolucency, sometimes triangular in shape, between the roots of teeth (Fig. 5.1). Occasionally, the radiolucent area is poorly defined or appears multilocular. Once such a lesion has been detected, thorough radiographic examination is required to exclude multiple tumors.

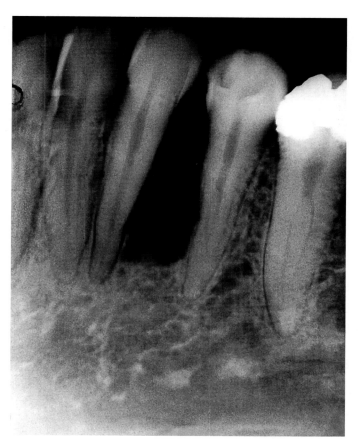

Fig. 5.1 Squamous odontogenic tumor. The tumor appears as an intrabony pocket between the canine and first premolar tooth.

MICROSCOPY

The characteristic features are multiple, circumscribed, rounded or more irregular islands of squamous epithelium in a moderately cellular fibrous stroma (Fig. 5.2). The islands are typically surrounded by flattened or round epithelial cells. The squamous cells forming the islands are often distorted by compression but, apart from mild pleomorphism, show no significant abnormality, and intercellular bridges are clearly seen (Fig. 5.3). Foci of keratin or parakeratin and calcifications, globular eosinophilic structures, or microcysts may form within the islands.

Occasionally, the tumor is continuous with and appears to be arising from the surface epithelium.

DIFFERENTIAL DIAGNOSIS

The histological appearances of squamous odontogenic tumor are

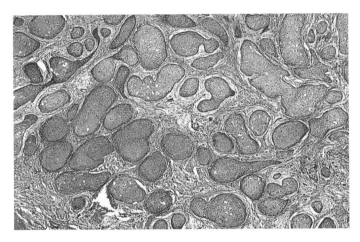

Fig. 5.2 Squamous odontogenic tumor. Rounded and more irregular islands of squamous epithelium with peripheral flattened epithelial cells are surrounded by fibrous stroma.

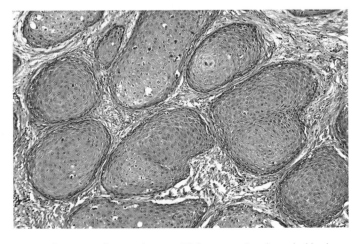

Fig. 5.3 Squamous odontogenic tumor. Higher power view shows the bland cytology.

distinctive, but morphologically identical areas have been reported by Wright[6] as mural thickenings in the walls of five odontogenic cysts. No evidence was found of development of solid squamous odontogenic tumors after conventional enucleation of these cysts. Other similar cases have been reported.[7–12]

This finding must be regarded as proliferation mimicking squamous odontogenic tumor, as there is no evidence of development of squamous odontogenic tumors from odontogenic cyst linings. In practical terms it seems that no more than careful follow-up is needed when this finding is made after enucleation of an odontogenic cyst.

Leider et al[13] suggest that, in the past, some cases of squamous odontogenic tumor were interpreted as acanthomatous ameloblastomas. Such a possibility seems unlikely now that these lesions are so well recognized and it is appreciated that the epithelial islands of squamous odontogenic tumor do not have a peripheral layer of palisaded columnar cells.

Occasionally, squamous odontogenic tumors have been mistaken for squamous cell carcinomas, but unlike the latter show a multiplicity of sharply demarcated islands of epithelium with borders of flattened cells and no significant atypia. There is no destructive invasion of surrounding tissues, and the stromal chronic inflammatory reaction typical of squamous cell carcinomas is also lacking.

HISTOGENESIS

The site of origin of squamous odontogenic tumors suggests that they arise from the rests of Malassez, but examples arising from embedded teeth suggests that they may sometimes arise from epithelial rests in the dental follicle. The rare extraosseous squamous odontogenic tumors seem likely to have arisen from the rests of Serres. However, Leider et al[13] and others have shown examples which appeared to be arising from the surface epithelium.

Squamous odontogenic tumor is firmly categorized as a benign neoplasm in the recent World Health Organization classification[14] and by Philipsen & Reichart[4] in their detailed analysis of reported cases. In favor of the idea that it is a hamartoma is the finding of multicentric examples, and particularly of familial multicentric squamous odontogenic tumors, as reported by Leider et al[13] in three siblings.

BEHAVIOR AND MANAGEMENT

This tumor is benign, although invasion of adjacent structures by maxillary lesions has been reported by Goldblatt et al.[15] Curettage or conservative resection and extraction of any involved teeth is usually effective. Out of the 33 cases analyzed by Baden et al,[5] the outcome was stated in 18, with periods of follow-up ranging from 18 months to 12 years. The only recurrence was among the first cases reported by Pullon et al,[1] when treatment was probably inadequate.

REFERENCES

1. Pullon PA, Shafer WG, Elzay RP, Kerr DA, Corio RL 1975 Squamous odontogenic tumor. Report of six cases of a previously undescribed lesion. Oral Surg 40: 616–630
2. Daley TD, Wysocki GP, Pringle GA 1994 Relative incidence of odontogenic tumors and jaw cysts in a Canadian population. Oral Surg Oral Med Oral Pathol 77: 276–280
3. Günhan O, Erseven G, Ruacan S et al 1990 Odontogenic tumours: a series of 409 cases. Austr Dent J 35: 518–522
4. Philipsen HP, Reichart PA 1996 Squamous odontogenic tumor (SOT): a benign neoplasm of the periodontium. A review of 36 reported cases. J Clin Periodontol 23: 922–926
5. Baden E, Doyle J, Mesa M, Fabie M, Lederman D, Eichen M 1993 Squamous odontogenic tumour. Report of three cases including the first extraosseous case. Oral Surg Oral Med Oral Pathol 75: 733–738
6. Wright JM 1979 Squamous odontogenic tumour-like proliferations in odontogenic cysts. Oral Surg 47: 354–358
7. Hodgkinson DJ, Woods JE, Dahlin DC, Tolman DE 1978 Keratocysts of the jaws. Cancer 41: 803–813
8. Fay JT, Baner J, Rothouse L, Kolas S, Klinger BJ, Sayers RJ 1981 Squamous odontogenic tumors arising in odontogenic cysts. J Oral Med 36: 35–38
9. Leventon GS, Happonen RP, Newland JR 1981 Squamous odontogenic tumour: report of two cases and review of the literature. Am J Surg Pathol 5: 671–677
10. Anneroth G, Hansen LS 1982 Variations in keratinizing cysts and tumors. Oral Surg Oral Med Oral Pathol 54: 530–546
11. Simon JH, Jenson JL 1985 Squamous odontogenic tumour-like proliferations in periapical cysts. J Endod 11: 446–448
12. Unal T, Gomel M, Gunel O 1987 Squamous odontogenic tumour-like islands in a radicular cyst: case report. J Oral Maxillofac Surg 45: 346–349
13. Leider AS, Jonker LA, Cook HE 1989 Multicentric familial squamous odontogenic tumour. Oral Surg Oral Med Oral Pathol 68: 175–181
14. Kramer IRH, Pindborg JJ, Shear M 1992 Histological typing of odontogenic tumours, 2nd edn. World Health Organization, Geneva
15. Goldblatt LI, Brannon RB, Ellis GL 1982 Squamous odontogenic tumor. Report of five cases and review of the literature. Oral Surg Oral Med Oral Pathol 54: 187–196

Calcifying epithelial odontogenic tumor

6

This tumor, with its bizarre cellular features, is often also referred to, for simplicity, as a Pindborg tumor, as Pindborg was the first to describe it in detail in 1958.[1] Though uncommon, this tumor is important, particularly because it has been mistaken for a poorly differentiated carcinoma.

INCIDENCE

Gender distribution

The most recently available data are those from Daley et al,[2] who found calcifying epithelial odontogenic tumors to account for 1.28% of 392 odontogenic tumors. Günhan et al[3] also found such tumors to comprise 1.5% of 403 odontogenic tumors. Although they formed fewer than 1% of 706 odontogenic tumors reported by Regezi et al,[4] this series included an unusually high number of odontomas. Franklin & Hindle[5] analyzed the relative frequency of ameloblastomas with calcifying epithelial odontogenic tumors on the basis of previously reported series.[6,7] They found that ameloblastomas predominated by a ratio of 17 : 1 in series from India and the USA and by 13 : 1 in an English series.

Hicks et al[8] have reported a clear cell variant of calcifying epithelial odontogenic tumor, and have tabulated the features of other variants from a review of 148 reported cases. Their findings largely confirm those of the analysis of 113 calcifying epithelial odontogenic tumors reported by Franklin & Pindborg,[9] but included additional information. Hicks et al[8] found an equal gender distribution for intraosseous tumors (mean age 40.3 years), but extraosseous tumors (mean age 31.8 years) were twice as frequent in females.

Intraosseous calcifying epithelial odontogenic tumors accounted for nearly 88% of all reported cases, while extraosseous tumors and those combined with adenomatoid odontogenic tumors accounted for 6% each.

Site distribution

Intraosseous calcifying epithelial odontogenic tumors analyzed by Hicks et al[8] involved the mandible twice as frequently as the maxilla, with a predilection for the molar region. By contrast, extraosseous tumors and mixed calcifying epithelial odontogenic tumor with adenomatoid odontogenic tumor had a predilection for the incisor–premolar region. Sixty-two per cent of the intraosseous tumors and 33% of the combined tumors were associated with an embedded tooth.

CLINICAL FEATURES

Symptoms are typically lacking until a slow-growing swelling becomes apparent. Franklin & Pindborg[9] were able to find reports of only eight cases where there had been pain. Other complaints were nasal stuffiness, epistaxis, and headaches, but in one case the tumor had caused proptosis.

RADIOGRAPHY

Radiographs may show a radiolucent area with well-defined margins, which can frequently mimic a dentigerous cyst. Alternatively, the margins are poorly defined and, although often unilocular in the early stages, the appearance later tends to become multilocular or honeycomb. Most characteristic are the diffuse radio-opacities within the lesion (Fig. 6.1), but they are variable in size. They are sometimes so extensive as to make the lesion relatively radio-opaque or, occasionally, so small as not to be seen in conventional radiographs. These radio-opacities are frequently uniformly distributed throughout the lesion to give a so-called 'driven snow' appearance.

MICROSCOPY

The appearances are variable but, typically, sheets or strands of pleomorphic, slightly eosinophilic epithelial cells lie in a connective tissue stroma. The epithelial cell membranes are typically distinct, and intercellular bridges may be clearly seen. A striking feature is the gross variation in nuclear size, including giant, frequently hyperchromatic nuclei and multinucleated cells. Though mitoses are rare, nucleoli are often prominent, so that there is an alarming resemblance to a poorly differentiated carcinoma. However, unlike most epidermoid carcinomas, abnormal mitoses and inflammatory infiltration of the stroma are usually absent.

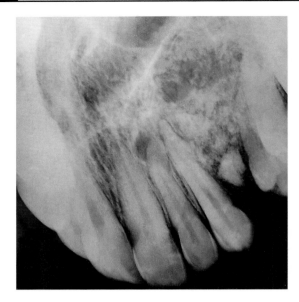

Fig. 6.1 Calcifying epithelial odontogenic tumor present for 18 months in a 28-year-old man. The normal trabecular pattern of the bone has been replaced by ill-defined radio-opacities, particularly at the site where the first premolar had been extracted, but the lesion involved the whole of the alveolar ridge in the angle between the nasal fossa and the antrum.

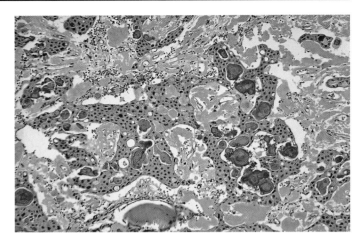

Fig. 6.2 Calcifying epithelial odontogenic tumor. Typical irregular islands of epithelial cells showing nuclear hyperchromatism and pleomorphism are interspersed with pinkish amyloid-like material and rounded calcifications.

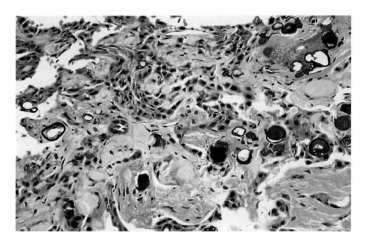

Fig. 6.3 Calcifying epithelial odontogenic tumor. Higher power view of the pleomorphic epithelial cells, amyloid-like deposits, and calcifications.

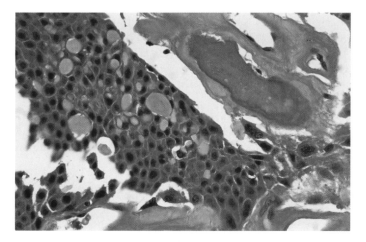

Fig. 6.4 Calcifying epithelial odontogenic tumor. Another view of the pleomorphic epithelial cells, with a suggestion of intercellar bridging, amyloid-like deposits, and calcifications.

Within the tumor, there are typically homogeneous hyaline areas, with the staining characteristics of amyloid, which may calcify. These calcifications form concentric masses (Liesegang rings) in and around the epithelial cells, particularly those which appear to be degenerating, and may form large masses. Rarely, dentine or tooth-like structures may form, but ameloblast-like cells are not seen (Figs 6.2–6.4).

The amyloid-like material seen in calcifying epithelial odontogenic tumors is by no means always present. Franklin & Pindborg[9] found that, of 113 reports, only 21 mentioned positive staining for amyloid and in eight others the staining was equivocal. Franklin et al[10] found by amino acid analysis that the major protein of this material shared similarities with tuft enamel protein, immune amyloid, and the variable light-chain component, but could not otherwise characterize it. According to Meenaghan et al,[11] amyloid or amyloid-like material can also be found in other odontogenic tumors, such as ameloblastomas, adenoameloblastomas, and ameloblastic odontoma.

Clear-cell variant of calcifying epithelial odontogenic tumor

Franklin & Pindborg (1976) noted the occasional presence of clear cells in some calcifying epithelial odontogenic tumors, and a clear-cell variant has been described by Schmidt-Westhausen et al,[12] who quoted reports of seven others. Hicks et al[8] analyzed the findings in nine cases, which represented 6% of all reported calcifying epithelial odontogenic tumors. The mean age of those affected was 46 years and the gender distribution was almost equal. Eighty-nine per cent of these tumors were intraosseous, and affected equally the anterior or posterior region of the mandible. Radiographically, 89% presented well-circumscribed radiolucencies, with focal calcifications in 55.6%. Eleven per cent each were associated with an unerupted tooth or widening of the periodontal ligament space.

Histologically, clear-cell calcifying epithelial odontogenic tumors have all the characteristics of the conventional type, including formation of amyloid-like material, polyhedral cells with distinct cell membranes, intercellular bridges and occasional calcified Liesegang rings. However, rounded, clear, or faintly eosinophilic cells, either isolated or in clusters, are present in many of the tumor islands or sheets but lack cellular and nuclear pleomorphism. They appear to develop from the tumor cells by accumulation, then loss of periodic acid/Schiff (PAS) positive material until they appeared empty. Hicks et al[8] also noted perineural invasion in their specimen.

It is important to distinguish clear-cell calcifying epithelial odontogenic tumors from the clear-cell odontogenic carcinoma (see Ch. 7).

BEHAVIOR AND MANAGEMENT

Calcifying epithelial odontogenic tumors are not encapsulated, are locally invasive, and their behavior is broadly similar to that of ameloblastomas. Hicks et al[8] found a recurrence rate of 14% after follow-up periods ranging from 1 to 31 years for the common type, but a 71.4% rate for nine clear-cell types after follow-up periods ranging from 13 to 48 months.

Once poorly differentiated carcinoma and clear-cell odontogenic carcinoma have been excluded, excision with a margin of normal bone is the current treatment of choice. As to the reported recurrences, the extent of the excisions has rarely been clear.

Basu et al[13] have reported a malignant counterpart of calcifying epithelial odontogenic tumor. This showed greater mitotic activity and abnormal mitoses and gave rise to nodal metastasis.

Hybrid calcifying epithelial odontogenic tumor and adenomatoid odontogenic tumor

Areas resembling calcifying epithelial odontogenic tumor in adenomatoid odontogenic tumor have been discussed in relation to the latter. These tumors have behaved like adenomatoid odontogenic tumors rather than calcifying epithelial odontogenic tumors, and none have as yet been reported to have recurred. Thus there seems little justification for the concept of a hybrid tumor.

REFERENCES

1. Pindborg JJ 1958 A calcifying epithelial odontogenic tumor. Cancer 2: 838–843
2. Daley TD, Wysocki GP, Pringle GA 1994 Relative incidence of odontogenic tumors and jaw cysts in a Canadian population. Oral Surg Oral Med Oral Pathol 77: 276–280
3. Günhan O, Ersevan G, Ruacon S et al 1990 Odontogenic tumours. A series of 409 cases. Aust Dent J 35: 518–522
4. Regezi JA, Kerr DA, Courtney RM 1978 Odontogenic tumors: analysis of 706 cases. J Oral Surg 36: 771–778
5. Franklin CD, Hindle MO 1976 The calcifying epithelial odontogenic tumour. Report of 4 cases, two with long term follow-up. Br J Oral Surg 13: 230–238
6. Doctor VM, Sirsat MV 1968 Calcifying epithelial odontogenic tumour (Pindborg tumour) in Indians. Ind J Cancer 5: 103–109
7. Vap DR, Dahlin DC, Turlington EG 1970 The so-called calcifying epithelial odontogenic tumor. Cancer 25: 629–636
8. Hicks MJ, Flaitz CM, Wong MEK, McDaniel RK, Cagle PT 1994 Clear cell variant of calcifying epithelial odontogenic tumour: case report and review of the literature. Head Neck 16: 272–277
9. Franklin CD, Pindborg JJ 1976 The calcifying epithelial odontogenic tumor. A review and analysis of 113 cases. Oral Surg 42: 753–765
10. Franklin CD, Martin MV, Clark A, Smith CJ, Hindle MO 1981 An investigation into the origin and nature of 'amyloid' in a calcifying epithelial odontogenic tumour. J Oral Pathol 10: 417–429
11. Meenaghan MA, Appel BN, Greene GW 1972 Amyloid-containing odontogenic tumors of man. Oral Surg 24: 908–919
12. Schmidt-Westhausen A, Philipsen HP, Reichart PA 1992 Clear cell calcifying epithelial odontogenic tumor. A case report. J Oral Maxillofac Surg 21: 47–49
13. Basu MK, Matthews JB, Sear AJ, Browne RM 1984 Calcifying epithelial odontogenic tumour: a case showing features of malignancy. J Oral Pathol 13: 310–319

Clear cell odontogenic carcinoma

7

This rare neoplasm, was first described by Hansen et al[1] as *clear cell odontogenic tumour with aggressive potential*. Lymph node and pulmonary metastases have been reported by Bang et al,[2] so that it has justifiably been renamed. Sadeghi & Levin[3] have reported a case and reviewed eight earlier ones. Seven of these were in females, but too few cases have been reported to gain any useful idea about the true overall or gender incidence of this neoplasm.

CLINICAL FEATURES

Most of these tumors have been in elderly patients (50–89 years) and have frequently caused loosening of teeth of either jaw and sometimes pain or tenderness as early symptoms. Expansion of the jaw and a ragged area of radiolucency are also produced.

MICROSCOPY

The tumor is poorly circumscribed and consists of sheets of cells with abundant clear cytoplasm. The cells are uniform in size with a central or eccentric nucleus and a delicate but well-defined cell membrane. They form islands or processes, which may show palisading in the relatively dense fibrous tissue septa (Figs 7.1–7.3).

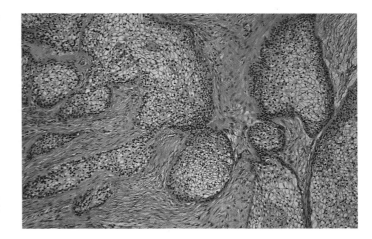

Fig. 7.2 Clear cell odontogenic carcinoma. Islands of tumor lack any ameloblast-like cells.

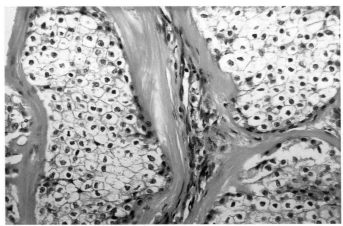

Fig. 7.3 Clear cell odontogenic carcinoma. Higher power view of the polygonal clear cells and lack of palisading.

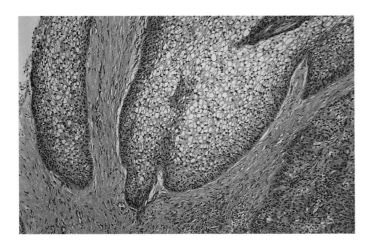

Fig. 7.1 Clear cell ameloblastoma. Processes of clear cells have palisades of ameloblast-like cells.

There may also be lesser, dense areas of small basaloid epithelial cells with scanty cytoplasm. Inflammatory cells are few or absent, but areas of hemorrhage may be seen. Nervous tissue may be enveloped and the tumor infiltrates the surrounding bone. In the case reported by Fan et al,[4] a follow-up biopsy after initiation of chemo- and immunotherapy showed nonkeratinizing squamous cells with intercellular bridges. Transition from clear cells could be seen in some areas.

A variable number of the epithelial cells may have a finely fibrillar rather than completely clear cytoplasm and may contain diastase-labile, periodic acid/Schiff (PAS) positive granules. There may be some nuclear pleomorphism, but no more than occasional mitoses. Intercellular bridges, calcifications, or amyloid-like material are not seen.

Fan et al[4] found that an aggressive clear cell odontogenic carcinoma showed raised levels of tumor markers such as squamous-cell-carcinoma-associated antigen TA-4, and carcinoembryonic antigen. Tumor cells were negative for mucicarmine, alcian blue, and oil red O stains. A few cells contained PAS-positive and diastase-labile cytoplasmic granules. Immunohistochemistry showed positive reactivity of some cells for keratin and epithelial membrane antigen (EMA), but negative reactions for S-100 protein, actin, vimentin, and myosin. Ultrastructurally, the tumor cells had abundant clear cytoplasm with sparse mitochondria, endoplasmic reticulum, lysosomal granules, and tonofilament bundles. The tumor cells were tightly interdigitated with microvilli, and intercellular desmosomes were frequently seen.

DIFFERENTIAL DIAGNOSIS

Some doubt may be felt as to whether the clear-cell variant of ameloblastoma and clear cell odontogenic carcinoma are distinct entities. However, by definition, clear cell ameloblastoma shows some features of typical ameloblastoma and a follicular or plexiform configuration. It also appears to be less aggressive with little or no tendency to metastasize.

Significant numbers of clear cells may also occasionally be found in calcifying epithelial odontogenic tumors, as described by Schmidt-Westhausen et al,[5] who noted this finding in seven earlier reports. However, calcifying epithelial odontogenic tumor has a considerably more pleomorphic cellular picture than clear cell odontogenic carcinoma, which also lacks the calcifications and amyloid formation typical of calcifying epithelial odontogenic tumor.

Intraosseous salivary gland tumors are a well-recognized entity of which mucoepidermoid tumor is the most common type. It too may contain clear cells, but not to such an extent as to mimic clear cell odontogenic carcinoma. Other clear cell salivary gland tumors do not appear to have been reported in the jaw. The most important tumor that needs to be distinguished from a clear cell odontogenic tumor is a metastasis of a renal cell carcinoma and, although this usually also involves the mandible rather than the maxilla, the differential diagnosis (see Ch. 52) needs to be considered as it so seriously affects the prognosis.

BEHAVIOR AND MANAGEMENT

Clear cell odontogenic carcinoma is aggressive. The example reported by Fan et al[4] massively invaded adjacent structures including the cranium and orbits, and metastasized to regional lymph nodes. However, this degree of spread did not appear until 11 years after the patient first noticed a painless swelling of the mandible. The tumor recurred after excision, chemotherapy, and immunotherapy, but there were no distant metastases when the patient was last seen, 2 years after the start of treatment. Of the nine cases analyzed by Sadeghi & Levin,[3] four recurred after variable periods of follow-up. Three metastasized to regional lymph nodes and one to the lungs.

Wide excision may be effective in the short term, but recurrences or metastases or both have sometimes been delayed for several years after treatment. Prolonged follow-up is therefore necessary.

REFERENCES

1. Hansen LS, Eversole LR, Green TL, Powell NB 1985 Clear cell odontogenic tumor – a new histologic variant with aggressive potential. Head Neck Surg 8: 115–123
2. Bang G, Koppang HS, Hansen LS et al 1989 Clear cell odontogenic carcinoma: report of three cases with pulmonary and lymph node metastases. J Oral Pathol Med 18: 113–118
3. Sadeghi EM, Levin S 1995 Clear cell odontogenic carcinoma of the mandible: report of a case. J Oral Maxillofac Surg 53: 613–616
4. Fan J, Kubota E, Imamura H, Shimokama T, Tokunaga O, Watanabe T 1992 Clear cell odontogenic carcinoma. A case report with massive invasion of neighboring organs and lymph node metastasis. Oral Surg Oral Med Oral Pathol 74: 768–775
5. Schmidt-Westhausen A, Philipsen HP, Reichart PA 1992 Clear cell epithelial odontogenic tumour. A case report. J Oral Maxillofac Surg 21: 47–49

Calcifying odontogenic cyst (odontogenic ghost cell cyst and tumor, Gorlin cyst)

8

The calcifying odontogenic cyst was recognized in the jaws by Gorlin et al in 1964.[1] Its cutaneous counterpart (*benign calcifying epithelioma of Malherbe* – currently termed a pilomatrixoma) was described in 1880. Though usually cystic, this lesion can rarely be solid and has some potential for continued growth. In an analysis of the variants of this tumor, Praetorius et al[2] came to the conclusion that there were two entities – a cyst and a neoplasm – with different histological morphology.

INCIDENCE

In their analysis of 392 odontogenic tumors, Daley et al[3] found 18 central calcifying odontogenic cysts. Hong et al[4] reviewed 92 cases in order to re-evaluate their nature as neoplasms. Buchner,[5] in an analysis of 215 reported cases, found an almost equal gender distribution (51.2% females). Patients ranged in age from 5 to 82 years (mean 31.6 years). The highest incidence was between the ages of 10 and 29 years, with 40% of cases appearing in the second decade. On average, males presented at a slightly later age (31.6 years) than females (29.1 years).

As for the variants discussed below, the mean age of patients with the cystic-type lesion was 34 years, with the odontoma-associated variant it was 17 years, and with the solid type it was 46 years.

Of 155 cases where racial origin was specified, Buchner[5] found that 48% were Asian and formed the largest single group. Whites formed 34%. Buchner[5] also noted that calcifying odontogenic cysts appeared to develop slightly more frequently in the maxilla and at an earlier age in Asians than in whites.

In the large series analyzed by Buchner,[5] the calcifying odontogenic cyst formed virtually equally frequently in the maxilla as in the mandible. The main differences were that 74% of the maxillary tumors affected the anterior (canine/incisor) region as opposed to 56% of the mandibular tumors, of which the remainder were in the premolar/molar regions. Most of the lesions associated with odontomas were in the incisor/canine regions and some of the cases, particularly those in the mandible, extended across the midline.

CLINICAL FEATURES

The calcifying odontogenic cyst gives rise to a painless swelling with expansion of the bone, which is occasionally perforated. In 58 cases where the size was stated, Buchner[5] found that it ranged from 0.5 to 12 cm in diameter, and that almost 60% were between 2 and 4 cm in size. He also noted that the mean delay between awareness of a lesion and presentation for treatment was 6 months, but ranged from 3 days to 9 years.

Radiographically, most calcifying odontogenic cysts appear as well-circumscribed, unilocular cyst-like areas of radiolucency, but are occasionally multilocular or appear less sharply circumscribed. A minority contain scattered radio-opacities, which range from mere flecks to large masses. Related teeth may sometimes be displaced or show root resorption.

Buchner[5] found that 32% of lesions were associated with unerupted teeth. The latter were more frequently maxillary lesions (63% of cases) than mandibular (37% of cases). In 24% the tumor was associated with an odontoma, particularly in younger patients. An associated odontoma is recognizable radio-

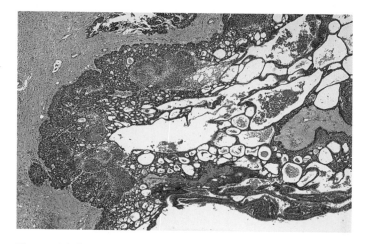

Fig. 8.1 Calcifying odontogenic cyst. In this example there are many microcysts and an apparent transition from a cystic- to a solid-type tumor.

graphically by its more densely radio-opaque tissues overlapping those of the calcifying odontogenic cyst.

MICROSCOPY

The calcifying odontogenic cyst, as its radiographic appearances imply, usually consists of a single cystic cavity or, less frequently, multiple smaller cavities (Fig. 8.1). The cyst wall consists of relatively thick fibrous tissue, while the epithelial lining is irregular in structure and variable in thickness. There are frequently foci where there is a well-defined basal cell layer, but, more characteristically, the basal layer consists of ameloblast-like cells with reversed polarity of their nuclei. Above this layer there is frequently a zone of loose edematous cells bearing some resemblance to stellate reticulum. However, the most striking and characteristic feature is the keratinized, anucleate (ghost) cells (Figs 8.2–8.6). The latter may form small foci within the epithelial lining or fuse

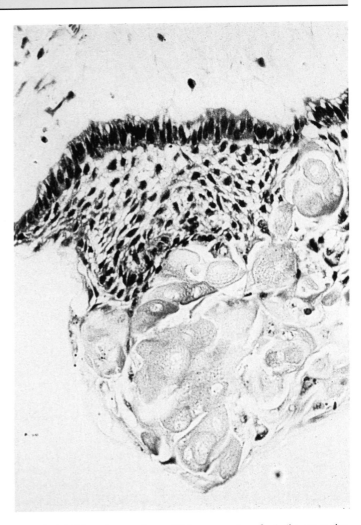

Fig. 8.4 Calcifying odontogenic cyst. Higher power view of a similar area to that shown in Figure 8.3.

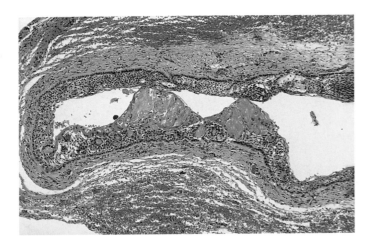

Fig. 8.2 Calcifying odontogenic cyst. Higher power view of the abnormal keratinization producing ghost cells and a few small calcifications.

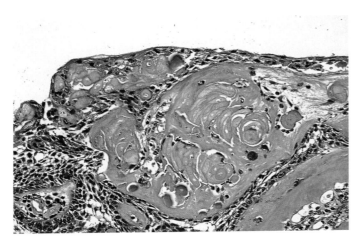

Fig. 8.3 Calcifying odontogenic cyst. Low-power view showing a cystic cavity with eosinophilic ghost cells protruding into it, and the palisaded basal layer with ameloblast-like cells.

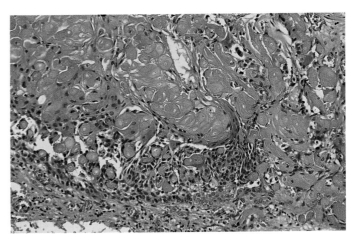

Fig. 8.5 Calcifying odontogenic cyst. Details of the abnormal keratinization (ghost cells) with outlines of nuclear remnants.

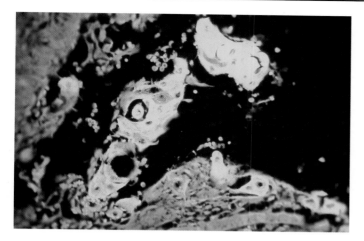

Fig. 8.6 Calcifying odontogenic cyst. Fluorescence microscopy shows thioflavin-T-positive ghost cells.

into large masses extending into or even filling the cyst lumen. The keratin masses may also extend into the underlying connective tissue and provoke a foreign body reaction. The ghost cells sometimes become mineralized to form calcified masses of variable size. Dentine-like material may sometimes also form.

SOLID (NEOPLASTIC TYPE) CALCIFYING ODONTOGENIC CYST

Buchner[5] found that 2% of so-called calcifying odontogenic cysts were solid tumors. The clinical features are similar to those of the cystic variant, but the solid type differs in its closer histologic resemblance to an ameloblastoma. Ameloblast-like cells surround strands or islands of epithelium, which sometimes resembles stellate reticulum. However, ghost cells are also present in variable amounts and there may be deposits of dentinoid. Cysts or slits are sometimes present in the epithelial islands which infiltrate a connective-tissue stroma.

HISTOGENESIS

There can be little doubt that the calcifying odontogenic cyst arises from some part of remnants of the dental lamina, but its morphological affinities with both the ameloblastoma and the pilomatrixoma leave more questions about its histogenesis than can be answered satisfactorily.

The categorization of this lesion is currently also less than satisfactory. While, as suggested by Praetorius et al,[2] only the solid variant of calcifying odontogenic cyst is a true neoplasm, it may be difficult to accept that the cystic type, which shares many histologic features, is a different entity. Moreover, it seems unnecessarily confusing to speak of a solid variant of the calcifying odontogenic cyst. But to term this solid variant a calcifying odontogenic tumor would also cause confusion with the calcify-

ing epithelial odontogenic tumor. Under the circumstances, the terms *epithelial odontogenic ghost cell cyst* and *epithelial odontogenic ghost cell tumor*, as proposed by Ellis & Shmookler,[6] have obvious advantages.

BEHAVIOR AND MANAGEMENT

It is widely accepted that the calcifying odontogenic cyst has a potential for continued growth. Nevertheless, Buchner[5] could find only eight reports of recurrence after treatment no more extensive than enucleation. The recurrences were detected 1–8 years after treatment. Unfortunately, the histology of the recurrent cases was documented in only three cases, but it appears that either the solid or cystic type can occasionally recur. Moreover, in the case reported by Wright et al[7] a mixed solid/cystic calcifying odontogenic cyst recurred as a purely cystic lesion. In the case reported by Slootweg & Koole,[8] both the primary lesion and the recurrence were cystic.

Kramer et al[9] state that calcifying odontogenic cysts that have ameloblastoma-like features may have an infiltrative pattern of growth. Nevertheless, the response of many calcifying odontogenic cysts to treatment does not, overall, seem to have been affected by the presence of ameloblast-like features. However, the behavior of calcifying odontogenic cysts that are associated with an ameloblastoma or other aggressive neoplasm is dominated by the latter, which should be treated appropriately.

Overall, therefore, wide excision of calcifying odontogenic cyst does not appear to be necessary, and the treatment of choice appears to be enucleation. However, more extensive surgery may be required if there is any doubt whether the lesion can otherwise be removed in its entirety. The possibility of recurrence must be borne in mind and, although recurrence is unusual, prolonged follow-up is required.

Peripheral (extraosseous) calcifying odontogenic cyst

The extraosseous variant of the calcifying odontogenic cyst is considerably more uncommon than the intraosseous type. However, Buchner et al[10] were able to review 45 cases.

INCIDENCE

The age distribution of the cases reviewed by Buchner et al[10] was scattered. Apparent peaks were seen in the age ranges 10–19 years (17.8%), 50–59 years (24.4%), and 70–79 years (15.5%). Overall, the highest incidence (49%) was in the sixth to eighth decades. At the extremes of life there were single cases at ages 9 and 92 years. Males and females were almost equally frequently affected, with 53% of cases being in females.

The most frequent site was the mandible (58% cases). The incisor/canine and premolar were most commonly affected.

CLINICAL FEATURES

Most lesions have appeared as painless, circumscribed, smooth swellings on the alveolar ridge or gingiva, and were usually 0.5–1 cm in diameter. The texture was described as firm in most cases, but some were soft and cystic. Saucerization of the underlying bone was seen in 25% of cases, but teeth were rarely displaced. The reported duration of the swelling in the series reported by Buchner et al[10] ranged from months to a remarkable 15 years in two cases.

MICROSCOPY

The morphology of peripheral calcifying odontogenic cyst is the same as that of the central type, with both solid and cystic types being represented. Unlike the central type, peripheral calcifying odontogenic cyst were solid in 36% of the cases analyzed by Buchner et al.[10]

All lesions contain ghost cells, and usually there is mineralization and dentinoid formation. Continuity between the lesion and the surface epithelium is occasionally seen.

HISTOGENESIS

The most probable origin of the peripheral calcifying odontogenic cyst is from remnants of the dental lamina known as the rests ('glands') of Serres. The peripheral ameloblastoma and gingival cyst of adults probably have similar origins, and Buchner et al[10] point out that all these peripheral lesions have a similar age distribution, with a mean of between 48 and 52 years. Despite continuity with the overlying epithelium seen in a minority of cases, it seems less likely that it retains any potential for odontogenic differentiation at so late an age and of originating an odontogenic tumor.

BEHAVIOR AND MANAGEMENT

Like the central type, peripheral calcifying odontogenic cyst is benign and responds to simple excision. Recurrence has rarely been reported.

Odontogenic ghost cell carcinoma

The malignant variant of the odontogenic ghost cell tumor is rare. Many authors, such as Ellis and Schmookler[6] who reported

the first examples, have been reluctant to term it a carcinoma and preferred the term *aggressive (malignant?) epithelial odontogenic ghost cell tumor*, despite its extension into muscle and other soft tissues. Scott & Wood[11] reported a recurrent tumor that had histological features of calcifying odontogenic cyst but had extended widely from the maxilla. However, they suggested that this might have been a variant of ameloblastoma.

Nevertheless, an odontogenic ghost cell tumor that metastasized to lungs and other sites to cause the death of the patient was reported by Grodjesk et al.[12] Those authors found that, at that time, five examples of aggressive behavior of these tumors had been reported. These cases included those already mentioned and one other reported by Ikemura et al.[13] Since then, McCoy et al[14] and Siar & Ng[15] have reported examples, although the tumor in the latter report in its initial form and first and second recurrences appeared to be a plexiform ameloblastoma.

CLINICAL FEATURES

Males have been mostly affected and the tumor appears to have a predilection for the maxilla. The ages of patients have ranged from 13 to 64 years.

This tumor grows relatively rapidly and typically causes painful expansion of the bone. Radiographs show an ill-demarcated area of radiolucency with variable degrees of destruction of the outer plates of bone.

MICROSCOPY

The appearances have been variable, but a prerequisite for the diagnosis is the presence of tissue typical of calcifying odontogenic cyst. However, in malignant ghost cell tumors the epithelial cells are pleomorphic. The nuclei are frequently hyperchromatic, show mitotic activity, and are retained in some of the ghost cells, and progressive transformation to squamous cell, basaloid, or undifferentiated carcinoma may be seen.

BEHAVIOR AND MANAGEMENT

Wide excision of odontogenic ghost cell carcinoma and careful follow-up is necessary, but the tumors are so rare there is as yet no definitive treatment protocol. An adequate period of follow-up was not possible in many of the reported cases, but two of the patients reported by Ellis & Shmookler[6] remained well for 6 years after treatment. By contrast, the patient reported by Grodjesk et al[12] died within a few months of the onset of symptoms. Despite extensive surgery, the maxillary mass rapidly recurred and spread. It failed to respond to radiotherapy, chest radiography strongly suggested the presence of metastases, and death quickly followed.

REFERENCES

1. Gorlin RJ, Pindborg JJ, Redman RS, Williamson JJ, Hansen LS 1964 The calcifying odontogenic cyst – a new entity and possible analogue of the cutaneous epithelioma of Malherbe. Cancer 17: 723–729
2. Praetorius F, Hjorting-Hansen E, Gorlin RJ, Vickers RA 1981 Calcifying odontogenic cyst; range variations and neoplastic potential. Acta Odontol Scand 39: 227–240
3. Daley TD, Wysocki GP, Pringle GA 1994 Relative incidence of odontogenic tumors and jaw cysts in a Canadian population. Oral Surg Oral Med Oral Pathol 77: 276–280
4. Hong SP, Ellis GL, Hartman KS 1992 Calcifying odontogenic cyst: a review of ninety-two cases with re-evaluation of their nature as neoplasms, the nature of ghost cells, and subclassification. Oral Surg Oral Med Oral Pathol 72: 56–64
5. Buchner A 1991 The central (intraosseous) calcifying odontogenic cyst: an analysis of 215 cases. J Oral Maxillofac Surg 49: 330–339
6. Ellis GL, Shmookler BM 1986 Aggressive (malignant?) epithelial odontogenic ghost cell tumor. Oral Surg Oral Med Oral Pathol 61: 471–478
7. Wright BA, Bhardwaj AK, Murphy D 1984 Recurrent calcifying odontogenic cyst. Oral Surg Oral Med Oral Pathol 58: 579–582
8. Slootweg PJ, Koole R 1980 Recurrent calcifying odontogenic cyst. J Maxillofac Surg 8: 143–146
9. Kramer IRH, Pindborg JJ, Shear M 1992 Histological typing of odontogenic tumours. World Health Organization/Springer-Verlag, Berlin
10. Buchner A, Merrell PW, Hansen LS, Leider AS 1991 Peripheral (extraosseous) calcifying odontogenic cyst. A review of forty-five cases. Oral Surg Oral Med Oral Pathol 72: 65–70
11. Scott J, Wood GD 1989 Aggressive calcifying odontogenic cyst – a possible variant of ameloblastoma. Br J Oral Maxillofac Surg 27: 53–59
12. Grodjesk JE, Dolinsky HB, Schneider LC, Dolinsky EH, Doyle JL 1987 Odontogenic ghost cell carcinoma. Oral Surg Oral Med Oral Pathol 63: 576–581
13. Ikemura K, Horie A, Tashiro H, Nandate M 1985 Simultaneous occurrence of a calcifying odontogenic cyst and its malignant transformation. Cancer 56: 2861–2864
14. McCoy BP, Carroll MKO, Hall JM 1992 Carcinoma arising in a dentinogenic ghost cell tumor. Oral Surg Oral Med Oral Pathol 74: 371–378
15. Siar CH, Ng KH 1994 Aggressive (malignant?) epithelial odontogenic ghost cell tumour of the maxilla. J Laryngol Otol 108: 269–271

Ameloblastic fibroma and fibrosarcoma 9

Ameloblastic fibromas have some histological resemblance to ameloblastomas, but are more benign in behavior and considerably more uncommon.

INCIDENCE

Among 392 odontogenic tumors analyzed by Daley et al,[1] there were six ameloblastic fibromas, which formed 1.5% of the sample. Among 706 odontogenic tumors analyzed by Regezi et al,[2] ameloblastic fibromas formed 2%, but this earlier series comprised fewer types of odontogenic tumor. In Turkey, by contrast, Günhan et al[3] found ameloblastic fibromas to account for 4.5% of odontogenic tumors. There may therefore be considerable racial differences in the incidence of ameloblastic fibroma, as in the case of ameloblastoma.

Trodahl[4] analyzed the findings in 36 acceptable cases of ameloblastic fibroma, and concluded that there was no significant gender difference in frequency. The ages of patients ranged from 18 months to 41 years, with a median of 15.5 years. No racial predilection could be confirmed. Later, Slootweg,[5] in an analysis of 55 cases, found that 60% of the tumors appeared after the age of 9 years and the mean age of those affected was 14.6 years. He also confirmed that there was little difference in the gender distribution, 52.7% being in males.

As to site, Trodahl[4] found that any site in the jaw could be affected, but that the mandible was involved in 88% of cases, usually in the posterior region. In the three cases affecting the maxilla, the anterior and posterior regions were equally frequently affected. These findings were confirmed by Slootweg,[5] in whose series 83% of tumors were in the mandible. Of these, 74% were in the posterior region.

CLINICAL FEATURES

Ameloblastic fibromas are slow growing and are usually asymptomatic apart from eventual expansion of the jaw. Trodahl[4] found that the presenting symptom in the majority (58%) was a swelling, but 17% were seen by chance on a routine radiograph. Two patients complained of pain and two of tenderness. Two noted failure of eruption of a tooth and one complained of a discharge.

RADIOGRAPHY

Radiographically, ameloblastic fibromas usually appear as multilocular radiolucencies with sclerotic margins, and typically range from 1 to 8 cm in diameter (Fig. 9.1). Small examples may appear unilocular, while large ones may extend through the cortices of the bone.

MICROSCOPY

Ameloblastic fibroma is a mixed odontogenic tumor and has distinctive epithelial and connective tissue components. It usually, but not invariably, has a dense fibrous capsule. The epithelium

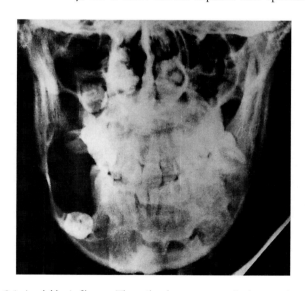

Fig. 9.1 Ameloblastic fibroma. The unilocular transparency in the posterior body of the mandible resembles a dentigerous cyst.

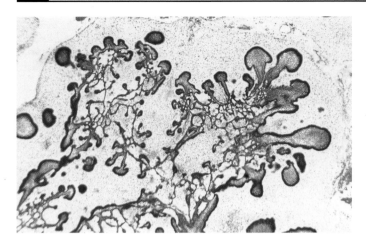

Fig. 9.2 Ameloblastic fibroma. Islands of odontogenic epithelium with peripheral ameloblast-like cells form typical cauliflower-like proliferations of epithelial cells in ectomesenchymal stroma resembling dental papilla.

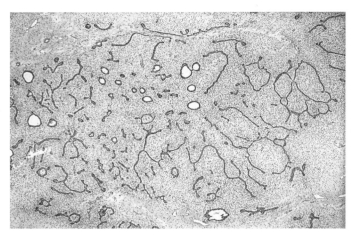

Fig. 9.4 Ameloblastic fibroma. Low-power view of another appearance with slender strands of odontogenic epithelium, lacking any stellate reticulum-like component, in a cellular ectomesenchymal stroma.

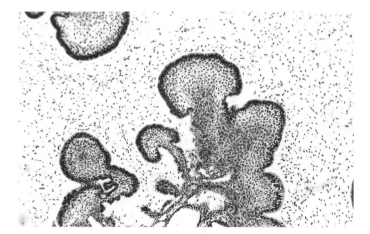

Fig. 9.3 Ameloblastic fibroma. Higher power view of the same tumor as shown in Figure 9.2.

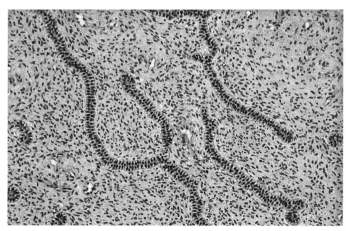

Fig. 9.5 Ameloblastic fibroma. Higher power view of double-layered strands of columnar cells in a more cellular stroma.

consists of ameloblast-like or more cuboidal cells surrounding others resembling stellate reticulum, or are sometimes more compactly arranged (Figs 9.2 and 9.3). The epithelium is sharply circumscribed by a basal membrane and forms islands, strands, or cauliflower-like proliferations in a loose but cellular, fibromyxoid connective tissue (Figs 9.4 and 9.5). The latter usually forms little collagen and resembles the immature dental papilla.

An exceedingly rare granular cell variant, in which large eosinophilic granular cells replace the fibromyxoid connective tissue component, has been described by Waldron et al[6] and termed *granular cell ameloblastic fibroma*. However, White et al,[7] after investigating four examples, concluded from electron microscopic studies that it was a distinct type of mesenchymal tumor.

HISTOGENESIS

Ameloblastic fibroma arises from odontogenic epithelial and

mesenchymal cells of the enamel organ and dental papilla, respectively. It appears to be a true mixed tumor and it is noticeable that, unlike the histologically somewhat similar-appearing ameloblastoma, malignant change in ameloblastic fibromas affects the mesenchymal component, not the epithelium.

Becker et al[8] investigated the distribution in four ameloblastic fibromas of collagen (types I, IV, and VI, and procollagen type III) and of undulin. Undulin is a glycoprotein associated with mature collagen fibrils and differentiated tissues. They found a previously undescribed organization of these matrix proteins. Collagen type VI clearly predominated over type I and procollagen type III. Undulin was not detectable in the neoplastic stroma, apart from weak expression around capillaries and highly cellular areas. There was thus a clear distinction between the tumor and the surrounding mesenchymes. A consequence of this finding is that epithelial tumor islands could be recognized as being outside the tumor stroma. The authors concluded that the epithelial cells of ameloblastic fibroma invade the surrounding normal mesenchyme, and might thereby induce de novo production of ectomesenchymal tumor stroma.

BEHAVIOR AND MANAGEMENT

Ameloblastic fibroma was termed *soft odontoma* in the past, as it was believed that it could mature into an odontoma. However, this change has never been seen in ameloblastic fibromas in older persons. Moreover, the mixed lesion, ameloblastic fibro-odontoma, shows a significantly different age and site distribution (see below). In particular, as shown by Slootweg,[5] ameloblastic fibro-odontoma is seen in a younger age group (mean age 8 years) than ameloblastic fibroma (mean age 14.6 years). The idea that a more highly differentiated lesion could form at an earlier mean age than the lesion from which it develops is clearly untenable. The belief that ameloblastic fibro-odontoma develops from an ameloblastic fibroma should, therefore, be dismissed.

Ameloblastic fibroma is a benign neoplasm. It is not a hamartoma and has considerable growth potential. Harrison et al,[9] for example, described an ameloblastic fibroma that filled the maxillary antrum, causing both an external swelling and obstruction of the ipsilateral nostril. Sawyer et al[10] reported an example that had been present for 23 years and weighed 2072 g. Despite its long duration, this tumor retained the immature character of the mesenchymal component. Ameloblastic fibroma also has a recognized proclivity for recurrence after excision. One of the tumors reported by Sawyer et al[10] recurred four times after the initial surgery. Trodahl,[4] in particular, reported a recurrence rate of 43.5% in 24 cases. Müller et al,[11] in their review of the literature, found a cumulative recurrence rate of 18.3%. However, reported recurrence rates inevitably depend on the completeness of excision.

Although ameloblastic fibromas may sometimes separate readily from their bony walls, conservative excision may be regarded as the treatment of choice. Nevertheless, approximately half the reported cases of ameloblastic fibrosarcoma have resulted from malignant change in ameloblastic fibromas, so that more radical excision may be justified for the benign stage of the tumor. Müller et al[11] particularly advise this more radical approach in view of their finding that 44% of ameloblastic fibrosarcomas had arisen in ameloblastic fibromas, as discussed below. Follow-up should also be prolonged.

Ameloblastic fibro-odontoma

Ameloblastic fibro-odontoma consists of an ameloblastic fibroma combined with an odontoma.

INCIDENCE

Slootweg,[5] in his extensive survey, was able to find reports of 50 ameloblastic fibro-odontomas, which had been seen over the period 1908 to 1980. This tumor is therefore more uncommon than the ameloblastic fibroma. As mentioned earlier, ameloblastic fibro-odontoma affects somewhat younger patients than ameloblastic fibroma and 62% of patients are younger than 10 years (mean age 8.1 years). It is also noticeable, as Slootweg[5] showed, that a higher proportion (48%) of ameloblastic fibro-odontomas form in the maxilla. This is more than twice as frequently as ameloblastic fibroma.

Like ameloblastic fibroma, ameloblastic fibro-odontoma shows little gender difference in incidence.

CLINICAL FEATURES

Ameloblastic fibro-odontoma, like an ameloblastic fibroma is typically asymptomatic, but radiographs typically show the opaque odontomatous tissues in a circumscribed, but otherwise radiolucent, area.

MICROSCOPY

Typical ameloblastic fibroma is associated with the calcifying or calcified dental tissues of an odontoma (Figs 9.6–9.8).

BEHAVIOR AND MANAGEMENT

The neoplastic component of an ameloblastic fibro-odontoma behaves in a similar manner to an ameloblastic fibroma. Therefore, conservative excision with a margin of sound bone appears to be the treatment of choice. However, it is possible that, once the tumor cells become functional and odontoma formation starts, the tumor may transform entirely into an odontoma. If so, more conservative treatment may be justified.

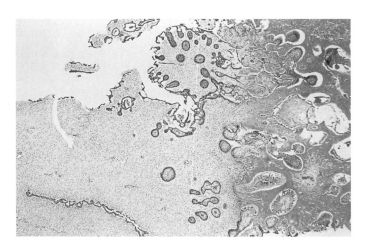

Fig. 9.6 Ameloblastic fibro-odontoma. Low-power view showing typical ameloblastic fibroma (left) merging with odontoma (right).

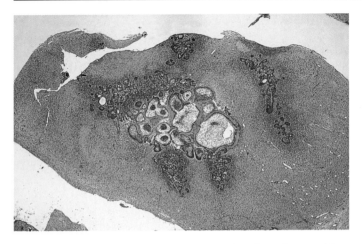

Fig. 9.7 Ameloblastic fibro-odontoma. Low-power view of an early stage with no more than a rimming of eosinophilic dental tissue.

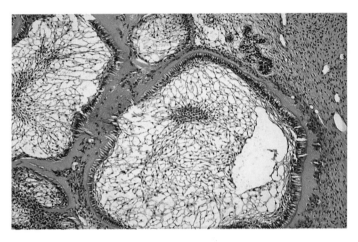

Fig. 9.8 Ameloblastic fibro-odontoma. High-power view of the same tumor as in Figure 9.9 showing induction of a thin rim of atubular dentine in the stroma by the ameloblast-like cells.

In the past there has been confusion between the ameloblastic fibro-odontoma and the odontoameloblastoma; as described earlier, the latter is an aggressive tumor for which more radical surgery is essential.

AMELOBLASTIC FIBRODENTINOMA

Ameloblastic fibrodentinoma can be regarded as a rare variant of ameloblastic fibro-odontoma. It consists of an ameloblastic fibroma in which the inductive effect of the epithelial component has resulted in deposition of dentine matrix or dentinoid. Ulmansky et al[12] were able to find 31 reported cases, added two more, and reviewed this tumor in detail. In most of the reported cases this tumor had been categorized as a *dentinoma*. Dentine forms only under the inductive action of odontogenic epithelium, so that the existence of a 'pure' dentinoma is no longer accepted.

Ameloblastic fibrosarcoma

Ameloblastic fibrosarcoma is the uncommon malignant counterpart of ameloblastic fibroma.

INCIDENCE

Wood et al,[13] from 44 cases, found that the mandible was twice as frequently affected as the maxilla. The reported age incidence ranged from 13 to 78 years, with an average of 26 years. Twenty-six males and 16 females were affected.

CLINICAL FEATURES

More than half the cases reviewed by Wood et al[13] appear to have arisen in ameloblastic fibromas or ameloblastic fibro-odontomas.[14–18] They initially have similar symptoms, but recur and become obviously aggressive. Others are clearly malignant from the start, grow rapidly, and cause either pain or swelling or both. Müller et al[11] reported five new cases and in reviewing the literature found reports of 51 more and also histologic evidence of an origin in ameloblastic fibromas in 44%.

RADIOGRAPHY

Typically, an ill-defined area of radiolucency may be associated in maxillary lesions, with extension into the antrum to produce an opacity as well as destruction of the walls.

MICROSCOPY

The essential features are islands of epithelium with the same features as those of the ameloblastic fibroma but surrounded by highly cellular and pleomorphic fibrous tissue (Figs 9.9 and 9.10). Pleomorphism may be gross and mitoses frequent, but there can be all grades of transition from the benign variant, so that it may be difficult to be certain, histologically, whether or not the mesenchymal component is malignant. Müller et al[11] found that one of their five ameloblastic fibrosarcomas was aneuploid, while all three of the ameloblastomas they studied were diploid. Unexpectedly, they found that one tumor with highly anaplastic stroma and bizarre tumor giant cells was diploid, and that in this small series there was no correlation between DNA ploidy with tumor grade.

In some areas, the sarcomatous element can overwhelm the epithelial component, but in the absence of epithelium the diagnosis cannot be confirmed. Dental hard tissues are occasionally present if the tumor has arisen in an ameloblastic fibro-odontoma and help to confirm the diagnosis.

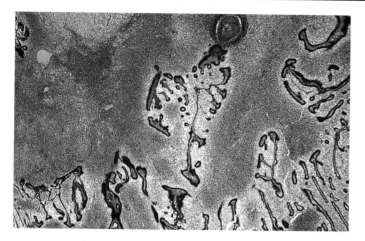

Fig. 9.9 Ameloblastic fibrosarcoma. Low-power view showing densely cellular and hyperchromatic stroma.

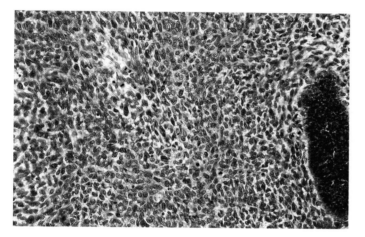

Fig. 9.10 Ameloblastic fibrosarcoma. Higher power view showing the densely cellular stroma with several mitoses.

BEHAVIOR AND MANAGEMENT

Ameloblastic fibrosarcomas are aggressive and will invade adjacent soft and hard tissues, including the base of the skull. Metastasis appears to be exceptional, and the case reported by Chomette et al[19] of pulmonary, followed by mediastinal, lymphatic and hepatic metastases appears to be the only documented example. This is in contrast to nonodontogenic fibrosarcomas of the head and neck, in which metastases may develop in approximately 25% (see Ch. 37). The presence of calcified dental tissues, implying origin from an ameloblastic fibro-odontoma or ameloblastic fibrodentinoma, probably does not affect the behavior. Wide radical excision seems to offer the most promising approach, as in many of the reported cases treated more conservatively there have been multiple recurrences, and sometimes death, from local spread of the tumor. Müller et al[11] found that, of 49 patients with ameloblastic fibrosarcoma with adequate follow-up, 20 died from their disease. Occasionally, such neoplasms are highly aggressive. A 17-year-old male reported on by Park et al[20] died from one such tumor within approximately 3 months of diagnosis, despite wide resection, adjuvant chemotherapy, and irradiation.

REFERENCES

1. Daley TD, Wysocki GP, Pringle GA 1994 Relative incidence of odontogenic tumors and jaw cysts in a Canadian population. Oral Surg Oral Med Oral Pathol 77: 276–280
2. Regezi JA, Kerr DA, Courtney RM 1978 Odontogenic tumors: analysis of 706 cases. J Oral Surg 36: 771–778
3. Günhan O, Erseven G, Ruacan S et al 1990 Odontogenic tumours: a series of 409 cases. Austr Dent J 35: 518–522
4. Trodahl JN 1972 Ameloblastic fibroma. A survey of cases from the Armed Forces Institute of Pathology. Oral Surg 33: 547–558
5. Slootweg PJ 1981 An analysis of the interrelationships of the mixed odontogenic tumors – ameloblastic fibroma, ameloblastic fibro-odontoma and the odontomas. Oral Surg 51: 266–276
6. Waldron CA, Thompson CW, Conner WA 1963 Granular cell ameloblastic fibroma. Oral Surg 16: 1202–1213
7. White DK, Sow-Yeh Chen BMD, Hartman KS et al 1978 Central granular-cell tumor of the jaws (the so-called granular-cell ameloblastic fibroma). A clinical and ultrastructural study. Oral Surg Oral Med Oral Pathol 45: 396–405
8. Becker J, Schuppan D, Philipsen HP, Reichart PA 1992 Ectomesenchyme of ameloblastic fibroma reveals a characteristic distribution of extracellular matrix proteins. J Oral Pathol Med 21: 156–159
9. Harrison WS, Sordill WC, Sciubba JJ, Liebers RM 1982 Ameloblastic fibroma: management of a patient with an extensive tumor. J Am Dent Assoc 104: 475–477
10. Sawyer DS, Nwoku AL, Mosadomi A 1982 Recurrent ameloblastic fibroma. Report of two cases. Oral Surg 53: 19–23
11. Müller S, Parker DC, Kapadia SB, Budnick SD, Barnes EL 1995 Ameloblastic fibrosarcoma of the jaws. A clinicopathologic and DNA analysis of five cases and review of the literature. Oral Surg Oral Med Oral Pathol 79: 469–477
12. Ulmansky M, Bodner L, Praetorius F, Lustman J 1994 Ameloblastic fibrodentinoma: report on two new cases. J Oral Maxillofac Surg 52: 980–884
13. Wood RM, Markle TL, Barker BF, Hiatt WR 1988 Ameloblastic fibrosarcoma. Oral Surg Oral Med Oral Pathol 66: 74–77
14. Chomette G, Aurio M, Guilbert F, Delcourt A 1983 Ameloblastic fibrosarcoma of the jaws – report of three cases. Pathol Res Pract 178: 40–44
15. Takeda Y, Kaneko R, Suzuki A 1984 Ameloblastic fibrosarcoma or ameloblastic fibrosarcoma. Virchows Arch I (Pathol Anat) 404: 253–357
16. Howell RM, Burkes EJ 1977 Malignant transformation of ameloblastic fibrodontoma to ameloblastic fibrosarcoma. Oral Surg Oral Med Oral Pathol 43: 391–401
17. Reichart PA, Zobl H 1978 Transformation of ameloblastic fibroma to fibrosarcoma – report of a case. Intl J Oral Surg 7: 503–507
18. Prein J, Remagen B, Speissl B, Schafroth U 1979 Ameloblastic fibroma and its sarcomatous transformation. Pathol Res Pract 166: 123–127
19. Chomette G, Aurio M, Guilbert F, Delcourt A 1983 Ameloblastic fibrosarcoma of the jaws – report of three cases. Pathol Res Pract 178: 40–44
20. Park HR, Shin KB, Sol MY, Suh KS, Lee SK 1995 A highly malignant ameloblastic fibrosarcoma. Report of a case. Oral Surg Oral Med Oral Pathol Oral Radiol Endod 79: 478–481

Odontogenic fibroma **10**

Odontogenic fibroma

The odontogenic origin of this rare endosteal tumor is confirmed by its formation only in the jaws and often by the presence of epithelial rests, sometimes in great numbers. However, rests are not always found.

INCIDENCE

Regezi et al[1] found no odontogenic fibromas among the 706 odontogenic tumors that they surveyed, but Daley et al[2] found them to form nearly 5% of 445 odontogenic tumors. In Turkey, Günhan et al[3] found odontogenic fibromas to comprise 4.5% of 403 odontogenic tumors. Among Hong Kong Chinese, Wu & Chan[4] found odontogenic fibromas to form 3.7% of their 82 odontogenic tumors.

Günhan et al[3] reported that, of their 18 cases, the mean patient age was 23.4 years (range 15–51 years); eight cases appeared in females and 10 in males. In this series, the majority (13 of 18) of cases were in the mandible, and particularly in the posterior region.

Handlers et al[5] found from an analysis of 39 cases that the mean patient age was 39.3 years and there was a female preponderance of 7.4 : 1. In contrast to earlier series, the tumor was slightly more frequently located in the maxilla (22 of 39 cases), and 21 of these 22 tumors were located anterior to the first molar. Most of the tumors were related to the roots of teeth.

CLINICAL FEATURES

Odontogenic fibroma forms a slow-growing, asymptomatic mass and usually remains unrecognized until a swelling becomes noticeable. Mobility of teeth may also become apparent. Alternatively, an odontogenic fibroma may be seen by chance on a radiograph

RADIOGRAPHY

Radiographically, odontogenic fibroma typically appears as a sharply defined, rounded area of lucency in a tooth-bearing area. Handlers et al[5] found that extensive root resorption was common and seen in 11 of 39 cases. Divergence of roots was occasionally seen. They also found that small lesions were usually unilocular (Fig. 10.1) while larger ones tended to show scalloping of the margins or multiloculation. All had sclerotic margins. Occasionally, there is patchy radio-opacity, which may rarely give a ground-glass appearance (Fig. 10.2).

MICROSCOPY

Gardner (1980)[6] suggested that odontogenic fibromas should be separated into a *simple* type, which resembles a dental follicle, and a *complex* type, as described in the 1971 World Health Organization (WHO) classification,[7] which typically contains more abundant epithelium and foci of dentinoid or cementum-like material.

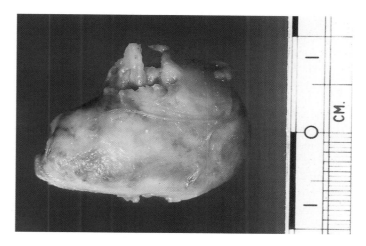

Fig. 10.1 Odontogenic fibroma. The gross specimen shows the smooth circumscribed outline of the tumor. The irregularity in the upper surface fitted the roots of the tooth to which it was related.

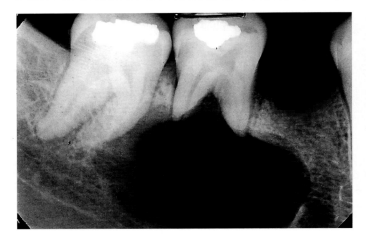

Fig. 10.2 Odontogenic fibroma. The area of radiolucency is rounded and well circumscribed. There is some resorption of the roots of the related tooth.

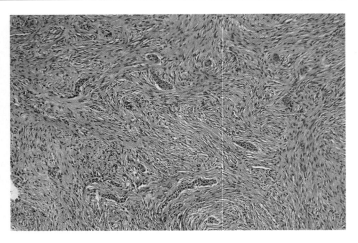

Fig. 10.4 Odontogenic fibroma. Serpentine strands and islands of inactive odontogenic epithelium surrounded by fibrous tissue with a fascicular configuration.

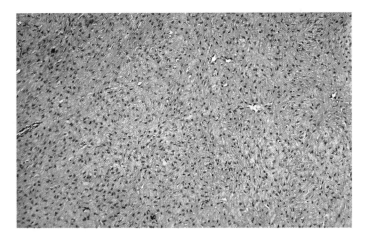

Fig. 10.3 Odontogenic fibroma, 'simple' type. This variant lacks odontogenic epithelium.

The simple type of odontogenic fibroma consists of relatively delicate fibrous tissue sometimes with a considerable amount of ground substance. Rests of odontogenic epithelium scattered throughout the fibrous mass may be lacking, but there may also be small calcifications (Fig. 10.3).

The complex type of odontogenic fibroma consists of relatively cellular mature fibrous tissue. The fibroblasts are spindle-shaped with variable amounts of collagen and are often arranged in distinct fascicles or interlacing bundles, which may have a whorled arrangement. Odontogenic epithelium is dispersed throughout as islands or strands (Fig. 10.4). It may be scanty or present in such large amounts as to be the most conspicuous feature. The epithelial cells are round or cuboidal with bland nuclei, and occasionally show vacuolation of the cytoplasm. Handlers et al[5] noted that, in one case, melanin pigmentation was seen within the epithelium. The mass is clearly circumscribed and encapsulation may be evident (Fig. 10.4). Cementum-like deposits of calcified material, often described as dentinoid, or (rarely) scanty trabeculae of woven bone are also seen.

Vincent et al[8] appear to have been the first to recognize a granular-cell variant of central odontogenic fibroma. Shiro et al[9] have described another variant in which there were sheets of cells with prominent cell membranes and containing eosinophilic granules. They found that, unlike the cells of a granular cell tumor, the granular cells of the odontogenic fibroma variant failed to stain for S-100 protein. Shiro et al[9] also identified from the literature 14 other cases, most of which had originally been categorized under other names, such as granular cell ameloblastoma.

Allen et al[10] have reported three cases of an otherwise typical odontogenic fibroma containing odontogenic epithelium, which also contained tissue with the appearances of a central giant cell granuloma (see Ch. 18). Where it was possible to see a junction between these two types of tissue, there was only a slight degree of intermingling. One tumor that recurred after curettage also showed both histologic components. It was not clear whether the giant cell tissue was reactive or the tumors represented combined lesions.

DIFFERENTIAL DIAGNOSIS

The main tumors from which a central odontogenic fibroma needs to be differentiated are the myxofibroma and the desmoplastic fibroma, both of which are more aggressively infiltrative and readily recur after limited excision. Radiographically, both are most frequently multilocular with a honeycomb or trabeculated appearance; less frequently, they are unilocular and the diffuse, infiltrative margins of desmoplastic fibroma may be seen. Myxofibromas have a poorly cellular myxoid stroma and usually lack any epithelial component. Desmoplastic fibroma (see Ch. 36) typically consists of fibrous tissue with abundant collagen or of highly cellular tissue consisting of tumor-like fibroblasts alone. The collagen fibers in the more fibrous specimens tend to form short bundles that lack the streaming patterns and are less well-defined than those of fibrosarcomas. However, tumor-like infiltration of surrounding tissues and envelopment of nerve and muscle fibers are characteristic features. No epithelial rests are present.

Hyperplastic dental follicles have sometimes been mistaken for odontogenic fibromas, as noted by Kim & Ellis[11] who found that, of 847 dental follicles or papilla referred to the Armed Forces Institute of Pathology, nearly 27 had been misdiagnosed as odontogenic tumors or cysts.

Dental follicles should readily be distinguishable by their envelopment of an unerupted tooth, usually a third molar, and a radiographic appearance resembling an embryonic dentigerous cyst. Histologically, dental follicles consist of sinuous fibrous connective tissue fibers and vary from being densely fibrous to myxomatous in appearance. An epithelial lining of variable character is present in 54% of cases. In most specimens small epithelial rests are present and around them the connective tissue may be hyalinized. Small foci of calcification are sometimes also seen.

BEHAVIOR AND MANAGEMENT

The odontogenic fibroma is benign and does not infiltrate the surrounding bone, which merely undergoes pressure resorption. From their review of 39 of these tumors, Heimdal et al[12] noted one that recurred 4 years after enucleation, but this had to be repeated 5 years later. By contrast, Dunlap & Barker[13] reported two cases with no evidence of recurrence at 9 and 10 years, respectively, after curettage. Prolonged follow-up information is scanty, but Handlers et al[5] concluded that the spectrum of histological patterns which they summarized appeared to have no correlation with clinical behavior. Only four of their own 19 cases reported by Handlers et al[5] had follow-up information. None of these showed any evidence of recurrence after curettage within periods of 3 months to 3 years. The histologic distinction between simple and complex types of odontogenic fibroma is also not accepted by the 1992 WHO classification[14] as being of value in predicting behavior.

Odontogenic fibromas usually shell out from the bone and are treated by enucleation or curettage. Recurrence appears to be no more than an occasional possibility. The recurrence may not appear until several years later, and is likely to be manageable by a further curettage.

Peripheral odontogenic fibroma

Clinically, the peripheral odontogenic fibroma has frequently been mistaken for a fibrous epulis and can only be recognized histologically by its content of odontogenic epithelial rests.

INCIDENCE

Peripheral odontogenic fibroma is usually regarded as rare, and in their review of the English literature Daley & Wysocki[15] could find reports of only 73 acceptable cases. However, Daley et al[2] found that in a Canadian population it accounted for 8.93% of 392 odontogenic tumors, and was almost twice as common as the central type. Daley & Wysocki[15] were, therefore, able to report 36 new cases. Earlier, Slabbert & Altini[16] had reviewed 30 cases, of which 93% were in blacks.

Daley & Wysocki[15] found that the peak incidence of peripheral odontogenic fibroma was between the ages of 20 and 29 years. Of 107 cases where the gender was stated, 48 were in males and 59 in females.

CLINICAL FEATURES

The peripheral odontogenic fibroma is clinically indistinguishable from the common fibrous epulis in that it forms a firm sessile or pedunculated mass on the attached gingiva, particularly of the anterior teeth. It is pink in color, unless traumatized.

MICROSCOPY

The appearances are variable. The fibrous tissue can be predominantly collagenous, highly cellular, or myxoid (Fig. 10.5). The epithelial content usually consists of small discrete strands or rests surrounded by a hyaline cuff, and sometimes includes clear cells (Figs 10.6 and 10.7). Calcifications may be present. Occasionally, epithelium is abundant, forming large follicles with palisading, as described by Slabbert & Altini[16] from a study of 30 cases. Granular cell and squamous cell variants were also reviewed by Daley & Wysocki.[15]

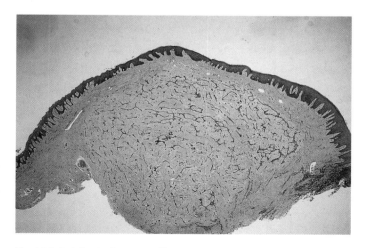

Fig. 10.5 Peripheral odontogenic fibroma. Low-power view shows amorphous calcifications in a fibrous stroma with an epithelial covering.

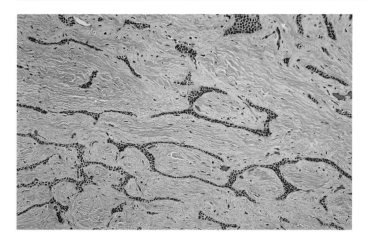

Fig. 10.6 Peripheral odontogenic fibroma. Higher power view of the same lesion as in Figure 10.5 shows fine strands of inactive odontogenic epithelium in a cellular fibrous stroma.

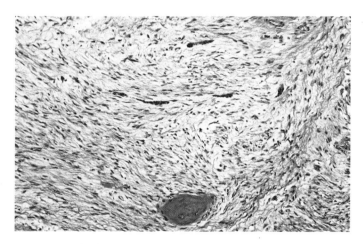

Fig. 10.7 Peripheral odontogenic fibroma. Only minute strands of odontogenic epithelium are surrounded by finely fibrillar fibrous tissue.

BEHAVIOR AND MANAGEMENT

The growth potential of peripheral odontogenic fibroma is thought to be limited, and excision is the treatment of choice. However, Daley & Wysocki[15] estimated that the recurrence rate might be as high as 39%. In some cases this was due to incomplete excision but others recurred as long as 4 years later.

REFERENCES

1. Regezi JA, Kerr DA, Courtney RM 1978 Odontogenic tumors: analysis of 706 cases. J Oral Surg 36: 771–778
2. Daley TD, Wysocki GP, Pringle GA 1994 Relative incidence of odontogenic tumors and jaw cysts in a Canadian population. Oral Surg Oral Med Oral Pathol 77: 276–280
3. Günhan O, Erseven G, Ruacan S et al 1990 Odontogenic tumours: a series of 409 cases. Austr Dent J 35: 518–522
4. Wu PC, Chan KW 1985 A survey of tumours of the jawbones in Hong Kong Chinese: 1963–1982. Br J Oral Maxillofac Surg 23: 92–102
5. Handlers JP, Abrams AM, Melrose RJ, Danforth R 1991 Central odontogenic fibroma: clinicopathologic features of 19 cases and review of the literature. J Oral Maxillofac Surg 49: 46–54
6. Gardner D 1980 The central odontogenic fibroma: an attempt at clarification. Oral Surg 50: 425–431
7. Pindborg JJ, Kramer IRH, Torloni H 1971 Histological typing of odontogenic tumors, jaw cysts and allied lesions. International classification of tumors, No. 5. World Health Organization, Geneva
8. Vincent SD, Hammond HL, Ellis GL, Juhlin JP 1987 Central granular cell odontogenic fibroma. Oral Surg Oral Med Oral Pathol 63: 715–721
9. Shiro BC, Jacoway JR, Mirmiran A, McGuirt WF, Siegal GP 1989 Central odontogenic fibroma, granular cell variant. Oral Surg Oral Med Oral Pathol 67: 725–730
10. Allen CM, Hammond HL, Stimson PG 1992 Central odontogenic fibroma, WHO* type. A report of three cases with an unusual associated giant cell reaction. Oral Surg Oral Med Oral Pathol 73: 62–66
11. Kim J, Ellis GL 1993 Dental follicular tissue: misinterpretation as odontogenic tumors. J Oral Maxillofac Surg 51: 762–767
12. Heimdal A, Isaacson G, Nilsson L 1980 Recurrent central odontogenic fibroma. Oral Surg Oral Med Oral Pathol 50: 140–144
13. Dunlap CL, Barker BF 1984 Central odontogenic fibroma of the WHO type. Oral Surg Oral Med Oral Pathol 57: 390–394
14. Pindborg JJ, Kramer IRH, Shear M 1992 Histological typing of odontogenic tumours, 2nd edn. World Health Organization/Springer-Verlag, Berlin
15. Daley TD, Wysocki GP 1994 Peripheral odontogenic fibroma. Oral Surg Oral Med Oral Pathol 78: 329–336
16. Slabbert H de V, Altini M 1991 Peripheral odontogenic fibroma: a clinicopathologic study. Oral Surg Oral Med Oral Pathol 72: 86–90

Odontogenic myxoma 11

Odontogenic myxoma, as its name implies, is peculiar to the jaws. Enzinger & Weiss[1] suggest that myxoid tumors elsewhere in the body arise from modified fibroblasts that produce excessive amounts of glycosaminoglycans, which in turn may inhibit polymerization of collagen. Myxomas of the jaws, by contrast, show a close structural resemblance to dental mesenchyme, occasionally contain epithelial rests, affect the tooth-bearing areas of the jaws, and a tooth is frequently absent.

INCIDENCE

Regezi et al[2] found myxomas to comprise 3% of 706 odontogenic tumors. Daley et al[3] found them to form 5.1% of 445 odontogenic tumors. In Turkey, Günhan et al[4] found myxomas to comprise 12.5% of 403 odontogenic tumors, but among Hong Kong Chinese Wu & Chan[5] found only 1% of their 82 odontogenic tumors to be myxomas.

With such small numbers in most series it is difficult to gain any reliable idea of the age, gender, and site distribution of odontogenic myxomas. Of the 51 examples reported by Günhan et al,[4] 38 (75%) were in females. The mean age of those affected was 32.3 years and the age range was 6–65 years. The 20 myxomas analyzed by Regezi et al[2] did not show a significantly different age distribution (mean 28 years, range 10–50 years). However, there was a considerably stronger female preponderance, with 19 (95%) of the 20 cases being in females. By contrast, only 66% of 21 odontogenic myxomas reported by Peltola et al[6] from Finland were in women. In Argentina, Keszler et al[7] found that myxomas were apparently more frequent there in children than in other reports. Of 80 myxomas, 12.5% were in children aged under 16 years, and 30% of these were in children below the age of 10 years.

There thus appear to be appreciable differences, particularly in the gender distribution of odontogenic myxomas, in different countries, but the relatively small numbers of these tumors in most series prevent confirmation of any definite racial trend.

In the series reported by Günhan et al,[4] 65% of 51 myxomas were in the maxilla, but there appeared to be no particular predilection for the anterior or posterior parts of the jaw. In the case of the 20 myxomas analyzed by Regezi et al,[2] the maxilla and mandible were equally frequently affected.

CLINICAL FEATURES

From the various series already described, it is clear that odontogenic myxomas predominantly affect females at a mean age of 28–30 years, but the possible age range is wide. A slow-growing, painless fusiform swelling of the jaw is the typical presentation. Harder,[8] in an analysis of the clinical findings in 15 cases, confirmed that loosening, displacement, or resorption of teeth are occasionally seen, but pain is rare.

RADIOGRAPHY

Radiographically, the appearances vary. Typically, there is a radiolucent area with scalloped margins or a soap-bubble appearance, which may be similar to that of an ameloblastoma (Fig. 11.1). However, Peltola et al[6] found that the radiolucent areas were as frequently unilocular as multilocular, and that the latter were more frequently in the posterior parts of the jaws. Intralesional trabeculation was seen in all the multilocular tumors but in only three of the unilocular ones.

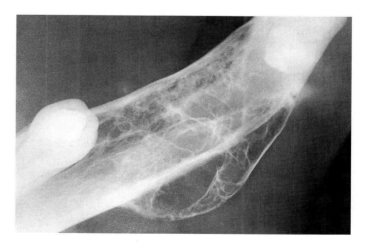

Fig. 11.1 Odontogenic myxoma. There is expansion of the mandible and a soap-bubble appearance.

MICROSCOPY

The cells are scantily distributed in loose mucoid intercellular material (Fig. 11.2), and are spindle-shaped or angular with long, fine, anastomosing processes (Fig. 11.3). Small amounts of collagen fibers may also be formed and there may be small, scattered epithelial rests. The tumor margins are ill-defined, and peripheral bone is progressively invaded and resorbed.

Occasional variations on these appearances are mainly due to formation of greater amounts of collagen, when the lesion may be termed a fibromyxoma (Fig. 11.4).

Harrison[9] and Handler et al,[10] among others, have carried out ultrastructural studies and concluded that the main tumor cells are fibroblast-like but not typical fibroblasts and that they show morphological variation. The epithelial inclusions were surrounded by a basement membrane and a clear zone. Well-developed cytoplasmic organelles suggested that they were metabolically active. Handler et al[10] confirmed the belief expressed by Harrison[9] that

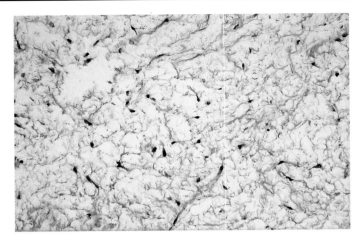

Fig. 11.3 Odontogenic myxoma. Higher power view showing typical loose myxomatous stroma with slender processes extending from the mesenchymal cells.

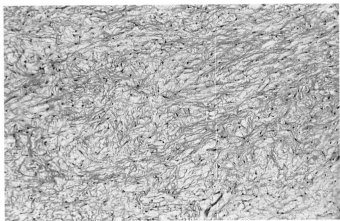

Fig. 11.4 Odontogenic fibromyxoma. The fibrous component is more prominent in this tumor.

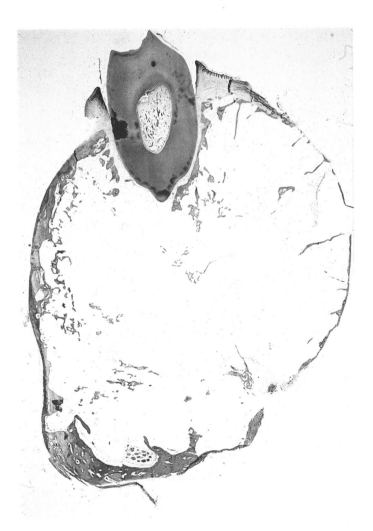

Fig. 11.2 Odontogenic myxoma. Low-power view of a section of the mandible with only a thin rim of bone surrounding the tumor. The inferior dental nerve has been displaced to the inferior border of the jaw.

the epithelial inclusions vary morphologically from a resemblance to rests of Malassez to widely separated cells resembling stellate reticulum.

Lombardi et al[11] demonstrated that the spindle cells of two odontogenic myxomas were keratin, nonspecific enolase, glial-specific protein, neurofilament, and factor- VIII-related antigen negative, but were strongly positive for S-100 protein. By contrast, Moshiri et al[12] reported the spindle-shaped cells to be vimentin and actin positive but S-100 negative; their ultrastructural studies also suggested that myxoma cells were myofibroblasts.

BEHAVIOR AND MANAGEMENT

Myxomas are benign, but can infiltrate widely. Recurrence after excision is common even after vigorous and repeated treatment, and residual tumor can persist in the jaws for many years. In spite of aggressive treatment, some tumors have been shown to persist for more than 30 years[13] after the original surgery. By this time the tumor may appear to be inactive and be symptomless.

Wide excision should be carried out in the hope of preventing recurrence, but this is not always successful. In the case of larger tumors, en bloc resection and reconstruction is probably advisable. Irradiation and other methods used to destroy residual tumor tissue have not proved to be of significant value.

Rare variants with a more cellular and pleomorphic microscopic picture can behave aggressively and may be categorized as myxo-sarcomas. However, though locally destructive, myxosarcomas appear to have little potential for metastasis.

REFERENCES

1. Enzinger FM, Weiss SW 1995 Soft tissue tumors, 3rd edn. CV Mosby, St Louis
2. Regezi JA, Kerr DA, Courtney RM 1978 Odontogenic tumors: analysis of 706 cases. J Oral Surg 36: 771–778
3. Daley TD, Wysocki GP, Pringle GA 1994 Relative incidence of odontogenic tumors and jaw cysts in a Canadian population. Oral Surg Oral Med Oral Pathol 77: 276–280
4. Günhan O, Erseven G, Ruacan S et al 1990 Odontogenic tumours: a series of 409 cases. Austr Dent J 35: 518–522
5. Wu PC, Chan KW 1985 A survey of tumours of the jawbones in Hong Kong Chinese: 1963–1982. Br J Oral Maxillofac Surg 23: 92–102
6. Peltola J, Magnusson B, Hopponen R-P, Borrman H 1994 Odontogenic myxoma – a radiographic study of 21 tumours. Br J Oral Maxillofac Surg 32: 298–301
7. Keszler A, Dominguez FV, Giannunzio G 1995 Myxoma in childhood: an analysis of 10 cases. J Oral Maxillofac Surg 53: 518–521
8. Harder F 1978 Myxomas of the jaws. Int J Oral Surg 7: 148–155
9. Harrison JD 1973 Odontogenic myxoma: ultrastructural and histochemical studies. J Clin Pathol 26: 570–582
10. Handler BH, Abaza NA, Quinn P 1979 Odontogenic myxoma. Surgical management and an ultrastructural study. Oral Surg 47: 203–217
11. Lombardi T, Kuffer R, Bernard J-P, Fiore-Donno G, Samson J 1988 Immunohistochemical staining for vimentin filaments and S-100 protein in myxoma of the jaws. J Oral Pathol 17: 175–177
12. Moshiri S, Oda D, Worthington P, Myall R 1992 Odontogenic myxoma: histochemical and ultrastructural study. J Oral Pathol Med 21: 401–403
13. Cawson RA 1972 Myxoma of the mandible with a 35 year follow-up. Br J Oral Surg 10: 59–63

Cementoblastoma

Cementoblastoma is a benign neoplasm that forms a mass of cementum-like tissue. It resorbs and becomes fused to the root of a tooth. Ulmansky et al[1] credit Norberg with first recognizing this tumor in 1930,[2] but Bouquot & Lense[3] give the credit to Rodriguez,[4] who in 1839 called it an exostosis. Though this tumor is sometimes termed *benign cementoblastoma*, there is no malignant counterpart.

INCIDENCE

Regezi et al[5] found cementoblastomas to represent fewer than 1% of their series of 706 odontogenic tumors, as did Daley et al[6] in Canada in their analysis of 392 odontogenic tumors. By contrast, Günhan et al,[7] in Turkey, found them to account for nearly 5.7% of their 403 odontogenic tumors. To what extent such differences represent racial variation or, as Günhan et al[7] suggest, diversity of histological criteria, is uncertain.

Jelic et al[8] analyzed the clinical findings in 15 cases. There was a virtually equal gender distribution: 66% of patients were aged between 15 and 30 years and only one was over 45 years old. In 14 cases where information was available, 12 were in the right mandibular molar or premolar region and only two were in the left molar region. The tumor was attached to the root of a molar tooth in 78% and to a premolar root in 14%.

In their analysis of 71 cases, Ulmansky et al[1] found that 49% of patients were below the age of 20 and 74% were below the age of 30 years. Females were slightly more frequently affected than men. In 78% of cases the tumor was in the mandible, with 90% of tumors occurring in the first molar or premolar region.

Though histologically similar, osteoblastoma has been regarded by some to be a separate entity, McLeod et al[9] have noted, in large series, that a disproportionately high number of osteoblastomas have arisen in the jaws.

CLINICAL FEATURES

The jaw is frequently expanded, and occasionally a cementoblastoma can cause gross bony swelling. Unlike most other odontogenic tumors, pain is a frequent complaint. It was recorded in 10 of the 15 cases studied by Jelic et al[8] and in 61% of the cases analyzed by Ulmansky et al.[1]

RADIOGRAPHY

Cementoblastomas give rise to a mass attached to the roots of a tooth. The mass is usually densely radio-opaque but may appear mottled, and has a thin but well-defined radiolucent rim. It is typically rounded, but may be more irregular, and at the periphery radiating trabecular of calcified tissue may be seen (Fig. 12.1). Resorption of the roots to which the mass is attached is common, but the tooth remains vital.

MICROSCOPY

The tumor resorbs and fuses to the root of a tooth and may even extend into the root canal (Fig. 12.2). Adjacent roots may also be resorbed without the tumor becoming fused to them.

At low power the mass may show radiating trabeculae of calcified tissue (Fig. 12.3). The cementum-like tissue typically contains many reversal lines, and has a pagetoid appearance (Fig. 12.4). Cells are enclosed within the hard tissue like osteocytes in bone,

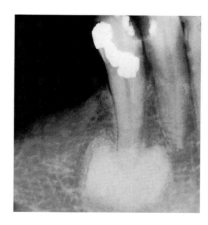

Fig. 12.1 Cementoblastoma. The rounded densely opaque mass is the attached to the apex of a tooth, and its radiolucent border can be seen in some areas.

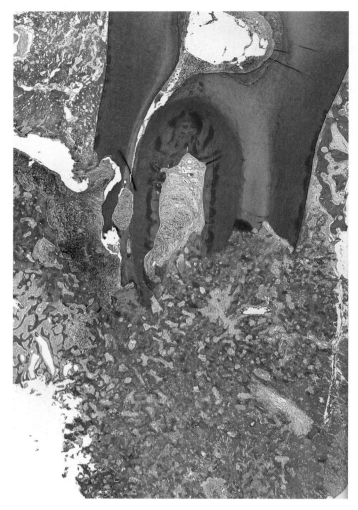

Fig. 12.2 Cementoblastoma. Low-power view shows a mass of irregular calcified tissue attached to the root of a tooth that has undergone extensive resorption.

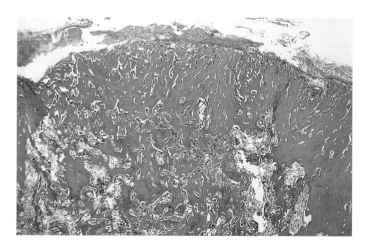

Fig. 12.3 Cementoblastoma. Low-power view shows a mass of irregular calcified tissue with a suggestion of a radial configuration at the periphery and traces of a fibrous capsule.

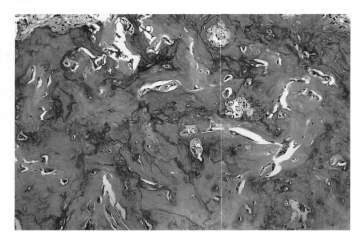

Fig. 12.4 Cementoblastoma. A densely calcified area showing a pagetoid pattern of reversal lines and cementocytes in lacunae.

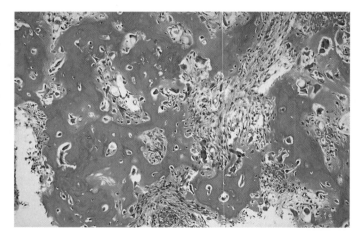

Fig. 12.5 Cementoblastoma. Higher power view of irregular deposits of cementum showing faint reversal lines, with an abundance of cementoblasts and cementoclasts giving it an osteoblastoma-like appearance.

while in the larger irregular spaces between the radiating trabeculae of calcified tissue, and particularly around the periphery, are many cementoblasts and cementoclasts (Fig. 12.5). These cells are sometimes plump, hyperchromatic, and pleomorphic. At the periphery and in areas of active growth there is a broad zone of unmineralized tissue and the mass has a fibrous capsule. The stroma is loose and vascular. Slootweg[10] has confirmed that the histological features of osteoblastomas and cementoblastomas are indistinguishable apart from the attachment of the cementoblastoma to the root of a tooth.

Initially a cementoblastoma may have an osteolytic phase followed by cementoblastic activity, but rarely, as reported by Eversole et al,[11] it may reach a large size before calcifying.

HISTOGENESIS

The relationship of the cementoblastoma to a root of a tooth and its cementoblast-like cells indicate that it arises from the perio-dontal membrane. However, the predilection of cementobla-stomas for the first molar or adjacent premolar region of the mandible is puzzling.

DIFFERENTIAL DIAGNOSIS

If not recognized by clinical and other features, the highly active cellular appearance, and pleomorphism of the cells, particularly at the periphery, a cementoblastoma may be mistaken for an osteosarcoma. However, cementoblastoma cells, though not readily distinguishable from osteoblasts and osteoclasts, do not show mitotic activity.

Though Slootweg[10] considered that a tumor should be cate-gorized as an osteoblastoma rather than a cementoblastoma even if related to, but not fused to, the root of a tooth. However, this seems an academic point as failure to detect fusion to a tooth root may not be evident until after operation, and management is therefore unaffected.

Focal sclerosing osteitis also affects patients below the age of 20 years and has the same site predilection as cementoblastoma. Unlike a cementoblastoma, the pulp of the tooth giving rise to sclerosing osteitis is inflamed or nonvital.

BEHAVIOR AND MANAGEMENT

Though Ulmansky et al[1] state that active growth of a cemento-blastoma is ultimately followed by a mature inactive state, it seems likely from the size of some reported tumors that cementoblastomas have continued growth potential. However, they are benign and, if the related tooth is extracted and the mass completely enucleated, recurrence is highly unlikely. If incompletely removed the mass will continue to grow. An aggressive variant, described for example by Langdon,[12] was painful, rapidly growing, and had cellular fea-tures suggestive of an osteosarcoma. However, it was readily enucleated and did not recur within the period of follow-up.

REFERENCES

1. Ulmansky M, Hjorting-Hansen E, Praetorius F, Haque MF 1994 Benign cementoblastoma. A review and five new cases. Oral Surg Oral Med Oral Pathol 77: 48–55
2. Norberg O 1930 Zur Kenntnis der dysontogenistischen Geschwulste der Kieferknochen. Z Zahnh 46: 321–355
3. Bouquot JE, Lense EC 1994 The beginning of oral pathology. Part I: First dental journal reports of odontogenic tumors and cysts, 1839–1860. Oral Surg Oral Med Oral Pathol 78: 343–350
4. Rodriguez BA 1839 Case of exostosis of the upper jaw. Am J Dent Sci 1: 88–89
5. Regezi JA, Kerr DA, Courtney RM 1978 Odontogenic tumors: analysis of 706 cases. J Oral Surg 36: 771–778
6. Daley TD, Wysocki GP, Pringle GA 1994 Relative incidence of odontogenic tumors and jaw cysts in a Canadian population. Oral Surg Oral Med Oral Pathol 77: 276–280
7. Günhan O, Erseven G, Ruacan S et al 1990 Odontogenic tumours: a series of 409 cases. Austr Dent J 35: 518–522
8. Jelic JS, Loftus MJ, Miller AS, Cleveland DB 1993 Benign cementoblastoma: report of an unusual case and analysis of 14 additional cases. J Oral Maxillofac Surg 51: 1033–1037
9. McLeod RA, Dahlin DC, Beabout JW 1976 The spectrum of osteoblastoma. Am J Roentgenol Radiat Ther Nucl Med 126: 321–335
10. Slootweg PJ 1992 Cementoblastoma and osteoblastoma: a comparison of histologic features. J Oral Pathol Med 21: 385–389
11. Eversole LR, Sabes WR, Dauchess VG 1973 Benign cementoblastoma. Oral Surg Oral Med Oral Pathol 36: 824–830
12. Langdon JD 1976 The benign cementoblastoma – just how benign? Br J Oral Surg 13: 239–249

Odontomas and related anomalies 13

Odontomas are hamartomas or malformations of dental tissues and not neoplasms. Like teeth, they do not develop further once fully calcified, but also like teeth may erupt into the mouth. Odontomas and mixed odontogenic tumors tend to form during the period of odontogenesis (up to the age of 20 years approximately). They may be discovered later but do not develop then.

INCIDENCE

Regezi et al,[1] in an analysis of 706 odontogenic tumors, found compound odontomas to account for 37% and complex odontomas to account for 30%. In Canada, Daley et al[2] found that compound and complex odontomas comprised 32.7% and 18.9%, respectively, of 392 odontogenic tumors.

In Turkey, Günhan et al[3] found that compound and complex odontomas each accounted for 9% of 403 benign odontogenic tumors. In Hong Kong Chinese, Wu & Chan[4] found both of them together to account for only 4% of 82 odontogenic jaw tumors.

Regezi et al[1] noted that 19% of odontomas were recognized before the age of 10 years and 51% between the ages of 10 and 20 years. Thereafter the frequency of finding odontomas rapidly declined, although an occasional example was found in the eighth decade. Males and females were approximately equally frequently affected.

Kaugars et al[5] have carried out a detailed analysis of the demography, site distribution, and other features of 351 odontomas, and have reviewed earlier surveys. Of the odontomas reviewed, 11.6% were recognized before the age of 10 years, 53.6% between the ages of 10 and 19 years, 19.6% between the ages of 20 and 29 years, and with decreasing frequency thereafter. The median age of those affected was 16 years. Females accounted for 51.5% of cases and males 48.5% Thirty-one per cent of odontomas were in blacks, although these accounted for only 15% of the biopsy material.

In the series reported by Regezi et al,[1] 59% of 396 odontomas were in the maxilla and 41% in the mandible. The single most common site (45% of cases) was the anterior maxilla, while 20% were found in the anterior mandible.

Of the 351 odontomas analyzed by Kaugars et al,[5] the maxilla was affected in 51% and the mandible in 49%. In the maxilla, 33.9% of odontomas were found in the anterior region and 7% in the premolar and 10% in the molar regions. In the mandible, 24.5% of odontomas were found in the anterior region and 12.7% in the premolar and 11.8% in the molar regions.

In this same series an association with an unerupted tooth was mentioned in 47.6%, and 27.6% of odontomas were found to be associated with dentigerous cysts. There were only two patients with multiple odontomas.

Odontomas are more frequently encountered in patients with Gardner's syndrome of intestinal polyposis, as noted by Korzcak[6] who reviewed its management. Other features of the syndrome are osteomas of the jaws, epidermoid cysts, desmoid tumors, and unerupted teeth or odontomas. It is the same entity as familial polyposis coli, and has the same high mortality from malignant change in the polyps.

CLINICAL FEATURES

Odontomas form hard masses that are usually painless. They may be detected by chance on a routine radiograph, or when they are large enough to cause a swelling of the jaw.

Odontomas tend to erupt, but once exposed to the saliva can become carious. Abscess formation can follow. Odontomas may also prevent normal teeth from erupting, or displace them. Cyst formation is another occasional complication. In the analysis carried out by Kaugars et al,[5] 15% of patients complained of pain, divergence of teeth, or suppuration.

RADIOGRAPHY

Odontomas are usually readily recognizable because of their dense opacity, particularly that of the areas of enamel. Also, like teeth, they develop within a dental follicle, which appears as a thin radiolucent rim. The irregular shape of a complex odontoma or the multiple denticles of a compound odontoma may also be distinguishable on a radiograph (Fig. 13.1). Should the mass become infected, the calcified tissues may be mistaken for a sequestrum or an area of sclerotic bone.

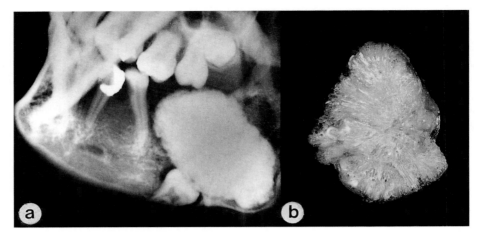

Fig. 13.1 a The well-circumscribed area of dense radio-opacity is typical of a complex odontoma. **b** The cut surface of the gross specimen shows the radial pattern.

BEHAVIOR AND MANAGEMENT

As already mentioned, odontomas have a strictly limited growth potential. The mass should be enucleated surgically as a potential source of obstruction to erupting teeth or as a possible focus for infection. Once erupted, a complex odontoma is particularly likely to become infected because of its many stagnation areas, which allow bacteria to proliferate undisturbed. Once dental caries has become established, infection can progress to kill the pulpal tissue and extend through the apex or apices to cause abscess formation.

As discussed below, odontogenic cells can very occasionally give rise to both an ameloblastoma and a composite odontoma (odontoameloblastoma). The behavior of this composite tumor is likely to be that of the ameloblastomatous component.

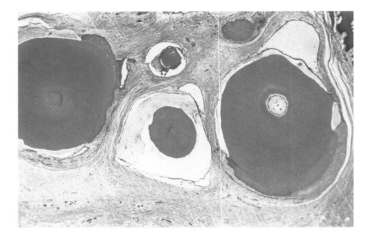

Fig. 13.2 Compound odontoma. Cross-section of multiple small tooth-like structures in a fibrous stroma.

Compound odontoma

Compound odontomas consist of many separate, small denticles. The malformation may be produced by repeated divisions of a tooth germ or by overgrowth of, and multiple budding-off from, the dental lamina, with the formation of many tooth germs (Fig. 13.2).

HISTOGENESIS

Histologically, the denticles have the structure of normal teeth, but are small and of simpler gross morphology. The denticles are embedded in fibrous connective tissue, and have a fibrous follicle (Fig. 13.3). Inflammatory or cystic changes may involve the mass.

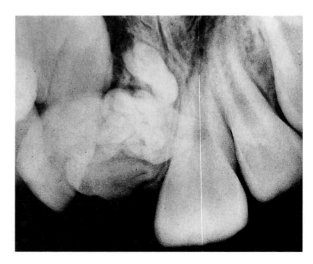

Fig. 13.3 Compound odontoma. The radiograph shows numerous small denticles.

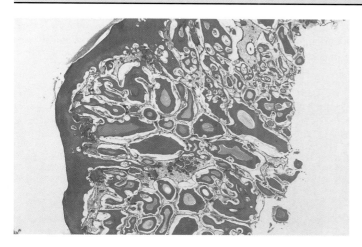

Fig. 13.4 Complex odontoma. There is totally irregular arrangement of dental tissues.

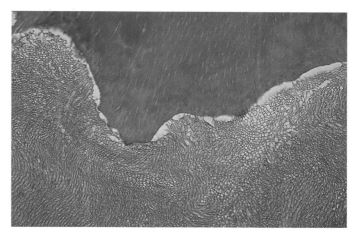

Fig. 13.6 Odontoma. Higher power view of tubular dentine and enamel matrix retaining the prismatic structure.

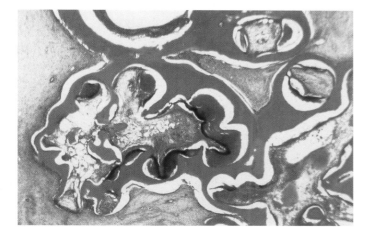

Fig. 13.5 Complex odontoma. At higher power, enamel matrix covering dentine, and pulp tissue within the dentine can be seen.

Complex odontoma

A complex odontoma consists of an irregular mass of hard and soft dental tissues, having no morphological resemblance to a tooth and frequently forming a cauliflower-like mass of hard dental tissues (Fig. 13.4).

Even when the morphology is thus grossly distorted, the pulp, dentine, enamel, and cementum form in appropriate anatomical relationship with one another and the mass is surrounded by a fibrous follicle (Fig. 13.5).

HISTOGENESIS

Histologically, the mass consists of enamel, dentine, and cementum, together with pulp and periodontal membrane in varying amounts. In decalcified specimens, any enamel matrix appears as hema-

toxyphilic fibrillar material due to persistence of prism sheaths, while the dentine matrix is eosinophilic and contains tubules (Fig. 13.6). The arrangement of these tissues is disordered, but frequently has a radial pattern. The pulp is usually finely branched so that the mass is perforated by small vascular channels like a sponge. If seen before calcification starts, the mass may be mistaken for one of the several types of odontogenic tumor.

Sedano & Pindborg[7] have shown that 20% of complex odontomas have foci of ghost cell keratinization. However, this does not affect their behavior.

Other types of odontoma

In the past, complex classifications have been devised to include such anomalies as dilated, gestant (invaginated), and geminated odontomas. Part of these malformations is obviously tooth-like, and they are currently regarded as malformed teeth. Dilated and gestant malformations arise by invagination of cells of the enamel organ or of the epithelial sheath of Hertwig, which actively proliferate to expand the developing tooth, or extend through the opposite pole. Gestant malformations range in severity from a singular pit in an otherwise normal upper lateral incisor to the so-called *dens in dente* or *dens invaginatus*.

These malformations must be removed as potential obstructions to the eruption of other teeth, as a focus for infection, or for cosmetic resions.

Enamel pearls ('enameloma')

Enamel pearls are uncommon, minor abnormalities, which are

formed on otherwise normal teeth by displaced ameloblasts or by proliferation of these cells beyond the normal limit of the amelocemental junction.

The pearl may consist only of a nodule of enamel attached to the dentine, or may have a core of dentine which sometimes contains a horn of pulp. Enamel pearls are usually rounded, a few millimeters in diameter, and often form near the bifurcation of first molar roots. An enamel pearl can cause a stagnation area at the gingival margin, but its removal may expose the pulp and necessitate extraction of the tooth.

'Dentinoma'

In the past, 'dentinomas' have been described, but it is now accepted that no anomaly consisting entirely of dentine exists. Dentine forms only under the influence of odontogenic epithelium, and cannot form in isolation.

REFERENCES

1. Regezi JA, Kerr DA, Courtney RM 1978 Odontogenic tumors: analysis of 706 cases. J Oral Surg 36: 771–778
2. Daley TD, Wysocki GP, Pringle GA 1994 Relative incidence of odontogenic tumors and jaw cysts in a Canadian population. Oral Surg Oral Med Oral Pathol 77: 276–280
3. Günhan O, Erseven G, Ruacan S et al 1990 Odontogenic tumours: a series of 409 cases. Austr Dent J 35: 518–522
4. Wu PC, Chan KW 1985 A survey of tumours of the jawbones in Hong Kong Chinese: 1963–1982. Br J Oral Maxillofac Surg 23: 92–102
5. Kaugars GE, Miller ME, Abbey LM 1989 Odontomas. Oral Surg Oral Med Oral Pathol 67: 172–176
6. Korzcak P 1990 The diagnostic significance and management of Gardner's syndrome. Br J Oral Maxillofac Surg 28: 80–84
7. Sedano HO, Pindborg JJ 1995 Ghost cell epithelium in odontomes. J Oral Pathol 4: 27–30

Fibro-osseous and giant cell lesions

Fibrous dysplasia 14

Waldron[1] classified fibro-osseous lesions essentially as follows:

I Fibrous dysplasia
   – Polyostotic
   – Monostotic
II Reactive (dysplastic) lesions in the tooth-bearing area, presumably of periodontal ligament origin
   – Periapical cemento-osseous dysplasia
   – Focal cemento-osseous dysplasia
   – Florid cemento-osseous dysplasia
III Fibro-osseous neoplasms
   – Cemento-ossifying fibroma.

This widely used classification encompasses a diverse group of lesions. It includes skeletal diseases such as fibrous dysplasia and others peculiar to the jaws such as cemento-osseous dysplasias. These diseases (apart from the neoplasm, *cemento-ossifying fibroma*) are probably developmental or reactive and lack a potential for progressive growth. Frequently the genetic disorder *cherubism* (see Ch. 17) is also included and, like the dysplasias, has limited growth potential.

Another common feature of most, but not all, fibro-osseous lesions is that they form bone or bone-like tissue in a benign connective tissue matrix. The 1992 World Health Organization classification[2] also includes simple (solitary) bone and aneurysmal bone cysts in this group (these are discussed in Chapter 25).

Nevertheless there are typically also considerable differences in the clinical and histologic features and behavior, so that the cemento-ossifying dysplasias and cemento-ossifying fibroma are discussed in the following chapters.

Fibrous dysplasia

Typical monostotic fibrous dysplasia is characterized by focal but poorly circumscribed fibro-osseous replacement of an area of bone. It forms a swelling that probably starts in childhood but usually undergoes arrest with maturation of the skeleton. The jaws, particularly the maxilla, are the most frequently affected sites in the head and neck region. Overall, these represent only 20–25% of cases overall, as the ribs and femur are considerably more frequently involved. Males and females are almost equally often affected.

Polyostotic fibrous dysplasia is more uncommon, but is histologically similar to monostotic disease. Several or many bones are involved. Females are affected more often, in a ratio of 3 : 1, and are likely to experience precocious puberty.

McCune–Albright's syndrome comprises polyostotic fibrous dysplasia, skin pigmentation, and sexual precocity. Lesions are typically unilateral or segmental.

The etiology of fibrous dysplasia is unknown. Unlike cherubism, there is no evidence of any genetic component.

CLINICAL FEATURES

Monostotic fibrous dysplasia is mainly seen in young adults at a mean age of about 25 years. Patients are occasionally seen as late as in their seventh decade and, as noted by Waldron & Giansanti,[3] may have been aware of the swellings for long periods, sometimes as long as 30 years. Polyostotic fibrous dysplasia is more frequent in childhood.

The lesion typically forms a painless, smoothly rounded swelling. Maxillary lesions frequently involve adjacent bones such as the zygoma or sphenoid. The mass may be large enough to cause disturbance of function in some sites. Displacement of teeth, for example, can cause malocclusion. Though the fibro-osseous mass weakens the bone, pathological fracture of the jaws is rare but relatively common in long bones.

Polyostotic fibrous dysplasia involves the head and neck region in up to 50% of cases. A jaw lesion may be the most conspicuous feature and the patient may appear initially to have monostotic disease. In a young girl particularly, a search for other skeletal lesions and pigmentation may be appropriate. Skin pigmentation consists of tan to brown macules, 1 cm or more across, with an irregular outline. Pigmentation frequently overlies affected bones, but has a predilection for the back of the neck, trunk, buttocks, or thighs. Though any skin area can be affected, pigmentation of the oral mucosa is very rare.

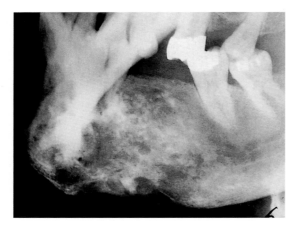

Fig. 14.1 Fibrous dysplasia. This example is heavily calcified but shows the lack of definable margins of the lesion.

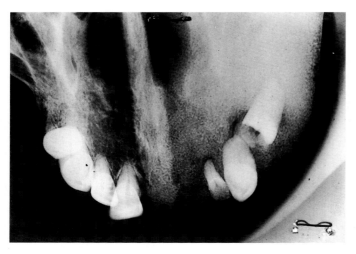

Fig. 14.2 Fibrous dysplasia. This occlusal radiograph shows the ground-glass appearance of some cases, as well as the lack of definable margins.

RADIOGRAPHY

The typical appearance is an area of lessened radiopacity, with a ground-glass or fine orange-peel texture. An important feature is that the lesion merges imperceptibly with surrounding normal bone (Figs 14.1 and 14.2). Maxillary lesions commonly extend into the antrum to obliterate its normal radiolucency. The outer surface may have an eggshell-thin cortex of expanded normal bone. However, a variety of appearances results from the degree of ossification. Predominantly fibrous lesions may mimic cysts or cystic tumors. More heavily ossified lesions may have a pagetoid pattern or a patchily sclerotic appearance.

Pierce et al[4] have reported an apparently unique example of fibrous dysplasia affecting two generations of a family and the findings after a 15-year follow-up. Though the lesions were histologically those of fibrous dysplasia, their distribution with steady bimaxillary expansion was more typical of cherubism. This had been the provisional clinical diagnosis in two of the three patients. Growth of the lesions stopped or slowed in the early teenage years and the bone became sclerotic. All three members of the family also showed a susceptibility to intraosseous infections.

MICROSCOPY

The typical appearance is of loose cellular fibrous tissue in which there are evenly distributed, irregular trabeculae of woven bone. The trabeculae are discrete and tend to be slender and arcuate or branched but very variable in shape. A fancied resemblance to Chinese writing in fact gives little idea of their appearance. Osteoblasts are scattered throughout the substance of the trabeculae. Osteoblastic rimming is less conspicuous than in ossifying fibroma, where the bone is typically also lamellar rather than woven. However, lamellar bone or calcified spherules can also be seen in fibrous dysplasia. The types and amount of bone vary considerably from case to case but more important is the lack of definable borders where the trabeculae of fibrous dysplasia merge indefinably into the surrounding normal bone and may involve the dental supporting tissues (Figs 14.3–14.10)

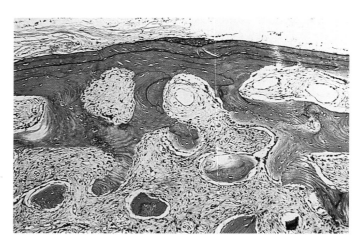

Fig. 14.3 Fibrous dyplasia. Low-power view shows lesional tissue merging with peripheral bone.

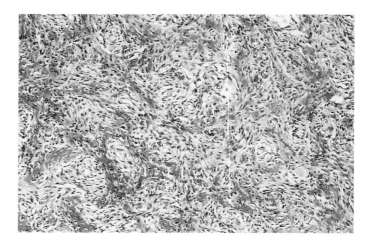

Fig. 14.4 Fibrous dysplasia. Early lesion shows cellular fibrous tissue with scanty bone formation.

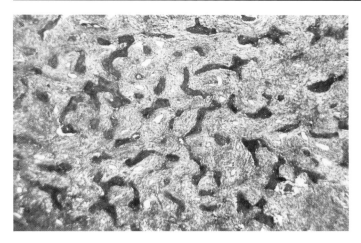

Fig. 14.5 Fibrous dysplasia. Irregular bone trabeculae in a fibrous stroma are typical.

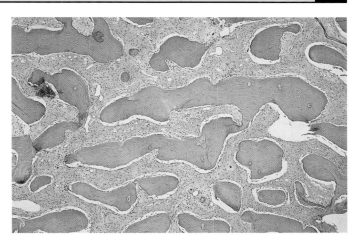

Fig. 14.8 Fibrous dysplasia. Mature specimen consisting of lamellar bone containing osteocytes.

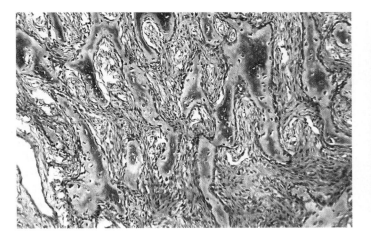

Fig. 14.6 Fibrous dysplasia. Higher power view showing irregular trabeculae of woven bone containing osteocytes and conspicuous osteoblastic rimming.

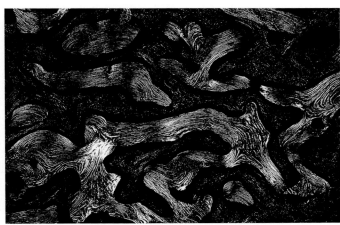

Fig. 14.9 Fibrous dysplasia. Polarized light microscopy confirms the lamellar structure of the bone seen in the previous specimen.

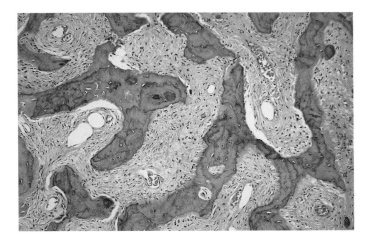

Fig. 14.7 Fibrous dysplasia. Mature specimen shows sparsely cellular bone with prominent reversal lines.

In addition to the mainly trabecular pattern, there may be myxoid areas or small foci of giant cells scattered in the fibrous stroma. These giant cells are not in such compact masses as those of giant cell lesions (Fig. 14.11).

BEHAVIOR AND MANAGEMENT

There is nothing as yet to suggest that different patterns of bone formation are of any value in predicting the behavior or response to treatment of fibrous dysplasia. The natural history is of steady progression until (very approximately) skeletal maturity is reached, when most lesions become static. Though the time of arrest is variable and there may be doubt as to whether this happens in all cases, there are undoubtedly numerous cases that have been followed for sufficient periods to confirm spontaneous arrest.

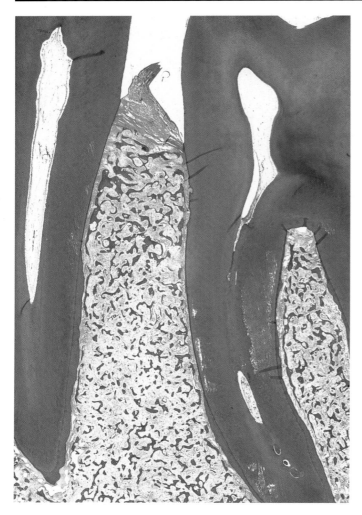

Fig. 14.10 Fibrous dysplasia. Involvement of the periodontal tissues has resulted in destruction of the lamina dura.

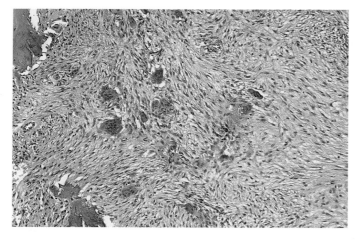

Fig. 14.11 Fibrous dysplasia. Typical small focus of scattered giant cells.

Treatment for fibrous dysplasia, when indicated, should be resection. This is only justifiable for disfiguring lesions or those that seriously interfere with function. Recurrence, usually within 2 or 3 years, may be expected in up to 30% of cases, largely because of the difficulty of defining the extent of and completely eradicating the disease. Occasionally, fibrous dysplasia involves the orbital region and can cause proptosis and, rarely, blindness. In such cases early radical excision and reconstruction is required. This may be undertaken via a transcranial approach planned with the help of three-dimensional computed tomograph reconstructions of the region.

Radiation is strictly contraindicated (as discussed below), but in all cases prolonged follow-up is required, particularly because of the small but real risk of sarcomatous change and, if that happens, the need for early intervention.

SARCOMATOUS CHANGE IN FIBROUS DYSPLASIA

The risk of sarcomatous change is greater in polyostotic disease and typically develops in early adult life. Ebata et al[5] identified 89 reported cases: the majority (61%) were osteosarcomas. The susceptibility to malignant change in fibrous dysplasia appeared to be related to the disease itself, but appoximately 30% of the reported cases had received radiation treatment. Ruggieri et al[6] found 28 sarcomas among 1122 cases of fibrous dysplasia. This represents an overall rate of malignant change of 2.5%. Nineteen of these sarcomas developed in monostotic disease and nine in polyostotic disease at a mean age of 40–46 years. Six of these sarcomas were in the maxilla, two were in the mandible, and in one both jaws were affected. The majority (19) of these neoplasms were high-grade osteosarcomas. The presenting symptoms were renewed swelling or pain, or both. Of these 28 sarcomas, Ruggieri et al[6] concluded that 46% were radiation induced and not necessarily related to the fibrous dysplasia. It therefore appears that there is a clear but small risk of spontaneous malignant change in fibrous dysplasia.

If sarcomatous change develops, wide radical excision is indicated, as for other sarcomas.

Atypical fibro-osseous lesions

As noted earlier, occasionally cases do not readily fit into the categories just described. Koury et al[7] have drawn attention to this problem with descriptions of five cases. These comprised multiple ossifying fibromas, osteosarcoma with concomitant multiple ossifying fibromas, a central low-grade osteosarcoma that had been diagnosed 20 years earlier as an atypical fibro-osseous lesion, juvenile or psammomatoid ossifying fibroma, and an unclassifiable fibro-osseous lesion. The last consisted of areas resembling ossifying fibroma, other areas resembling a fibromxyoma, and foci of giant cells. All had histological features in common, but differed widely in behavior. Causes for concern, emphasized by Koury et al,[7] when the histological features are inconclusive are persistent growth of the lesion, particularly in an older person, rapid or destructive growth and pain, and rapid recurrence after resection.

REFERENCES

1. Waldron CA 1993 Fibro-osseous lesions of the jaws. J Oral Maxillofac Surg 51: 828–835
2. Pindborg JJ, Kramer IRH, Shear M 1992 Histological typing of odontogenic tumours, 2nd edn. World Health Organization Springer-Verlag, Berlin
3. Waldron CA, Giansanti JS 1973 Benign fibro-osseous lesions of the jaws. Part I: Fibrous dysplasia of the jaws. Oral Surg Oral Med Oral Pathol 35: 190–201
4. Pierce AM, Sampson WJ, Wilson DF, Goss AN 1996 Fifteen year follow-up of a family with inherited fibrous dysplasia. J Oral Maxillofac Surg 54: 780–786
5. Ebata K, Usami T, Tohnai, Kaneda T 1992 Chondrosarcoma and osteosarcoma arising in polyostotic fibrous dysplasia. J Oral Maxillofac Surg 50: 761–764
6. Ruggieri P, Sim FH, Bond JR, Unni KK 1994 Malignancies in fibrous dysplasia. Cancer 73: 1411–1424
7. Koury ME, Regezi JA, Perrott DH, Kaban LB 1995 'Atypical' fibro-osseous lesions: diagnostic challenges and treatment concepts. Int J Oral Maxillofac Surg 24: 162–169

Cemento-ossifying fibroma   15

No practical distinction can be made between so-called cementifying and ossifying fibroma and they are categorized together as cemento-ossifying fibroma in the 1992 World Health Organization classification.[1] It appears to be peculiar to the jaws and is not recognized as an entity in other parts of the skeleton by Fechner & Mills[2] and others.

INCIDENCE

This tumor can affect patients over a wide age range, but most commonly appears between 20 and 40 years of age. In 64 of these tumors analyzed by Eversole et al,[3] females were five times as frequently affected as males but in the 45 cases analyzed by Summerlin & Tomich,[4] females were twice as frequently affected as males.

CLINICAL FEATURES

This uncommon tumor is well circumscribed and undergoes slow expansile growth, usually in the mandibular premolar or molar region. The most common complaint is a painless swelling, unless seen by chance on a routine radiograph.

Van Heerden et al[5] have described eight examples of giant ossifying fibroma (8–15 cm diameter) in Africa. Focal areas of aneurysmal bone cyst formation was noted in the majority.

RADIOGRAPHY

The tumor has well-defined margins and is radiolucent, with varying degrees of calcification (Fig. 15.1). Calcifications tend to be concentrated at the center of the lesion and some specimens appear largely radio-opaque with a narrow radiolucent rim. Sometimes there is divergence or occasionally there is resorption of related roots. Large mandibular tumors are rare but can cause a characteristic downward bowing of the lower border of the jaw.

MICROSCOPY

Cemento-ossifying fibromas have well-defined capsules. They

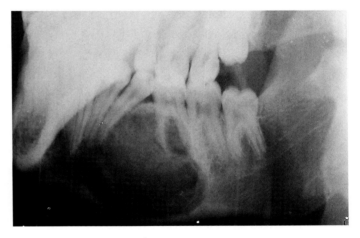

Fig. 15.1 This example of an unusually large cemento-ossifying fibroma has well-defined margins and scattered calcifications in the predominantly radiolucent area.

consist of stellate or spindle-shaped fibroblasts, with a widely variable degree of cellularity. Some specimens show moderate amounts of collagen, while others may have less intercellular matrix and the cells may be in whorled or storiform patterns.

The types of calcification within the tumor also vary widely, as described by Sciubba & Younai.[6] Trabeculae of woven bone with osteoblastic rimming are often prominent and frequently form an interconnecting reticular pattern. Thicker trabeculae of lamellar bone as well as dystrophic calcifications may also be seen. Some specimens have a predominance of acellular ovoid or spherical calcifications resembling cementicles (Figs 15.2–15.9). These nodules are minute at first, but gradually grow, fuse, and ultimately form a dense mass. Similar cementicle-like calcifications can be found in fibro-osseous lesions of the skull or other bones far distant from any odontogenic tissue, and most so-called cementifying fibromas show admixed spherical calcifications and bone trabeculae, so that the different patterns of calcification are clearly only minor variants of the same pathologic process.

DIFFERENTIAL DIAGNOSIS

Histologically, cemento-ossifying fibroma may be indistinguishable

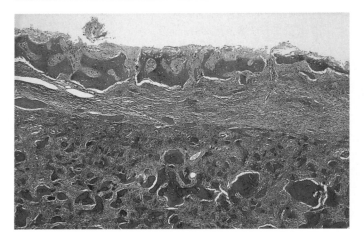

Fig. 15.2 Cemento-ossifying fibroma. Low-power view shows the capsule and surrounding normal bone.

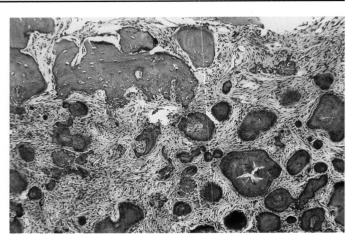

Fig. 15.5 Cemento-ossifying fibroma. There is a mixed picture of acellular globular deposits and irregular bone trabeculae in a highly cellular stroma.

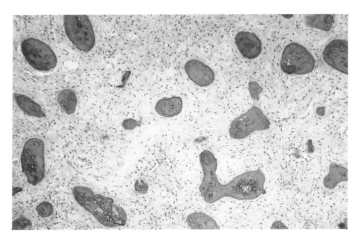

Fig. 15.3 Cemento-ossifying fibroma. Rounded deposits of cemento-osseous material lie in a cellular stroma.

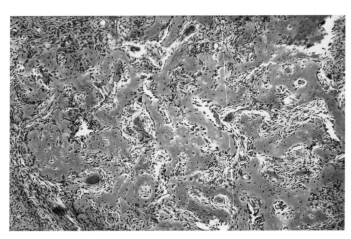

Fig. 15.6 Cemento-ossifying fibroma. In this example, immature bone trabeculae contain many osteocytes and have osteoblastic rimming, and are more prominent than the cellular stroma.

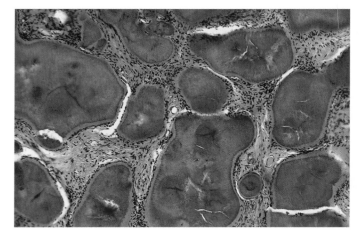

Fig. 15.4 Cemento-ossifying fibroma. Higher power view shows globular deposits of mainly acellular cementum.

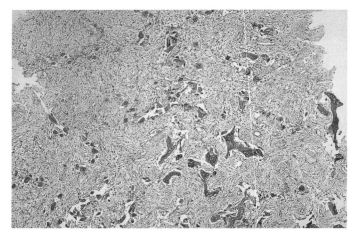

Fig. 15.7 Cemento-ossifying fibroma, juvenile aggressive type. A cellular fibrous stroma contains scanty irregular trabeculae of bone and aggregates of giant cells.

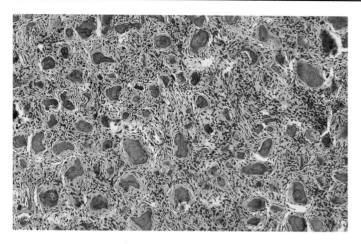

Fig. 15.8 Cemento-ossifying fibroma, juvenile aggressive type. Calcifications consist of small globules of cementum-like material in a highly cellular stroma.

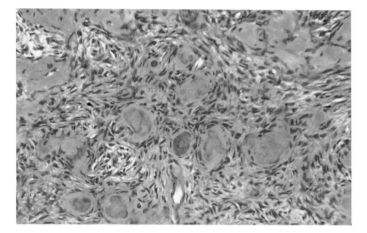

Fig. 15.9 Cemento-ossifying fibroma, juvenile aggressive type. Higher power view shows the globular calcifications and highly cellular stroma.

from many cases of fibrous dysplasia, except by the clinical and radiographic findings. Important differences are that cemento-ossifying fibroma more frequently affects the mandible, is well circumscribed, and can have a fibrous capsule. Fibrous dysplasia, by contrast, merges with normal bone at its margins. It can also extend to the alveolar margin, but in so doing does not fuse with or otherwise distort the roots of teeth.

Microscopically, the trabeculae in fibrous dysplasia, though variably shaped, tend to be slender and arcuate or branched with osteoblasts throughout their substance. This contrasts with the more conspicuous osteoblastic rimming typical of cemento-ossifying fibroma, where the bone is typically lamellar rather than woven.

Some areas of a cemento-ossifying fibroma also may not be distinguishable microscopically from periapical cemental dysplasia or from other focal cemento-osseous dysplasia, but overall it is better circumscribed and poorly vascular. Cemento-ossifying fibroma typically also appears radiographically as a well-

demarcated radiolucent area with a sclerotic rim and can cause bowing of the lower border of the mandible.

BEHAVIOR AND MANAGEMENT

As noted by Sciubba & Younai,[6] the patterns of calcified tissue formation have no effect on the behavior of the tumor. Cemento-ossifying fibromas may have a definable capsule and, unlike the fibro-osseous dysplasias, can be readily enucleated. Occasionally, large tumors that have distorted the jaw require local resection and bone grafting. The prognosis is good and recurrence rare. However, if an associated tooth is extracted, a densely calcified cemento-ossifying fibroma can become a focus for chronic osteomyelitis. If this happens, wide excision becomes necessary.

Juvenile active ('aggressive') ossifying fibroma

This designation is given to some rarely reported ossifying fibromas, mainly found in the maxilla of younger patients. Some have been locally aggressive and showed a tendency to recur. However, Slootweg & Müller[7] restricted use of the term 'juvenile ossifying fibroma' to those tumors that mainly affected patients of 15 years or younger and which histologically showed a highly cellular but loose fibroblastic stroma containing strands of osteoid with entrapped osteoblasts. However, some more cellular ('active') variant of ossifying fibroma may be difficult to distinguish from an osteoblastoma, and should probably be categorized as such. However, there are no definitive histologic criteria for distinguishing these tumors from more typical cemento-ossifying fibromas Despite the cellular ('active') appearance of the juvenile ossifying fibromas reported by Slootweg & Müller,[7] all were cured by conservative surgery (see Figs 15.7–15.9).

Peripheral ossifying fibroma

Buchner & Hansen[8] have described in detail the types of calcification and bone formation in these gingival lesions, but emphasize that they are reactive and not the peripheral counterpart of central cemento-ossifying fibroma.

REFERENCES

1. Pindborg JJ, Kramer IRH, Shear M 1992 Histological typing of odontogenic tumours, 2nd edn. World Health Organization/Springer-Verlag, Berlin

2. Fechner RE, Mills SE 1992 Tumors of the bones and joints. Atlas of tumor pathology. Armed Forces Institute of Pathology, Washington, DC, Third series, fascicle 8

3. Eversole LR, Leider AS, Nelson K 1985 Ossifying fibroma: a clinicopathologic study of sixty four cases. Oral Surg Oral Med Oral Pathol 60: 505–511

4. Summerlin DJ, Tomich CE 1994 Focal cemento-osseus dysplasia; a clinicopathologic study of 221 cases. Oral Surg Oral Med Oral Pathol 78: 611–620

5. Van Heerden WFP, Raubenheimer EJ, Weir RG, Kreidler J 1989 Giant ossifying fibroma: a clinicopathologic study of 8 tumors. J Oral Pathol Med 18: 506–509

6. Sciubba JJ, Younai F 1989 Ossifying fibroma of the mandible and maxilla: review of 18 cases. J Oral Pathol Med 18: 315–321

7. Slootweg PJ, Müller HJ 1990 Juvenile ossifying fibroma. Report of four cases. J Cranio Max Fac Surg 18: 125–129

8. Buchner A, Hansen LS 1987 The histomorphologic spectrum of peripheral ossifying fibroma. Oral Surg Oral Med Oral Pathol 63: 452–461

Cemento-osseous dysplasias 16

Periapical cemento-osseous dysplasia

INCIDENCE

Periapical cemento-osseous dysplasia affects women, particularly the middle-aged, 10–15 times more frequently than men. It is also more common in blacks. It usually affects the mandibular incisor region, but can involve several sites or be generalized.

CLINICAL FEATURES

The condition is asymptomatic and is usually seen by chance in routine radiographs

RADIOGRAPHY

Periapical cemento-osseous dysplasia can be seen in radiographs in its early stages as rounded radiolucent areas simulating periapical granulomas; the related teeth are vital. Increasing radio-opacity starts centrally until the masses become densely radio-opaque, and all stages of development may be seen in multiple lesions.

MICROSCOPY

The appearances resemble those of cemento-ossifying fibroma. In the early stages, cellular fibrous tissue contains foci of cementum-like tissue that grows and fuses to form a solid, bone-like mass (Figs 16.1–16.3).

BEHAVIOR AND MANAGEMENT

Periapical cemento-osseous dysplasia does not appear to have any potential for continued growth. The main consideration is to distinguish early lesions from periapical granulomas by routine dental investigation. Once this has been confirmed, further treatment is usually unnecessary.

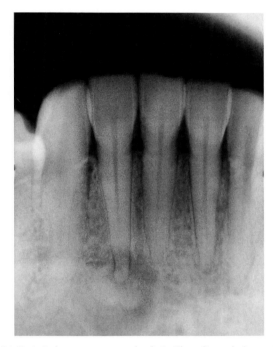

Fig. 16.1 Periapical cemento-osseous dysplasia. The radiograph shows a localized area of sclerosis at the apex of a vital mandibular incisor. It leaves the periodontal ligament space intact and has a surrounding area of ill-defined radiolucency.

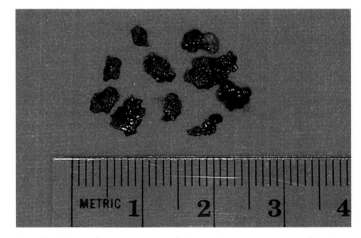

Fig. 16.2 Periapical cemento-osseous dyplasia. Macroscopic specimen showing the gritty fragments of bone surrounded by vascular connective tissue.

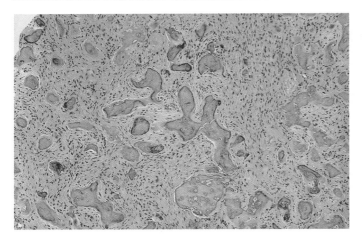

Fig. 16.3 Periapical cemento-osseous dyplasia. Multiple foci of cemento-osseous tissue lie in a moderately cellular fibrous stroma.

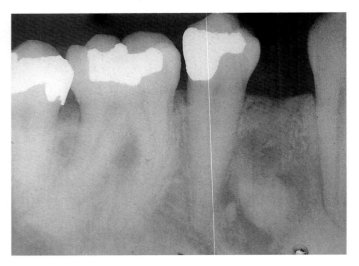

Fig. 16.4 Focal cemento-osseous dysplasia. A localized area of sclerosis has a surrounding area of ill-defined radiolucency.

Focal cemento-osseous dysplasia

Waldron[1] suggests that this may be the most commonly encountered fibro-osseous dysplasia, but that it has received disproportionally scanty attention. It is not recognized as a distinct entity in the 1992 World Health Organization classification[2] of odontogenic tumors, but Summerlin & Tomich[3] have presented the findings in 221 cases. Focal cemento-osseous dysplasia resembles the florid type histologically, but differs in its radiographic and clinical features.

INCIDENCE

The average age at presentation of the patients described by Summerlin & Tomich[3] was 37, and 88% of them were females. Blacks accounted for only 32% of these patients and, overall, accounted for only 7% of their surgical accessions. The posterior mandible was the site of predilection in 77%.

CLINICAL FEATURES

The lesions are, with rare exceptions, asymptomatic and discovered by chance on routine radiographs. Slight swelling of the jaw may occasionally be seen.

RADIOGRAPHY

Focal cemento-osseous dysplasia appears as a moderately well-defined, mottled radiolucent/opaque or more sclerotic area, usually less than 2 cm in diameter, sometimes with a sclerotic rim. Lesions are sometimes related to teeth, but some are present in edentulous areas. A simple bone cyst is sometimes associated (Fig. 16.4).

MICROSCOPY

The lesion consists of cellular fibrous tissue containing many small blood vessels, trabeculae of woven bone or cementum-like calcifications, and, sometimes, scattered foci of giant cells interspersed by scanty fibrous tissue. Summerlin & Tomich[3] frequently also noted large areas of hemorrhage at the periphery of lesions.

BEHAVIOR AND MANAGEMENT

Dental infection should be excluded by examination. The nature of the lesion is confirmed by biopsy. Unlike cemento-ossifying fibroma, lesional material is not readily separated from the surrounding bone and is gritty and hemorrhagic. Whether thorough curettage to remove an symptomatic lesion is justified seems doubtful, especially as Waldron[1] reports that residual tissue left after biopsy does not seem to progress or cause symptoms. Summerlin & Tomich[3] encourage prolonged follow-up after confirmation of the diagnosis, as two of their patients progressed to florid cemento-osseous dysplasia. Any associated bone cysts tend to resolve more slowly than those seen in isolation.

Florid cemento-osseous dysplasia and gigantiform cementoma

Thirty-four cases of florid cemento-osseous dysplasia were described by Melrose et al.[4] Middle-aged or elderly women, particularly blacks, are affected. The calcifications are symmetrical, may involve all four quadrants, and are asymptomatic unless infected. There is a rare familial type for which the title *giganti-*

form cementoma may be reserved. The disorder is strictly localized to tooth-bearing areas and not associated with any other skeletal disease.

RADIOGRAPHY

Florid cemento-osseous dysplasia appears as radio-opaque, irregular or lobulated masses without radiolucent borders interspersed with ill-defined radiolucent/radio-opaque areas. In the past, these calcifications have been interpreted as chronic diffuse sclerosing osteomyelitis. However, any infection of these lesions is a secondary event, but can result from exposure of the calcified masses to the mouth. Simple bone cysts are occasionally associated (Fig. 16.5).

MICROSCOPY

Florid cemento-osseous dysplasia consists of masses of densely calcified material resembling secondary cementum. They contain few lacunae and are sometimes fused to the roots of teeth (Fig. 16.6).

BEHAVIOR AND MANAGEMENT

Diagnosis is by the clinical and radiographic features. Biopsy is not indicated because of the risk of infection.

In the absence of symptoms, observation by regular follow-up with radiographs at intervals is appropriate. Complete removal of

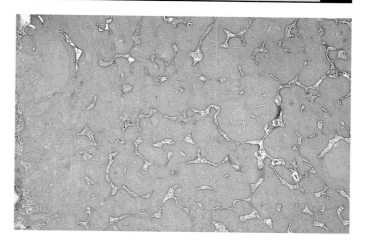

Fig. 16.6 Florid cemento-osseous dysplasia. Fused sclerotic masses of cemento-osseous tissue are interspersed with scanty fibrous tissue.

these lesions is likely to require extensive surgery and is not normally justified. If infection supervenes, as a result of extraction of an associated tooth or from any other source, chronic osteomyelitis can develop in the densely calcified tissue. In such circumstances the mass may eventually sequestrate or the entire lesion may need to be excised to allow the infection to resolve.

Although supervention of infection in florid cemento-osseous dysplasia can cause chronic osteomyelitis, this should not be confused with chronic diffuse sclerosing osteomyelitis. The latter as pointed out by Schneider & Mesa[5] is a primary condition. It affects whites as frequently as blacks, is painful, unilateral and shows a single area of diffuse sclerosis containing small, ill-defined osteolytic areas and having indistinct borders. Also, unlike florid cemento-osseous dysplasia it extends into the body of the mandible and may involve the ramus. However, the two conditions are unlikely to be distinguishable histologically if a specimen is taken from infected florid cemento-osseous dysplasia during a symptomatic period.

REFERENCES

1. Waldron CA 1993 Fibro-osseous lesions of the jaws. J Oral Maxillofac Surg 51: 828–835
2. Pindborg JJ, Kramer IRH, Shear M 1992 Histological typing of odontogenic tumours, 2nd edn. World Health Organization/Springer-Verlag, Berlin
3. Summerlin D-J, Tomich CE 1994 Focal cemento-osseous dysplasia: a clinicopathological study of 221 cases. Oral Surg Oral Med Oral Pathol 78: 611–620
4. Melrose RJ, Abrams AM, Mills BG 1976 Florid osseous dysplasia. A clinicopathologic study of thirty-four cases. Oral Surg Oral Med Oral Pathol 41: 62–68
5. Schneider LC, Mesa ML 1990 Differences between florid osseous dysplasia and chronic diffuse sclerosing osteomyelitis. Oral Surg Oral Med Oral Pathol 70: 308–312

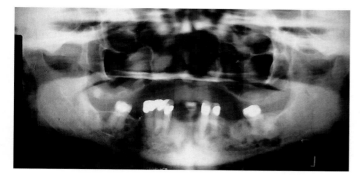

Fig. 16.5 Florid cemento-osseous dysplasia. Radiography shows multiple ill-defined areas of sclerosis and radiolucency on both sides of the mandible.

Cherubism

Cherubism is an autosomal dominant disease (formerly known as *familial fibrous dysplasia*) with variable expressivity. It was originally described by Jones,[1] who reported on a remarkable family with severe manifestations of the disease. Due to weaker penetrance of the trait in females, the phenotype is approximately twice as common in males.[2] Like other genetic diseases, many nonfamilial cases appear as a result of new mutations. Commonly, only isolated cases are seen, but Peters[3] reported a family with no fewer than 20 affected members. Like other genetic diseases, many nonfamilial cases appear as a result of new mutations. However, Zohar et al[4] were able to trace, in an unbroken line through four generations, family members who showed either fibrous dysplasia or cherubism, though this association is not otherwise recognized. A high rate of chromosomal breakage was noted in cytogenetic analysis.

The disorder appears to be recognized worldwide, but though seen in Japan appears to be rare there.[5]

The characteristic abnormalities are multiple, symmetrical masses in the jaws. These, which appear cyst-like radiographically, form in infancy or childhood and give the face an excessively chubby or, less frequently, a so-called cherubic appearance. Partial or complete resolution of the lesions with skeletal maturation is the general rule.

CLINICAL FEATURES

The onset is typically between the ages of 6 months to 7 years,[6] but, rarely, manifestations are delayed until 10 or more years later into late teenage.[7] Symmetrical mandibular swelling is the most common presentation. Radiographic changes may be seen considerably earlier than clinical signs. The time of the onset of clinically evident disease and the rapidity of its progress are both variable and, rarely, the facial deformity does not appear until after puberty.[8]

Frequently, only the mandible, particularly the region of the angles, is involved. Maxillary involvement is usually associated with widespread mandibular disease. Extensive maxillary lesions cause the eyes to appear to be turned heavenward; this, together with the plumpness of the face, is the cause of these patients being likened to cherubs. The appearance of the eyes is due to such factors as the maxillary masses pushing the floors of the orbits and eyes upwards, with the result that the sclera below the pupils becomes exposed. Expansion of the maxillae may also cause stretching of the skin and some retraction of the lower lids. Rarely, destruction of the infra-orbital ridges weakens support for the lower lid.

The alveolar ridges are expanded and the mandibular swelling may be sometimes be so gross lingually as to interfere with speech, swallowing, or even breathing. Maxillary involvement can cause the palate to become an inverted V shape. Teeth are frequently displaced and may be loosened.

Despite the lack of inflammation, there is frequently cervical lymphadenopathy, due to reactive hyperplasia and fibrosis. This is typically seen in the early stages and may have completely subsided by puberty.[9]

RADIOGRAPHY

Defects are usually more extensive than the clinical swelling. The angles of the mandible are bilaterally involved and the process extends towards the coronoid notch and sometimes also forwards along a considerable part of the body of the mandible (Fig. 17.1). Panoramic radiographs are necessary to determine the extent of the disease, but Bianchi et al[10] have also described its appearances on computed tomography scanning and followed its development.

The lesions simulate multilocular cysts as a result of fine bony septa extending between the soft tissue masses. Progressive expansion of the latter reduces the bony cortices to eggshell thickness.

Maxillary involvement is shown by diffuse rarefaction of the bone, but spread of the soft tissue masses can cause opacity of the sinuses. A distinctive radiographic sign described by Cornelius & McClendon[11] is exposure of the posterior part of the hard palate in lateral skull films, as a result of forward displacement of the teeth. In severe cases, upward bulging of the orbital floor and destruction of part of the infraorbital ridges may be seen. Even after complete clinical resolution of the facial swelling, bone defects may be evident radiographically.

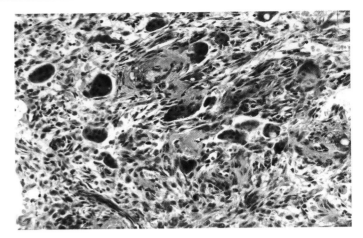

Fig. 17.2 Cherubism. Multiple giant cells are surrounded by a vascular stroma

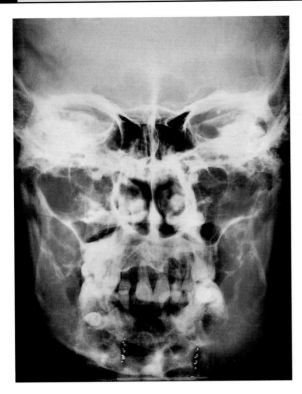

Fig. 17.1 Cherubism. The radiograph shows the bilateral expansion of the mandible in the region of the mandible and the cyst-like appearance of the areas of radiolucency. There is almost complete absence of mandibular permanent teeth.

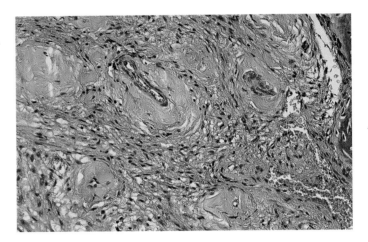

Fig. 17.3 Cherubism. Typical vascular cuffing in a fibrous area.

MICROSCOPY

The soft-tissue masses consist of highly cellular and vascular fibrous tissue containing many giant cells. The fibrous tissue may be loose and relatively delicate in some areas but dense in others. Blood vessels are numerous and are typically surrounded by a cuff of eosinophilic fibrin-like material, but this appears to be perivascular collagen[12] (Figs 17.2 and 17.3).

The giant cells have variable numbers of nuclei and may be in compact foci or scattered. There may also be small irregular bone trabeculae of which some are probably metaplastic, but others are remnants of normal bone undergoing resorption. Occasionally, epithelial remnants of teeth the development of which has been aborted by the disease may be seen. Chomette et al[13] have described a high level of acid phosphatase in the early stages of osteolysis. This was followed by fibroblastic proliferation with raised leucine aminopeptidase activity. Finally, osteogenesis was associated with high alkaline phosphatase and ATPase in the lesions.

A limited biopsy of cherubism tissue may be indistinguishable microscopically from some areas of fibrous dysplasia, but overall the many giant cells and scanty bone of cherubism are in contrast with the pattern of bone trabeculae but scanty giant cells which are typical of fibrous dysplasia. More important are the clinical presentation and distinctive radiographic features. In particular, the early onset and symmetric distribution of the lesions distinguishes cherubism from fibrous dysplasia and from other giant cell lesions. A positive family history helps to confirm the diagnosis.

BEHAVIOR AND MANAGEMENT

Most cases can be allowed to progress to spontaneous resolution and the parents reassured accordingly. Occasionally, examples of total restoration of a normal facial appearance, despite persistence of radiographic changes, have been illustrated.[14] Exceptionally, treatment may be necessary for extensive lesions that interfere with function (particularly when sight becomes impaired as a result of displacement of the orbit) or are disfiguring. Surgery is the only feasible method of treatment, as the possible complications of radiotherapy in a child preclude its use. Treatment ranging from conservative curettage, repeated as necessary, to more aggressive resection and filling the void with autogenous bone chips has been used from time to time. Nevertheless, if carried out while the disease is still active, surgery is equally likely to be followed by recurrence and further bone destruction. Any surgery should be delayed, if possible until the disease is becoming quiescent in adolescence. However, most cases can probably be relied upon to regress without treatment.[15] Occasionally, the change from significant childhood facial deformity to a totally normal facial appearance has been illustrated.[16] Nevertheless, in this latter case, despite complete clinical resolution, a dental extraction provoked renewed activity of residual bone lesions and fungation of lesional material from the socket. There should thus be caution in surgery to the jaws until radiographic resolution has also been achieved.

CHERUBISM IN NOONAN'S SYNDROME

Giant cell lesions of the jaws and other sites have been described in Noonan's syndrome (see Ch. 18), and cherubism itself has also been reported in this genetic anomaly.[17,18]

REFERENCES

1. Jones WA 1933 Familial multilocular cystic disease of the jaws. Am J Cancer 17: 946–950
2. Talley DB 1952 Familial fibrous dysplasia of the jaws. Oral Surg 5: 1012–1019
3. Peters WJN 1979 Cherubism: a study of twenty cases in one family. Oral Surg Oral Med Oral Pathol 47: 307–311
4. Zohar Y, Grausbord R, Shabtai F, Talmi Y 1989 Fibrous dysplasia and cherubism as an hereditary disease. Follow-up of four generations. J Cran Maxill Fac Surg 17: 340–344
5. Hitomi G, Nishide N, Mitsui K 1996 Cherubism: diagnostic imaging and review of the literature in Japan. Oral Srug Oral Med Oral Pathol Radiol Endod 81: 623–628
6. Hamner JE, Ketcham AS 1969 Cherubism: an analysis of treatment. Cancer 23: 720–726
7. Dukart RC, Kolodny SC, Polte HW, Hooker SP 1974 Cherubism. Oral Surg 37: 722–727
8. Kuepper RC, Harrigan WF 1978 Treatment of mandibular cherubism. J Oral Surg 36: 638–641
9. Topazian RG, Sostich ER 1965 Familial fibrous dysplasia of the jaws (cherubism). J Oral Surg 23: 559–556
10. Bianchi SD, Boccardi A, Mela F, Romognoli R 1987 The computed tomographic appearances of cherubism. Skeletal Radiol 16: 6–10
11. Cornelius EA, McClendon JL 1969 Cherubism – hereditary fibrous dysplasia of the jaws. Roentgenographic features. Am J Roentgenol 106: 136–143
12. Hamner JE, Schofield HH, Cornryn J 1977 Benign fibrosseous jaw lesions of periodontal membrane origin. Cancer 22: 861–878
13. Chomette G, Auriol M, Guilbert F, Vaillant JM 1988 Cherubism. Histo-enzymological and ultrastructural study. Intl J Oral Maxillofac Surg 17: 219–223
14. Cawson RA, Binnie WH, Eveson JW 1995 Color atlas of oral disease. Mosby-Wolfe, London, p 8.9
15. Katz JO, Dunlap CL, Ennis RL 1992 Cherubism: report of a case showing regression without treatment. J Oral Maxillofac Surg 50: 301–303
16. Cawson RA, Binnie WH, Eveson JW 1994 Color atlas of oral disease, 2nd edn. Mosby-Wolfe, London
17. Dunlap C, Neville B, Vickers RA et al 1989 The Noonan syndrome/cherubism association. Oral Surg Oral Med Oral Pathol 67: 698–705
18. Addante RR, Breen GH 1996 Cherubism in a patient with Noonan's syndrome. J Oral Maxillofac Surg 54: 210–213

Central giant cell granuloma 18 and other giant cell lesions

Central giant cell granuloma

Most central giant cell lesions of the jaws appear to be hyperplastic. They were formerly, and still sometimes are, termed *giant cell reparative granulomas*, as they were thought to represent a reparative process when first described in the jaws by Jaffe.[1] However, the name is misleading in that there is no granuloma formation in the histological sense. There is also little evidence that these lesions represent a reparative process.

Though general acceptance of the term *central giant cell granuloma* implies that the jaw lesion is not a neoplasm, it may grow rapidly and and be mildly destructive. A few lesions pursue a more aggressive course, so that there is some doubt of whether it is a separate entity from the giant cell tumor ('osteoclastoma'). As discussed below, this issue has been given some impetus by the conclusions reached by Whitaker & Waldron.[2] Overall, however, giant cell granulomas of the jaws follow a far more benign course than giant cell tumors, which tend to be widely destructive and can metastasize despite a benign histological appearance.

INCIDENCE

Central giant cell lesions of the jaws are uncommon. They formed 0.17% of 20 000 oral biopsies reported by Waldron & Shafer.[3] Wu & Chan[4] noted one central giant cell lesion among 114 tumors of the jaws among Hong Kong Chinese. Other series mentioned in earlier chapters include only odontogenic tumors.

Whitaker & Waldron,[2] in their review of 142 cases, confirmed a female preponderance (63% of cases); this preponderance was almost 3 : 1 in the age group 11–30 years. Sixty-four per cent of lesions were seen before the age of 30 years.

The most frequent site is the mandible. However, Kaffe et al,[5] have found, in a review of 80 reports, that in contrast to the traditional view that giant cell granulomas predominantly affected the deciduous tooth-bearing area, 53% were in the posterior mandible or extended up into the ramus. Nevertheless, of 18 new cases that they presented, all except three were in the premolar or canine regions. About 25% are in the maxilla, usually in the anterior part.

CLINICAL FEATURES

The majority of lesions are painless swellings, which sometimes displace teeth. Only 6% of those in Whitaker & Waldron's series[2] caused pain or paresthesia, but behavior such as perforation of cortical bone or root resorption was seen in 40% and categorized by them as 'aggressive.'

Radiographically, central giant cell lesions give rise to rounded radiolucent areas, which are usually well delineated and have some resemblance to an ameloblastoma. Sixty-one per cent of cases reported by Whitaker and Waldron (1993) appeared multilocular on radiographs but 39% were monolocular (Figs 18.1–18.3). Of 18 new cases presented by Kaffe et al,[5] seven were multilocular and 11 had ill-defined margins. In their review

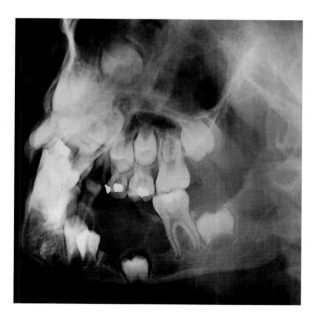

Fig. 18.1 Central giant cell granuloma in a 7½-year-old boy. The radiograph shows a multilocular area of radiolucency expanding the mandible.

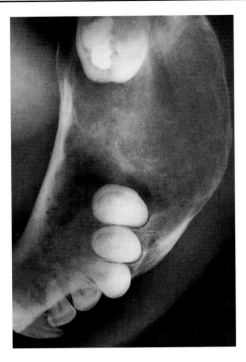

Fig. 18.2 Central giant cell granuloma in a 31-year-old woman. An occlusal radiograph shows predominantly buccal expansion of the mandible and a faint suggestion of a soap-bubble pattern.

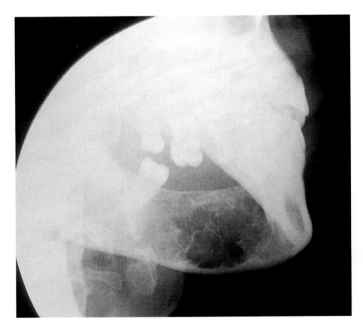

Fig. 18.3 Central giant cell granuloma. An extensive rounded area of radiolucency in the body of the mandible shows scalloped margins and a soap-bubble appearance.

they found that only 6% crossed the midline. Confirmation of the diagnosis depends on biopsy, but needs to be supplemented by blood chemistry to exclude hyperparathyroidism, as discussed later.

MICROSCOPY

Giant cell granuloma forms a lobulated mass of proliferating connective tissue containing many giant cells. It is frequently highly vascular, so that signs of bleeding and deposits of hemosiderin are seen. Giant cells are frequently gathered in focal aggregations around areas of hemorrhage. In some cases there is considerable fibroblastic proliferation, while in others there is prominent osteoid and bone formation, particularly near the periphery. Occasionally the stromal cells are ovoid, resembling those of a giant cell tumor, and there is little fibroblastic activity. The giant cells vary in size and density, ranging from widely separated small or irregular giant cells to evenly distributed, large giant cells with 20 or more nuclei, resembling those of a giant cell tumor. In the latter case osteoid formation may be absent. Overall however, Franklin et al[6] have shown that in giant cell granulomas the giant cells are smaller and contain fewer nuclei than those of giant cell tumors of the axial skeleton (Figs 18.4–18.6).

There are no changes in blood chemistry, but the histological features are indistinguishable from those of hyperparathyroidism.

HISTOGENESIS

The earlier name giant cell 'reparative' granuloma derives from Jaffe's unproven hypothesis[1] (also applied to simple bone cysts) that they were a reaction to trauma that had caused intramedullary hemorrhage. No evidence supports this idea and giant cell hyperplasia does not follow bleeding into bone after a fracture or enucleation of a cyst. Moreover, these lesions often grow rapidly, and far from being reparative are locally destructive.

The giant cells have been shown by Flanagan et al[7] by their response to calcitonin, their activity in tissue culture, and by osteoclast-specific monoclonal antibodies to be indistinguishable from osteoclasts. However, the view that central giant cell granulomas originated from hyperplasia of giant cells responsible for

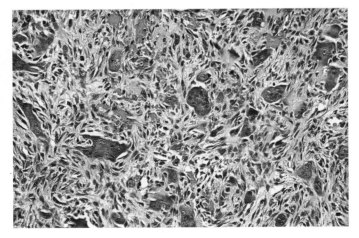

Fig. 18.4 Central giant cell granuloma. Irregular giant cells of varying size are surrounded by a cellular and vascular fibrous stroma.

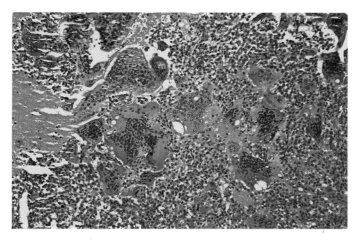

Fig. 18.5 Giant cell granuloma. The unusually large multinucleate giant cells causes the lesion to resemble a giant cell tumor.

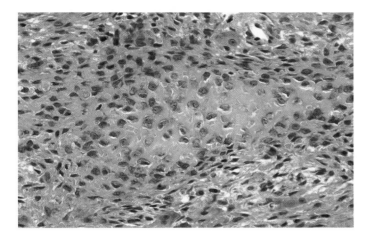

Fig. 18.6 Giant cell granuloma. Osteoid formation is a typical feature.

resorption of the teeth does not appear to be consistent with their sites of predilection, as discussed earlier.

Whether giant cell granulomas of the jaw represent the benign end of the spectrum of giant cell tumors remains a matter for speculation. Giant cell tumor (osteoclastoma) affects long bones, but may not be distinguishable with certainty, by microscopy alone, from a giant cell granuloma.

Giant cell tumors of long bones have an almost equal gender incidence, with only a slight female preponderance, and are usually painful and fast growing. In 10%, pathological fracture is the first sign. Microscopically, diagnosis of giant cell tumor is made on the background of mononuclear cells. The latter are rounded or polygonal and resemble normal histiocytes but sometimes show numerous mitotic figures.

Auclair et al[8] carried out a histomorphologic comparison between 49 giant cell granulomas of the jaws and 42 giant cell tumors of long bones. The mean age of patients with giant cell granulomas was 21 years and that of patients with giant cell tumors was 25 years. However, the only statistically significant histologic differences

between the lesions were the greater number of nuclei in the giant cells of giant cell tumors. Nevertheless, 10% of the giant cell granulomas were histologically similar to most giant cell tumors.

Whitaker & Waldron[2] described six patients aged from 30 months to 67 years who had lesions showing microscopic features typical of giant cell tumor of long bones. In the four cases where follow-up data were available, one was well 2 years after a second curettage, one remained well 1 year after four curettages, another remained well 2 years after curettage followed by resection, while one remained well 8 years after extensive resections. Whitaker & Waldron[2] concluded that lesions which recurred more frequently showed evenly distributed giant cells, mitotic activity, and absence of osteoid formation. They found an overall recurrence rate of 16% in 47 cases where follow-up data were available. In those six lesions that had the histological appearance of giant cell tumors, follow-up data were available for only four, and in two of these the response to a second curettage appeared to be good with the patients being alive and well 1 and 2 years later. Resections were carried out after failure to respond to curettage in two patients. Both patients were alive and well 2 and 8 years later. Thus, even those lesions resembling giant cell tumors histologically behaved considerably less aggressively than typical long bone tumors.

It would be unwise to state categorically that giant cell granulomas of the jaws and giant cell tumors of the long bones are distinct entities. However, there are usually major differences between the two conditions. Giant cell granulomas of the jaw tend to affect a younger age group, and even those categorized as 'aggressive' are far less destructive than giant cell tumors. The most aggressive of the giant cell lesions of the jaws recorded by Whitaker & Waldron[2] was in the maxilla. Though it recurred twice, it must be appreciated that the thin maxillofacial bones allow such lesions to spread relatively easily through them. Nevertheless, these same authors concluded that giant cell lesions of the maxilla had less tendency to recur than those in the mandible.

In contrast to these jaw lesions, Fechner & Mills[9] quote a recurrence rate of up to 60% for giant cell tumors. Wold et al[10] also consider that giant cell reparative granulomas of the small bones of the hands and feet are reactive lesions and different entities from giant cell tumors of the same bones. They differed microscopically from giant cell tumors in that there was osteoid formation in 100%, stromal hemorrhage in 93%, clustering of giant cells in 73%, and a stromal storiform pattern in 20% of their 30 cases. All these were lacking in giant cell tumors of the same bones apart from hemorrhage in 44%, and Fechner & Mills[9] have maintained this stance. The possibility that a giant cell tumor could develop in the jaws cannot be disputed, but it must be an exceptionally rare event, and the behavior and response to treatment of giant cell granulomas of the jaws suggests that, from a practical viewpoint, they are separate entities.

BEHAVIOR AND MANAGEMENT

Other causes of giant cell lesions of the jaws must be excluded, as discussed below. The histologic and radiographic findings may provide a general guide to likely behavior. Whitaker & Waldron[2] found that nonaggressive/nonrecurrent lesions showed small, irregularly shaped and distributed giant cells, osteoid formation, and fewer mitoses than recurrent or aggressive lesions. The site of the lesion also appeared to bear some relation to behavior. Whitaker & Waldron[2] found that lesions in the mandibular molar region were significantly more frequently aggressive or recurrent than were those in the mandibular ramus. A higher proportion of nonrecurrent to recurrent lesions was also found in the anterior maxilla, though the most aggressive lesion that they followed up was in this site. Though, as mentioned earlier, Whitaker & Waldron[2] believed that central giant cell granulomas and giant cell tumors formed a continuous spectrum, aggressive behavior typical of a giant cell tumor is not seen in the jaws. Whitaker et al[11] have shown that the nucleolar organizer region (AgNOR) counts of five recurrent giant cell lesions were significantly higher (1.73 ± 0.15) than those from four nonaggressive and nonrecurrent lesions (1.33 ± 0.14) but only higher than the counts from five aggressive lesions (1.54 ± 0.21) in the mononuclear and giant cell nuclei. However, they were diffident about concluding that AgNOR quantification was as yet a reliable guide to giant cell lesion behavior. Unfortunately, the follow-up data on a sufficient number of these lesions were not available in order to test the overall value of these findings in predicting the optimal line of treatment. There is also so much overlap in the findings between the recurrent and nonrecurrent lesions as to make prediction difficult in individual cases.

Curettage is usually therefore the first line of treatment and is frequently adequate. Small fragments that may be left behind do not necessarily require further treatment, and sometimes appear to resolve spontaneously. A minority of these tumors are more aggressive and recurrence follows incomplete removal; however, frequently, further curettage appears to be adequate. Wide excision is occasionally required for otherwise uncontrollable lesions.

Harris[12] confirmed the finding of Flanagan et al[7] that some central giant cell granulomas regress with calcitonin treatment. Four patients aged 11–59 years who received subcutaneous calcitonin daily showed complete regression of the lesions and no recurrence during follow-up of up to 4 years. Potentially mutilating surgery was thus avoided and though calcitonin treatment had to be continued for 6–24 months, there were no disturbances of blood chemistry or other adverse effects.

In the cases reported by Harris[12] the response to calcitonin was not correlated with the histology in terms of giant cell size and density, but the lesions were aggressive in terms of bone destruction.

Giant cell tumors (osteoclastomas) occasionally form in such bones as the temporal or sphenoid, and as discussed earlier Whitaker & Waldron[2] believe that benign giant cell granulomas and aggressive giant cell tumors form the ends of a continuous spectrum. If this is the case then the name 'giant cell *granuloma*' is particularly inappropriate. In their report of a primary malignant giant cell tumor of the jaw, Mintz et al[13] claimed it to be the first documented case. This tumor metastasized to the lungs and a lymph node. However, this is quite exceptional, and even those giant cell lesions of the jaws that resemble giant cell tumors histologically and recur may respond to a second curettage.

Other giant cell lesions

GIANT CELL TUMOR

As already discussed, some believe that giant cell granulomas and giant cell tumors form the ends of a continuous spectrum, and occasionally the histological appearances are so similar as to make an absolute distinction difficult. However, Fechner & Mills[9] point out that giant cell tumors show more uniformly distributed giant cells which can be large, sometimes with more than 50 nuclei. The stroma consist of round or oval mononuclear cells and frequently resemble normal histiocytes. Mitotic activity in these cells is common. Fibrous tissue is only occasionally present, and reactive osteoid or bone is likely only to be present at the margins.

By contrast, giant cell granulomas typically contain smaller giant cells, which tend to be irregularly distributed but are often aggregated around foci of hemorrhage. The stroma is generally fibroblastic, and mitotic activity is scanty or absent. In the majority of cases there are trabeculae of osteoid or bone within the lesion.

HYPERPARATHYROIDISM

Bone lesions of hyperparathyroidism cannot be reliably distinguished histologically from nonendocrine central giant cell granulomas. Blood chemistry analysis should be carried out, and raised serum, calcium, alkaline phosphatase, and parathormone levels indicate hyperparathyroidism in which giant cell lesions are frequently multiple.

CHERUBISM

The microscopic features may be indistinguishable from giant cell granuloma, but lesions are symmetrical and young children are affected (see Ch. 17).

FIBROUS DYSPLASIA

A limited biopsy may show foci of giant cells, but the radiographic appearances, histological features, and behavior are distinctive (see Ch. 14).

ANEURYSMAL BONE CYSTS

Aneurysmal bone cysts may contain many giant cells but their other histological features (see Ch. 25), in particular the multiple blood-filled spaces, should enable the distinction to be made readily.

OSTEOSARCOMA

Some osteosarcomas contain many giant cells, but show far more cellular pleomorphism, hyperchromatism, and a variety of other cells often of indeterminate appearance as described below.

GIANT CELL GRANULOMAS OF PAGET'S DISEASE

Giant cell granulomas are well recognized as a complication of Paget's disease. They tend to affect the skull or facial skeleton, but are even more uncommon than osteosarcomas in Paget's disease. They usually become evident early in the course of severe disease and develop only in pagetic bones. Upchurch et al[14] concluded that the giant cell lesions of Paget's disease resembled giant cell 'reparative' granulomas rather than giant cell tumors. Bhambhani et al[15] described involvement of the mandible in a 59-year-old man with aggressively active Paget's disease. The microscopic appearances were similar to those of a giant cell granuloma or benign giant cell tumor.

These lesions are so uncommon that there is no definitive protocol for treatment. Treatment with bisphosphonates is likely to be the first choice, but the response of the patient reported by Bhambhani et al[15] to high-dose pamidronate was poor. Cure of the jaw lesion was only achieved by wide excision.

Noonan-like, multiple giant cell lesion syndrome

Cohen & Gorlin[16] described this uncommon syndrome of which the main features are short stature, low intelligence or delayed development, neck webbing, ocular hypertelorism, prominent ears, pectus excavatum, pulmonary stenosis and giant cell lesions of bones joints or soft tissues. Betts et al[17] have reported another patient with Noonan's syndrome where multiple giant cell lesions of the jaw and of the left index finger developed. Van Damme & Mooren[18] added a somewhat similar case in whom Noonan-like syndrome was associated with occult hyperparathyroidism.

If this syndrome is recognized, the chief oral problem is the multiplicity of giant cell lesions and their tendency to recur. A poor long-term prognosis in some cases may preclude repeated surgery.

Giant cell epulis (peripheral giant cell granuloma)

This lesion forms on the gingiva and, though it resembles a giant cell granuloma histologically, it is probably reactive and not related to the central giant cell granuloma.

CLINICAL FEATURES

Giant cell epulides form, as the term implies, on the gingival margins, usually in or near the anterior part of the mouth. They are typically soft and reddish purple in color, but cannot be distinguished reliably clinically from other hyperplastic nodules. They are usually approximately 1 cm in maximum dimension. Slight saucerization of the underlying bone may be seen radiographically, but this is not a distinctive feature. Almost any age can be affected and they are more frequent in females. Giansanti & Waldron[19] reviewed 720 examples, while Katsikeris et al[20] presented 224 new cases and reviewed no fewer than 956 reported examples.

MICROSCOPY

The nodule consists of multinucleated giant cells of varying size in a vascular stroma of ovoid and spindle-shaped fibroblasts. The giant cells carry the markers of macrophages. There is a covering of mucosal epithelium which is separated from the lesional tissue by a layer of dense fibrous connective tissue (Figs 18.7–18.10).

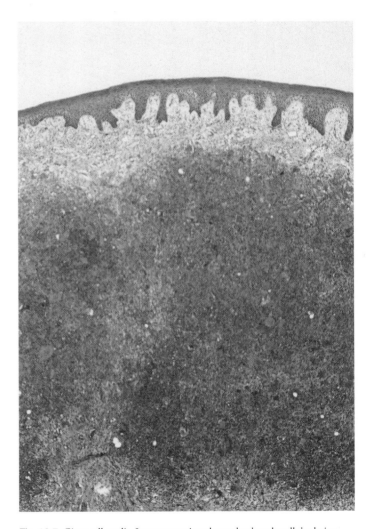

Fig. 18.7 Giant cell epulis. Low-power view shows the densely cellular lesion separated from the epithelial covering by the lamina propria.

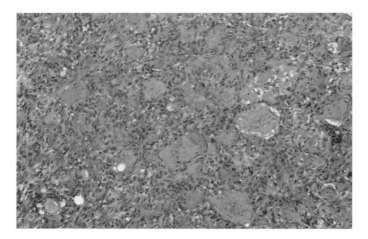

Fig. 18.8 Giant cell epulis. Higher power view shows the giant cells with varying numbers of nuclei in a vascular stroma of plump spindle cells.

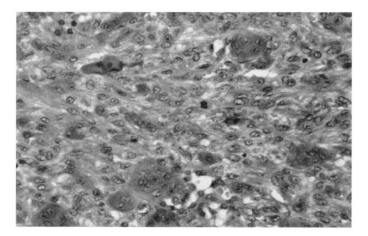

Fig. 18.9 Giant cell epulis. Mitoses are occasionally seen among the stromal cells, but do not appear to affect behavior.

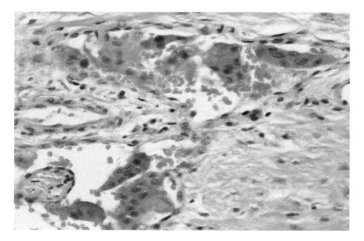

Fig. 18.10 Giant cell epulis. Giant cells may sometimes be seen in lymphatics; this is of no prognostic significance.

Hemorrhage into the mass frequently leaves deposits of hemosiderin. Ulceration of the surface is associated with inflammatory cells infiltrating the mass. In some cases there is considerable fibrous proliferation leaving a small central focus of giant cells. This appears to be a healing reaction.

Despite histologic similarities the giant cell epulis appears to bear no relationship to the central giant cell granuloma as mentioned earlier, and does not behave like the latter. However central giant cell granulomas can rarely erode through the bone to appear on the alveolar ridge, but then appear as a broad-based sessile, purplish-red elevation of the mucosa, with an extensive area of radiolucency beneath. Rarely also a giant cell epulis is due to hyperparathyroidism[21] and is then likely to be associated with other lesions in bones and changes in the blood chemistry.

BEHAVIOR AND MANAGEMENT

Giant cell epulides respond to simple excision with removal of any source of local irritation. Recurrence is uncommon but Katsikeris et al[20] considered from their analysis of reports that it might be between 5% and 10%. However the completeness of the excisions in such cases may possibly be questioned.

REFERENCES

1. Jaffe HL 1953 Giant cell reparative granuloma, traumatic bone cysts and fibrous (fibro-osseous) dysplasia of the jaw-bones. Oral Surg Oral Med Oral Pathol 6: 159–175
2. Whitaker SB, Waldron CA 1993 Central giant cell lesions of the jaws. A clinical, radiologic and histopathologic study. Oral Surg Oral Med Oral Pathol 75: 199–208
3. Waldron CA, Shafer WG 1966 The central reparative giant cell reparative granuloma of the jaws. Am J Clin Pathol 45: 437–447
4. Wu PC, Chan KW 1985 A survey of tumours of the jawbones in Hong Kong Chinese: 1963–1982. Br J Oral Maxillofac Surg 23: 92–102
5. Kaffe I, Ardekian L, Taicher S, Littner MM, Buchner A 1996 Radiologic features of central giant cell granuloma of the jaws. Oral Surg Oral Med Oral Pathol Oral Radiol Endod 81: 720–726
6. Franklin OD, Craig GT, Smith CJ 1979 Quantitative analysis of histologic parameters in giant cell lesions of the jaws and long bones. Histopathology 3: 511–522
7. Flanagan AM, Tinkler AMB, Horton MA, Williams DM, Chambers TJ 1988 The multinucleate cells in giant cell granulomas of the jaws are osteoclasts. Cancer 62: 1139–1145
8. Auclair PL, Cuenin P, Kratochvil FJ, Slater LJ, Ellis GL 1988 A clinical and histomorphologic comparison of the central giant cell granuloma and the giant cell tumor. Oral Surg Oral Med Oral Pathol 66: 197–208
9. Fechner RE, Mills SE 1992 Tumors of the bones and joints. Atlas of tumor pathology. Armed Forces Institute of Pathology, Washington, DC, third series, fascicle 8
10. Wold LE, Dobyns JH, Swee RG, Dahlin DC 1986 Giant cell reaction (giant cell reparative granuloma) of the small bones of the hands and feet. Am J Surg Pathol 10: 491–496
11. Whitaker SB, Vigneswaram N, Budnick SD, Waldron CA 1993 Giant cell granulomas of the jaws: evaluation of nucleolar organiser regions in lesions of varying behaviour. J Oral Pathol Med 22: 402–405
12. Harris M 1993 Central giant cell granulomas regress with calcitonin therapy. Br J Oral Maxillofac Surg 31: 89–94
13. Mintz GA, Abrams AM, Carlsen GD, Melrose RJ, Fister HW 1981 Primary malignant giant cell tumor of the mandible. Report of a case. Oral Surg Oral Med Oral Pathol 51: 164–171
14. Upchurch KS, Lee SS, Schiller AL, Rosenthal DI, Campion EW, Krane SM 1983 Giant cell reparative granuloma of Paget's disease: a unique clinical entity. Ann Intern Med 98: 35–40
15. Bhambhani M, Lamberty BGH, Clements MR, Skingle SJ, Crisp AJ 1992 Giant cell tumours in mandible and spine: a rare complication of Paget's disease of bone. Ann Rheumat Dis 51: 1335–1337

16. Cohen MM, Gorlin RJ 1991 Noonan-like giant cell lesion syndrome. Am J Med Genet 40: 159–166

17. Betts NJ, Stewart JCB, Fonseca RJ, Scott RF 1993 Multiple central giant cell lesions with a Noonan-like phenotype. Oral Surg Oral Med Oral Pathol 76: 601–607

18. Van Damme Ph A, Mooren RECM 1994 Differentiation of multiple giant cell lesions, Noonan-like syndrome, and (occult) hyperparathyroidism. Int J Oral Maxillofac Surg 23: 32–36

19. Giansanti JS, Waldron CA 1969 Peripheral giant cell granuloma: review of 720 cases. J Oral Surg 17: 787–791

20. Katsikeris N, Kakarantza-Angelopoulou E, Angelopoulos AP 1988 Peripheral giant cell granuloma: clinicopathologic study of 224 new cases and review of 956 reported cases. Int J Oral Maxillofac Surg 17: 94–99

21. Smith BR, Fowler CB, Svane TJ 1988 Primary hyperparathyroidism presenting as a 'peripheral' giant cell granuloma. J Oral Maxillofac Surg 46: 65–69

Odontogenic cysts

Cysts of the jaws: general considerations

19

With few exceptions, jaw cysts fulfil the criteria of being pathologic, fluid-filled cavities lined by epithelium. Cysts are common in the jaws because of the presence of epithelium involved in tooth development and, in particular, of epithelial rests remaining in the jaws afterwards. The latter give rise to radicular cysts (see Ch. 23), which account for approximately 55% of all jaw cysts. Only a few (simple and aneurysmal bone cysts) lack an epithelial lining or fluid contents. Cysts are the most common cause of chronic swellings of the jaws, but few pose significant diagnostic or management difficulties for competent surgeons.

The great majority of jaw cysts are odontogenic and usually radicular. They can be recognized by the history, and clinical and radiographic features. It is only rarely that the microscopic findings fail to confirm this assessment. However, it must always be borne in mind that, radiographically, ameloblastoma (see Ch. 3) is the great deceiver. The classification of jaw cysts is shown in Table 19.1.

RELATIVE FREQUENCY OF DIFFERENT TYPES OF CYST

The analysis by Ahlfors et al[1] of the relative frequency of the different types from a sample of 5914 jaw cysts is shown in Table 19.2. Shear's series[2] of 2616 jaw cysts showed the distribution given in Table 19.3. This latter series included both odontogenic and nonodontogenic cysts and other cyst-like lesions, but this last group was so small as not to bias the figures significantly. It was also based on a population with a large African component and Shear (1992) quotes the relative incidence of individual types of jaw cyst in the different populations.

A more recent series reported by Kreidler et al[3] was based on 367 lesions in a European population (Table 19.4). It includes other entities such unicystic ameloblastomas, but excludes many other types of cyst that were included by Shear.[2]

In earlier series, odontogenic keratocysts show a wide variation in incidence because of differences in the diagnostic criteria used.

The majority of cysts of the jaw show a similar pattern of slow expansive growth. They differ mainly in their relationship to a

Table 19.1 Classification of jaw cysts

Odontogenic cysts
Developmental
Dentigerous
Eruption
Gingival cysts:
– dental lamina cyst
– adult gingival cyst
Lateral periodontal, botryoid, and glandular odontogenic cysts
Odontogenic keratocysts
Inflammatory
Periodontal (radicular) and residual
Paradental
Neoplastic
Cystic ameloblastomas.
Calcifying odontogenic cyst
Neoplasia developing in pre-existing cysts
Nonodontogenic cysts
Nasopalatine duct cyst
Globulomaxillary cyst
Nasolabial (soft tissue cyst)
Midline cysts
Pseudocysts
Simple (solitary) bone cyst
Aneurysmal bone cyst
Stafne bone cavitieson

Table 19.2 Percentage distribution of 5914 jaw cysts (after Ahlfors et al[1])

Cyst type	%
Radicular	58.2
Juxtaradicular	0.5
Residual	12.0
(Total radicular cysts	70.7)
Unspecified	0.1
Keratocyst	5.4
Follicular	18.6
Lateral periodontal	0.8
Globulomaxillary	0.3
Nasopalatine	3.5
Median palatine	0.05
Aneurysmal bone cyst	0.05
Traumatic bone cyst	0.5

Table 19.3 Percentage distribution of 2616 jaw cysts (after Shear[2])

Cyst type	%
Radicular/residual	52.3
Dentigerous	16.6
Keratocyst	11.2
Nasopalatine	11.0
Paradental	2.5
Solitary	1.0
Calcifying odontogenic	1.0
Eruption	0.8
Lateral periodontal	0.7
Nasolabial	0.7
Globulomaxillary	0.5
Gingival cyst of adults	0.5
Inflammatory collateral	0.5
Aneurysmal bone cyst	0.5
Postoperative maxillary	0.2
Mucosal cyst of maxillary antrum	0.1

Table 19.4 Relative frequency of the major different types of cystic lesions of the jaws (after Kreidler et al[3])

Cyst type	%
Radicular and residual cysts	56.9
Dentigerous cysts	21.3
Odontogenic keratocysts	10.6
Unicystic ameloblastomas	4.1
Nasopalatine duct cysts	2.7
Glandular odontogenic cysts	1.6
Paradental, traumatic, calcifying odontogenic and lateral periodontal cysts	> 1

Table 19.5 Differential diagnosis of radiolucent cyst-like lesions of the jaws

1. Cysts:
   Odontogenic
   Nonodontogenic

2. Tumors
   Odontogenic
   Nonodontogenic (including metastases)

3. Tumor-like lesions (giant cell granuloma)

4. Hyperparathyroidism

5. Cherubism

6. Stafne bone cavity

7. Solitary bone cyst

8. Aneurysmal bone cyst

9. Anatomical structures (antrum, nasal airways, incisive canal fossa)

Table 19.6 Major characteristics of jaw cysts*

Cyst type	Typical site/ relationship to teeth	Male/ female ratio	Age range (years)	Radiographic features
Radicular periodontal	At apex of nonvital tooth	3 : 2	20–50	Unilocular
Residual	Causative tooth exracted	Equal	≥ 50	Unilocular
Paradental	Related to inflamed third molar follicle	4 : 1	20–29	Unilocular, over roots of third molar
Dentigerous	Upper 3s. Lower 8s	2 : 1	10–40	Unilocular. Contains crown of tooth
Keratocyst (parakeratinized)	Frequently molar region. Impacted tooth in 50%±	2 : 1	40± (mean)	Multilocular
Keratocyst (orthokeratinized)	Frequently molar region	3 : 2	34± (mean)	Usually unilocular. 'Dentigerous' in 40%±
Nasopalatine	Midline. Anterior maxilla	Almost equal	40± (mean)	Unilocular. Sometimes heart-shaped
Nasolabial	Soft tissues, deep to alae nasi, but may saucerize underlying bone	1 : 4	30–50 (peak)	Unilocular depression of bone of labial surface of maxilla
Calcifying odontogenic cyst	Majority in incisor–canine region	?	?	Unilocular. Sometimes flecked with calcifications. Teeth vital. Associated odontoma in 25%

*So-called globulomaxillary and median mandibular cysts are excluded due to a lack of evidence that they are separate entities.

Demography

The age, gender and site distribution of cysts is discussed exhaustively by Shear.[2] It is considerably complicated by such factors as apparent racial differences, differences in the incidence of the same cyst at different ages in males and females, and the sources of the data. Such data will therefore be only briefly summarized in the following sections.

tooth: this and the radiographic features are usually an adequate guide as to their nature (Tables 19.5 and 19.6). Even if it is impossible to decide the precise nature of a cyst this rarely affects treatment. However, it is essential to distinguish odontogenic keratocysts and cystic ameloblastomas from radicular or dentigerous cysts. These occasionally have identical radiographic appearances and diagnosis ultimately depends on microscopy.

REFERENCES

1. Ahlfors E, Larsson A, Sjögren S 1984 The odontogenic keratocyst: a benign cystic tumour? J Oral Maxillofac Surg 42: 10–19
2. Shear M 1992 Cysts of the oral regions, 3rd edn. Wright, Bristol
3. Kreidler JF, Raubenheimer EJ, van Heerdem WFP 1993 A retrospective analysis of 367 cystic lesions of the jaws – the Ulm experience. J Cranio-Maxillo-Fac Surg 21: 339–341

Odontogenic keratocysts 20

These cysts, which were given the name odontogenic keratocysts by Philipsen,[1] are uncommon but important because of their peculiarly infiltrative mode of growth and strong tendency to recur after removal. The earlier term *primordial cyst* was retained by Hoffman et al[2] for a lesion that they regarded as a distinct entity, but has otherwise been discarded.

INCIDENCE

The quoted frequency of odontogenic keratocysts varies widely, probably as a result in variations in the criteria used for diagnosis. In large series they have formed 5–11% of jaw cysts.[3,4] The frequency in other published series has ranged from 1.5%[3], to 17.4% of odontogenic cysts.[5,6]

Rachanis & Shear[7] have calculated age-standardized incidence rates for odontogenic keratocysts in the Witwatersrand of South Africa. The results were remarkably consistent, with rates of 0.67 to 0.61 per million for black males, 0 for black females, 4.78 to 5.37 per million for white males, and 3.5 to 3.64 per million for white females. Earlier, Brannon,[3] from an analysis of 312 odontogenic keratocysts from 283 patients, found the male/female ratio to be 1.35 : 1, and Haring & van Dis[8] from their 60 cases also found a male/female ratio of 1.3 : 1. By contrast, Ahlfors et al,[4] from their series of 255 odontogenic keratocysts, found males to be affected twice as frequently as females.

Keratocysts are seen over a wide age range. In an analysis of 106 cases, Shear[9] found the ages to range from 10 to 79 years, with a peak between 10 and 39 years. However, the age-specific morbidity rates that he calculated for the Witwatersrand (1965–1974) showed a bimodal distribution, with peaks in the age ranges 10–29 years and 50–64 years, with the highest rate being in the older age group. Ahlfors et al[4] also found a major peak of frequency in the age range 25–34 years and a smaller one at 55–64 years for 225 keratocysts, while Haring & van Dis[8] from their 60 cases also found a striking bimodal distribution, with peaks at ages 21–30 years and 61–70 years.

Woolgar et al[10] found that in 60 patients with the basal cell naevus (Gorlin–Goltz) syndrome the peak incidence was at age 19–29 years, with a sharp decline thereafter. The inclusion of such cases partly accounts for the bimodal age distribution seen in several series, but Rippin & Woolgar[11] confirmed that in 379 non-syndrome patients there were broad peaks of incidence between the ages of 19 and 49 years and again between 59 and 79 years.

A more recently evaluated variable that apparently affects age and gender distribution is the type of keratinization in the cyst. The analysis of 449 cases by Crowley et al[12] showed that the mean age of those with parakeratinized cysts was 39.6 years while that for the orthokeratinized type was 33.8 years. The analysis confirmed the considerably higher overall frequency of odontogenic keratocysts among whites and males, who acccounted for 61.8% of cases.

Among 319 keratocysts analyzed by Ahlfors et al,[4] parakeratinized cysts were more than twice as frequent in males as females, but for the 11 orthokeratinized cysts males and females were virtually equally represented. Among 49 odontogenic keratocysts analyzed by Crowley et al,[12] males also accounted for 61.8% of cases, but for orthokeratinized cysts males accounted for only 56.6%.

Between 70% and 75% of keratocysts have been in the mandible. Overall, the angle is the most frequent site and the cyst typically extends for variable distances into the ramus and forwards into the body. Extension of the cavity up the ramus, even into the neck of the condyle, is characteristic.

The only significant difference in site of predilection between para- and orthokeratinized cysts analyzed by Crowley et al[12] was that 16.3% of the orthokeratinized but only 5.7% of the parakeratinized type were in the midline.

CLINICAL FEATURES

The lack of significant symptoms arising from odontogenic keratocysts gives no warning of the difficulties of managing them. They are typically symptomless until the bone has expanded or they become infected. The main difference from the more common odontogenic cysts is that expansion of the jaw is much less than would be expected from the radiographic extent of the lesion. Hence there are often no clinical signs until the cyst is well advanced, and occasionally extensive cysts are found by chance on routine radiographs in asymptomatic patients.

Occasional effects of odontogenic keratocysts include pain, discharge, and paresthesiae.

RADIOGRAPHY

Keratocysts appear as well-defined radiolucent areas. Parakeratotic cysts are typically multilocular or rounded with a scalloped margin. Orthokeratotic keratocysts are frequently unilocular, as were all but one of the 12 reported by Vuhahala et al.[13] A multilocular keratocyst may be difficult to differentiate from an ameloblastoma radiographically, but the bony wall of a keratocyst is typically sclerotic and appears as a more sharply demarcated cortex.

Sometimes a keratocyst may envelop an unerupted tooth and simulate a dentigerous cyst. In the series analyzed by Crowley et al,[12] 75.5% of the orthokeratinized but only 47.8% of parakeratinized cysts were associated with impacted teeth. They also found that 40% of orthokeratinized cysts but only 22.5% of parakeratinized cysts had appeared radiographically as dentigerous cysts. Sixteen of their 449 odontogenic keratocysts had appeared to be lateral periodontal cysts. Nine of the 12 orthokeratinized cysts reported by Vuhahala et al[13] had been interpreted radiographically as dentigerous cysts (Fig. 20.1).

As they enlarge, keratocysts tend to displace the roots of adjacent teeth.

MICROSCOPY

Odontogenic keratocysts can be categorized as *orthokeratotic* or *parakeratotic*. The latter, which form over 85% of keratocysts, have a considerably higher recurrence rate.

Despite the term 'odontogenic keratocyst' the majority of keratocysts, namely the parakeratotic type, fail to form significant amounts of keratin. Even radicular or dentigerous cysts can occasionally show metaplastic keratinization, but they lack any tendency to recur after enucleation.

The wall of odontogenic keratocysts is thin and the lining has the following characteristic features (Figs 20.2–20.9):

- The epithelium is of uniform thickness, typically about 7–10 cells thick without rete ridges.

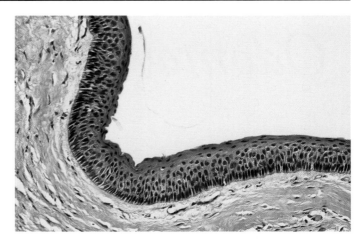

Fig. 20.2 Odontogenic keratocyst, parakeratinized type. The lining is of uniform thickness with a prominent basal cell layer.

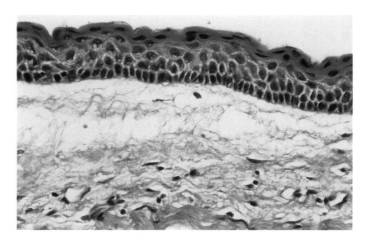

Fig. 20.3 Odontogenic keratocyst, parakeratinized type. Higher power view confirms the uniform thickness of the epithelial lining, the prominent columnar basal cell layer, the thin eosinophilic parakeratin, and the tenuous attachment to the fibrous wall.

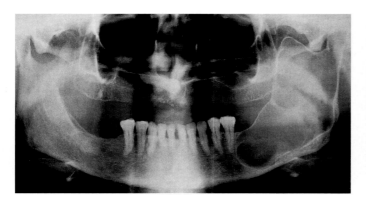

Fig. 20.1 Odontogenic keratocyst. This example shows an extensive radiolucent area with a well-defined anterior margin, and extends from the premolar region into the condyle and coronoid processes. The appearance is readily mistaken for that of an ameloblastoma.

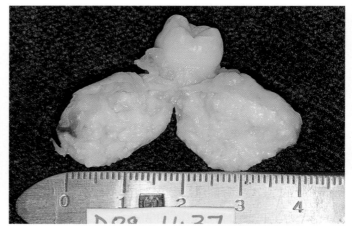

Fig. 20.4 Odontogenic keratocyst, orthokeratinized type with dentigerous relationship. The specimen has been bisected to show the solid keratinous contents.

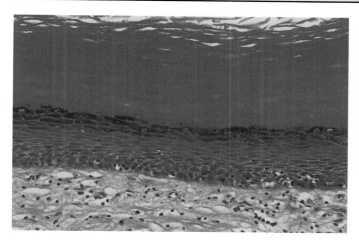

Fig. 20.5 Odontogenic keratocyst, orthokeratinized type. The flattened lining has a prominent granular cell layer and many layers of laminated keratin.

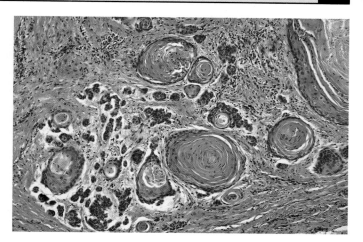

Fig. 20.8 Odontogenic keratocyst. Higher power view of daughter cysts containing keratin whorls and numerous small islands of odontogenic epithelium.

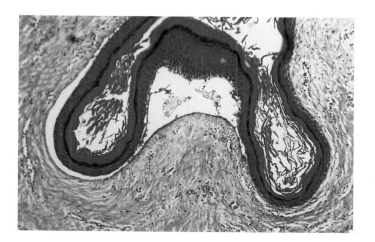

Fig. 20.6 Odontogenic keratocyst. The convolutions of the lining and its separation from the fibrous wall are common findings.

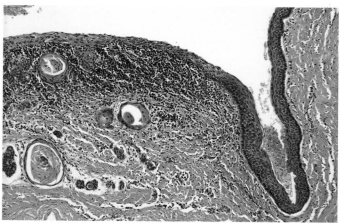

Fig. 20.9 Odontogenic keratocyst, parakeratinized type. Inflammation has destroyed the characteristic features of part of the lining.

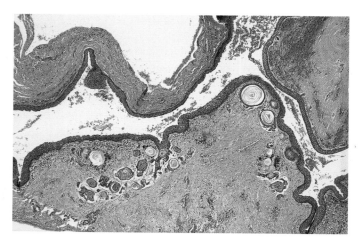

Fig. 20.7 Odontogenic keratocyst. Multiple daughter microcysts are present.

- The squamous epithelium has a clearly defined, palisaded layer of tall basal cells in the parakeratotic type, and a prickle cell layer, which forms the bulk of the epithelium, which is often much folded. In the orthokeratotic type, the basal cell layer is cuboidal or flattened.
- Keratin formation amounts to no more than a thin eosinophilic layer of parakeratin in the parakeratotic variant. In the orthokeratotic variant there is a well-defined granular cell layer, and keratin formation may be so abundant as to fill the cyst cavity with semi-solid material.
- The epithelial lining, particularly of parakeratotic cysts, frequently appears to be thrown up into folds.
- The fibrous wall is thin and often loose or myxoid. Unlike other odontogenic cysts, the epithelial lining is weakly attached to and readily separates from the underlying connective tissue.

Table 20.1 Important features of keratocysts

	Parakeratotic cyst	Orthokeratotic cyst
Relative frequency (approx.) (%)	88	12
Gender* (%)		
Male	62	57
Female	38	43
Mean age at presentation (years)	34	40
Association with impacted tooth (%)	48	76
Midline location (%)	6	16
Pain (%)	15	9
Radiographic appearance	Usually multilocular	Frequently monolocular
Recurrence (%)	43	4

* Overall: M, 61.5%; F, 38.5%.

- Occasionally, daughter cysts or epithelial islands are present in the cyst wall, particularly when the patient has the jaw cysts, naevoid basal cell carcinoma (Gorlin–Goltz) syndrome.
- Inflammatory cells are typically absent or scanty. If significant inflammation is superimposed, the characteristic appearances of the epithelium are lost, so that the lining resembles that of a radicular cyst. Confirmation then depends on finding uninflamed areas of typical epithelium.

Dysplasia in the lining of odontogenic keratocysts has been reported by Ruud & Pindborg[14] and by Ahlfors et al.[4]

The chief clinical and radiographic features of these two types of cyst are summarized in Table 20.1, but in essence the main differences are in the microscopic appearances and in the fact that the parakeratotic variant appears to have the strongest tendency to recur.

The microscopic appearance of odontogenic keratocysts is, incidentally, closely similar if not identical to that of cholesteatomas. This is not to suggest that cholesteatomas are aberrant odontogenic keratocysts, but, rarely, other dental anomalies such as an odontoma have been described in the ear,[15,16] as has an ameloblastoma.[17]

HISTOGENESIS

Keratocysts are thought to have arisen from parts of the dental lamina. Nevertheless, if this is so, it is difficult to reconcile the frequent appearance of keratocysts in late middle age unless their growth is quite remarkably slow. The factors determining the development of these cysts are also unknown. In particular, keratocysts differ from other cysts in that proliferation of their lining rather than hydrostatic pressure is the main determinant of growth. Li et al[18] found that the index of proliferation of suprabasal cells of keratocysts was significantly higher (94.4 ± 22.7 proliferating cell nuclear antigen positive (PCNA+) cells/mm) than that of radicular cysts (11.0 ± 4.1 PCNA+ cells/mm) and was similar to that of oral

mucosal epithelium (80.8 ± 20.6 PCNA+ cells/mm). Toller,[19] using radioactive labeling of cyst lining explants to estimate mitotic activity, also found mean labeling indices of 13% for keratocysts, 1.7% for nonkeratotic jaw cysts, and 7% for human oral mucous membrane. He therefore suggested that, despite their slow growth, the lining may be proliferating more actively than cells of the oral mucosa. Possibly as a consequence of this high proliferative activity, keratocysts also tend to extend by finger-like processes along the lines of least resistance, namely the cancellous spaces. Hence these cysts may be of considerable size before they expand the jaw and cause a swelling. To accommodate this overgrowth, the cyst lining becomes greatly folded. This epithelial proliferation is probably a factor determining the frequency with which keratocysts recur and the difficulties in eradicating them, particularly if they are allowed to extend into the soft tissue. As a consequence, the lesion has been likened to a benign cystic neoplasm by Toller[20] and Ahlfors et al,[4] among others.

The possibility that p53 expression in keratocyst lining might be correlated with behavior has been explored, most recently by Lombardi et al (1995)[19]. They found overall, that staining was weak and speckled and that it bore no correlation with recurrence rates.

BEHAVIOR AND MANAGEMENT

Behavior

The overriding clinical problem with keratocysts is their strong tendency to recur after treatment. Shear,[9] in his meticulous survey of earlier reports, found recurrence rates ranging from 62% to 3%. Inevitably these figures reflect differences in the degree of rigor in the treatment of these cysts and the duration of follow-up, but there is, broadly speaking, a decline in the reported recurrence rates over the period 1963–1988 covered by Shear's survey. However, these earlier series take no account of differences in behavior between the ortho- and parakeratinized cysts. In a survey of 24 orthokeratotic cysts, Wright[21] found only a single recurrence and that the parakeratotic variant was more likely to recur. His conclusions were abundantly confirmed by Ahlfors et al,[4] who reported that all of their 105 parakeratinized but none of their orthokeratinized cysts recurred.

Crowley et al[12] found a recurrence rate of at least 46% in 387 parakeratinized cysts and only a single recurrence among 55 orthokeratinized cysts. They also found that 2.2% of the 449 cysts had linings that were partly orthokeratinized and partly parakeratinized, and these cysts had a similar recurrence rate to that of the entirely parakeratinized cysts.

Possible factors contributing to recurrence include the following.

- Keratocyst fibrous walls are thin and fragile and, particularly when the cysts are large, are very difficult to enucleate intact.
- The lining is weakly attached to the fibrous wall, readily separates from it, and may not be entirely removed with it.
- Extension of the cyst into cancellous bone increases the difficulty of removing the lining.

- Keratocysts may have in their periphery satellite daughter cysts, which may be left behind after enucleation of the main cyst.
- Evidence that the epithelial lining, particularly of parakeratinized cysts, is more vigorously proliferative than that of other cyst linings suggests that if a few epithelial cells remain they can readily form another cyst after enucleation of the main lesion.
- If, as seems likely, keratocysts develop from remnants of dental lamina, then other remnants of dental lamina might contribute to the formation of a second lesion that appears to be recurrent. The fact that recurrences have occasionally appeared several decades after the original operation suggests that new lesions of this sort can develop.

The reasons for the higher recurrence rate of parakeratinized cysts are not clear. However the fact that cysts with mixed-type linings have a recurrence rate consistent with the parakeratinized component suggests that the proliferative capacity of the latter is a major determinant.

The time of recurrence is very variable. It is typically within the first 5 years, but may, as already mentioned, be after many years.

Management

The diagnosis should preferably be confirmed before operation, in order to exclude an ameloblastoma. The quickest and most reliable method is by biopsy. Once the lesion has been opened, careful inspection will confirm whether the lesion is cystic, but is unlikely that it will be possible to differentiate an odontogenic keratocyst enclosing a tooth from a unicystic ameloblastoma with the same feature. However, the prognosis of these lesions is somewhat similar.

The consensus is that the more conservative the enucleation the greater the likelihood of recurrence. Once the diagnosis has been confirmed, treatment should be by complete enucleation, but this is usually difficult. The lining is friable (particularly if inflamed) and the cyst outline usually complex. However, treatment should be vigorous to try to ensure that every fragment of cyst lining has been removed, but this is difficult. Recommendations have ranged from simple enucleation with prolonged follow-up, to jaw resection and reconstruction.

Conservative treatment as advocated by Meiselman[22] is appropriate. The cyst should be opened widely and the bony margins cut back by at least 5 mm all round, to enable complete enucleation of the lining and fibrous wall. The bony wall can also be abraded with bone burs in an attempt to insure removal of traces of cyst lining. The overlying mucosa can also be excised to remove possible remnants of dental lamina which, though the possibility is controversial, might give rise to recurrences. El Haji & Anneroth,[23] who also noted an improvement in recurrence rates with the passage of time, found that 22% of nine keratocysts where adherent overlying mucosa had been removed, recurred, but 34% of 38 cysts recurred after adherent lining had been dissected from overlying mucosa. They also noted recurrence of 39% of keratocysts that had been removed piecemeal, but of only 27.5% of those

removed in one piece. Higher recurrence rates were noted in cases where enucleation was supplemented by cryosurgery than when enucleation alone was used, but presumably done more carefully. Though the orthokeratotic variant is less likely to recur, there is probably no justification for less thorough conservative treatment than for the parakeratotic type. However, resection is not required.

Vigorous treatment and, whenever possible, removal intact of every trace of the lining, is therefore advocated. However, there is no absolute certainty of a complete cure. Rarely, keratocysts have recurred in bone grafts after excision, as reported by DeGould & Goldberg[24] who reviewed four reports.

Keratocysts that have penetrated the cortex of the jaw can also continue to grow in the soft tissues, and are then even more difficult to eradicate. An even greater danger is that of penetration of the skull base, as happened in three cases reported by Jackson et al.[25]

Clearly, it is important to warn patients of the possible need for further operations and that they should have regular radiological examinations at intervals for an indefinite period. Any recurrences should be treated in a similar manner when they develop. However, by such methods, the morbidity is low and most teeth in relation to the cyst can be conserved.

Williams & Connor[26] advocate an aggressive approach because of the risk of extension, particularly of maxillary keratocysts, into soft tissues, because of the possibility of intracranial penetration. However, their procedure is largely similar to that of Meiselman,[22] apart from treating the bony walls, after enucleation and curettage with a fixative (Carnoy's solution) for 3 min.

Resection involves greater morbidity, tooth loss, and longer hospital stay, but needs to be considered for the rare large keratocysts of the posterior maxilla and those that have destroyed the lower border of the mandible. Williams & Connor[26] also advise resection for recurrent keratocysts.

Peripheral odontogenic keratocyst

Only a few examples of these lesions have been reported.[27,28] They have resembled adult gingival cysts clinically, and occasionally cause saucerization and focal fenestration of the underlying bone. Follow-up data were available for only one of these cases, which recurred 7 years after removal.

Naevoid basal cell carcinoma syndrome multiple jaw cysts, skeletal anomalies, and multiple basal cell carcinomas

This syndrome, often called the *Gorlin–Goltz syndrome*, is inherited as an autosomal dominant trait and includes the following main features:

- Multiple keratocysts of the jaws in approximately 85% of patients.
- Multiple, early onset basal cell carcinomas of the skin in over 50% of patients.
- Skeletal anomalies (usually of a minor nature), such as bifid ribs and abnormalities of the vertebrae.
- Characteristic facies with frontal and temporoparietal bossing and a broad nasal root in about 70% of cases.
- Intracranial anomalies frequently include a characteristic lamellar calcification of the falx cerebri, an abnormally shaped sella turcica, and occasionally intracranial tumors.

Many other findings have been reported (Table 20.2). The overall effects on the patient depend on the predominant manifestations. Thus in some cases there are many basal cell carcinomas, which can be disfiguring or troublesome in other ways. Though termed 'naevoid,' these tumors differ from typical basal cell carcinomas only in their early onset, and have even been seen in a 2-year-old child. In other patients the main problem is the many jaw cysts, which necessitate repeated operations.

Rippin and Woolgar[11] studied 60 patients with basal cell naevus syndrome, and found women to suffer odontogenic keratocysts slightly more frequently than men. Furthermore, in their survey of the literature they concluded that 4–5% of all patients with keratocysts had multiple cysts and other features of the syndrome,

and that a further 1% had other features of the syndrome but only a single keratocyst.

Bale et al[30] have demonstrated a chromosome 9q deletion in a patient, and genetic-linkage studies in a large kindred have indicated that the naevoid basal cell carcinoma syndrome gene maps to precisely the same location lost in tumors. These findings show that tumors arise as a result of homozygous inactivation of the gene, and imply that the normal gene has a tumor suppressor function.

MICROSCOPY

The cysts are usually of the parakeratotic type. Woolgar et al,[10] from a study of 164 syndrome cysts, found that 54% had satellite cysts and 34% had islands of epithelium in the walls, but of 164 nonsyndromal keratocysts only 11% and 8%, respectively showed these features.

BEHAVIOR AND MANAGEMENT

Patients should be warned of the possible need for repeated operations to remove jaw cysts and of other lesions typical of the syndrome. Referral to a dermatologist or other specialists may also be necessary.

The cysts must be managed like other keratocysts and enucleated intact if possible. If large, preliminary marsupialization to allow shrinkage of the cyst before enucleation has been recommended. If neglected, these cysts can give rise to any of the complications of other jaw cysts.

Table 20.2 Findings in adults with naevoid basal cell carcinoma syndrome (from Gorlin[29])

Features showing a frequency of ≥ 50%	Features showing a frequency of ≤14% but not random
Enlarged occipitofrontal circumference	Medulloblastoma (true frequency unknown)
Mild ocular hypertelorism	Inguinal hernia (?)
Multiple basal cell carcinomas	Meningioma
Odontogenic keratocysts of jaws	Lymphomesenteric cysts
Epidermal cysts of skin	Cardiac fibroma
Palmar and/or plantar pits	Fetal rhabdomyoma
Calcified ovarian cysts (probably overestimated frequency)	Ovarian fibrosarcoma
Calcified falx cerebri	Marfanoid build
Rib anomalies (splayed, fused, partially missing, bifid, etc.)	Agenesis of corpus callosum
Spina bifida occulta of cervical or thoracic vertebrae	Cyst of septum pellucidum
Calcified diaphragma sellae (bridged sella, fused clinoids)	Cleft lip and/or palate
Hyperpneumatization of paranasal sinuses	Polydactyly, postaxial (hands or feet)
	Sprengel deformity of scapula
Features showing a frequency of 15–49%	Congenital cataract, glaucoma, coloboma of iris, Medullated retinal nerve fibers
Calcification of tentorium cerebelli and petroclinoid ligament	Subcutaneous calcifications of skin (possibly underestimated frequency)
Short fourth metacarpals	Minor kidney malformations
Kyphoscoliosis or other vertebral anomalies	Hypogonadism in males
	Mental retardation

Mandibular cysts with sebaceous differentiation

Occasional reports have alluded to sebaceous differentiation in jaw cysts, and Brannon[3] mentioned that 33 of 312 odontogenic keratocysts contained sebaceous glands. The earliest detailed account was provided by Craig et al,[31] who termed the lesion a dermoid cyst of the mandible.

Christensen & Propper[32] presented another case and reviewed earlier reports. In their case, the cyst was lined mainly by keratinizing stratified squamous epithelium, with a flat epitheliomesenchymal junction and a generally well-defined basal cell layer. It was largely of uniform thickness, like an odontogenic keratocyst, but sometimes thicker in the regions of sebaceous tissue. Sebaceous tissue was scattered along the length of the lining, either in contact with or immediately subjacent to it, opening into the cyst cavity.

Sebaceous glands are common in the oral mucosa, but are not normally present within the jaws. It is uncertain, therefore, whether a jaw cyst containing sebaceous glands should be categorized as a variant of an odontogenic keratocyst or as a dermoid cyst.

REFERENCES

1. Philipsen HP 1956 Om Keratocytes (kolesteatomer) i kaeberne. Tandlaegebladet 60: 963–980
2. Hoffman S, Jacoway JR, Krolls SO 1987 Intraosseous and parosteal tumors of the jaws. Atlas of tumor pathology. Armed Forces Institute of Pathology, Washington, DC, second series Fascicle 24
3. Brannon RB 1976 The odontogenic keratocyst. A clinicopathologic study of 312 cases. Part I. Clinical features. Oral Surg Oral Med Oral Pathol 42: 54–72
4. Ahlfors E, Larsson A, Sjögren S 1984 The odontogenic keratocyst: a benign cystic tumour? J Oral Maxillofac Surg 42: 10–19
5. Hoffmeister B, Härle F 1985 Zysten im Kiefer-Gesichtbereich – eine katamnestiche. Studie an 3353 Zysten. Deutsche Zahnärtzl Zschrft 40: 610–614
6. Radden BG, Reade PC 1973 Odontogenic cysts. A review and clinicopathological study of 368 odontogenic cysts. Austr Dent J 18: 218–225
7. Rachanis CC, Shear M 1978 Age-standardised incidence rates of primordial (keratocyst) on the Witwatersrand. Comm Dent Oral Epidemiol 6: 296–299
8. Haring JI, van Dis ML 1988 Odontogenic keratocysts: a clinical, radiographic and histopathologic study. Oral Surg Oral Med Oral Pathol 66: 145–153
9. Shear M 1992 Cysts of the oral regions, 3rd edn. Wright, Bristol
10. Woolgar JA, Rippin JW, Browne RM 1987 A comparative histological study of odontogenic keratocysts in basal cell naevus syndrome and control patients. J Oral Pathol 16: 75–80
11. Rippin JW, Woolgar JA 1991 In Browne RM (ed) Investigative pathology of odontogenic cysts. CRC Press, Boca Raton, FL
12. Crowley TE, Kaugars GE, Gunsolley JC 1992 Odontogenic keratocysts: a clinical and histologic comparison of the parakeratin and orthokeratin variants. J Oral Maxillofac Surg 50: 22–26
13. Vuhahala E, Nikai H, Ijuhin N et al 1993 Jaw cysts with orthokeratinization: analysis of 12 cases. J Oral Pathol Med 22: 35–40
14. Rud J, Pindborg JJ 1969 Odontogenic keratocysts: a follow-up study of 21 cases. J Oral Surg 323–330
15. Bellucci RJ, Zizmore J, Goodwin RE 1975 Odontoma of the middle ear. Arch Otolaryngol 101: 571–573
16. Prasad S, Hirsch B, Kamerer DB, Curtin H 1991 Odontoma of the middle ear cleft. Am J Otol 12: 452–454
17. Klinger KI, McManis JC 1969 Soft tissue ameloblastoma. Oral Surg 28: 266–270
18. Li T-J, Browne RM, Matthews JB 1994 Quantification of PCNA+ cells within odontogenic jaw cyst epithelium. J Oral Pathol Med 23: 184–189
19. Toller PA 1971 Autoradiography of explants from odontogenic cysts. Br Dent J 131: 57–61
20. Toller PA 1967 Origin and growth of cysts of the jaws. Ann R Coll Surg 40: 306–336
21. Wright JM 1981 The odontogenic keratocyst: orthokeratinized variant. Oral Surg Oral Med Oral Pathol 51: 609–618
22. Meiselman F 1994 Surgical management of the odontogenic keratocyst: conservative approach. J Oral Maxillofac Surg 520: 960–963
23. El Haji G, Anneroth G 1996 Odontogenic keratocysts – a retrospective clinical and histological study. Intl J Oral Maxillofac Surg 25: 124–129
24. DeGould MD, Goldberg JS 1991 Recurrence of an odontogenic keratocyst in a bone graft. Report of a case. Intl J Oral Maxillofac Surg 20: 9–11
25. Jackson IT, Potparie Z, Fasching M, Shievink WI, Tidstrom K, Hussain K 1993 J Cranio Max Fac Surg 21: 319–325
26. Williams TP, Connor FA 1994 Surgical management of the odontogenic keratocyst: aggressive approach. J Oral Maxillofac Surg 520: 964–966
27. Dayan D, Buchner A, Gorsky M, Harel-Raviv M 1988 The peripheral odontogenic keratocyst. Intl J Oral Maxillofac Surg 17: 81–83
28. Chehade A, Daley TD, Wysocki GP, Miller AS 1994 Peripheral odontogenic keratocyst. Oral Surg Oral Med Oral Pathol 77: 494–497
29. Gorlin RJ 1987 Naevoid basal cell carcinoma syndrome. Medicine 66: 98–113
30. Bale AE, Gailani MR, Leffel DJ 1994 Nevoid basal cell carcinoma syndrome. J Invest Dermatol 103: 126S–130S
31. Craig GT, Holland CS, Hindle MO 1980 Dermoid cyst of the mandible. Br J Oral Surg 18: 237–239
32. Christensen RE, Propper RH 1982 Intraosseous mandibular cyst with sebaceous differentiation. Oral Surg 53: 591–595

Follicular cysts 21

Dentigerous cysts

A dentigerous cyst surrounds the crown of an unerupted tooth. It is attached to the neck of the tooth and is, in effect, an expanded follicle.

INCIDENCE

Dentigerous cysts account for approximately 18% of jaw cysts (see Tables 19.1–19.3). Shear & Singh[1] showed that dentigerous cysts were considerably more frequent among whites than blacks and more frequent in white males than white females. They showed that the age-standardized incidence rates for dentigerous cysts on the Witwatersrand, South Africa, per million per year, ranged from 1.09 to 1.22 for black males, 1.18 to 1.39 for black females, 9.92 to 10.83 for white males, and 7.26 to 8.04 for white females.

The higher frequency of dentigerous cysts in whites than blacks seems to be related to the higher frequency of impacted teeth in whites. In a radiographic study, Brown et al[2] showed that impacted teeth were present in 22.2% of blacks but in 34.8% of whites.

Although dentigerous cysts can be seen in early childhood the incidence rises progressively, reaching a peak in the decade 30–39 years. It then declines gradually, but dentigerous cysts are still occasionally seen in the eighth decade.

As mentioned above, the frequency of dentigerous cysts is slightly greater in males than females in South Africa and also in Europe.[3,4]

The location of dentigerous cysts varies with the age of the patients, but overall the great majority surround a mandibular third molar and somewhat fewer involve a maxillary canine. Among 184 dentigerous cysts analyzed by Shear,[5] 122 were in the mandible and 62 were in the maxilla. Eighty-four involved a mandibular third molar, 36 involved a maxillary canine, 23 involved a mandibular premolar, and other teeth were only occasionally affected.

CLINICAL FEATURES

Like other cysts, if uncomplicated, dentigerous cysts cause no symptoms until the swelling becomes obtrusive or infection supervenes. Frequently, dentigerous cysts are detected by chance on radiographs or when the cause of a missing tooth is sought. Infection causes the usual symptoms of pain and greater swelling.

RADIOGRAPHY

The appearance is characteristic; namely, a well-defined radiolucent cystic area surrounding the crown of an unerupted and displaced tooth (Fig. 21.1). The cavity is rounded and unilocular, but occasionally, trabeculation or ridging of the bony wall appears as pseudoloculation. The slow, regular growth of these cysts usually results in a sclerotic bony outline and a well-defined cortex. The affected tooth is often displaced a considerable distance; a third

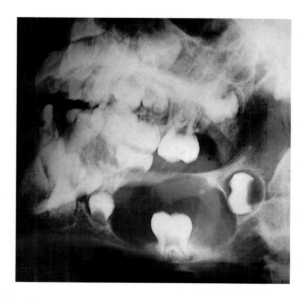

Fig. 21.1 Dentigerous cyst. The rounded area of well-defined radiolucency extends the full depth of the mandible and has displaced the enclosed molar tooth to the lower border. The attachment of the cyst to the cervical region of the tooth can be seen.

molar, for example, may be pushed to the lower border of the mandible or, more rarely, into the neck of the condyle. Occasionally, the tooth within a dentigerous cyst is a supernumerary. A dentigerous cyst in the lower third molar region may become very large and extend into the coronoid process and condylar neck. Occasionally, a keratocyst may envelop the crown of the tooth, as may an ameloblastoma, and either may produce a radiographic appearance simulating exactly a dentigerous cyst. Microscopy of the cyst lining is therefore essential.

MICROSCOPY

Browne[6] has described in detail the histological features. The lining typically consists of flattened or cuboidal epithelium, usually about five cells thick, attached to the neck of a tooth. Mucous (goblet) cells are present in about 40% of cases, and sometimes are so numerous as to form a continuous layer in part of the lining. Ciliated cells may also very occasionally be seen. The epithelium may, rarely, undergo metaplastic keratinization. The connective tissue capsule is moderately cellular and sometimes contains a few chronic inflammatory cells. It usually also contains epithelial rests, which are typically more numerous close to the attachment of the cyst to the tooth. Cholesterol clefts may also be seen (Figs 21.2–21.6).

HISTOGENESIS

Dentigerous cysts arise as a result of cystic change in the remains of the enamel organ after enamel formation is complete. Occasionally, the division between the remnants of the internal enamel epithelium and the external enamel epithelium forming the main cyst lining can be seen microscopically at the attachment

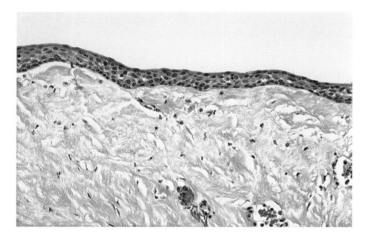

Fig. 21.2 Dentigerous cyst. Higher power view of the thin, regular lining of nonkeratinized squamous epithelium.

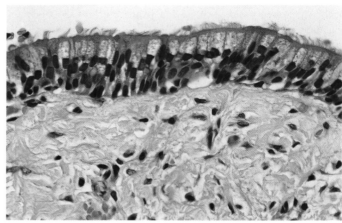

Fig. 21.4 Dentigerous cyst. Ciliated epithelium is sometimes present.

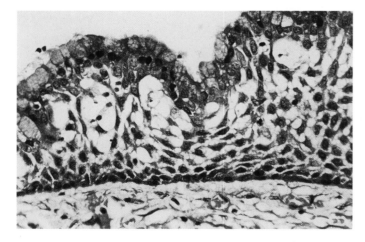

Fig. 21.3 Dentigerous cyst. Extensive mucous metaplasia in the lining is a frequent finding.

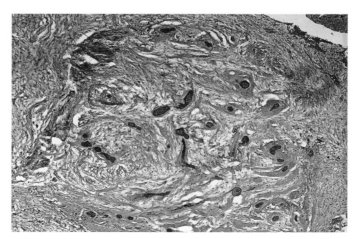

Fig. 21.5 Dentigerous cyst. Numerous inactive epithelial rests are present in the cyst wall.

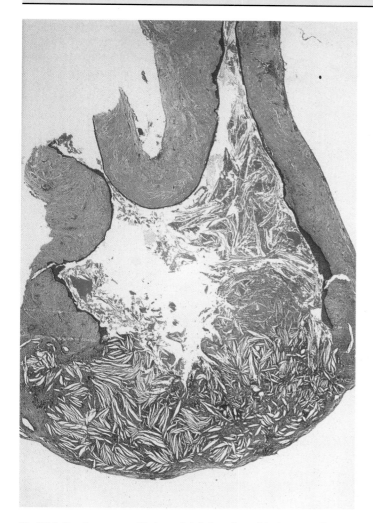

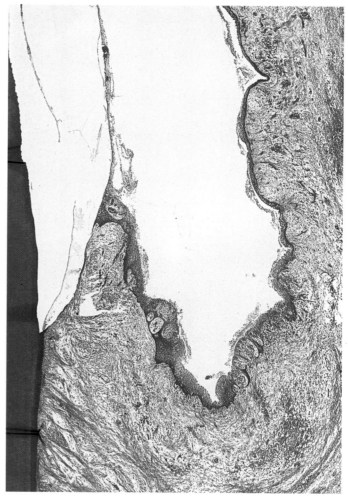

Fig. 21.6 Dentigerous cyst. Cholesterol clefts have formed in the cyst wall as a result of breakdown of blood cells, and have extended into the cyst cavity.

Fig. 21.7 Dentigerous cyst. Reduced enamel epithelium separates the enamel space (left) from the cyst cavity (right).

of the cyst to the neck of the tooth (Figs 21.7 and 21.8). Though such a cyst appears to form between the layers of the reduced enamel epithelium, the layer that remains attached to the surface of the enamel is usually of negligible thickness and the enamel is in direct contact with the cyst contents. The cyst lining originates from the major part of the reduced enamel epithelium, and progressive growth of the cyst leads to dilatation of the dental follicle.

Immunohistochemistry has not as yet contributed greatly to determining the histogenesis of dentigerous cysts, but it has shown some differences in the keratin patterns between these and other odontogenic cysts. Hormia et al[7] showed that keratocysts, radicular cysts, and most dentigerous cysts lacked high-molecular-weight keratins typical of keratinizing squamous epithelia. Only dentigerous cysts, like some ameloblastomas, expressed cytokeratin 18, so that there might be a histogenetic variant of dentigerous cysts distinct from those that arise by splitting of the reduced enamel epithelium. Matthews et al[8] demonstrated that keratins 13 and 19 were sufficiently consistently expressed by dentigerous cysts, odontogenic keratocysts, and radicular cysts to be useful

markers of odontogenic epithelium. Seven examples of dentigerous cysts also stained positively for pankeratin, CEA, EMA, and rat liver antigen (RLA). The numbers of nuclei expressing Ki67 indicated proliferative activity intermediate between that of odontogenic keratocysts and radicular cysts. They suggested that the more heterogeneous, weak reactivity for keratin 19 reported by Hormia et al[7] was probably due to the choice of monoclonal antibody. MacDonald & Fletcher[9] claimed that the epithelium of dentigerous cysts could be distinguished from that of odontogenic keratocysts by LP34 reactivity. They showed that nine examples of dentigerous cyst epithelium stained strongly positive for keratins of intermediate molecular weight with LP34, while none of a similar number of odontogenic keratocysts did so.

Maeda et al[10] demonstrated that the linings of most odontogenic cysts, unlike nonodontogenic cysts, failed to express keratins RGE53.

Li et al,[11] investigating the proliferative activity of jaw cysts using antibody to proliferating cell nuclear antigen (PCNA), found that the proliferative activity of radicular and dentigerous cyst lining

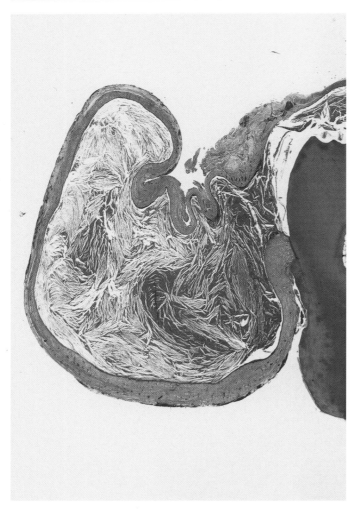

Fig. 21.8 Dentigerous cyst. The attachment of the cyst lining to the neck of a tooth can be seen.

epithelium was low in comparison with that of odontogenic keratocysts and normal oral mucosal epithelium, and in particular that the index of proliferation (5.1 ± 3.0 PCNA$^+$ cells/mm) for dentigerous cysts was lower than that of radicular cysts (11.0 ± 4.1 PCNA$^+$ cells/mm). Such findings confirm that dentigerous cyst growth is slow.

The factors that initiate dentigerous cyst development are not known. Inflammation does not play a significant role, but there is a strong association between the failure of eruption of teeth and the formation of dentigerous cysts. It is not merely that a dentigerous cyst may prevent a tooth from erupting, but dentigerous cysts predominantly affect maxillary canines and mandibular third molars, which are particularly prone to failure of eruption.

BEHAVIOR AND MANAGEMENT

Once the diagnosis has been established it may occasionally be preferable to marsupialize a dentigerous cyst to allow the tooth to erupt if it is in a favorable position and space is available. Alternatively, the tooth can be transplanted to the alveolar ridge or extracted, as appropriate, and the cyst enucleated. In most cases, enucleation (see radicular cysts, Ch. 23) with removal of the tooth and primary closure is carried out.

Eruption cysts

An eruption cyst occasionally forms in the gingiva overlying a tooth about to erupt. Eruption cysts are extraosseous, but are probably superficial dentigerous cysts.

CLINICAL FEATURES

Eruption cysts are seen in children and only very rarely in adults. They most frequently involve teeth anterior to the first permanent molars and appear as a soft, rounded, pink or bluish swelling in the gingiva overlying the unerupted tooth. Fluctuation may be detectable. Eruption cysts are painless unless infected, and many probably burst spontaneously and unnoticed.

MICROSCOPY

An eruption cyst is lined by thin, poorly formed stratified squamous epithelium and is separated from the oral mucosa by connective tissue (Fig. 21.9).

BEHAVIOR AND MANAGEMENT

The tissue overlying the crown of the tooth may be removed.

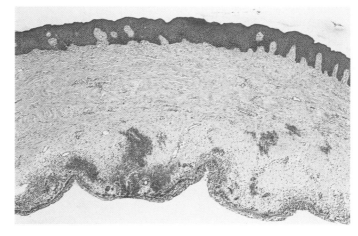

Fig. 21.9 Eruption cyst. The oral mucosa above is separated from the roof of the cyst below.

However, these cysts do not obstruct eruption of affected teeth, and most probably burst spontaneously as the tooth erupts.

REFERENCES

1. Shear M, Singh S 1978 Age-standardized incidence rates of ameloblastoma and dentigerous cyst on the Witwtersrand, South Africa. Common Dent Oral Epidemiol 6: 195–199
2. Brown LH, Berkman S, Cohen D, Kaplan AL, Rosenberg M 1982 A radiological study of the frequency and distribution of impacted teeth. J Dent Assoc S Africa 37: 627–630
3. Mourshed F 1964 A roentgenographic study of dentigerous cysts. I. Incidence in a population sample. Oral Surg Oral Med Oral Pathol 18: 47–53
4. Roggan R, Donath K 1985 Klinik und Pathomorphologie odontogener follikulärer Zysten – Nachuntersuchung von 239 Fallen. Deutsche Zahnärtzl Ztschr 40: 536–540
5. Shear M 1992 Cysts of the oral regions, 3rd edn. Wright, Bristol
6. Browne RM (ed) 1991 Investigative pathology of odontogenic. CRC Press, Boca Raton, FL
7. Hormia M, Ylipaavalniemi P, Nagle RB, Virtanen I 1987 Expression of cytokeratins in dontogenic jaw cysts: monoclonal antibodies reveal distinct variation between different cyst types. J Oral Pathol 16: 338–346
8. Matthews JB, Mason GI, Browne RM 1988 Epithelial markers and proliferating cells in odontogenic cysts. J Pathol 156: 283–290
9. MacDonald AW, Fletcher A 1989 Expression of cytokeratin in the epithelium of dentigerons cysts and odontogenic keratocysts: an aid to diagnosis. J Clin Pathol 42: 736–739
10. Maeda Y, Hirota J, Yonedi K, Osaki I 1990 Immunohistochemical study of jaw cysts: different existence of keratins in odontogenic and non-odontogenic epithelial linings. J Oral Pathol Med 19: 289–294
11. Li T-J, Browne RM, Matthews JB 1994 Quantification of PCNA· cells within odontogenic jaw cyst epithelium. J Oral Pathol Med 23: 184–189

Gingival and lateral periodontal cysts

22

Gingival cysts

Two types of gingival cyst are recognized: infantile (dental lamina cyst of the newborn) and adult types.

DENTAL LAMINA AND MIDPALATAL RAPHE CYSTS OF INFANCY

Small nodules of epithelium (Bohn's nodules) or cysts, which have arisen from epithelial rests of Serres, from the dental lamina, are found on the buccal or lingual aspects of the alveolar ridge in the gingiva. They involute spontaneously or rupture through the gingiva, and are rarely found after the age of 3 months.

Similar lesions (Epstein's pearls) in the region of the junction of the hard and soft palates arise from nonodontogenic epithelium of the midpalatal raphe. Either of these cysts may enlarge sufficiently to appear as creamy colored swellings a few millimeters in diameter. Most rupture spontaneously and heal in a matter of months.

Extensive surveys[1,2] have shown Bohn's nodules or Epstein's pearls to be present in up to 80% of neonates.

MICROSCOPY

Dental lamina cysts are lined by thin stratified squamous epithelium a few cells thick and contain layers of desquamated keratin (Fig. 22.1).

GINGIVAL CYSTS OF ADULTS

Adult gingival cysts account for approximately 0.5% of jaw cysts. Several small series have been reported.[3–5] Adult gingival cysts appear, from the combined totals from these reports, to affect males slightly more frequently than females. Most patients are over the age of 40 years, and the peak incidence is at between 50 and 59 years.

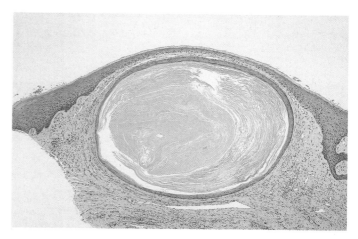

Fig. 22.1 Dental lamina cyst. A well-defined, keratin-filled cyst is lined by thin, stratified squamous epithelium.

CLINICAL FEATURES

Adult gingival cysts form painless, slowly enlarging, dome-shaped swellings, usually less than 1 cm in diameter, in the free or attached gingiva of the labial or buccal aspect of the alveolar ridge. The mandible, particularly the premolar–canine region, is more frequently affected than the maxilla. These cysts may sometimes superficially erode the underlying bone.

MICROSCOPY

The epithelial lining is variable in character. The cysts may be lined by flattened squamoid or low cuboidal epithelium (one or a few cells thick), or, entirely or in part, by nonkeratinizing stratified squamous epithelium. Among the low cuboidal cells, isolated clear cells are sometimes present and occasionally are numerous. Dome-shaped thickenings of squamoid cells protruding into the cyst lumen or indenting the underlying connective tissue are more typical of botryoid odontogenic cysts, as discussed below (Figs 22.2 and 22.3).

133

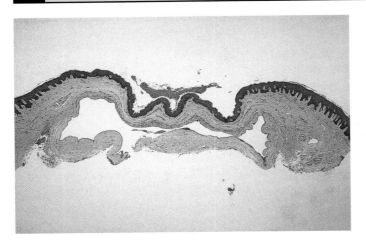

Fig. 22.2 Gingival cyst. Oral mucosa overlies the collapsed cyst cavity, which shows small thickenings of the epithelial lining.

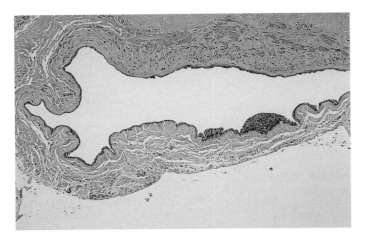

Fig. 22.3 Gingival cyst. Higher power view shows the thin epithelial lining with focal thickenings.

HISTOGENESIS

Adult gingival cysts probably arise from the rests of Serres, but their late appearance is difficult to explain. It seems reasonable to regard them as the extraosseous counterparts of lateral periodontal cysts, as Wysocki et al[5] have proposed. These cysts have similar age and site distributions and share the histological features, particularly the localized thickenings of the epithelium, that are characteristic of botryoid odontogenic cysts. Like the latter, adult gingival cysts are occasionally multilocular.

The suggestion that adult gingival cysts could result from traumatic implantation of superficial epithelium is no more than a theoretical possibility, and has not been substantiated.

BEHAVIOR AND MANAGEMENT

Adult gingival cysts grow slowly and respond to local excision.

However, if they are multilocular and botryoid histologically, it is possible that they have a similar propensity to recur as the botryoid odontogenic cyst.

Lateral periodontal cysts

These uncommon cysts are intraosseous and form beside a vital tooth. The term 'lateral periodontal cyst,' excludes lateral odontogenic keratocysts and lateral radicular cysts. However, earlier reports of lateral periodontal cysts included these different entities. As discussed below, botryoid odontogenic cysts and glandular odontogenic cysts are frequently regarded as variants of the lateral periodontal cyst, though they differ in their biological behavior. However, too few cases have been reported as yet to be certain whether they are distinct entities.

INCIDENCE

Lateral periodontal cysts formed 0.7% of the 2616 cysts described by Shear.[6] Pooled data from this and other surveys[7,8] showed patients' ages to range widely, but the majority were aged between 40 and 69 years, with a peak between 50 and 59 years.

The small numbers of patients in each study preclude any firm indication of whether males or females are predominantly affected.

Lateral periodontal cysts are most frequently located in the mandible anterior to the molar region. Approximately 10% of lateral periodontal cysts are found in the maxilla, usually in the canine–incisor region.

CLINICAL FEATURES

Lateral periodontal cysts are symptomless, unless infected, and are frequently found on routine radiographs. If the cysts erode through the bone and extend into the gingiva they form soft bluish, fluctuant swellings. Associated teeth are vital.

RADIOGRAPHY

Lateral periodontal cysts appear as round or ovoid radiolucent areas with sclerotic margins, between the roots of the related teeth, approximately midway between their apices and the alveolar margin. Most cyst are 3–7 mm in diameter, and only rarely do they exceed 10 mm.

The radiographic appearance is similar to that of other odontogenic cysts, apart from their position beside a tooth, near the crest of the alveolar ridge.

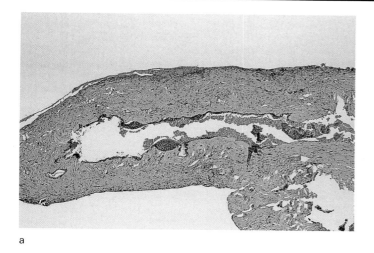

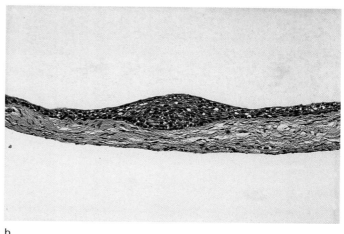

a

b

Fig. 22.4 a Lateral periodontal cyst. The lining is similar to that of the gingival cyst shown in Figure 22.3. **b** Higher power view shows one of the focal thickenings in the epithelial lining.

MICROSCOPY

Lateral periodontal cysts are lined by squamous or cuboidal epithelium, frequently only one or two cells thick, but sometimes with focal thickenings resembling a gingival cyst. Some of these cells may have clear cytoplasm and resemble those seen in the dental lamina. Approximately two-thirds of clear and other cells are glycogen rich[9] (Fig. 22.4).

BEHAVIOR AND MANAGEMENT

Lateral periodontal cysts grow slowly and do not appear to have the same propensity for recurrence as botryoid and glandular odontogenic cysts. They respond to enucleation, and related teeth should be retained if possible.

BOTRYOID ODONTOGENIC CYSTS

This uncommon entity was described by Weathers & Waldron,[10] who gave it this term because of the gross appearance of the specimen which, being polycystic, had a fancied resemblance to a bunch of grapes. They regarded it as a multilocular variant of the lateral periodontal cyst, which showed proliferation of the lining epithelium to form nodules or plaques. However, Shear,[11] among others, believes that the botryoid odontogenic cyst may be a different entity from the lateral periodontal cyst, particularly because of its propensity for recurrence.

CLINICAL FEATURES

Botryoid odontogenic cysts typically affect adults over the age of 50 years. There appears to be no significant gender distribution. Demographic, clinical, microscopic, and radiographic features of

33 previously unreported cases were described by Gurol et al,[12] who concluded that fewer than 40 other cases had been reported. They found the mandibular premolar to canine region to be the main site. Some examples have affected the mandibular incisor to canine region or extended across the midline, as discussed below. The cysts frequently cannot be distinguished clinically from simple lateral periodontal cysts.

RADIOGRAPHY

Botryoid odontogenic cysts can be considerably larger than conventional lateral periodontal cysts, and multilocularity may be clearly seen. However, histologically confirmed botryoid odontogenic cysts may appear unilocular in radiographs.[13]

Botryoid odontogenic cysts may also differ in their location from lateral periodontal cysts. Kaugars[14] reported two botryoid odontogenic cysts, one of which extended towards the periapical region of the premolars, while the other involved a considerable area of the periapical region in the midline of the mandible. Heikinheimo et al[15] also reported a botryoid odontogenic cyst, which extended from the right first molar region to the left second premolar and was close to the lower border of the mandible in places.

MICROSCOPY

Botryoid odontogenic cysts consist of loculi lined by flattened nonkeratinized epithelium. All the 33 cases analyzed by Gurol et al[12] were histologically multilocular, despite the fact that 15 of them appeared unilocular radiographically. The loculae are separated by fine fibrous septa. However, histologic multilocularity should not be considered a criterion of diagnosis because of possible distortion of the configuration during surgery or laboratory processing.

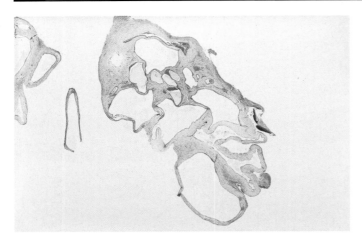

Fig. 22.5 Botryoid odontogenic cyst. An almost completely intact specimen shows the multiple cysts separated by fibrous septa, giving the so-called 'bunches of grapes' appearance.

The distinctive feature is the sporadic bud-like, nodular, or plaque-like proliferations protruding into the cavity. These proliferations may bud off to become islands, which may become cystic. Interspersed among the epithelial cells are clear, glycogen-containing cells. Clusters of epithelial odontogenic rests, largely consisting of clear cells, may be seen in the surrounding connective tissue. A discrete hyalinized zone may be seen immediately subjacent to the basal epithelial layer. This zone may promote separation of the epithelium from the capsule (Fig. 22.5).

HISTOGENESIS

Heikinheimo et al[15] have shown that botryoid odontogenic cyst epithelium strongly expresses cytokeratin 18, which is absent from gingival epithelium but present in some dentigerous cysts and focally in ameloblastomas. Cytokeratin 19, which is also a major component of odontogenic epithelium, was also expressed by all the cells of the botryoid odontogenic cyst epithelium. Heikinheimo et al were, therefore, convinced that, as their location also suggests, these cysts were odontogenic.

Botryoid odontogenic cysts may thus arise from remnants of the dental lamina, from remnants of the reduced enamel epithelium, or from the root sheath of Hertwig, but it is not possible to speculate further to any great purpose. However, proliferation and cystic change in several epithelial rests may give rise to the polycystic character of botryoid odontogenic cysts.

The determinants of the propensity for botryoid odontogenic cysts to recur are also obscure, but it may not always be possible to remove every lobule intact. Lynch & Madden,[16] for example, showed an example with an extension joined to the main body of the lesion by a thin stalk, and with discrete microcysts in the cyst wall. As mentioned earlier, rests of odontogenic epithelium may also be seen in the surrounding connective tissue. Any of these rests, if left after excision, might proliferate to form additional

cysts. The delay of many years typically seen before recurrence may suggest that proliferation of the parent odontogenic epithelium has formed a new lesion, but the fact that recurrences have been in the site of the original cyst indicates that it is the tissue of the latter that is responsible.

BEHAVIOR AND MANAGEMENT

Botryoid odontogenic cysts have an undoubted propensity for recurrence. Kaugars[14] reported three cases that recurred 9 years after initial surgical removal. Three of the 10 cases reported by Greer & Johnson[13] recurred 8 years, and two cases recurred 10 years after removal. Heikinheimo et al[15] reported an exceptionally large botryoid odontogenic cyst which recurred four times over a period of 9 years. Semba et al[17] summarized the frequency of recurrence of 17 cases for which follow-up information was available of 21 cases reported to that date. Six of these cysts had recurred after periods of 17 months to 10 years. The remaining 11 cases showed no evidence of recurrence, but the periods of follow-up were brief, ranging from 2 months to 2 years.

Because of surgical difficulties in removing botryoid odontogenic cysts entire, they should be excised rather than enucleated. Wide excision with sacrifice of teeth does not seem to be justified if it can be certain that prolonged radiographic follow-up can be maintained. Any recurrence can then be controlled by a further limited excision before the cyst reaches a large size. However, knowledge of the potentialities of these lesions is, as yet, limited.

GLANDULAR ODONTOGENIC CYSTS (SIALO-ODONTOGENIC CYSTS)

The glandular odontogenic cyst was first described by Padayachee et al,[18] who reported two examples of a cyst with features of both a botryoid odontogenic cyst and a central muco-epidermoid tumor.

Gardner et al,[19] on the basis of eight cases, defined this entity more precisely and termed it a glandular odontogenic cyst. Hussain et al[20] presented four new cases and reviewed 13 others. There was an approximately equal gender distribution. The mean age of patients was 51 years (range 19–85 years) and 56% were between the ages of 40 and 60 years. Hussain et al confirmed that the main features of these cysts were that they formed slow-growing swellings that were painless in 75% of cases. Eighty-eight per cent of cysts were in the anterior mandible, nine of the 17 cases appeared multilocular radiographically, and 14 crossed the midline. Only two of the 17 cysts were in the maxilla.

Glandular odontogenic cysts were found by Kreidler et al[21] to be more frequent than lateral periodontal cysts (see Table 19.1), but this finding may be biased by the small numbers involved.

Clinically and radiographically, glandular odontogenic cysts cannot be reliably distinguished from lateral periodontal or botryoid odontogenic cysts.

MICROSCOPY

Glandular odontogenic cysts can be multi- or unilocular. Takeda[22] specifically mentioned that the glandular odontogenic cyst he observed was unicystic, while the one reported by Semba et al[17] was multicystic. The latter also commented that a major distinction between glandular odontogenic and botryoid odontogenic cysts is the different frequency of multilocularity.

Glandular odontogenic cysts typically show (Figs 22.6–22.8):

- An epithelial lining frequently much thicker than that of a botryoid odontogenic cyst, but also of highly variable thickness. It has a flat lower border.
- An irregular or even papillary lumenal surface to the epithelium, with a superficial layer of eosinophilic cuboidal cells and some ciliated cells.
- Pools of mucicarmine-positive material and mucous cells in variable numbers within the epithelium.
- Whorls, nodules, or duct-like structures of epithelial cells ('epithelial spheres') that may protrude into the cyst cavity as in a botryoid odontogenic cyst. The fibrous wall is sometimes highly vascular and may contain a few scattered inflammatory cells.

Histologically, Hussain et al[20] illustrated exceptionally clearly the multiplicity of small discrete cysts in one example, and the infiltrative pattern of growth. Mucus-secreting cells were numerous in the mainly stratified squamous epithelial lining. The lining also showed plaque-like thickenings, which usually projected into the cyst lumen, but sometimes into the fibrous capsule, and sometimes had a whorled pattern. The mucus-secreting cells were mostly in the surface layer of the lining, but some lined crypt-like spaces within the epithelium.

DIFFERENTIAL DIAGNOSIS

Waldron & Koh[23] discussed possible relationships between intraosseous mucoepidermoid carcinoma and glandular odontogenic cyst. As noted earlier, Padaychee & van Wyk[18] reported two cystic lesions with features of both botryoid odontogenic cyst and mucoepidermoid carcinoma, which they concluded were glandular odontogenic cysts. Ficarra et al[24] also reported a glandular odontogenic cyst where an initial diagnosis of mucoepidermoid carcinoma had been made. Sadeghi et al[25] went further, and suggested the term 'mucoepidermoid odontogenic cyst' for the glandular odontogenic cyst. Though descriptive, this term is also likely to perpetuate confusion between the cyst and the tumor.

Glandular odontogenic cysts may show areas of squamous epithelium containing prominent mucin-positive cells, and thus resemble in part a mucoepidermoid carcinoma. However, the latter is unlikely to be multilocular with cysts largely lined by flattened squamoid epithelium. This lining also shows foci of proliferation to form whorled nodules or plaques, and there may also be foci of columnar and ciliated cells, as already described. The overall appearances are therefore considerably different from

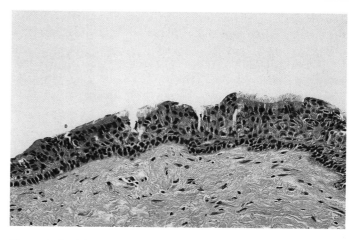

Fig. 22.6 Glandular odontogenic cyst. The lining of squamous epithelium is of irregular thickness. It lacks distinctive features, but shows a small area of ciliated cells.

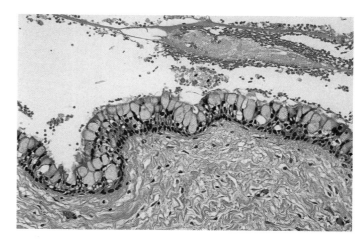

Fig. 22.7 Glandular odontogenic cyst. Numerous mucous cells are prominent in this area of the lining.

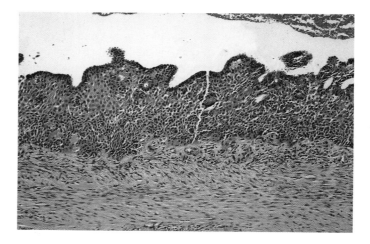

Fig. 22.8 Glandular odontogenic cyst. In this thickened area of epithelial lining are several duct-like structures lined by cells similar to those seen at the surface.

those of a mucoepidermoid carcinoma. In particular, there is no true invasion of the surrounding tissues that the latter frequently shows.

Other odontogenic cysts and, in particular, dentigerous cysts frequently contain mucous cells in their lining, but again the overall appearance is quite different from that of a glandular odontogenic cyst.

HISTOGENESIS

There are too few data to establish whether and to what degree the histogenesis of glandular odontogenic cysts differs from that of botryoid odontogenic cysts. Semba et al[17] have shown the surface and suprabasal layers of the epithelium to be strongly positive for cytokeratins 10 and 11 (KL1+). Cytokeratins 8, 18, and 19, which are characteristic of simple epithelium, were only weakly expressed in all layers. A negative reaction for EMA in the area of the glandular structures and mucous cells suggested that they were not of true glandular origin. Semba et al[17] concluded that glandular odontogenic cysts were probably odontogenic, that the mucous cells were metaplastic, and that the EMA negativity was a further feature distinguishing glandular odontogenic cysts from mucoepidermoid carcinoma.

BEHAVIOR AND MANAGEMENT

Glandular odontogenic cysts have a propensity for recurrence. Semba et al[17] summarized the frequency of recurrence of 12 reported cases. Three had recurred after periods of 3 years to 3 years 8 months. There was no sign of recurrence in the remaining nine cases, where the periods of follow-up ranged from 6 months to 20 years. In view of the small numbers of glandular odontogenic cysts and botryoid odontogenic cysts on which follow-up information is available, it cannot yet be said that the recurrence rates of these two cyst types are significantly different. However, a few glandular odontogenic cysts have not recurred after periods of 10–20 years.

Follow-up information was incomplete in the series reviewed by Hussain et al,[20] but nine of the 17 glandular odontogenic cysts that had been treated conservatively (curettage or enucleation) showed a recurrence rate of 55%. There was a long interval before recurrence (average 4.9 years, range 1.5–9 years).

It is important, therefore, to ensure that all traces of a glandular odontogenic cyst lining are removed. In practical terms

the diagnosis is likely only to be confirmed by microscopy after operation. However, if the cyst is found to be multilocular, resection may be advisable. The patient should be warned of the possibility of recurrence, particularly if treatment has been conservative, and follow-up should be prolonged.

REFERENCES

1. Monteleone L, McLellan MS 1964 Epstein's pearls (Bohn's nodules) of the palate. J Oral Surg 22: 301–304
2. Fromm A 1967 Epstein's pearls, Bohn's nodules and inclusion cysts of the oral cavity. J Dent Children 34: 275–287
3. Reeve CM, Levy BP 1968 Gingival cysts: a review of the literature and a report of four cases. Periodontics 6: 115–117
4. Buchner A, Hansen LS 1979 The histomorphologic spectrum of the gingival cyst of the adult. Oral Surg Oral Med Oral Pathol 48: 523–539
5. Wysocki GP, Brannon RB, Gardner DG, Sapp P 1980 Histogenesis of the lateral periodontal cyst and the gingival cyst of the adult. Oral Surg Oral Med Oral Pathol 50: 327–334
6. Shear M 1992 Cysts of the oral regions, 3rd edn. Wright, Bristol
7. Cohen DA, Neville BW, Dammm DD, White DK 1984 The lateral periodontal cyst. J Periodontol 55: 230–234
8. Rasmusson LG, Magnusson BC, Borrman H 1991 The lateral periodontal cyst. A histopathological and radiographic study of 32 cases. Br J Oral Maxillofac Surg 29: 54–57
9. Altini M, Shear M 1992 The lateral periodontal cyst: an update. J Oral Pathol Med 21: 245–250
10. Weathers DR, Waldron CA 1973 Unusual multilocular cysts of the jaws (botryoid odontogenic cysts). Oral Surg Oral Med Oral Pathol 36: 235–241
11. Shear M 1994 Developmental odontogenic cysts. An update. J Oral Pathol Med 23: 1–11
12. Gurol M, Burkes J, Jacoway J 1995 Botryoid odontogenic cyst: analysis of 33 cases. J Periodontol 66: 1069–1073
13. Greer RO, Johnson M 1988 Botryoid odontogenic cyst: clinicopathologic analysis of ten cases with three recurrences. J Oral Maxillofac Surg 46: 574–579
14. Kaugars GE 1986 Botryoid odontogenic cyst. Oral Surg Oral Med Oral Pathol 62: 555–559
15. Heikinheimo K, Happonen R-P, Forssell K, Kuusilehto A, Virtanen I 1989 A botryoid odontogenic cyst with multiple recurrences. Int J Oral Maxillofac Surg 18: 10–13
16. Lynch DP, Madden CR 1985 The botryoid odontogenic cyst. Report of a case and review of the literature. J Periodontol 56: 163–167
17. Semba I, Kitano M, Mimura T, Sonoda S, Miyawaki A 1994 Glandular odontogenic cyst: analysis of cytokeratin expression and clinicopathological features. J Oral Pathol Med 23: 377–382
18. Padayachee A, van Wyk CW 1987 Two cystic lesions with features of both the botryoid odontogenic cyst and the central mucoepidermoid tumour: sialo-odontogenic cyst. J Oral Pathol Med 16: 499–504
19. Gardner DG, Kessler HP, Morency R, Schaffner DL 1988 The glandular odontogenic cyst: an apparent entity. J Oral Pathol 17: 359–366
20. Hussain K, Edmondson HD, Browne RM 1995 Glandular odontogenic cysts. Diagnosis and treatment. Oral Surg Oral Med Oral Pathol 79: 593–603
21. Kreidler JF, Raubenheimer EJ, van Heerdem WFP 1993 A retrospective analysis of 367 cystic lesions of the jaws – the Ulm experience. J Cranio Max Fac Surg 21: 339–341
22. Takeda Y 1994 Glandular odontogenic cyst mimicking a lateral periodontal cyst: a case report. Int J Oral Maxillofac Surg 23: 96–97
23. Waldron CA, Koh ML 1990 Central mucoepidermoid carcinoma of the jaws: report of four cases with analysis of the literature and discussion of the relationship to mucoepidermoid, sialodontogenic and glandular odontogenic cysts. J Oral Maxillofac Surg 48: 871–877
24. Ficarra G, Chou L, Panzoni E 1990 Glandular odontogenic cyst (sialo-odontogenic cyst). Int J Oral Maxillofac Surg 19: 331–333
25. Sadeghi EM, Weldon LL, Kwon PH 1991 Mucoepidermoid odontogenic cyst. Int J Oral Maxillofac Surg 20: 142–143

Radicular and paradental cysts 23

Radicular (apical periodontal) cysts

The term 'radicular cyst' avoids possible confusion with the different types of periodontal cysts. Bouquot & Lense[1] give credit to Brown[2] for the first description in 1839.

INCIDENCE

Radicular cysts are the most common cause of chronic major jaw swellings and by far the most common type of cyst of the jaws. They comprised 70.7% of 5914 jaw cysts analyzed by Ahlfors et al,[3] but approximately 55% of other large series (see Ch. 19). The reasons for the difference in the findings of Ahlfors et al[3] from others are unclear.

Radicular cysts are rarely seen before the age of 10 years and are most frequent between the ages of 20 and 60 years. Shear[4] found that, in South Africa, for 558 radicular cysts the peak frequency was between the ages of 20 and 29 years, while in a series of 161 English patients there was a steady rise in frequency after the age of 10 years but the peak was not reached until the age of 40–49 years. It seems likely that this difference is the result of neglect of dental caries among blacks in South Africa at that time. Though Shear also found that radicular cysts were approximately twice as frequent among white as black patients in South Africa, this probably reflects different referral rates.

Radicular cysts are only rarely associated with deciduous teeth. It is likely that because these teeth, whether vital or not, are naturally exfoliated, any incipient cyst formation is aborted. Oehlers[5] has demonstrated that cysts resolve spontaneously when the inflammatory stimulus is removed.

Radicular cysts are more common in men than women, in the proportion of approximately 3 : 2.

Shear,[4] in his analysis of the sites of 789 radicular cysts in South Africa, found that approximately 60% of cysts were in the maxilla and 40% in the mandible. The maxillary incisor teeth are by far the most frequently affected. These teeth are highly susceptible to dental caries and to trauma, which can kill the pulp.

Certain types of nonmetallic restorations ('silicates') used in the past for these teeth were also toxic to the pulp.

CLINICAL FEATURES

A dead tooth which has led to cyst formation is (by definition) present and its relationship to the cyst is usually obvious in radiographs.

The vast majority of radicular cysts, like other cysts of the jaws, cause slowly progressive painless swellings. There are no symptoms until the cyst becomes obtrusive. Smaller cysts may be found when radiographs are taken of nonvital teeth. If infected, cysts frequently become painful and may swell more rapidly, partly due to peripheral inflammatory edema.

Any swelling is rounded and, at first hard. Later, thinning of the bone may give rise to eggshell cracking on palpation. Finally, part of the wall can be resorbed entirely, leaving a soft, fluctuant, bluish swelling beneath the mucous membrane.

RESIDUAL CYSTS

These are periapical cysts that have persisted after extraction of the causative tooth. Cysts of the jaws in older persons are usually residual cysts, which are one of the most common causes of swelling of the edentulous jaw. The cysts can cause trouble by interfering with the fit of dentures.

Progressive thinning or even disappearance of residual cyst linings is seen. This probably represents a stage in slow spontaneous regression, as shown by Oehlers.[5]

LATERAL RADICULAR CYSTS

Lateral radicular cysts are rare. They form at the side of the tooth as a result of the opening of a lateral branch of the root canal. Also rarely, the tooth is vital and the cyst appears to have resulted from inflammation in an adjacent gingval pocket; it then may be regarded as a type of paradental cyst.

RADIOGRAPHY

A radicular cyst appears as a rounded, clearly radiolucent area with a sharply defined outline, intimately related to the apex of a tooth (Fig. 23.1). There is sometimes a condensed peripheral radio-opaque rim, but only if growth has been very slow, and this is usually only seen in older patients.

The dead tooth from which a radicular cyst has arisen can be seen and may show an obvious carious cavity (Fig. 23.2). Adjacent teeth usually remain vital but may be displaced a little or, occasionally, be slightly mobile. Very large cysts in the maxilla may extend in any available direction, become irregular in shape, and can cross the midline.

Infection causes the cyst outline to become hazy as a result of increased vascularity and resorption of the surrounding bone.

MICROSCOPY

All stages can be seen, from a periapical granuloma containing a few strands of proliferating epithelium to an enlarging cyst with a hyperplastic epithelial lining and dense inflammatory infiltrate (Figs 23.3 and 23.4).

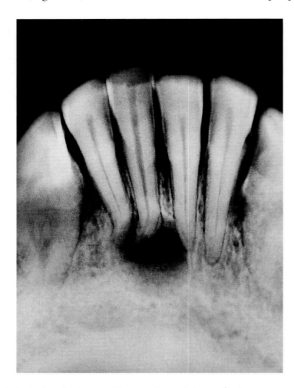

Fig. 23.1 Early radicular cyst. The typical rounded area of radiolucency is at the apex of a tooth. The latter is not carious, but the pulp has probably been killed by trauma severing the apical vessels.

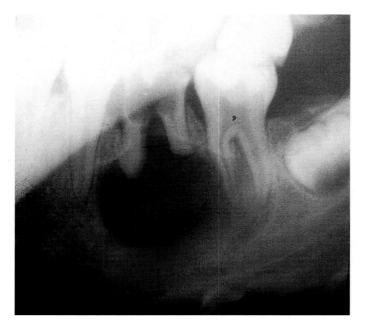

Fig. 23.2 Radicular cyst. This larger example shows the well-circumscribed appearance of the cyst at the apex of a grossly carious tooth.

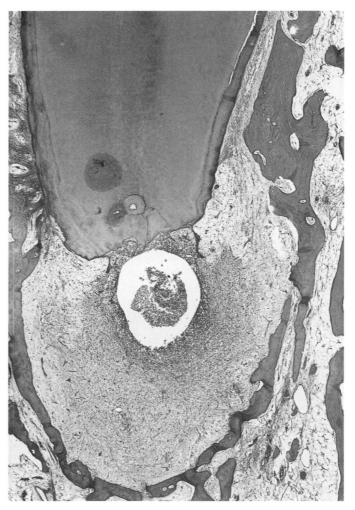

Fig. 23.3 Apical granuloma at the apex of a nonvital tooth, showing mild inflammation, an incipient cyst cavity, and resorption of the surrounding bone to accommodate it.

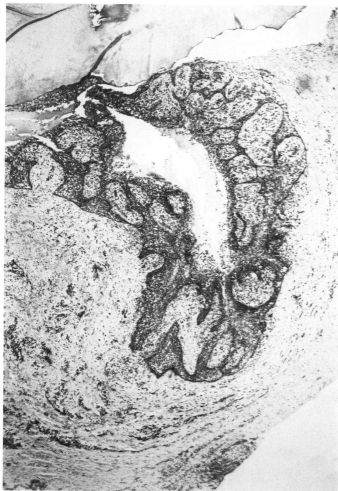

Fig. 23.4 Apical granuloma showing more prominent epithelial proliferation as a result of stimulation of the epithelial rests of Malassez and early arcaded configuration of the epithelium.

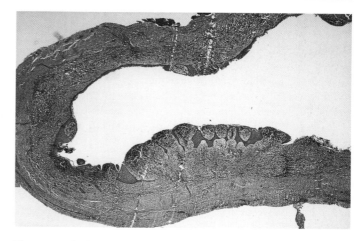

Fig. 23.5 Radicular cyst. Early stage showing intense inflammatory reaction and irregular epithelial lining.

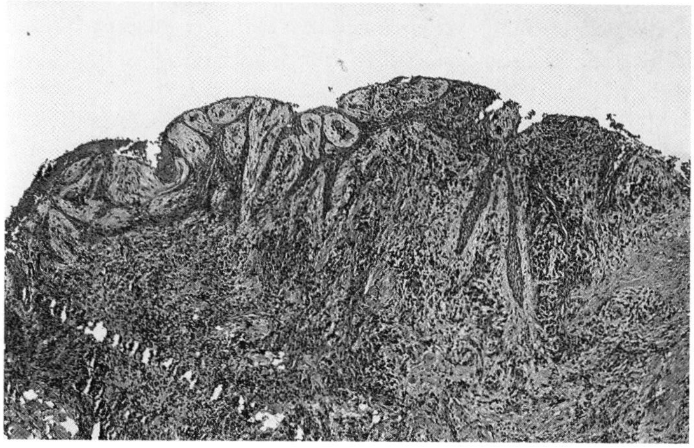

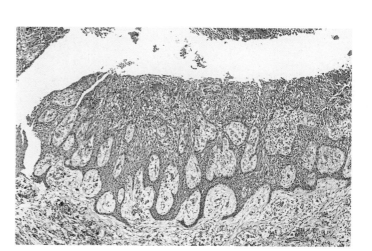

Fig. 23.6 Radicular cyst. Higher power view shows mildly hyperplastic nonkeratinized squamous epithelial lining.

The epithelial lining

The lining consists of stratified squamous epithelum of variable thickness and is sometimes incomplete. Early, active proliferation of the lining epithelium is associated with inflammation, and the epithelium may then be thick, irregular, and hyperplastic or form rings and arcades, giving a net-like appearance (Figs 23.5–23.7). Similar arcading of the epithelium is seen when inflammation is imposed on the lining of an odontogenic keratocyst.

As radicular cysts mature, the epithelial lining becomes thinner and flatter and inflammatory cells become progressively fewer.

Though the epithelium is stratified squamous in type, it is somewhat poorly formed and lacks a defined basal cell layer. Browne,[6] from an analysis of 402 radicular cysts, found mucous cells in 39.6% of them, and their frequency increased with the age of the patient. However, these cells are present only in modest numbers and are usually isolated or in small groups. Ciliated cells were present in 0.7% and keratinization in 2% of

Fig. 23.7 Radicular cyst. Typical arcaded pattern often seen in the epithelial lining.

cysts. Hyaline bodies were seen in 6.7% and mineralized bodies in the fibrous walls of 2.5%.

Ciliated cells were always accompanied by mucous cells. Ciliated cells are more frequent in maxillary cysts, and it has usually been possible to show that there had been an opening into the maxillary antrum. However, ciliated epithelium can also occasionally be seen in radicular cysts of the mandible, as reported by Redman.[7] This ciliated epithelium is probably metaplastic, but is of no practical significance.

Mucous cell hyperplasia in association with Muir–Torre syndrome

As mentioned earlier, mucous cells are frequently found in the linings of dentigerous cysts. They are relatively few in radicular cysts, but Swerdloff et al[8] have reported an isolated example of mucous cell hyperplasia in a radicular cyst associated with the Muir–Torre syndrome: this is believed to be the first documented report. The cyst was histologically conspicuous for the many goblet cells, staining positively with the periodic acid/Schiff (PAS) reagent, and was widely distributed in the superficial layer of the entire lining. When mucous cells are numerous in the lining of a radicular cyst, Muir–Torre syndrome should possibly be suspected.

Muir–Torre syndrome is inherited as an autosomal dominant trait with high penetrance and expressivity. Cutaneous sebaceous tumors of any type are associated with gastrointestinal neoplasms, most frequently of the colon. The latter are of low grade and are associated with long survival.

Rushton bodies

In a minority of radicular cysts, the epithelium contains foci of hyaline refractile material, often referred to as Rushton bodies,[9] although they had been described by Dewey in 1918.[10] This material assumes linear, circinate, hairpin, or more irregular forms (Fig. 23.8). Its nature remains controversial. Its presence in the epithelium suggests that it is an epithelial product and it resembles the refractile epithelial cuticle, which attaches the gingival epithelium to cementum in the floor of periodontal pockets. However, numerous studies have failed to confirm that Rushton bodies are an epithelial product. Alternative theories of a hematogenous origin for Rushton bodies also remain unconfirmed.

The cyst wall

The capsule consists of collagenous fibrous connective tissue. During active growth the capsule is vascular and shows a moderately heavy inflammatory infiltrate adjacent to and infiltrating the proliferating epithelium.

Plasma cells are often prominent or predominant, and produce antibodies against microbial products leaking from the tooth. Mast cells are usually also present, but are rarely conspicuous.

Around the capsule there is osteoclastic activity and resorption of the bone of the cyst wall. Beyond the zone of resorption there is usually active bone replacement. The net consequence is that the cyst expands but retains a bony shell, even after it has extended beyond the normal contours of the jaw (Fig. 23.9). Nevertheless,

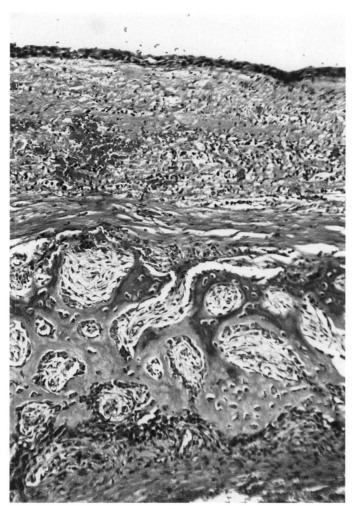

Fig. 23.9 Radicular cyst, showing the process of expansion of the bony cyst wall with resorption above and apposition below.

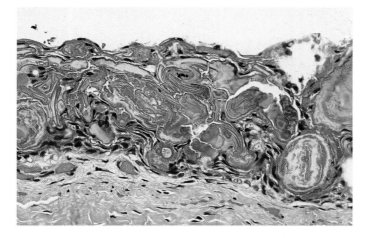

Fig. 23.8 Radicular cyst. Hairpin-like and other configurations of hyaline (Rushton) bodies in the lining.

resorption outpaces apposition to cause the bony wall to become progressively thinner until it forms a mere eggshell. The wall finally disappears altogether and the cyst starts to distend the soft tissues. Long-standing cysts are often characterized by a thin flattened epithelial lining, a thick fibrous wall, and minimal inflammatory infiltrate.

Clefts

Within the cyst capsule or contents there are often needle-shaped spaces or clefts left by cholesterol that dissolved out during specimen preparation. Clefts form in the cyst wall, but frequently extend into the cyst cavity. Small clefts are enclosed within attenuated foreign body giant cells and are associated with extravasated red cells and blood pigment. Breakdown of blood cells is indicated by deposits of hemosiderin and positive (Perl) staining for iron in the surrounding tissues (Figs 23.10 and 23.11).

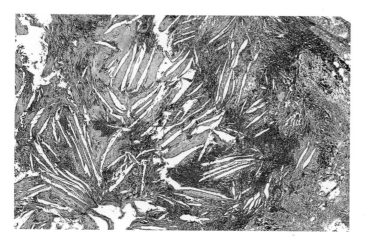

Fig. 23.10 Radicular cyst. Cholesterol clefts and hemosiderin deposits.

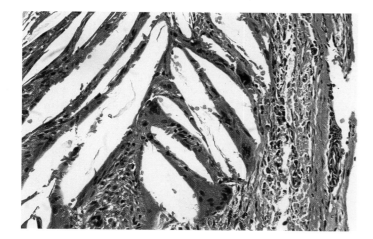

Fig. 23.11 Radicular cyst. Cholesterol clefts showing their origin within giant cells. Hemosiderin deposits are associated.

Cyst fluid

The fluid is usually watery and opalescent, but sometimes may be thicker, more viscid, and yellowish. Cholesterol crystals may give it a shimmering appearance and their characteristic notched rhomboidal shape may be seen by microscopy in a smear of the fluid. In sections, the protein content of the fluid is usually seen as amorphous eosinophilic material, often containing broken-down leucocytes, foam cells distended with fat globules, and clefts left by dissolved-out cholesterol.

PATHOGENESIS

The pathogenesis of odontogenic cysts has been reviewed in detail by Browne & Smith.[11] The main factors responsible for cyst development include the following in varying degree:

- proliferation of the epithelial lining and connective tissue capsule
- accumulation of fluid within the cavity
- resorption of the surrounding bone and incomplete compensatory repair.

Epithelial proliferation

Radicular cysts develop from epithelium-containing periapical granulomas, which form at the apices of nonvital teeth. The sequence of events is that death of the dental pulp, usually as a sequel to dental caries, is followed by infection of the necrotic tissue. Leakage of antigenic material through the tooth apex leads to a chronic inflammatory reaction and proliferation of granulation tissue to form a nodule, usually about 55 mm in diameter, known as a periapical granuloma. Some of these granulomas contain odontogenic epithelium, which can proliferate and line a central cavity. Miniature radicular cysts are thus formed. In human jaws obtained at autopsy, all stages in development of radicular cyst formation from periapical granulomas can be seen.

Young cysts, in particular, often show thick irregular epithelium, suggestive of active proliferation. The potential of epithelial rests of Malassez to proliferate appears to vary widely between individuals. In any series of apical granulomas the epithelial content varies from apparent absence to a thick apparently vigorous layer. Binnie & Rowe[12] were able to find periapical epithelial remnants in only 37% of beagle dogs. If this finding also applies to humans, it may explain the variation in individual susceptibility to radicular cyst formation. Clinically, it is not uncommon also to find in neglected mouths, teeth that have decayed away to the gingival margin and have therefore been nonvital for a considerable period. Nevertheless, they have given rise only to periapical granulomas, but not dental cysts. Such cases suggest either the absence of odontogenic rests or a weak potential of this epithelium to proliferate.

It seems clear, therefore, that infection from the pulp chamber is the stimulus to epithelial proliferation and ultimately of radicular cyst formation in susceptible individuals. As mentioned earlier,

Oehlers[5] confirmed that the majority of radicular cysts, regardless of size, would regress without surgical treatment once infection had been eliminated from the root canal or the tooth extracted.

However, epithelial proliferation in radicular cysts appears to be slow. As mentioned in Chapter 20, Li et al,[13] investigated the proliferative activity of jaw cyst epithelium, using antibody to proliferating cell nuclear antigen (PCNA). They found that the proliferative activity of radicular cyst epithelium was low in comparison with that of odontogenic keratocysts and normal oral mucosal epithelium. However, the index of proliferation for radicular cyst epithelium (11.0 ± 4.1 PCNA$^+$ cells/mm) was twice as high as that of dentigerous cyst epithelium (5.1 ± 3.0 PCNA$^+$ cells/mm).

Hydrostatic effects of cyst fluids

Radicular and many other types of cyst tend to grow expansively in a balloon-like manner. The hydrostatic pressure within cysts appears to be about 70 cmH$_2$O, and is therefore higher than the capillary blood pressure.

Earlier views were that cyst fluid contained mainly low-molecular-weight proteins and that the cyst wall, by acting as a semi-permeable membrane, maintained osmotic tension high enough to cause cyst expansion. More recent experiments have shown that cyst fluid is largely inflammatory exudate containing high concentrations of proteins, some of which, such as immunoglobulins, are of high molecular weight, together with cholesterol, breakdown products of erythrocytes, inflammatory cells, exfoliated epithelial cells, and fibrin. These findings are consistent with the usual presence of inflammation in cyst walls, as a consequence of which the capillaries in the cyst wall are more permeable and exude fluid into the cavity. The net effect is that hydrostatic pressure causes expansion of the cyst cavity.

Lombardi & Morgan[14] identified an inner subepithelial and an outer bone-facing zone containing fibroblasts, which stained positively for α-smooth muscle actin in all 51 radicular, dentigerous, residual, and keratocysts, and less frequently in some other types of cyst that they examined. They suggested that these myofibroblasts could contribute to cyst-wall elasticity and constrain cyst expansion.

Bone resorbing factors

In vitro, cyst tissue in culture can be induced to release bone resorbing factors. These are predominantly prostaglandins E$_2$ and E$_3$. Various cysts and tumors possibly differ in the quantities of prostaglandins produced, but it is uncertain to what extent this affects the mode of growth of cysts. Collagenase may be found in the walls of keratocysts, but its contribution to cyst growth is also unclear.

DIFFERENTIAL DIAGNOSIS

Radiolucent lesions that must be considered in the differential diagnosis of cysts have been summarized in Table 19.1. The main practical consideration is to differentiate radicular and dentigerous cysts from unilocular keratocysts or ameloblastomas, as discussed earlier.

Resorption of the apices of adjacent teeth suggests a neoplasm rather than a cyst, but is not diagnostic. Rarely, a metastatic deposit may produce a sharply defined radiolucency instead of an ill-defined and irregular area. Tumors also tend to be painful and to grow more rapidly than cysts. Nevertheless, it may be difficult or impossible to distinguish them from an infected cyst in radiographs, until at operation the solid nature of a tumor becomes obvious and microscopy confirms the diagnosis.

Aspiration

The cystic nature of a radiolucent area can be confirmed by aspirating its contents by a needle inserted through the wall under aseptic conditions. However, this fluid will not distinguish one cyst from another, or a cystic neoplasm from a true cyst. The presence of cholesterol crystals is of little diagnostic value. Rarely, a keratocyst may be filled with a semi-solid mass of squames and no aspirate is obtainable through a thin needle.

BEHAVIOR AND MANAGEMENT

The clinical and radiographic findings yield a reliable diagnosis in the great majority of cases. It is usually only after removal and microscopy that a cyst is found to be a unilocular keratocyst or ameloblastoma. However, this is so infrequent that preliminary biopsy or aspiration is rarely carried out.

Despite differences in detail between the various techniques for treatment of cysts, they all depend on one of two basic principles: enucleation with primary wound closure, or marsupialization (or occasionally marsupialization followed by enucleation).

However, only enucleation and primary closure, without bone grafting, is commonly carried out, and in competent hands this technique is completely satisfactory. Marsupialization into the antrum may be used for large maxillary cysts with incomplete bony walls separating them from the antrum. Radicular cysts are slow growing and, if enucleated complete or even if marsupialized, have no potential for recurrence.

Though residual cysts may eventually regress spontaneously, in practical terms, patients are more quickly relieved of them by surgical enucleation.

Paradental cysts

The paradental cyst is an uncommon inflammatory odontogenic cyst, first described by Craig,[15] who presented 48 cases. Ackerman et al[16] reported 50 further examples. Fowler & Brannon[17] carried out a clinicopathological study on six new cases and reviewed the literature. Vedtofte & Praetorius[18] have reviewed in detail the findings in 29 paradental cysts, but presented slightly different criteria of diagnosis.

INCIDENCE

In Shear's series of 2616 jaw cysts,[4] paradental cysts formed 3.5%, and in the series analyzed by Ackerman et al[16] they formed 3% of 1852 odontogenic cysts. By contrast, Daley et al[19] found paradental cysts to account for only 0.48% of 6847 odontogenic cysts.

The series reported by Craig,[15] Ackerman et al,[16] and Fowler & Brannon[17] agree on the peak age of frequency of 20–29 years and of a preponderance of males. In Craig's series and that of Fowler & Brannon, the male female ratio was 5 : 1, while in the series reported by Ackerman et al it was 2.3 : 1.

Paradental cysts usually form on the buccal and distal aspects of a partially erupted third molar tooth and are associated with pericoronitis. The latter was present in all cases reported by Craig,[15] Ackerman et al,[16] and Fowler & Brannon.[17] However, Vedtofte & Praetorius[18] described a relationship with the mandibular third molar in only 52% of cases, with the second molar in 24% and the first molar in 17%. Most of these cysts were, therefore, in the category described as *mandibular buccal infected cyst* by Shear[4] and form on the buccal aspect of first molars in children between the ages of 6 and 8 years. The remainder were associated with either the maxillary second molar (3.4%) or the canine and lateral incisor (3.4%). The 1992 World Health Organization criteria[20] do not regard the paradental cyst as described by Craig[15] as a single entity but, like others such as Vedtofte & Praetorius,[18] describe as 'paradental' a variety of inflammatory cysts developing beside a tooth. Inflammatory collateral cysts and mandibular infected buccal cysts are therefore grouped together under the heading 'paradental cyst.'

CLINICAL FEATURES

Pain and swelling are the most frequent symptoms. There is typically obvious inflammation round the affected tooth.

RADIOGRAPHY

Paradental cysts can be seen to be superimposed on the buccal and distal aspect of an intact third molar. The periodontal ligament space is of normal width and the apical lamina dura remains intact.

Infected buccal cysts can be seen to be superimposed on the lateral aspect of the affected tooth in lateral and occlusal radiographs, and can sometimes extend to involve an adjacent tooth.

MICROSCOPY

Paradental cysts are attached to the amelocemental junction of a vital tooth, usually on the buccal aspect of a third molar, which in many cases has an enamel projection. They rarely exceed 2 cm in diameter.

There is an intense inflammatory reaction in the cyst wall; otherwise the microscopic features do not differ from those of many radicular cysts, but the tooth is vital.

Paradental cysts probably originate from the reduced enamel epithelium after unilateral expansion of the follicle as a result of inflammatory destruction of the adjacent alveolar bone.

BEHAVIOR AND MANAGEMENT

Enucleation is the treatment of choice and is not followed by recurrence.

REFERENCES

1. Bouquot JE, Lense EC 1994 The beginning of oral pathology. Part I: First dental journal reports of odontogenic tumors and cysts, 1839–1860. Oral Surg Oral Med Oral Pathol 78: 343–350
2. Brown AM 1839 Reviewe of Burdell and Burdell's observations on the structure, physiology, anatomy and diseases of the teeth. Am J Dent Sci 1: 19–24
3. Ahlfors E, Larsson A, Sjogren S 1984 The odontogenic keratocyst: a benign cystic tumor? J Oral Maxillofac Surg 42: 10–19
4. Shear M Cysts of the oral regions, 3rd edn. Wright, Bristol
5. Oehlers FAC 1970 Periapical lesions and residual dental cysts. Br J Oral Surg 8: 103–113
6. Browne RM 1972 Metaplasia and degeneration in odontogenic cysts in man. J Oral Pathol 1: 145–158
7. Redman RS 1989 Respiratory epithelium in an apical periodontal cyst of the mandible. Oral Surg Oral Med Oral Pathol 67: 77–80
8. Swerdloff M, Archard HO, Krimsky PK 1990 Mucous cell hyperplasia in an odontogenic cyst from a patient with Muir–Torre syndrome. J Oral Maxillofac Surg 48: 1334–1337
9. Rushton MA 1955 Hyaline bodies in the epithelium of dental cysts. Proc R Soc Med 48: 407–409
10. Dewey KW 1918 Cysts of the dental system. Dent Cosmos 60: 555–570
11. Browne RM, Smith AJ 1991 In Browne RM (ed) Investigative pathology of odontogenic cysts. CRC Press, Boca Raton, FL
12. Binnie WH, Rowe AHR 1974 The incidence of epithelial rests, proliferation and apical periodontal cysts following root canal treatment in young dogs. Br Dent J 137: 56–70
13. Li T-J, Browne RM, Matthews JB 1994 Quantification of PCNA· cells within odontogenic jaw cyst epithelium. J Oral Pathol Med 23: 184–189
14. Lombardi T, Morgan PR 1995 Immunohistochemical characterisation of odontogenic cysts with mesenchymal and myofilament markers. Oral Pathol Med 24: 170–176
15. Craig GT 1976 The paradental cyst. A specific inflammatory odontogenic cyst. Br Dent J 141: 9–14
16. Ackerman GL, Cohen M, Altini M 1987 The paradental cyst: a clinicopathological study of 57 cases. Oral Surg Oral Med Oral Pathol 64: 308–312
17. Fowler CB, Brannon RB 1989 The paradental cyst: a clinicopathologic study of six new cases and review of the literature. J Oral Maxillofac Surg 47: 243–248
18. Vedtofte P, Praetorius F 1989 The inflammatory paradental cyst. Oral Surg Oral Med Oral Pathol 68: 182–188
19. Daley TD, Wysocki GP, Pringle GA 1994 Relative incidence of odontogenic tumors and oral and jaw cysts in a Canadian population. Oral Surg Oral Med Oral Pathol 77: 276–280
20. Pindborg JJ, Kramer IRH, Shear M 1992 Histological typing of odontogenic tumours, 2nd edn. World Health Organization/Springer-Verlag, Berlin

Nonodontogenic cysts

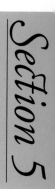

Nasopalatine duct, incisive canal and related cysts 24

These uncommon cysts form in the midline of the anterior part of the maxilla. The nasopalatine, median palatine, palatine papilla, and median alveolar cysts are variants, but differ slightly in their relation to the postulated line of the incisive canal.

INCIDENCE

Nasopalatine duct cysts formed 11% of 2616 jaw cysts analyzed by Shear.[1] Swanson et al[2] found the mean age at presentation of 344 cysts to be 42.5 years, with a range of 9–84 years. Fifty-four per cent of patient were male and 46% female. Shear's 157 patients[1] included 82 blacks in whom the male/female ratio was 5.3 : 1. Among whites with nasopalatine duct cysts the ratio was 2 : 1, and for all 157 patients it was 3 : 1, but other series have shown an equal gender distribution.

CLINICAL FEATURES

Nasopalatine duct cysts are slow growing and resemble other jaw cysts clinically, apart from their site. The most common symptom is swelling of the palate in the midline, just posterior to the central incisors. Complaints noted by Swanson et al[2] were swelling in 52%, discharge in 25%, pain in 20%, and a combination of these symptoms in 70%. Any discharge is usually intermittent, with a salty or, occasionally, foul taste. Growth of a nasopalatine duct cyst can displace the roots of the incisors.

If neglected, nasopalatine duct cysts can cause swelling of most of the hard palate or perforate the palate anteriorly and form a swelling of the alveolar ridge behind the lip. If very superficial these cysts give rise to the so-called palatine papilla cyst.

RADIOGRAPHY

Radiography shows a well-defined rounded, ovoid or occasionally heart-shaped radiolucent area, and often there is sclerotic margin in the anterior part of the midline of the maxilla (Fig. 24.1). These cysts are usually symmetrical, but may be slightly larger to one side. The related incisor teeth are vital unless diseased, and it

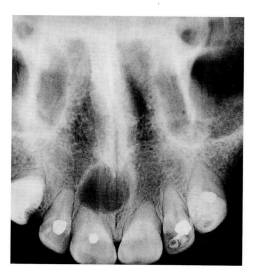

Fig. 24.1 Nasopalatine duct cyst. The rounded area of radiolucency is close to the midline of the anterior maxilla.

should be possible, in an occlusal view, to see that their apices are separated from the margin of the cyst and that the lamina dura is intact. Computed tomography is useful for visualizing the extent of large nasopalatine duct cysts.

The anterior palatine fossa must be distinguished from a small nasopalatine duct cyst. The maximum size of a normal fossa is 6 mm according to Roper-Hall,[3] but Swanson et al[2] found that, although the mean size of nasopalatine duct cysts was 17.1 mm, 6.4% were less than 6 mm in diameter. In such cases, operative interference is only justified by complaint of symptoms.

MICROSCOPY

The lining of nasopalatine cysts is variable, but usually consists of either stratified squamous epithelium or ciliated columnar (respiratory) epithelium, or both together. Mucous glands are often also present. A few scattered chronic inflammatory cells are often seen in some parts of the cyst wall, but are not a prominent feature. In the series analyzed by Swanson et al,[2] respiratory epithelium alone was seen in only 10% of cases, but was seen in combination with other types of epithelium in 18%. Squamous, columnar, cuboidal, or a combination of these types of epithelia, but without respiratory epithelium, was seen in 72%.

A characteristic feature is the frequent presence of neurovascular bundles in the wall. These are the long nasopalatine nerve and vessels, which pass through the nasopalatine canal and are often removed with the cyst (Figs 24.2 and 24.3).

PATHOGENESIS

Incisive canal cysts arise from the epithelium of the nasopalatine ducts in the incisive canal. In cats, for example, there is an organ of smell communicating with the mouth through the palatine canal, and they inhale through the mouth when identifying an odor. In man, only vestiges of a primitive organ of smell in the incisive canal can be found in the form of incomplete epithelium-lined ducts, cords of epithelial cells, or merely epithelial rests.

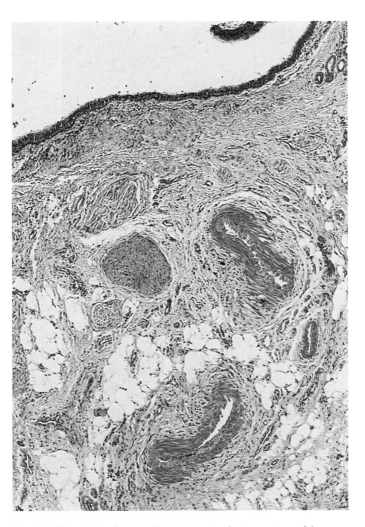

Fig. 24.2 Nasopalatine duct cyst. Low-power view showing sections of the nasopalatine artery and nerve in the cyst wall.

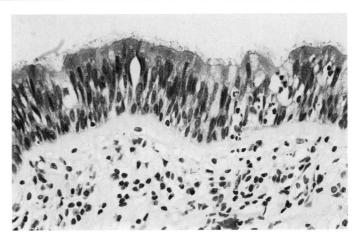

Fig. 24.3 Nasopalatine duct cyst. Part of the lining consists of pseudostratified ciliated epithelium.

BEHAVIOR AND MANAGEMENT

Nasopalatine cysts should be enucleated. Enucleation of exceptionally large examples carries the risk of perforation of the nasal floor or formation of a palatal fistula. The site of these cysts also makes possible damage to the nerve supply of the anterior palate with resulting anesthesia or devitalization of the anterior teeth.

Swanson et al[2] noted that 2% of nasopalatine duct cysts recurred after periods of 3 months to 6 years after operation.

THE 'GLOBULOMAXILLARY CYST'

The term 'globulomaxillary cyst' has been applied to a cyst of the anterior maxilla between the roots of the lateral incisor and canine teeth. Wysocki & Goldblatt[4] ascribe the first description to Thoma in 1937.[5] The latter described it as a 'fissural entity' and believed it to be due to proliferation of sequestered epithelium along the line of fusion of embryonic processes. This view was widely accepted until Christ[6] pointed out, as is generally accepted, that this view of embryological development is incorrect and there is no evidence that epithelium becomes buried in this fashion. Christ[6] critically examined reports of globulomaxillary cysts published during the period 1920–1969, and found them to be lateral periodontal, lateral dentigerous, or odontogenic keratocysts. As a result, the concept of the globulomaxillary cyst has been discarded

Moreover, as Wysocki & Goldblatt[4] point out, both the radiograph and photomicrograph shown by Thoma[5] are typical of a radicular cyst associated with a nonvital central incisor teeth.

MEDIAN MANDIBULAR CYST

Rarely, a cyst forms in the midline of the anterior mandible, associated with vital teeth. These cysts are so uncommon that they are not listed in the large series of jaw cysts cited earlier.

The median mandibular cyst was thought to be a fissural cyst that originated from entrapped epithelium during fusion of the halves of the mandible or a developmental cyst that resulted from inclusion of epithelium trapped in the central groove of the mandibular process in the 10–14 mm embryo. These concepts are untenable. The mandible forms as a single unit within the mandibular process, there is no fusion, and it is not possible for epithelium to become entrapped.

There are only isolated case reports of median mandibular cysts. Gardner[7] examined 20 such reports and concluded that all were probably odontogenic cysts. Therefore, the precise diagnosis is unlikely to be made until microscopy has been carried out.

The treatment of choice is enucleation, but care must be taken not to endanger the vitality of related anterior teeth. Histology will then show whether any further treatment is necessary and how the patient should be advised. If the cyst is exceptionally large, marsupialization may be necessary.

NASOLABIAL CYST

This soft tissue cyst is described in Chapter 26.

REFERENCES

1. Shear M 1992 Cysts of the oral regions, 3rd edn. Wright, Bristol
2. Swanson KS, Kaugars GE, Gunsolley JC 1991 Nasopalatine duct cyst: an analysis of 334 cases. J Oral Maxillofac Surg 49: 268–271
3. Roper-Hall HT 1938 Cysts of developmental origin in the premaxillary region, with special reference to their diagnosis. Br Dent J 65: 405–436
4. Wysocki GP, Goldblatt LI 1993 Invited commentary. The so-called 'globulomaxillary cyst' is extinct. Oral Surg Oral Med Oral Pathol 76: 185–186
5. Thoma K 1937 Facial cleft or fissural cysts. Int J Orthod 23: 83–89
6. Christ TF 1970 The globulomaxillary cyst: an embryologic misconception. Oral Surg Oral Med Oral Pathol 30: 515–526
7. Gardner DG 1988 An evaluation of reported cases of median mandibular cysts. Oral Surg Oral Med Oral Pathol 65: 208–213

Simple and aneurysmal bone cysts (pseudocysts) of the jaws

25

Simple and aneurysmal bone cysts have been categorized among the fibro-osseous lesions in the 1992 World Health Organization (WHO) classification,[1] but seem to have little in common with them. Traditionally, these pseudocysts have been included among other jaw cysts as in Shear's monograph[2] but, unlike other jaw cysts, are more frequent in other parts of the skeleton.

Simple (solitary, 'traumatic', 'hemorrhagic') bone cysts

'Simple bone cyst' is a preferable term to 'solitary bone cyst,' as these cyst can occasionally be multiple. They are bone cavities, but have no epithelial lining and often no fluid content. Lucas,[3] in 1929, was probably the first to describe simple bone cysts, and in 1949 Rushton[4] delineated their major characteristics.

INCIDENCE

In two very large samples,[5,6] simple bone cysts accounted for 0.5% and 0.6% of jaw cysts, and in Shear's series of 2616 jaw cysts they accounted for 1%.[2] In Japan, Saito et al[7] found them to account for 1.2% of 1283 jaw cysts.

Fifty-five to 70% of simple bone cysts form between the ages of 11 and 20 years.[8,9] Relatively few cases are seen in earlier life or after the age of 21 years, but exceptionally they can be found up to the age of 75 years. Males and females are equally or almost equally as frequently affected.

These findings were essentially confirmed by Kuroi[10] in his analysis of 225 cases, apart from the fact that 59% of the patients were male.

At least 90–95% simple bone cysts affect the mandible. However, among 66 cases, Hansen et al[11] found 23% to be in the maxilla.

CLINICAL FEATURES

Simple bone cysts are usually asymptomatic, but Hansen et al,[11] for example, found that pain was experienced by 9% and sensitive teeth or tenderness by 3% of patients. The remainder (14%) had only vague and nonspecific symptoms. Therefore, simple bone cysts are frequently found by chance on routine (especially panoramic) radiographs, as were all the cases surveyed by Saito et al.[7] Significant expansion of the jaw is unusual even with large simple bone cysts, and related teeth are typically vital.

RADIOGRAPHY

These cavities form rounded, radiolucent areas. They usually tend to be less sharply defined than odontogenic cysts, and have three distinctive features (Figs 25.1 and 25.2):

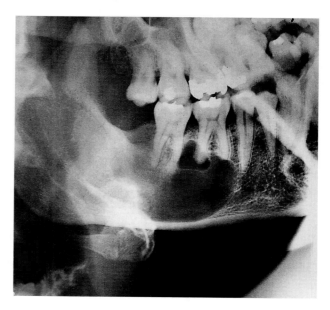

Fig. 25.1 Simple bone cyst. The radiograph shows a well-defined area of radiolucency in the posterior mandible. It extends between the roots of the molar teeth, almost to the crest of the alveolar ridge.

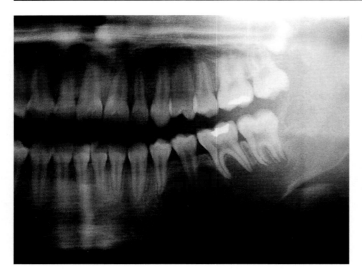

Fig. 25.2 Simple bone cyst. The characteristic upward extension of the lesion between the roots of several teeth is shown, but downward expansion of the lower border of the mandible is unusual.

- the area of radiolucency is typically much larger than the size of any swelling suggests
- the cavity can arch up between the roots of the teeth and, as a consequence, may be first seen on a bite-wing radiograph
- the outline is typically irregular

Simple bone cysts can also extend across the midline of the anterior mandible. Forssell et al[12] have provided schematic diagrams from the radiographs of the outlines of 23 simple bone cysts, showing these features and the variety of shapes.

MICROSCOPY

The cavity has a rough bony wall, and such lining as there is may be thin connective tissue or there may be only a few red cells, blood pigment, or osteoclasts adhering to the surface of the bone (Fig. 25.3).

There are often no cyst contents, but there may sometimes be a little fluid. In Howe's series,[13] 58% had no visible lining, while in the remainder a thin membrane, granulation tissue, or blood clot was seen adhering to the bony wall of the cavity. Hansen et al[11] noted that 50% of simple bone cysts were described at operation as being dry empty cavities, 38% contained fluid that ranged from straw-colored to bloody, 3% were described as cavities with fat lobules, and 7.5% were described as cavities with granulation tissue. In the analysis by Kuroi,[10] the cavity was empty or contained fluid in 94% of 237 cases, and 96% of 135 lesions had no lining or only connective or granulation tissue in the wall.

Simple bone cysts are occasionally associated with florid cemento-osseous dysplasia, as noted by Melrose et al.[14]

PATHOGENESIS

The pathogenesis of simple bone cysts is unknown. According to

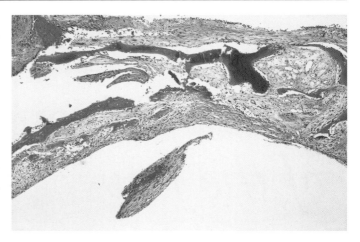

Fig. 25.3 Simple bone cyst. The bony wall has a thin lining of fibrous tissue of nondescript appearance.

Olech et al,[15] these cysts ('traumatic' or 'hemorragic' bone cysts) resulted from injury to and hemorrhage within the bone of the jaw. Hemorrhage was alleged to be followed by failure of organization of the clot and of bony repair. However, there is no evidence that a blow, insufficient to cause a fracture, can cause extensive bleeding within the bone, or that anything other than normal repair would follow. Blood-filled bone cavities in the jaws are left by the enucleation of cysts, but simple bone cysts do not arise as a complication. Furthermore, a common form of treatment for simple bone cysts is to open them and to allow bleeding into the cavity. Normal healing usually follows, and so it is difficult to accept that bleeding within the jaw can both cause simple bone cysts and also cause them to resolve. That aside, only a minority of patients with simple bone cysts have a history of trauma, which is also unlikely to have affected the high proportion of affected females.

In view of the age of most patients and the behavior of simple bone cysts, it seems likely that they are a developmental anomaly.

BEHAVIOR AND MANAGEMENT

Simple bone cysts are slow growing. Friedrichsen[16] observed one to enlarge slowly over a period of 9 years. Clearly, simple bone cysts do not spring full-grown from the start, but whether they continue to grow beyond a certain size is less clear. Giant simple bone cysts in older patients or pathologic fractures from such a cause do not appear to have been seen.

Spontaneous resolution therefore seems to be a distinct possibility, and has been reported.[17–20] This view was also accepted by Saito et al,[7] who noted that new bone was forming in two simple bone cysts that had been excised. In the words of Hall,[21] 'treatment by surgical intervention is almost universally agreed upon'; as a result, simple bone cysts are unlikely to be allowed to complete what may be a limited life-cycle.

The main reason for opening the cavity is to confirm the diagnosis. The characteristic lack of cyst fluid and the unlined bony wall are then usually enough to provide the diagnosis, but it is preferable, if possible, to remove some of the connective tissue lining for confirmatory purposes. Opening the cavity is followed by healing, either as a result of bleeding or because of spontaneous resolution.

Despite the evidence for spontaneous resolution, there is no doubt that simple bone cysts in the jaws can recur but, unlike their counterparts in long bones, rarely do so. Multiple simple bone cysts with recurrences have been reported by Feinberg et al,[22] while Kuttenberger et al[23] were the first to report a recurrence in a bone graft after excision. However, they also accepted that this apparent recurrence might have been an independent lesion developing in the rib used for the reconstruction.

It must be emphasized that recurrence of simple bone cysts is so rare that it is not an argument for radical treatment.

Aneurysmal bone cyst

Although categorized with fibro-osseous and giant cell lesions in the WHO classification,[1] Fechner & Mills[24] believe that there is considerable evidence of a vascular origin for aneurysmal bone cysts.

These cysts were first described by Jaffe & Lichtenstein in 1942.[25] The use of the term 'aneurysmal' was intended to refer to rapid distension of the bony cavity, rather than to describe the vascular pathology.[26] Bernier & Bhaskar[27] are credited with reporting the first example in the jaw.

INCIDENCE

Age and gender distribution

According to El Deeb et al,[28] aneurysmal bone cysts account for 1.5% of nonepithelial-cyst-like lesions of the jaws. In Shear's series,[2] they accounted for 0.5% of 2126 of all types of jaw cyst.

Of 238 aneurysmal bone cysts (all skeletal sites) reviewed by Vergel et al,[29] 54% were in females and ages ranged from 18 months to 69 years (mean 16.1 years). Of these, 24% of patients were in their first decade and 55% were in their second. Struthers & Shear[30] found from their survey of 46 aneurysmal bone cysts of the jaws that 93% were seen in the first three decades, with a peak between the ages of 10 and 19 years. Females accounted for 62% overall, but males and females were almost equally frequently affected in the peak age group.

Site distribution

Aneurysmal bone cysts most frequently form in the long bones, pelvis, or vertebrae. Among 238 aneurysmal bone cysts reviewed by Vergel et al,[29] only five were in or close to the jaws. In the case of jaw lesions, 55–60% are in the mandible, mostly in the molar region and sometimes extending into the ramus.

CLINICAL FEATURES

The main manifestation is usually a painless swelling, which may sometimes expand rapidly.

RADIOGRAPHY

Radiographic appearances are variable, but typically consist of a radiolucent area, which may be balloon-like, sometimes with a suggestion of trabeculation or loculation (Fig. 25.4). Areas of bone resorption and apposition may sometimes simulate an osteosarcoma.

MICROSCOPY

Aneurysmal bone cysts are covered by a thin layer of bone and periosteum. When removed, venous blood seeps out and the gross specimen appears as livid, friable material in which blood-filled spaces may be discernible.

The lesion consists of a highly cellular mass containing blood-filled cavities, which has been likened to a blood-filled sponge. Despite this appearance, the vascular spaces lack an endothelial lining identifiable by immunohistochemistry or electron microscopy. Alles & Schulz[31] therefore suggest that the appearance is due to extravasation of red cells from the septal capillaries, which lack a basal membrane to their endothelium. Larger, thin-walled

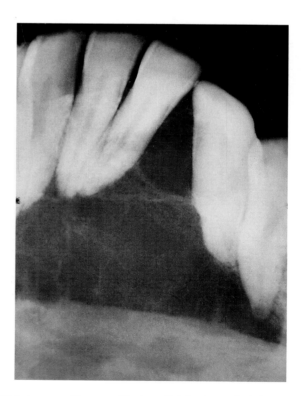

Fig. 25.4 Aneurysmal bone cyst. The large, ill-defined area of radiolucency with a finely trabeculated pattern has tilted the incisor teeth.

vessels are sometimes prominent in the septa. Other areas are more solid and contain varying numbers of giant cells, which have a tendency to cluster round a vascular space. In other such areas, osteoid formation may be prominent.

Extreme cellularity, mitotic activity, and the frequent presence of giant cells may lead to confusion with a sarcoma. This belief may be reinforced by lesions that grow rapidly or show radiographic appearance suggestive of osteosarcoma (Figs 25.5–25.10).

ASSOCIATED LESIONS

In 123 aneurysmal bone cysts outside the head and neck region, Martinez & Sissons[32] found that 36 were part of another bone lesion, particularly a giant cell tumor or chondroblastoma. Other lesions that have been associated include simple or dentigerous cysts, fibrous dysplasia, nonosteogenic fibroma, osteosarcoma, cemento-ossifying fibroma, and hemangioma. Aneurysmal bone cysts have also been reported in association with fractures or other bone injuries,[33] but coincidence is difficult to exclude.

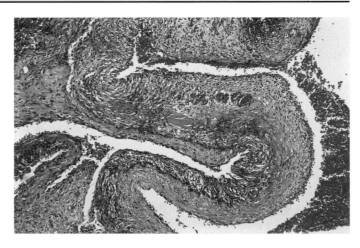

Fig. 25.7 Aneurysmal bone cyst. The spongy fibrovascular tissue and extravasated blood are a typical appearance.

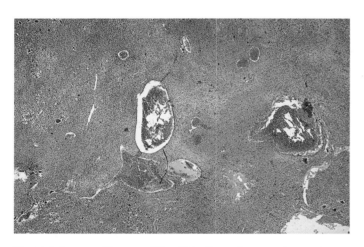

Fig. 25.5 Aneurysmal bone cyst. The cellular fibrous tissue contains prominent cyst-like vascular spaces.

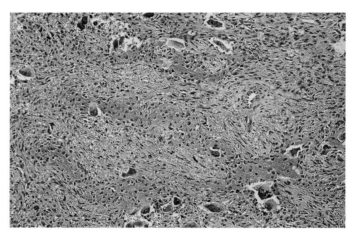

Fig. 25.8 Aneurysmal bone cyst. Osteoid formation is prominent in this area.

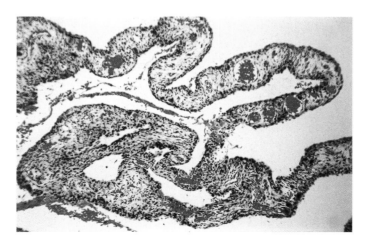

Fig. 25.6 Aneurysmal bone cyst. Another area shows the spongy fibrous tissue containing prominent blood vessels.

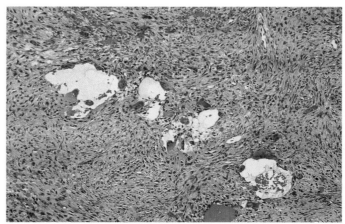

Fig. 25.9 Aneurysmal bone cyst. The vascular spaces clearly lack any endothelial lining, and giant cells form part of their walls.

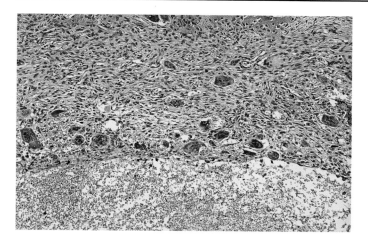

Fig. 25.10 Aneurysmal bone cyst. Higher power view confirms the lack of endothelial lining of the vascular spaces and the presence of multiple giant cells.

HISTOGENESIS

The nature of aneurysmal bone cysts remains controversial. Shear[2] has examined the problem in great detail from his own experience, from the work of Struthers[34] and of Struthers & Shear,[35,36] and from a detailed review of the literature. The many theories about their origin have been reviewed by Hernandez et al.[37]

That aneurysmal bone cysts are not neoplastic is shown by those cysts that undergo spontaneous resolution, as noted by and Hernandez et al[37] and others.[38,39] Aneurysmal bone cysts also develop in association with, or are secondary to, other bone lesions or tumors, as mentioned earlier. Biesecker et al[40] proposed that aneurysmal bone cysts originated from a pre-existing arteriovenous aneurysm and, as mentioned earlier, Fechner & Mills[24] present evidence that strongly suggests a vascular origin.

Thus nothing is known for certainty about the pathogenesis aneurysmal bone cyst. Although the most obvious possibility is that the aneurysmal bone cyst is a vascular malformation, Hernandez et al[37] suggest that there is a moderate degree of consensus that it is a non-neoplastic, fibrodysplastic lesion.

BEHAVIOR AND MANAGEMENT

Diagnosis from the clinical and radiographic findings may be difficult. Computed tomography scanning will define the extent of the lesion more precisely. Aspiration is likely to yield venous blood, unlike aspiration from a central hemangioma, which can also be excluded by angiography. Biopsy is essential, particularly if radiographs suggest an osteosarcoma.

Once the diagnosis has been confirmed, treatment usually consists of thorough curettage, as advocated by Motamedi & Yazdi,[41] who reported the findings and treatment of 11 examples in the jaws. Excision may be preferable, as the lesion occasionally recurs. The blood appears to be static, and severe bleeding is

uncommon. Any recurrences can be treated by more extensive curettage or by block excision, but are far less frequent in jaw lesions than elsewhere in the skeleton.

Cryotherapy is an alternative approach, but experience of its value is limited. Radiotherapy has also been used, either in association with curettage or to deal with recurrences. However, Vergel et al[29] noted that, of 13 patients so treated, three developed sarcomas.

In contrast to such practices, the reports of spontaneous resolution suggest that an expectant approach may be worth consideration, provided that the biopsy diagnosis is certain.

REFERENCES

1. Pindborg JJ, Kramer IRH, Shear M 1992 Histological typing of odontogenic tumours, 2nd edn. World Health Organization Springer-Verlag, Berlin
2. Shear M 1992 Cysts of the oral regions, 3rd edn. Wright, Bristol
3. Lucas CD 1929 Do all cysts of the jaws originate from the dental system? J Am Dent Assoc 16: 659–661
4. Rushton MA 1946 Solitary bone cysts in the mandible. Br Dent J 81: 37–49
5. Ahlfors E, Larsson A, Sjögren S 1984 The odontogenic keratocyst: a benign cystic tumour? J Oral Maxillofac Surg 42: 10–19
6. Hoffmeister B, Härle F 1985 Zysten im Kiefer-Gesichtbereich – eine katamnestiche Studie an 3353 Zysten. Deutsche Zahnärztl Zschrft 40: 610–614
7. Saito Y, Hoshina Y, Nagamine T, Nakajima T, Suzuki M, Hayashi T 1992 Simple bone cyst. A clinical and histopathologic study of fifteen cases. Oral Surg Oral Med Oral Pathol 74: 487–491
8. Howe GL 1965 'Haemorrhagic' cysts of the mandible. Br J Oral Surg 3: 77–91
9. Hansen IS, Sapone J, Sproat RC 1979 Traumatic bone cysts of jaws. Report of sixty-six cases. Oral Surg Oral Med Oral Pathol 37: 899–910
10. Kuroi M 1980 Simple bone cyst of the jaw: review of the literature and report of a case. J Oral Surg 38: 456–459
11. Hansen LS, Sapone J, Sproat RC 1979 Traumatic bone cysts of the jaws. Oral Surg Oral Med Oral Pathol 37: 399–310
12. Forssell K, Forssell H, Happonen R-P, Neva M 1988 Simple bone cyst. Review of the literature and anlysis of 23 cases. Intl J Oral Maxillofac Surg 17: 21–24
13. Howe GL 1965 'Haemorrhagic cysts' of the mandible. Br J Oral Surg 3: 55–75
14. Melrose RJ, Abrams AM, Mills BG 1976 Florid osseous dysplasia: a clinical-pathologic study of thirty-four cases. Oral Surg 41: 62–82
15. Olech E, Sicher H, Weinmann JP 1951 Traumatic mandibular bone cysts. Oral Surg Oral Med Oral Pathol 4: 1160–1172
16. Friedrichsen SW 1993 Long-term progression of a traumatic bone cyst. A case report. Oral Surg Oral Med Oral Pathol 76: 421–424
17. Blum T 1955 An additional report on traumatic bone cysts. Oral Surg 8: 917–939
18. Szerlip L 1966 Traumatic bone cysts. Resolution without surgery. Oral Surg 21: 201–204
19. Cowan CG 1980 Traumatic bone cysts of the jaws and their presentation. Int J Oral Surg 9: 287–291
20. Killey HC, Kay LW, Seward GR 1977 Benign cystic lesions of the jaws, their diagnosis and treatment. Churchill Livingstone, Edinburgh
21. Hall AM 1976 The solitary bone cyst. Report of two cases. Oral Surg 42: 164–168
22. Feinberg SE, Finkelstein MW, Page HL, Dembo JB 1989 Recurrent 'traumatic' bone cysts of the mandible. Oral Surg 57: 418–422
23. Kuttenberger JJ, Farmand M, Stöss H 1992 Recurrence of a solitary bone cyst of the mandible in a bone graft. Oral Surg Oral Med Oral Pathol 74: 550–556
24. Fechner RE, Mills SE 1992 Tumors of the bones and joints. Atlas of tumor pathology. Armed Forces Institute of Pathology, Washington, DC, third series, fascicle 8
25. Jaffe HL, Lichtenstein L 1942 Solitary unicameral bone cyst with emphasis on the roentgen picture, the pathologic appearance and pathogenesis. Arch Surg 44: 1004–1025
26. Jaffe HL 1958 Aneurysmal bone cyst. Tumors and tumorous conditions of the bones and joints, 1st edn. Lea & Febiger, Philadelphia
27. Bernier J, Bhaskar S 1958 Aneurysmal bone cyst of the mandible. Oral Surg 11: 1018–1022
28. El Deeb, Sedano HO, Waite DE 1980 Aneurysmal bone cyst of the jaw. Intl J Oral Surg 9: 301–311
29. Vergel AM, Bond JR, Shives TC, McLeod RA, Unni KK 1992 Aneurysmal bone cyst. A clinicopathologic study of 228 cases. Cancer 69: 2921–2931
30. Struthers PJ, Shear M 1984 Aneurysmal bone cyst of the jaws. I. Clinicopathological features. Intl J Oral Surg 13: 85–89
31. Alles JU, Schulz A 1986 Immunocytochemical markers (endothelial and histiocytic) and ultrastructure of primary aneurysmal bone cysts. Hum Pathol 17: 39–45
32. Martinez V, Sissons HA 1988 Aneurysmal bone cyst. A review of 123 cases including primary lesions and those secondary to other bone pathology. Cancer 61: 2291–2304

33. Struthers PJ, Shear M 1984 Aneurysmal bone cyst of the jaws. II. Pathogenesis. Intl J Oral Surg 13: 92–100

34. Struthers PJ 1980 Aneurysmal bone cyst. M Dent Dissertation. University of Witwatersrand, Johannesburg

35. Struthers PJ, Shear M 1984 Aneurysmal bone cyst of the jaws. I. Clinicopathological features. Intl J Oral Surg 13: 85–89

36. Struthers PJ, Shear M 1984 Aneurysmal bone cyst of the jaws. II. Pathogenesis. Intl J Oral Surg 13: 92–100

37. Hernandez GA, Castro A, Castro G, Amador E 1993 Aneurysmal bone cyst versus hemangioma of the mandible. Report of a long-term follow-up of a self-limiting case. Oral Surg Oral Med Oral Pathol 76: 790–796

38. Waitzkin ED, de Luca SA 1986 Aneurysmal bone cyst. Am Family Physic 33: 137–138

39. Malghem J, Maldague B, Essenlinckx W, Noel H, De Nayer P, Vincent A 1989 Spontaneous healing of aneurysmal bone cysts: a report of three cases. J Bone Joint Surg Br 71: 645–650

40. Biesecker JL, Margrove RC, Huvos AG, Miké V 1970 Aneurysmal bone cyst: a clinicopathologic study of 66 cases. Cancer 26: 615–625

41. Motamedi MHK, Yazdi E 1994 Aneurysmal bone cyst of the jaws: analysis of 11 cases. J Oral Maxillofac Surg 52: 471–475

Oral and perioral soft tissue cysts

26

Nasolabial cyst

This uncommon cyst forms in the soft tissues, deep to the naso-labial fold. Roed-Petersen[1] analyzed the data on 111 reported nasolabial cysts and added five more. Further series of 51 and 45 cases have also been reported.[2,3]

INCIDENCE

Nasolabial cysts formed 0.7% of the 2616 cysts described by Shear;[4] all (141) of them were in females and the ages of those affected ranged from 12 to 75 years, with a peak frequency in the fourth and fifth decades.

CLINICAL FEATURES

Nasolabial cysts cause swelling of the upper lip in the canine region, may obliterate the nasolabial fold, and may distort the nostril, which in extreme cases can become obstructed. There may be shallow saucerization of the underlying bone. These cysts are usually unilateral, but 10% are bilateral.

MICROSCOPY

The fibrous cyst wall is typically lined entirely or, more frequently, in part by pseudo-stratified columnar epithelium, sometimes ciliated (Figs 26.1 and 26.2). Some goblet cells and metaplastic areas of stratified squamous epithelium are also sometimes present. Rarely, the cyst is lined by cuboidal epithelium. In addition, any combination of these types of epithelia may be present. The fibrous wall may contain mucous glands and is sometimes highly vascular. The wall may occasionally contain a layer of cartilage.

BEHAVIOR AND MANAGEMENT

Nasolabial cysts expand slowly and cause no complications other than those already mentioned. Rarely, the cyst perforates the nasal mucosa and discharges into the nose.

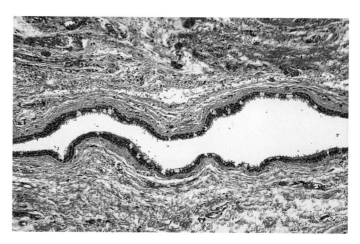

Fig. 26.1 Nasolabial cyst. Thin, regular lining of bilayered epithelium.

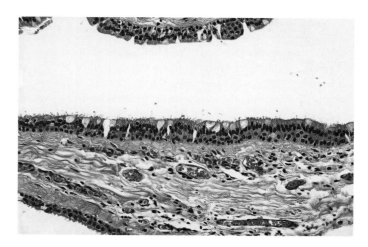

Fig. 26.2 Nasolabial cyst. Higher power view showing the ciliated lining with goblet cells.

Conservative enucleation is the treatment of choice.

HISTOGENESIS

Nasolabial cysts probably arise from remnants of the lower part of the embryonic lacrimal duct. Consistent with this view are the facts that these cysts are usually lined, like the nasolacrimal duct, by pseudostratified columnar epithelium, and that they are sometimes bilateral.

MUCOCELES

Mucoceles usually result from damage to the duct and obstruction to the drainage of a minor salivary gland. The common sites are the lower lip, and the retromolar pad and cheek, from occlusal trauma from erupting upper wisdom teeth. Rarely, mucoceles form in the palate after trauma by sharp bones or crusts. The mechanism of production of these cysts is tearing of the duct wall, which leads to leakage of saliva into the superficial tissues.

MICROSCOPY

Mucoceles are usually mucous extravasation cysts. In the early stages, pools of extravasated mucus surrounded by an inflammatory reaction form in the submucosal connective tissue. These pools coalesce to produce a macroscopic cyst with a wall of compressed but cellular connective tissue, and the inflammatory reaction progressively subsides. Occasionally, such cysts form immediately beneath the epithelium to form a pemphigoid-like bulla.

Occasionally, obstruction causes the duct to become distended, and the result is a true retention cyst lined by duct epithelium, sometimes containing mucous cells (Figs 26.3–26.7).

MANAGEMENT

Untreated mucoceles eventually burst and discharge spontaneously. However, recurrence typically follows as a result of healing of the overlying epithelium and further accumulation of secretion. Complete excision of the cyst with its minor gland of origin is

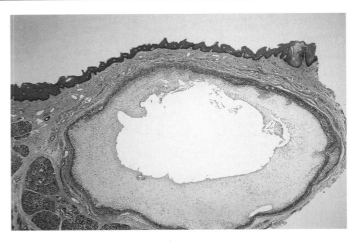

Fig. 26.4 Mucous extravasation cyst. Submucosal cyst with fibrous tissue lining and adjacent salivary tissue.

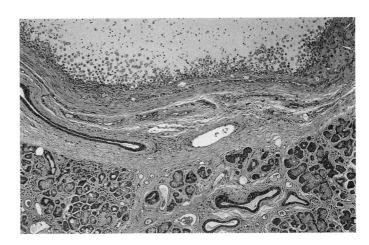

Fig. 26.5 Mucous extravasation cyst. Higher power view shows the compressed fibrous tissue forming a capsule, macrophages leaking into the cyst lumen and adjacent salivary gland lobules.

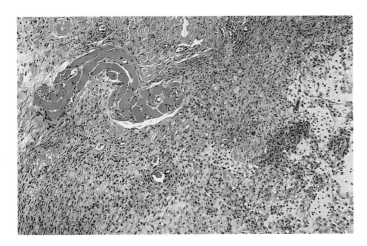

Fig. 26.3 Mucous extravasation cyst. In this early stage, saliva has infiltrated muscle and provoked an inflammatory reaction.

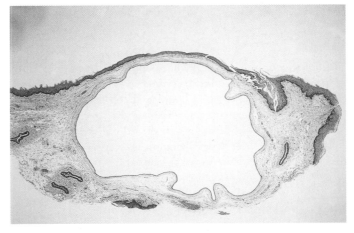

Fig. 26.6 Mucous retention cyst. Low-power view shows the highly circumscribed appearance of the epithelial-lined cyst due to gross dilatation of the minor gland duct.

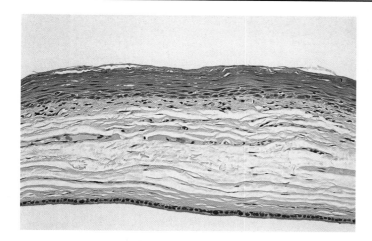

Fig. 26.7 Mucous retention cyst. The lining of cuboidal epithelium is just deep to the lamina propria.

therefore indicated. This is done through a linear incision through the overlying mucosa. Occasionally, mucoceles recur after surgery, either because the affected glandular tissue has not been completely excised or because operation has caused further scarring that blocks adjacent glands. In this situation cryosurgery or diathermy is often curative.

RANULA

Occasionally, damage to the duct of the sublingual gland causes the formation of a mucous extravasation cyst appearing as a tense bluish (frog's belly) swelling in the anterior floor of the mouth just to one side of the midline. Such a ranula is submucosal, but lies entirely above the mylohyoid muscle. It may reach 3 or 4 cm in diameter and impede speech.

A deep ranula lies entirely within the submental space, or it may be plunging and hour-glass in shape. It then lies partly superficial and partly deep to the mylohyoid muscle, having passed through a developmental dehiscence in the latter. The lining of an extensive ranula is difficult to excise and usually ruptures during surgery. However, this is unimportant, as permanent cure is achieved by excision of the affected sublingual gland, with little regard to the ranula itself. In the case of a plunging ranula, Mizuno & Yamaguchi[5] recommend transoral drainage in addition. (See Figs 26.3–26.7.)

OTHER SALIVARY CYSTS

Congenital cysts are occasionally seen, and lymphoepithelial (branchial cleft) cysts can extend into the parotid area.

Benign lymphoepithelial parotid cysts, which are often bilateral and are seen on computed tomography scanning in association with cervical lymphadenopathy, are strongly suggestive of infection, with human immunodeficiency virus (HIV).

So-called 'branchial cleft cysts' are well recognized. However, lymphoepithelial cysts can also develop within the oral cavity and are of more controversial origin. Toto et al[6] concurred with earlier views that lymphoepithelial cysts are pseudocysts and that the epithelium could be of salivary duct or tonsillar crypt origin. Buchner & Hansen[7] have described the clinicopathologic findings in 38 cases.

Clinically, intraoral lymphoepithelial cysts usually form in the floor of the mouth or tongue, but occasionally occur in other sites, such as the soft palate. In most cases the cysts are symptomless, range from 1 to 10 mm in size, and form round or oval submucosal swellings that are freely mobile and occasionally discharge. A wide age range can be affected, but the peak incidence is in the third decade. Men are affected almost twice as frequently as women.

MICROSCOPY

Intraoral lymphoepithelial cysts are usually lined by a flat layer of stratified squamous epithelium, which may be parakeratinized. A few are lined by pseudostratified columnar epithelium, which is sometimes ciliated and may contain goblet cells. Others may be lined by simple flat or cuboidal epithelium. In most cases, lymphoid tissue entirely surrounds the cyst, and in the majority of cases contains germinal follicles (Figs 26.8 and 26.9).

BEHAVIOR AND MANAGEMENT

Conservative surgical excision is adequate.

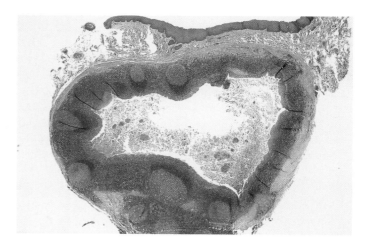

Fig. 26.8 Intraoral lymphoepithelial cyst. This submucosal cyst has an incomplete lining of stratified squamous epithelium, with prominent lymphoid follicles in the wall.

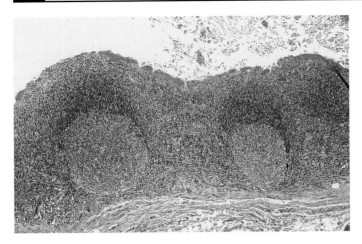

Fig. 26.9 Intraoral lymphoepithelial cyst. Higher power view shows the incomplete epithelial lining and normal germinal centers in the lymphoid follicles.

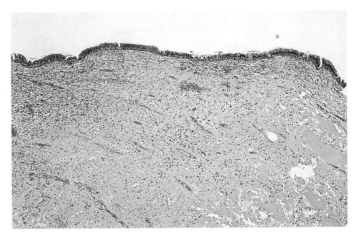

Fig. 26.10 Antral mucous cyst. This retention type is lined by pseudostratified columnar (respiratory) epithelium.

Benign mucosal cysts of the antrum

The benign mucosal cyst of the antrum is sometimes referred to as a mucocele or retention cyst. Kwapis & Whitten[8] point out that widespread use of panoramic radiography indicates that these cysts are more common than previously thought. Myall et al[9] from examination of 1429 orthopantomograms, found mucosal cysts in 5% of them, while Rhodus[10] found, from panoramic radiographs of 1249 patients, 4.3% to be affected. Their main oral importance is to distinguish them from odontogenic cysts extending into the maxilla. The peak incidence is between the ages of 21 and 30 years, and males account for 68% of cases.

Symptoms are usually absent until the patient becomes aware of a sensation of fullness of the side of the face, numbness, or nasal obstruction.

RADIOGRAPHY

Antral cysts are usually single and appear as smooth, spherical, or dome-shaped opacities with a narrow or broad base. They vary in size from less than 10 mm to occasional lesions that fill the antral cavity. The thin cortical line of the antral floor persists intact and is not displaced, and so antral cysts should be readily distinguishable from maxillary odontogenic cysts.

MICROSCOPY

Antral mucous cysts may either be secretory (retention) cysts and lined by respiratory or less well-differentiated epithelium, or nonsecretory and, like oral mucous extravasation cysts, be lined by fibroblasts (Fig. 26.10).

BEHAVIOR AND MANAGEMENT

Radiographic follow-up shows that some of these cysts can persist unchanged for long periods, while others slowly enlarge or resolve spontaneously.

Because of the possibility of spontaneous regression and absence of symptoms in most cases, there is probably little justification for surgical intervention. If there are symptoms that can be ascribed to an antral cyst, the cyst can be cannulated and drained. Alternatively, it can be removed via a Caldwell–Luc approach.

POSTOPERATIVE MAXILLARY CYST (SURGICAL CILIATED CYST OF THE MAXILLA)

This subgroup of maxillary antral cysts has mainly been reported from Japan where it appears to be a far more frequent phenomenon than in Europe, America, or southern Africa. Shear[4] saw only four cases among 2616 cysts over a 32-year period. By contrast, Maeda et al[11] reported on 100 examples seen over a 5-year period in Japan. These high figures have been attributed to the many Caldwell–Luc operations carried out in Japan just after the Second World War, before antibiotics became available. However, this theory does not seem to correlate sufficiently closely with the reported ages of those affected.

CLINICAL FEATURES

Postoperative maxillary cysts are seen in patients aged 20 years or older, the peak incidence occurring between the ages of 30 and 39 years; occasional examples are seen in the eighth decade.

In virtually all cases there is a history of surgical intervention or trauma to the maxillary antrum, but there is a delay of one or more decades before the onset of symptoms. In the series reported by Yamamato & Takagi[12] the shortest latent period was 4 years and the longest was 49 years.

Symptoms include pain or discomfort, or swelling of the face or palate, and there may be discharge of pus.

RADIOGRAPHY

Radiographically, a postoperative maxillary cyst appears as a well-defined radiolucent area related to the sinus. The area is usually unilocular and there may be sclerosis of at least part of the surrounding bone. There is no communication with the antrum, although the cyst may appear to encroach on it. Later, as the cyst enlarges, bone destruction becomes evident and it may perforate the antral wall and expand beyond its margins.

MICROSCOPY

Postoperative maxillary cysts are lined by ciliated columnar epithelium, which undergoes squamous metaplasia in inflamed areas or becomes ulcerated. Other residua of inflammation, such as cholesterol clefts, foam cells, or hemosiderin, may also be seen. The cyst wall consists of dense fibrous tissue, which is sometimes infiltrated by inflammatory cells.

BEHAVIOR AND MANAGEMENT

Enucleation is usually possible, but there is a risk of recurrence if the cyst is infected or has perforated the bony wall so that the cyst wall is thin and firmly adherent to surrounding tissues. In such cases, marsupialization is the treatment of choice.

CLINICAL FEATURES

Oral dermoid cysts are uncommon. Gibson & Fenton,[15] in a search of the English literature for the preceding 30 years, found only 30 cases, while Howell[16] found only five examples that had been seen in oral surgical units in England over a period of 9 years. Sublingual dermoid cysts form swellings of the floor of the mouth and neck. They are probably present at birth, but treatment is not usually sought before the age of 45 years. Dermoids are painless and asymptomatic until they become large enough to interfere with function. They are soft or doughy in consistency if filled with keratin. Ultimately, a sublingual dermoid can interfere with speech or swallowing and, if infected, rapid expansion can be life-threatening by obstructing the airway, as reported by Cortezzi & de Albuquerque.[17] Remarkably, patients sometimes tolerate these cysts until they are so large as to protrude from the mouth and prevent it from closing.[18]

MICROSCOPY

Sublingual dermoids have a fibrous wall lined by stratified squamous epithelium, which is thinly or heavily keratinized (Fig. 26.11). In the latter case the cyst is filled with keratin. Hair follicles and other skin adnexae may be seen in the wall.

BEHAVIOR AND MANAGEMENT

A sublingual dermoid cyst should be the first possibility considered when a midline submucosal swelling is seen in the anterior floor of the mouth. The diagnosis is almost certain if the mass has a putty-like consistency due to keratin accumulation. Aspiration should be avoided because of the risk of introducing infection but, if necessary, can be carried out immediately preoperatively.

Sublingual dermoid and epidermoid cysts

Dermoid cysts are lined by epidermis. Epidermoid cysts also contain skin appendages, but many sections may have to be examined before they are found. Frequently, therefore, either type may be referred to indifferently as a dermoid. They are an occasional finding in the anterior floor of the mouth in the midline, sometimes associated with a swelling in the neck. Rarely, other sites such as the palate can be affected. Concomitant sublingual and submental dermoid cysts have been reported in infants by Calderon & Kaplan[13] and Worley & Laskin.[14] Although it has been postulated that they arise from epithelium trapped between the two lingual swellings that enlarge backwards from the mandibular arch to form the anterior two-thirds of the tongue, this seems unlikely, as such epithelium is endodermal and would not be expected to produce skin and its adnexae.

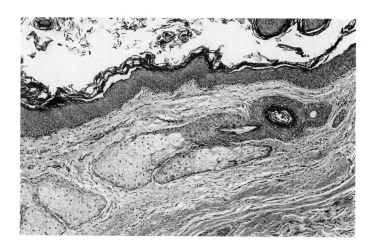

Fig. 26.11 Dermoid cyst. The lining of keratinized squamous epithelium overlies sebaceous tissue

Enucleation is curative and recurrence is rare. If infection has supervened and the airway is threatened, intubation if possible or, failing that, tracheostomy is necessary.

Thyroglossal duct cyst

The anlage of the median lobe of the thyroid gland originates as a diverticulum from a site that will become the foramen caecum at the junction of the anterior two-thirds and the posterior third of the tongue. This tissue remains attached to the base of the tongue, but migrates down the neck anterior to the hyoid bone to its adult position. By the sixth or seventh week of development the duct closes and normally involutes, but in a few patients complete involution is not achieved.

Vestiges of thyroglossal duct tissue can give rise to cysts or sinuses, and be the site of infection, cosmetic defects, or, rarely, of carcinoma.

The great majority of thyroglossal duct cysts form in or very close to the midline below the hyoid bone. They are usually only a few centimeters in diameter and are symptomless unless infected, when they give rise to fistula formation. Otherwise they form soft, sometimes fluctuant swellings and gradually enlarge. Typically, but not invariably, they rise during swallowing or protrusion of the tongue. Rarely, thyroglossal duct cysts form in the floor of the mouth or beneath the foramen cecum, and can then give rise to dysphonia or dyspnea, particularly if infection intervenes.

MICROSCOPY

Thyroglossal duct cysts and are lined by respiratory or squamous epithelium, but this may be destroyed by infection, leaving only granulation or fibrous tissue. Mucous glands may be present, but thyroid tissue is rarely seen (Fig. 26.12).

BEHAVIOR AND MANAGEMENT

Thyroglossal duct cysts should be excised. The tract should be traced down from its source to the pyramidal lobe of the thyroid gland and removal of a 1 cm block of surrounding tissue and a 1–2 cm segment of the center of the hyoid bone is advised to ensure complete elimination of duct tissue. Van der Wal et al[15] reported no recurrences in eight of 16 patients thus treated, but in the remaining untreated patients the cyst remained unchanged in one, shrank in three, and completely disappeared in four.

Anterior midline lingual cyst (intralingual cyst of foregut origin)

Anterior midline lingual cysts are rare and of controversial histo-

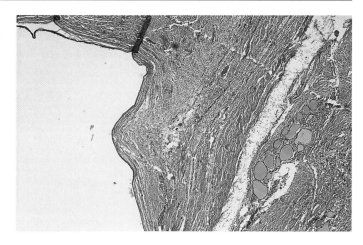

Fig. 26.12 Thyroglossal cyst. This cyst is lined by flattened squamous epithelium and has a thick fibrous wall with colloid-containing thyroid follicles nearby.

genesis. As reviewed by Shear,[4] they are present at birth but may not become evident until infancy, when they appear as a soft swelling in the anterior part of the midline of the tongue. They can sometimes become so large as to cause difficulty with eating or, occasionally, respiratory obstruction.

Histologically anterior midline lingual cysts can be lined by stratified squamous or pseudostratified columnar epithelium, which may be ciliated.

Anterior midline lingual cysts should be excised and are unlikely to recur.

Heterotopic oral gastrointestinal cysts

These rare cysts are discussed in Chapter 54.

Thymic cysts

Thymic cysts in the neck are particularly uncommon. Their nature is unlikely to be recognized until established by microscopy. Strome & Eraklis[20] found fewer than 60 cases of cervical thymic cysts in the world literature.

Thymic cysts probably arise from remnants of the thymopharyngeal duct, which mainly originates from the third branchial arch. They are twice as common in males as females, and nearly 70% are seen in the first decade. Thymic cysts typically form in or adjacent to the carotid sheath and can therefore be found anywhere from the angle of the mandible to the midline. They cause a slowly enlarging mass, which is sometimes painful and can occasionally swell rapidly due to intracystic hemorrhage.

MICROSCOPY

Thymic cysts are round or tubular with thick or thin fibrous walls. The lining consists of cuboidal, columnar, or stratified squamous epithelium, unless this is replaced by granulation tissue. Diagnosis depends on finding thymic tissue in the wall, but many sections may have to be examined.

BEHAVIOR AND MANAGEMENT

The diagnosis is unlikely to be suspected clinically and excision could lead to removal of contiguous thymic tissue. This must obviously be avoided in young patients because of the risk of endangering immunologic development. The main clue to the nature of a thymic cyst is the finding of a thin fibrous cord or an extension of the cyst to the thymic region of the mediastinum. Analysis of preoperative frozen sections is therefore desirable in order to confirm the diagnosis.

REFERENCES

1. Roed-Petersen B 1969 Nasolabial cysts. Br J Oral Surg 7: 84–95
2. Wesley RK, Scannell T, Nathan LE 1984 Nasolabial cyst: presentation of a case with a review of the literature. J Oral Maxillofac Surg 42: 188–192
3. Van Bruggen AP, Shear M, du Preez IJ, van Wuk DP, Beyers D, Leeferink GA 1985 Nasolabial cysts. A report on 10 cases and a review of the literature. J Dent Assoc S Africa 40: 15–19
4. Shear M 1992 Cysts of the oral regions, 3rd edn. Wright, Bristol
5. Mizuno A, Yamaguchi K 1993 The plunging ranula. Intl J Maxillofac Surg 22: 113–115
6. Toto PD, Wortel JP, Joseph G 1982 Lymphoepithelial cysts and associated immunoglobulins. Oral Surg Oral Med Oral Pathol 54: 59–65
7. Buchner A, Hansen LS 1980 Lymphoepithelial cysts of the oral cavity. Oral Surg 50: 441–449
8. Kwapis BW, Whitten JB 1971 Mucosal cysts of the maxillary sinus. J Oral Surg 29: 561–566
9. Myall RWT, Eastep PB, Silver JG 1974 Mucous retention cysts of the maxillary antrum. J Am Dent Assoc 89: 1338–1342
10. Rhodus NL 1990 The prevalence and significance of maxillary sinus mucous retention cysts. Ear Nose Throat J 69: 82–90
11. Maeda Y, Osaki T, Yibeda K, Hirota J 1987 Clinico-pathologic studies on postoperative maxillary cysts. Int J Oral Maxillofac Surg 16: 682–687
12. Yamamato H, Takagi M 1986 clinicopathologic study of the postoperative maxillary cyst. Oral Surg Oral Med Oral Pathol 62: 544–548
13. Calderon S, Kaplan I 1993 Concomitant sublingual and submental epidermoid cysts. J Oral Maxillofac Surg 51: 790–792
14. Worley CM, Laskin DM 1993 Conicidental sublingual and submental epidermoid cysts. J Oral Maxillofac Surg 51: 787–790
15. Gibson WS, Fenton NA 1982 Congenital sublingual dermoid cyst. Arch Otolaryngol 108: 745–748
16. Howell CJT 1985 The sublingual dermoid cyst. Report of five cases and review of the literature. Oral Surg Oral Med Oral Pathol 66: 578–580
17. Cortezzi W, de Albuquerque EB 1994 Secondarily infected epidermoid cyst in the floor of the mouth causing a life-threatening situation. J Oral Maxillofac Surg 52: 762–764
18. Mathur SK, Menon PRN 1980 Dermoid cyst of the tongue. Report of a case. Oral Surg 51: 217–218
19. Van der Wal N, Wiener JD, Allard RHB, Henzen-Logmans SC, van der Waal I 1987 Thyroglossal duct cysts in patients over 30 years of age. Int J Oral Maxillofac Surg 16: 416–419
20. Strome M, Eraklis A 1977 Thymic cysts in the neck. Laryngoscope 87: 1645–1649

Nonodontogenic (primary) tumors of the jaws

Tumors of bone 27

It is not always possible to be certain whether some tumors of the jaws are of osseous or dental origin, but such a distinction is usually of little practical significance. Many of these tumors are rarely seen in the jaws and are considerably more common in other parts of the skeleton.

Osteoma and other bony overgrowths

Neoplasms of either compact or cancellous bone are less common than localized overgrowths (exostoses). Exostoses consist of lamellae of compact bone (Fig. 27.1). Exceptionally large specimens may have a core of cancellous bone. Small exostoses may form irregularly on the surface of the alveolar processes, and specific variants develop on the palate (torus palatinus) or mandible (torus mandibularis). The latter differ from other exostoses only in their characteristic sites of development and their symmetrical shape.

Torus palatinus. This tumor may start to develop in early adult life, but is not usually noticed until middle age. The common site is towards the posterior of the midline of the hard palate, and the swelling is rounded and symmetrical, sometimes with a midline groove. If the swelling is large enough to interfere with the fitting of a denture or is otherwise obtrusive, it should be removed.

Tori mandibularis. This tumor forms on the lingual aspect of the mandible opposite the mental foramen (Fig. 27.2). They are typically bilateral, forming hard, rounded swellings (Fig. 27.3). Their behavior and management is the same as that of torus palatinus.

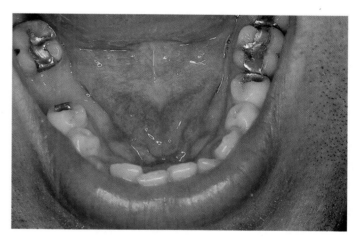

Fig. 27.2 Tori mandibularis. These tumors have the same structure as their palatine counterparts, but are bilateral, affect the lingual aspect of the mandibular premolar region, and are less common.

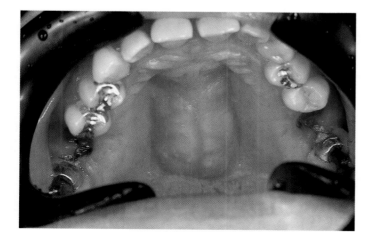

Fig. 27.1 Torus maxillaris. Histologically this resembles a compact osteoma, but it is in fact a developmental anomaly in this palatal site.

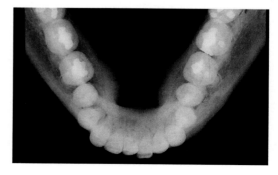

Fig. 27.3 Tori mandibularis. The radiograph clearly shows the symmetrical outgrowths of bone from the lingual aspects of the mandible.

COMPACT AND CANCELLOUS OSTEOMA

Compact osteomas are very slow growing. They consist of dense lamellae of bone that are sometimes arranged like the layers of an onion, with occasional blood vessels, but no Haversian systems (Figs 27.4 and 27.5).

Cancellous osteomas consist of trabeculae of bone, between which are marrow spaces, surrounded by a lamellated cortex (Figs 27.6–27.8).

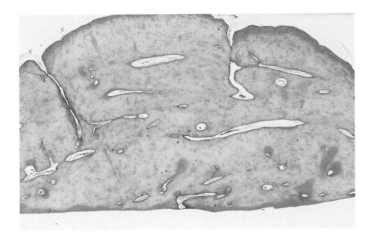

Fig. 27.4 Osteoma, compact type consisting of densely laminated bone.

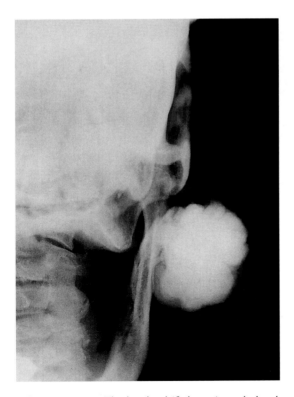

Fig. 27.5 Compact osteoma. The densely calcified mass is attached to the outer aspect of the ramus of the mandible.

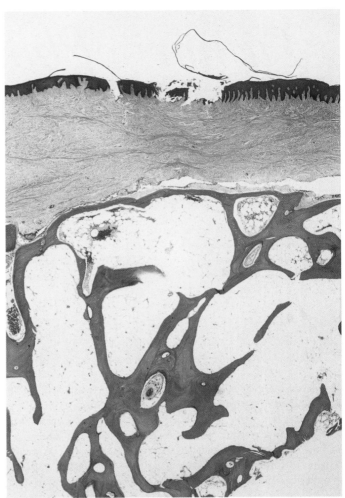

Fig. 27.6 Osteoma, cancellous type.

Osteomas should be excised only if they become large enough to cause symptoms or make the fitting of a denture difficult.

GARDNER'S SYNDROME

Gardner's syndrome is an important marker of internal malignancy. It comprises multiple osteomas of the jaws, polyposis coli with a high malignant potential, and often other abnormalities such as dental defects and epidermal cysts. The syndrome is inherited as an autosomal dominant trait.

The osteomas of the jaws are typically multiple and may be ranged along the alveolar ridge, along the borders of the mandible, or form endosteal radio-opacities (Fig. 27.9). However, the importance of this syndrome is that most of those affected die of bowel cancer by the age of 50 years. Although some members of the family do not have polyposis coli, the finding of multiple osteomas of the jaws should prompt examination for bowel disease.

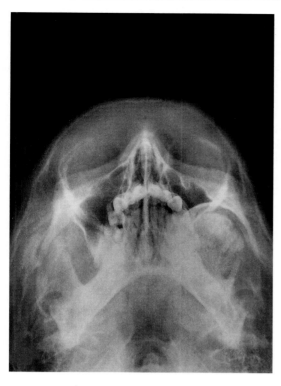

Fig. 27.7 Cancellous osteoma. The rounded mass is attached to the neck of the condyle and extends to the anterior part of the zygomatic arch.

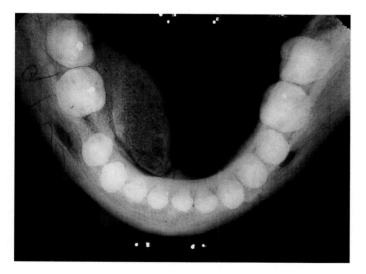

Fig. 27.8 Cancellous osteoma. This unusually large tumor has been molded forward from its pedicle between the molar teeth by the tongue muscles. Its cancellous nature can be seen.

OSTEOCHONDROMA (CARTILAGE-CAPPED OSTEOMA)

This bony overgrowth grows by ossification beneath a cartilaginous cap. Osteochondromas are rare in the maxillofacial skeleton, but in this area the condyle and coronoid process are most frequently

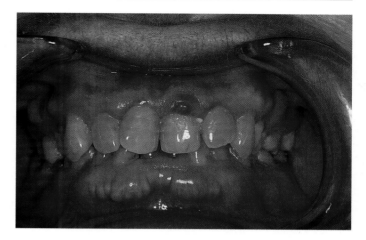

Fig. 27.9 Gardner's syndrome. Multiple osteomas protrude from the alveolar bone of both jaws.

affected. There, it can interfere with joint function and limit opening of the mouth. The bony overgrowth will be seen on radiographs, but the cartilaginous cap may not be obvious. Almost any age can be affected, but the mean age of patients is in the fifth decade.

MICROSCOPY

The appearance is not unlike that of an epiphysis with a cap of hyaline cartilage overlying slowly proliferating bone (Fig. 27.10). The cartilage cells are sometimes regularly aligned, but the cartilage is sometimes more irregular and may contain minute foci of ossification. As age advances the cartilaginous cap becomes progressively thinner and the mass consists increasingly of bone, which is usually mostly cancellous and contains fatty or hemopoietic marrow. The cortex and medulla of the mass are continuous with those of the underlying bone.

BEHAVIOR AND MANAGEMENT

It is unclear whether osteochondromas are true neoplasms or developmental anomalies. Those that arise from the condyle cannot readily be distinguished from condylar hyperplasia. Typically, but not invariably, growth of the tumor ceases with skeletal maturation. Complete excision together with the overlying periosteum is curative, but Henry et al[1] found that in the axial skeleton approximately 3% of tumors underwent sarcomatous change.

MULTIPLE OSTEOCHONDROMATOSIS

This rare genetic anomaly is an autosomal dominant trait, but males are somewhat more frequently affected than females.

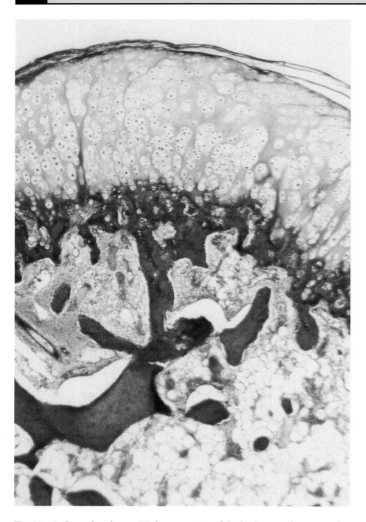

Fig. 27.10 Osteochondroma. High-power view of the hyaline cartilage cap and endochondral ossification (below).

Osteochondromas usually appear in early infancy, particularly on the limbs, and may eventually be numbered in hundreds, but the face and jaws are usually spared. Growth of the lesions stops at the end of puberty, but chondrosarcomatous change later in life may take place in 10–25% of cases.

SOFT TISSUE OSTEOCHONDROMAS

The tongue is the site most frequently affected by these rare tumors, where they form firm painless swellings. They respond to excision.

Ossifying (cemento-ossifying) fibroma

No distinction is drawn between ossifying and cementifying fibroma, as discussed in Chapter 26.

'JUVENILE ACTIVE (AGGRESSIVE)' OSSIFYING FIBROMA

This designation has been given to some rarely reported ossifying fibromas that are mainly found in the maxilla of younger patients. They can locally aggressive and show a tendency to recur. A more cellular ('active') variant of ossifying fibroma may be difficult to distinguish from an osteoblastoma, and should probably be categorized as the latter. However, there are no definitive criteria for distinguishing these tumors from more typical cemento-ossifying fibromas.

Osteoid osteoma and osteoblastoma

These tumors or tumor-like lesions are not histologically distinguishable. They differ clinically and radiographically but may merely be variants of the same disorder. They are both rare in the jaws and more common in other bones. Most patients are below the age of 30 years, and males are affected twice as often as females.

OSTEOID OSTEOMA

The mandible is affected approximately twice as frequently as the maxilla. The typical complaint is of pain, which is characteristically worse at night, but is variable in nature and severity; it is usually troublesome rather than disabling. The pain may be relieved by aspirin, and can occasionally precede radiologically detectable changes. Osteoid osteomas that are less than 2 cm in diameter appear to have limited growth potential.

RADIOGRAPHY

Osteoid osteoma is considerably more frequently cortical than medullary in site, and typically shows a nidus of radiolucency surounded by densely sclerotic bone. In a minority the nidus becomes calcified.

MICROSCOPY

Diagnosis depends on finding the nidus, although this may be no more than 1–2 mm in diameter. If the whole specimen is available, the nidus may be identifiable, by the naked eye, as a greyish or reddish core that may be soft or granular. The nidus consists of osteoid and woven bone, which is in trabeculae of irregular length and width, and rimmed by osteoblasts (Fig. 27.11). The trabeculae may also show a pagetoid (jig-saw puzzle or 'mosaic') pattern of reversal lines. The connective-tissue matrix is highly vascular, with many small, thin-walled vessels and fibroblasts.

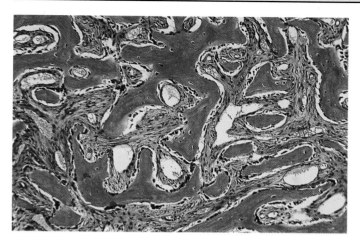

Fig. 27.11 Osteoid osteoma. Trabeculae of bone show prominent osteoblastic rimming.

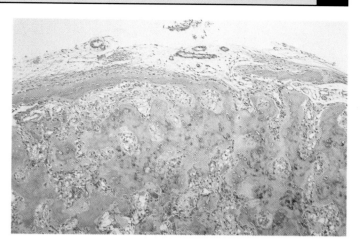

Fig. 27.12 Osteoblastoma showing the well-circumscribed periphery.

BEHAVIOR AND MANAGEMENT

Excision of the complete nidus, although usually minute, is necessary, otherwise recurrence is likely. The problem of finding the nidus is made easier by the small size of the whole mass, which can be removed entire. The condition is benign and surgical excision is curative.

OSTEOBLASTOMA

Osteoblastomas are even more uncommon than osteoid osteomas, particularly in the head and neck region, but in this area the mandible is also the most frequent site. Among 306 osteoblastomas reported by Lucas et al,[2] 11% were in the jaws. Males outnumbered females by a ratio of 2 : 1. Like osteoid osteoma those aged under 30 years are affected; Lucas et al[2] found the mean age to be 20.4 years. The chief complaint is of dull aching pain, which is traditionally said to be unresponsive to aspirin. More important is that osteoblastomas have a potential for progressive growth, can cause swelling of the jaw, and may loosen adjacent teeth.

RADIOGRAPHY

Radiographically, an osteoblastoma appears as a rounded area of radiolucency, usually in the medulla and containing variable amounts of mineralization. Unlike osteoid osteoma, nidus tissue forms the bulk of the lesion and perilesional sclerosis is usually slight. The mass is also larger (2–10 cm diameter). However, the radiographic features are variable, can mimic osteosarcoma or other malignant tumors in up to 25% of cases, and show a sunray appearance or Codman's triangles.

MICROSCOPY

Osteoblastomas are well circumscribed (Fig. 27.12). 'Giant osteoid

osteoma,' an earlier name for osteoblastoma, indicates the similarities of their appearance, and osteoblastoma cannot reliably be distinguished from the nidus of osteoid osteoma. However, the osteoblasts can sometimes be large and epithelioid in appearance. Five of the jaw tumors reported by Lucas et al[2] had an epithelioid-predominant histological pattern of large osteoblasts, and were multifocal with numerous niduses of active growth, which could be mistaken for infiltrative growth (Fig. 27.13). Some of these osteoblastomas with an epithelioid-predominant pattern had earlier been misdiagnosed as osteosarcomas. With regard to the sometimes difficult differential diagnosis between osteoblastoma and osteosarcoma, Lucas et al[2] concluded that both could have a trabecular osteoid pattern and show cartilaginous matrix formation (Fig. 27.14). However, in osteosarcomas, the malignant osteoblasts tended to form compact clusters with no intervening matrix, and to show nuclear hyperchromatism and greater mitotic activity. By contrast, in osteoblastomas the cells between the trabeculae had a looser more polymorphic pattern and the tumor as a whole had a sharp interface with the host tissue. Though some areas of osteo-

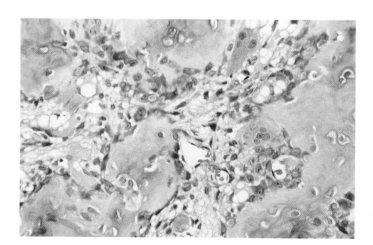

Fig. 27.13 Osteoblastoma showing the cellular appearance, with the nuclei having prominent nucleoli.

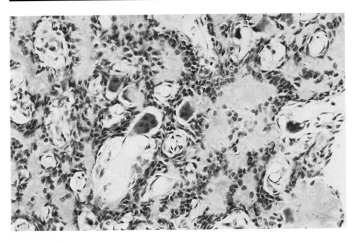

Fig. 27.14 Osteoblastoma. Another area shows highly cellular tissue with numerous osteoblasts and osteoid formation.

blastomas were indistinguishable from osteosarcoma, only the latter showed destructive permeation of surrounding tissue, with irregular extensions between host trabeculae.

BEHAVIOR AND MANAGEMENT

Although the large series reported by Lucas et al[2] confirmed that osteoblastomas are otherwise benign, they do have a potential for progressive and sometimes aggressive growth. There have been isolated reports of malignant change in osteoblastoma, but Lucas et al[2] considered that in several such cases there was doubt as to the original microscopic diagnosis. However, two (in the tibia and thoracic vertebra) of their 306 cases, which were clearly histologically benign at first, later underwent malignant change.

The risk of malignant change is therefore very small and conservative excision is the treatment of choice, but recurrence is possible if this is inadequate. Nevertheless, other examples of these tumors apparently regress after subtotal excision.

As mentioned earlier, cementoblastoma is also histologically similar to, and can be regarded as a counterpart of, osteoblastoma. If related to the root of a tooth and the microscopic findings are appropriate, it seems reasonable to regard the tumor as a cementoblastoma. In addition, a cementoblastoma may be distinguishable microscopically by peripheral, radiating columns of cementum surrounded by large cementoblasts.

Osteosarcoma

This highly malignant tumor, the most common *primary* (*nonodontogenic*) neoplasm of bone, is overall rare. Approximately 7% of osteosarcomas may be found in the jaws and, according to Garrington et al,[3] their annual incidence in the USA is 1 per 1.5 million persons.

Most cases of osteosarcoma have no identifiable cause, except for those that have followed irradiation, as reviewed by Zachariades et al[4] who quote an estimated 10% of cases. A high proportion of these patients had been treated for fibrous dysplasia but with the growing concern about the dangers of irradiation to benign disease this hazard should diminish, and reports of post-irradiation osteosarcoma of the jaws are few. In south China, where there is a high incidence of nasopharyngeal carcinoma, Dickens et al[5] reported four cases of osteosarcoma of the maxilla out of 1000 patients treated with radiotherapy for nasopharyngeal carcinoma. They regarded this risk as so small as not to be a contraindication to this form of treatment.

Osteosarcoma is also a recognized complication of Paget's disease of bone but hardly ever in the jaws. In the 114 Japanese patients reported by Tanzawa et al,[6] none had a history of trauma, any antecedent benign tumor or Paget's disease. One patient had previously had fibrous dysplasia and three others had received radiotherapy.

In a review of 66 patients with osteosarcoma of the jaws, Clark et al[7] found the mean age to be 34.2 years (range 12–79 years). Sixty-four per cent of the patients were male, and 36% were females. Fifty-one per cent of the tumors were in the maxilla and 49% in the mandible.

Vege et al[8] found that of 34 patients with craniofacial osteosarcoma seen in Bombay, India, over a 19-year period, the mean age was 30.9 years, with a major peak of frequency between the ages of 21 and 30 years. Nineteen of the patients were male, and 15 were female. The mandible was affected in 19 cases and the maxilla in 32.

In Japan, Tanzawa et al[6] in their analysis of 116 osteosarcomas of the maxillofacial region reported during the preceding 60 years, found the average age to be 36 years with a range of 5–82 years, and the highest incidence being in the third decade. The frequency of mandibular tumors showed a sharp peak between the ages of 20 and 30 years, especially in females, while maxillary tumors showed a more even distribution without any sharp peak. Apparently peculiar to Japan, the number of females affected (68) exceeded that of males (46). Sixty-seven of these osteosarcomas were in the mandible, 43 were in the maxilla, three were in the ethmoid, and one was in the temporal bone.

CLINICAL FEATURES

Swelling and pain for an average of 3 months before consultation were the most frequent symptoms reported by Clark et al.[7] In 89 patients surveyed by Tanzawa et al,[6] swelling was by far the most frequent single complaint. Pain was noted in only 3.4% of patients with a mandibular tumor, and a similar number experienced tenderness. Reddening of the skin was noted in 2.2% of both mandibular and maxillary tumors.

A typical picture is that of a firm swelling, which grows in a few months and becomes painful. The teeth may become loosened and there may be paresthesia or anesthesia in the mental nerve area. Metastases to the lungs may develop early. However, the fact that some patients have symptoms long before diagnosis suggests that some of these tumors are slow growing. Among the patients reported by Tanzawa et al,[6] the longest delay between onset of symptoms and start of treatment was 6 years in the case of maxillary tumors and 8 years for mandibular tumors.

RADIOGRAPHY

The appearances are varied. In the early stages there may be only subtle changes, with only slight variation in the trabecular pattern, but an early feature may be symmetrical widening of the periodontal ligament space around one or several teeth as a result of tumor infiltration (Figs 27.15 and 27.16).[3] This finding is not specific, but if it is associated with pain, swelling, or other radiographic changes is highly suggestive of osteosarcoma. Lindquist et al,[9] in an analysis of 16 cases of osteosarcoma of the mandible, regarded widening of periodontal ligament spaces, widening of the inferior dental canal, and the sun-ray effect as almost pathognomonic of osteosarcoma.

Later, irregular bone destruction usually predominates over bone formation. Bone formation in a soft-tissue mass is characteristic of osteosarcoma. A sun-ray appearance at the surface or Codman's triangles at the margins due to elevation of the periosteum and neoplastic new bone formation may be seen on appropriate radiographs, but are uncommon and are not specific

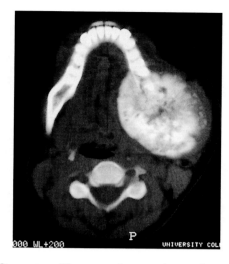

Fig. 27.16 Osteosarcoma. The computed tomography scan shows a more extensive tumor, which causes gross medial and lateral expansion of the mandible with irregular areas of osteosclerosis.

to osteosarcoma. The extent of the tumor can be shown by computed tomography scanning.

MICROSCOPY

Osteosarcomas originate from bone cells, and this can produce a highly pleomorphic picture in which bone formation does not necessarily predominate. The tumor cells are variable in size and shape, many are large and hyperchromatic, and mitotic figures may be prominent, particularly in the more highly cellular areas (Figs 27.17–27.20). Cells resembling osteoblasts, fibroblasts and cartilage cells can be recognized; giant cells may be conspicuous, but many cells are of indeterminate appearance.

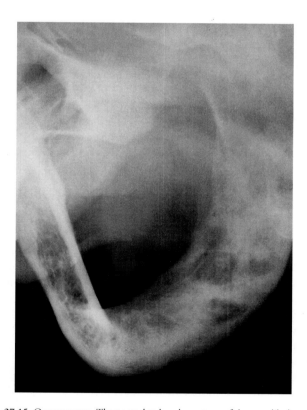

Fig. 27.15 Osteosarcoma. The normal trabecular pattern of the mandibular bone has been replaced by multiple irregular areas of radiolucency and radio-opacity in this early osteosarcoma.

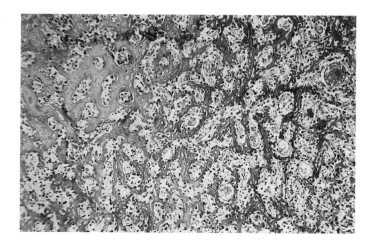

Fig. 27.17 Osteosarcoma. Interlacing strands of osteoid are surrounded by neoplastic osteoblasts.

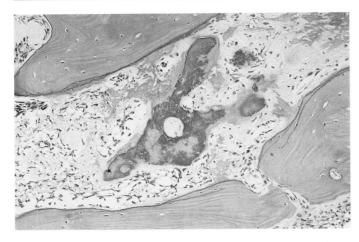

Fig. 27.18 Osteosarcoma. Angular tumor osteoblasts and neoplastic osteoid are infiltrating normal bone.

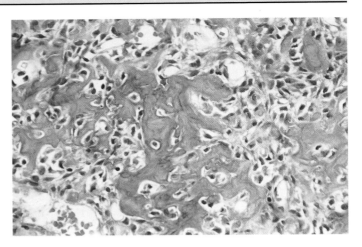

Fig. 27.20 Osteosarcoma. Higher power view of neoplastic osteoid and numerous pleomorphic and hyperchromatic osteosarcoma cells.

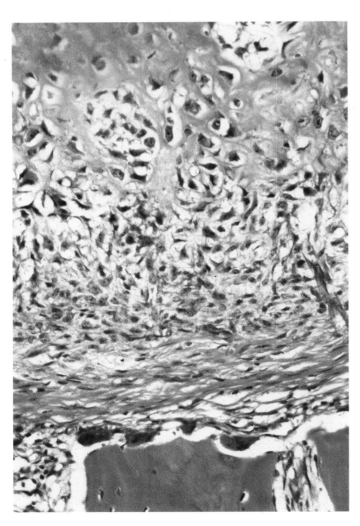

Fig. 27.19 Osteosarcoma. Higher power view of neoplastic osteoid and tumor cells (above) and active destruction of normal bone (below).

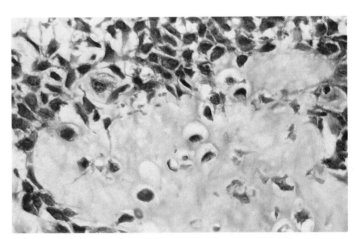

Fig. 27.21 Osteosarcoma. High-power view of an area of chondroid metaplasia.

Formation of osteoid, however small the amount may be, is the criterion of diagnosis of osteosarcoma, as enunciated by Liechtenstein & Jaffe[10] (Figs 27.17–27.20). Inability to detect osteoid appears to be a factor limiting the value of aspiration cytology. Cartilage and fibrous tissue are usually also present (Fig. 27.21). Predominantly fibroblastic variants appear to have a somewhat better prognosis than the more common osteoblastic type.

The amount of these tissues may vary widely in different parts of the tumor, but in jaw osteosarcomas there is frequently extensive cartilage formation and limited areas of osteoid formation. Malignant cartilage as the main finding in a small biopsy can lead to a mistaken diagnosis of chondrosarcoma. Overall, the general picture is one of uncontrolled and irregular cell activity.

A rare variant, *small-cell osteosarcoma*, has a close resemblance to Ewing's sarcoma but for the fact that it forms osteoid. Another uncommon variant appears histologically to be a low-grade tumor and consists largely of spindle-shaped cells and limited osteoid formation. Low-grade intramedullary osteosarcomas are difficult to differentiate histologically from benign lesions such as fibrous dysplasia, desmoblastic fibroma, or ossifying fibroma. However, they are infiltrative and destructive and pursue a relentless course.

James et al[11] have emphasized the difficulties of differential diagnosis in such cases. In a 6-year-old boy in whom a diagnosis of desmoplastic fibroma had been made, the tumor continued to grow slowly for 12 years and then rapidly, to produce a swelling 17 cm across and weighing 1500 g. Microscopy showed an osteoblastic osteosarcoma with osteoid production only in the center of the tumor.

BEHAVIOR AND MANAGEMENT

Diagnosis depends on biopsy, which may need to be repeated if there is any doubt. Chest radiographs must also be taken, as secondary deposits may be present when the patient is first seen (Fig. 27.22). Fine-needle aspiration has been reported by White

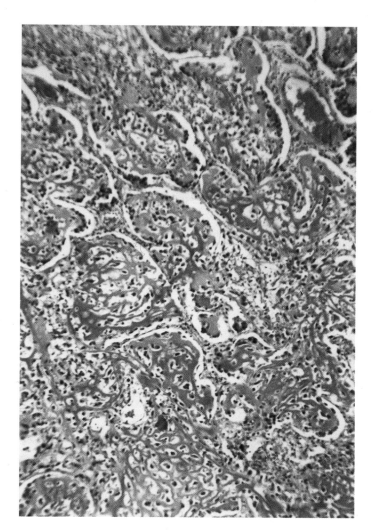

Fig. 27.22 Osteosarcoma. Pulmonary metastasis showing remnants of alveolar structure.

et al[12] to give an 80% accuracy in the diagnosis of osteosarcoma. Serum alkaline phosphatase levels are raised in about 50% of cases, particularly in those tumors where new bone formation predominates.

Osteosarcomas of the jaws are rapidly invasive but tend to metastasize to the lungs less frequently or later than those of the axial skeleton. Metastasis to regional nodes may be seen in fewer than 10% of cases. Nevertheless, approximately 50% of osteosarcomas of the jaw recur locally within a year of initial treatment. Only four of 66 patients reported by Clark[14] developed metastases, but most died from uncontrollable local disease. Regezi et al[14] analyzed the results of treatment of 16 osteosarcomas of the jaws treated initially with excision or resection. The longest survival without recurrence was 14 years and the shortest was 6 months. Five other patients developed recurrences from which one patient died within 2 years, but data were incomplete in the remainder.

With aggressive surgery supplemented as necessary by radiotherapy and sometimes chemotherapy, Tran et al[15] claimed a 49% 10-year survival rate for 15 osteosarcomas (mainly of the maxilla or mandible), but deaths continued even after a decade.

Early radical excision of osteosarcoma of the jaws is the first requirement. This involves mandibulectomy or maxillectomy, together with wide excision of any soft-tissue extensions of the tumor. However, osteosarcomas often extend within the medulla for some distance beyond the radiographic margins, so that recurrence of the tumor in the excision margins is a major problem. Excision may be combined with pre- or postoperative radiotherapy by such means as high-dose interstitial needling, and adjuvant chemotherapy is increasingly widely used. Immunotherapy has proved to be disappointing.

The prognosis depends mainly on the extent and site of the tumor at operation, and deteriorates with spread to the soft tissues, lymph nodes, or the base of the skull, or with recurrence after excision, which may happen in over 50% of cases.

JUXTACORTICAL OSTEOSARCOMA

Juxtacortical osteosarcoma is a rare variant which, like endosteal osteosarcoma, mainly affects the limbs, but can occasionally involve the jaws. Its chief importance is its better prognosis as reviewed by Banerjee,[16] who also reported a case, and by Millar et al,[17] who reported four cases and reviewed eight previous reports.

CLINICAL FEATURES

Juxtacortical osteosarcoma typically affects the mandible, and the average age of patients is about 35 years. The tumor forms a slow-growing mass on the surface of the jaw or in the adjacent parosteal tissue, and is typically rounded with a broad base. It may cause dull aching pain.

RADIOGRAPHY

Radiographically, juxtacortical osteosarcoma characteristically has an opaque base and is more radiolucent superficially. The pattern of and amount of opacity and radiolucency vary widely.

MICROSCOPY

Juxtacortical osteosarcoma characteristically shows a deep zone of benign-looking, parallel trabeculae of bone separated by fibrous tissue; mitotic activity and cellular abnormalities are frequently difficult to find. The more superficial and, in particular, the radiolucent zones are likely to show more obvious neoplastic activity and cellular pleomorphism consistent with osteosarcoma. A minority of specimens show obviously sarcomatous features throughout.

The terms *periosteal osteosarcoma* and *parosteal osteosarcoma* result from an attempt to subdivide the variants of this tumor, when affecting the long bones, on the basis of differing radiographic and microscopic features. Some believe that the periosteal type is a separate entity and tends to be a high-grade tumor with more obviously malignant features (Figs 27.23 and 27.24). Even so, its prognosis is appreciably better than that for endosteal osteosarcoma. However, this subclassification does not appear as yet to be justifiable for jaw tumors.

BEHAVIOR AND MANAGEMENT

The first essential is to establish the diagnosis firmly as early as possible by adequate biopsy of the superficial radiolucent areas.

Wide excision, including underlying bone, is desirable, although recurrence has even followed hemimandibulectomy. Of the four cases reported by Millar et al[17] all were disease-free 1–16 years

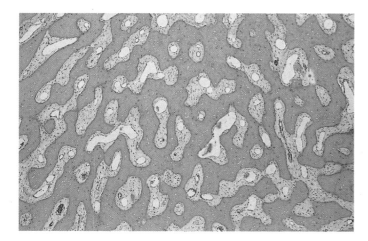

Fig. 27.23 Parosteal osteosarcoma. Relatively well-formed trabeculae of bone without great numbers of neoplastic osteoblasts are interspersed with fibrous stroma. The picture is in-keeping with the better prognosis than that of endosteal tumors.

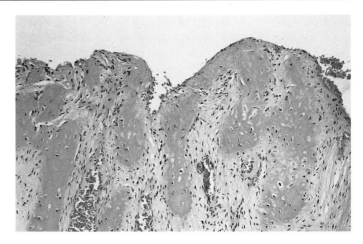

Fig. 27.24 Parosteal osteosarcoma. Higher power view of the periphery shows some foci of chondroid differentiation that are typical of this tumor

later, and of the eight earlier cases five were recurrence-free for periods of 6–11 years.

Extraskeletal osteosarcoma, chondrosarcoma and Ewing's sarcoma

These sarcomas can develop in the soft tissues but only do so very rarely. They must be distinguished from a variety of pseudosarcomatous lesions or other sarcomas.

Extraskeletal osteosarcoma afflicts patients of greater age (typically middle-aged) than its skeletal counterparts. Four cases of osteosarcoma of the tongue have been reported[18] and all happen to have affected the left side.

Histologically, extraskeletal osteosarcomas do not differ from their osseous counterparts, and form osteoid and sometimes bone. They are usually high-grade tumors. Despite aggressive treatment, the outcome with tumors more than 5 cm across or with nodal metastases appears always to be fatal.[19]

REFERENCES

1. Henry CH, Granite EL, Rafetto LK 1992 Osteochondroma of the mandibular condyle: report of a case and review of the literature. J Oral Maxillofac Surg 50: 1102–1108
2. Lucas DR, Unni KK, Mc Leod RA, O'Connor MI, Sim FH 1994 Osteoblastoma: a clinicopathologic study of 306 cases. Hum Pathol 25: 117–134
3. Garrington GE, Scofield HH, Cornyn J, Hooker SP 1967 Osteosarcoma of the jaws. Analysis of 56 cases. Cancer 20: 377–391
4. Zachariades N, Patrinou C, Benetos S, Xpolyta A, Keleki I 1988 Post-irradiation osteogenic sarcoma. J Oral Maxillofac Surg 43: 267–299
5. Dickens P, Wei WI, Sham JST 1990 Osteosarcoma of the maxilla in Hong Kong Chinese postirradiation for nasopharyngeal carcinoma. Cancer 66: 1924–1926
6. Tanzawa H, Uchiyama S, Sato K 1991 Statistical observation of osteosarcoma of the maxillofacial region in Japan. Analysis of 114 Japanese cases reported between 1930 and 1989. Oral Surg Oral Med Oral Pathol 72: 444–448
7. Clark JL, Unni KK, Dahlin DS, Devine KD 1983 Osteosarcoma of the jaws. Cancer 51: 2311–2316
8. Vege DS, Birges AM, Aggrawal K 1990 Osteosarcoma of the craniofacial bones. Craniomaxillofac Surg 19: 90–93
9. Lindquist C, Teppo L, Sane J, Holmstrom T, Wolf J 1986 Osteosarcoma of the mandible: analysis of nine cases. J Oral Maxillofac Surg 44: 759–764

10. Lichtenstein L, Jaffe HL 1943 Chondrosarcoma of bone. Am J Pathol 19: 553–589

11. James PL, O'Regan MB, Speight PM 1990 Well differentiated osteosarcoma of the mandible of a six-year-old child. J Laryngol Otol 104: 335–340

12. White VA, Fanning CV, Ayala AG et al 1988 Osteosarcoma and the role of fine-needle aspiration biopsy. A study of 51 cases. Cancer 62: 1238–1246

13. Clark JL, Unni KK, Dahlin DC, Devine KD 1983 Osteosarcoma of the jaw. Cancer 51: 2311–2316

14. Regezi JA, Zarbo RJ, McClatchey KD, Courtney RM, Crissman JD 1987 Osteosarcomas and chondrosarcomas of the jaws. Immunohistochemical correlations. Oral Surg Oral Med Oral Pathol 64: 302–307

15. Tran LM, Mark R, Meier R, Calcaterra TC, Parker RG 1992 Sarcomas of the head and neck. Prognostic factors and treatment strategies. Cancer 70: 169–177

16. Banerjee SC 1981 Juxtacortical osteosarcoma of the mandible review of the literature and report of a case. J Oral Surg 39: 535–538

17. Millar BG, Browne RM, Flood TR 1990 Juxtacortical osteosarcoma of the jaws. Br J Oral Maxillofac Surg 28: 73–79

18. Loyzaga JM, Machin PF, Sala J 1996 Osteogenic sarcoma of the tongue. Case report and review of the literature. Pathol Res Pract 191: 75–78

19. Jundt G 1996 Critical commentary to 'Osteogenic sarcoma of the tongue.' Pathol Res Pract 192: 79

Cartilaginous tumors

28

Chondroma and chondrosarcoma

CHONDROMA

Chondromas are particularly uncommon in the jaws. Many so-called chondromas of the jaws ultimately prove to be malignant, and a significant proportion of chondrosarcomas in this area were originally mistaken for chondromas.

CLINICAL FEATURES

Chondromas are far more often found (but are still rare) in the nose or nasal sinuses, and hence can occasionally be found in the maxilla. True chondromas are small and likely to be no more than chance findings as firm, smooth-surfaced nodules.

MICROSCOPY

Chondromas consist of hyaline cartilage. The cells may be irregular in size and distribution, but the distinction between chondromas and low-grade chondrosarcomas is notoriously difficult. Calcification or ossification may develop within the cartilage. Batsakis et al[1] suggest that, for all cartilaginous tumors: (a) all those proximal to the hands and feet are suspect for malignancy; (b) multiple blocks should be examined because areas diagnostic of a chondrosarcoma may be only focal; (c) the size may be a final determinant, with 3.0 cm being the maximum size expected for a chondroma; (d) dedifferentiation of a benign or low-grade cartilaginous tumor is always possible; and (e) an adequate margin of normal tissue is mandatory for excisions.

MANAGEMENT

Treatment is by wide excision. This is necessary to help to distinguish benign from malignant tumors by providing adequate margins for examination, and to take into account the probabi-

lity that a chondroid tumor is malignant. Even when the microscopy appears benign, careful, prolonged follow-up is essential.

CHONDROSARCOMA

There is wide variation in the reported, relative frequency of chondrosarcomas and osteosarcomas of the jaws. These differences probably result from the use of different histological criteria for distinguishing chondrosarcomas from chondrogenic osteosarcomas. Also as described by Garrington & Collett,[2] chondrosarcomas were not clearly distinguished from osteosarcomas until Lichtenstein & Jaffe[3] laid down clear diagnostic criteria. From a practical viewpoint this distinction may be important, as chondrosarcomas of the jaws appear to have a worse prognosis than osteosarcomas.[4]

In the latter survey, the mean age of 36 patients was 33.3 years, with a peak incidence between the ages of 21 and 30 and a range of 16–67 years. Twenty-nine patients were male and eight were female, but this was largely the result of the predominantly male intake at the Armed Forces Institute of Pathology. The mandible was the site of 20 tumors and the maxilla of 16. Two of the 37 patients related a history of the death of immediate family members from bone tumors, and the offspring of a third patient died from a possible bone tumor.

CLINICAL FEATURES

Pain, swelling, or loosening of teeth associated with an area of greater or lesser radiolucency are typical.

RADIOGRAPHY

Radiographically, chondrosarcomas are osteolytic with poorly defined borders. Calcifications are frequently present in the radiolucent area, and occasionally calcification of the neoplastic cartilage may become widespread and dense (Figs 28.1 and 28.2). Occasionally, a chondrosarcoma may appear multilocular and, if lacking calcifications, may mimic an ameloblastoma. Hackney et

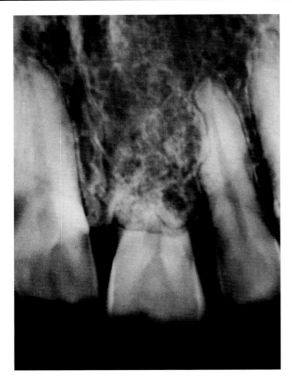

Fig. 28.1 Chondrosarcoma. Radiographically the tumor appears lobulated and has caused extensive resorption of the related teeth.

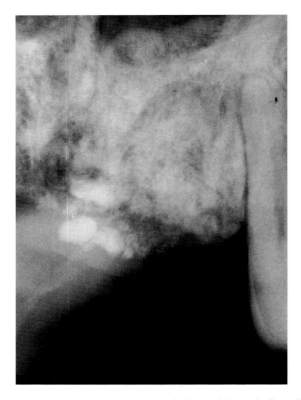

Fig. 28.2 Chondrosarcoma. This specimen, which extended into the floor of the left nasal fossa, shows extensive calcifications.

al[5] point out that symmetrical widening of the periodontal ligament space around affected teeth may be a distinctive feature. Ormiston et al[6] have reported two cases in which chondrosarcomas mimicked periodontal lesions, and which as a result of biopsy allowed exceptionally early treatment.

The radiographic margins are an unreliable guide to the extent of the tumor, which can infiltrate between bone trabeculae without resorbing them.

MICROSCOPY

The product of the neoplastic chondrocytes ranges from comparatively well-formed cartilage (grade I) to myxoid tissue (grade III). Grade I tumors are the most frequent type found in the jaws. The chondrocytes show the pleomorphism characteristic of these sarcomas; they may be binucleate, but show no mitotic activity in grade I tumors (Figs 28.3 and 28.4). Grade II tumors

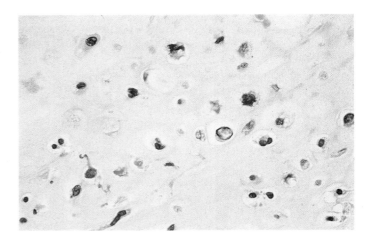

Fig. 28.3 Chondrosarcoma. Hyaline matrix with pleomorphic neoplastic chondrocytes, including a binucleate cell, in lacunae.

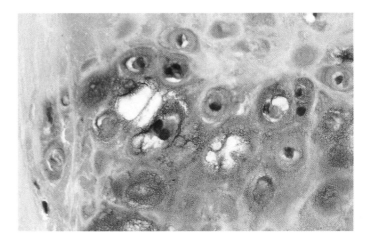

Fig. 28.4 Chondrosarcoma. Binucleate malignant chondrocytes in a hyaline stroma are undergoing basophilic change.

form myxoid tissue as well as cartilage, and there are occasional mitoses among the chondrocytes. The amount of calcification corresponds with the radiographic appearances and can be punctate or loose and fluffy in appearance (Figs 28.5–28.7).

BEHAVIOR AND MANAGEMENT

Maxillofacial chondrosarcomas are aggressively invasive (Fig. 28.8); local recurrence or persistent tumor is the main cause of death. Fewer than 10% of these tumors (usually grade III) metastasize; the lungs or other bones are then the usual targets. Metastasis to lymph nodes is very rare.

Chondrosarcomas must be excised as early and as widely as possible. A 2–3 cm margin is usually advised. The first operation is critical, as inadequate excision is likely to lead to recurrences beyond the original area of operation, with inevitable problems of management. As mentioned earlier, a major difficulty is the

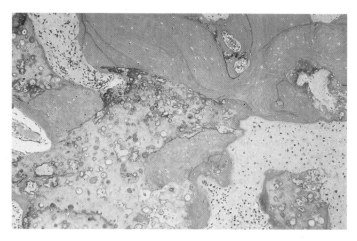

Fig. 28.7 Chondrosarcoma. Normal bone is being invaded by malignant chondroid tissue, part of which has undergone calcification.

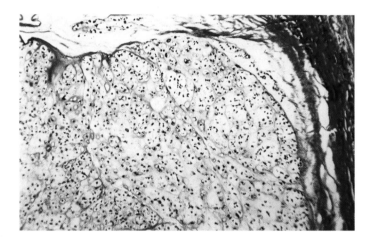

Fig. 28.5 Chondrosarcoma. Multiple malignant chondrocytes have formed a lacy stroma of faintly basophilic chondroid tissue.

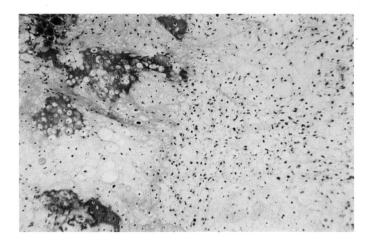

Fig. 28.6 Chondrosarcoma. Partial calcification of the malignant chondroid matrix.

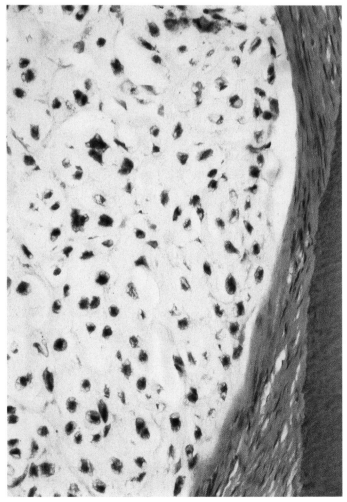

Fig. 28.8 Chondrosarcoma. Invasion of periodontal ligament.

ability of the tumor to extend along cancellous spaces a considerable distance beyond the radiographic margins. Another is the ability of chondroid tumors to seed and grow in the soft tissues of the operation site. Chondrosarcomas only occasionally respond to radiotherapy, and chemotherapy appears to be of little value.

The prognosis of chondrosarcomas of the maxillofacial region is generally worse than that for other sites because of the difficulties of adequate excision in this area. The 5-year survival rate is 40–60%, and depends on the tumor stage and grade, and on the extent of the original excision. Maxillary tumors have an even worse prognosis than mandibular ones, but in the 37 cases reported by Garrington & Collett[4] there were no survivors from chondrosarcoma of either jaw after 15 years. The two cases mimicking periodontal lesions described by Ormiston et al[6] survived for 3.5 and 3 years after limited en bloc marginal resections.

CHONDROSARCOMA VARIANTS

Mesenchymal chondrosarcoma and clear cell chondrosarcoma show considerable differences in their prognoses from conventional chondrosarcomas.

MESENCHYMAL CHONDROSARCOMA

This tumor is considerably more uncommon than conventional chondrosarcoma, but a relatively high proportion (15–35%) are in the craniofacial region. A minority form in the soft tissues.

CLINICAL FEATURES

Mesenchymal chondrosarcoma patients show a wide age distribution. The tumor presents no specific signs or symptoms, but rapidly developing pain and swelling, sometimes with loosening of teeth, are typical.

RADIOGRAPHY

Radiographically, an area of radiolucency, usually speckled with calcifications, is typical. There is only partial circumscription and no peripheral sclerosis.

MICROSCOPY

The overall appearance is that of a highly cellular tumor in which only small foci of tissue are recognizable as poorly formed cartilage.

Typically, the bulk of the tumor consists of sheets of irregularly ovoid, or sometimes spindle-shaped, darkly staining cells, with little cytoplasm and with occasional or numerous mitoses. Scattered about are generally small, poorly circumscribed foci of cartilage in which there may be calcification (Figs 28.9 and

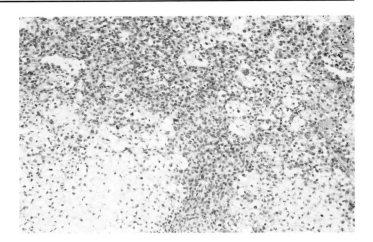

Fig. 28.9 Mesenchymal chondrosarcoma. Concentrations of malignant cells with small areas of chondroid tissue.

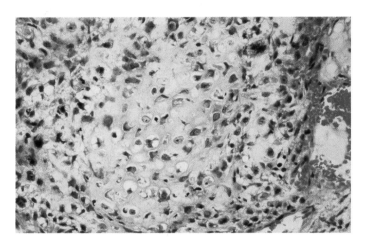

Fig. 28.10 Mesenchymal chondrosarcoma. Higher power view of more typical chondroid tissue and numerous pleomorphic chondrocytes with conspicuous nucleoli and some binucleate forms.

28.10). These foci may be scanty or occasionally form the bulk of the tumor and some areas of the tumor may be highly vascular.

Striking variations in the histological picture may be seen. Hemangiopericytoma-like mesenchymal chondrosarcoma is a variant that consists of sheets of small mesenchymal cells surrounding cleft-like vascular spaces (Fig. 28.11). Cartilage can sometimes be very scanty in such tumors, and the overall appearance can suggest a blood vessel rather than a chondroid tumor. In another variant the vascular component forms sinusoids within the tumor.

BEHAVIOR AND MANAGEMENT

Mesenchymal chondrosarcoma is highly malignant and the frequency of metastases is high. Spread, usually to the lungs but sometimes to lymph nodes, frequently follows local recurrences.

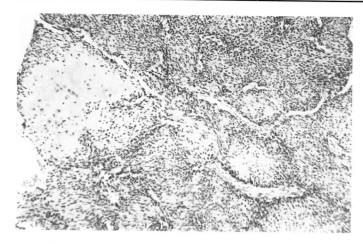

Fig. 28.11 Mesenchymal chondrosarcoma, hemangiopericytoma-like variant. There is a striking resemblance to a hemangiopericytoma, but with a small focus of malignant cartilaginous stroma.

Early radical surgery followed by combined chemotherapy is therefore required. However, its value is as yet uncertain, and either local recurrences or metastases can appear 10 or more years after treatment. There are no reliable microscopic guides to prognosis.

CLEAR CELL CHONDROSARCOMA

Clear cell chondrosarcoma is a rare variant with a slow rate of growth. Slootweg[7] reported an example in the maxilla which he believed to be the first case reported in this region. It consists of closely packed, monomorphic clear cells with small nuclei and distinct cytoplasmic borders and little intervening matrix. Transitions can be traced from these cells to those lying in lacunae in a chondroid matrix and showing hyperchromatism, pleomorphism, and multiple nuclei. Transitions may also be seen between clear cells and spindle-shaped mesenchymal cells. Extragnathic clear cell chondrosarcomas have also been reported.[8,9]

BEHAVIOR AND MANAGEMENT

Wide en bloc excision is the treatment of choice.

Chondromyxoid fibroma (fibromyxoid chondroma)

This rare tumor occasionally forms in the mandible. Lustman et al[10] found 10 earlier reports and added three more. Twelve of these were in the mandible, and Damm et al[11] reported another example in the maxilla. Zillmer & Dorfman[12] found one example in the mandible among 36 chondromyxoid fibromas, and dis-

cussed the clinicopathologic findings in detail. Lingen & Polverini,[13] in reviewing the disease, noted that only 18 cases involving the jaws had been reported at that time. Of these, only four were in the maxilla. The importance of this tumor is that, although benign, it can be mistaken microscopically for a chondrosarcoma.

CLINICAL FEATURES

Most patients are less than 30 years of age, and symptoms are frequently slight or absent. However, chondromyxoid fibroma can sometimes simulate a malignant tumor by causing pain, swelling of the jaw, or loosening of teeth.

RADIOGRAPHY

Radiographically it is likely to appear as a radiolucent area with irregular but, typically, sclerotic margins and trabeculation or an appearance suggesting loculation. Opacities are rarely seen in the tumor area. In the unusual example reported by Lingen & Polverini,[13] the tumor caused a gingival swelling in the canine region of the mandible and an ill-defined area of radiolucency between the canine and second incisor in a 10-year-old boy.

MICROSCOPY

The appearances are variable, but typical features are lobules of myxoid and chondroid tissue, with more cellular and compact peripheries and separated by fine but highly vascular fibrous tissue septa. In excision specimens the surrounding bone may be seen to be sclerotic.

The cells of the myxoid areas are variable in shape, but many are angular or stellate with long slender processes, or may be within lacunae. The more closely packed peripheral cells tend to be more rounded and may have an epithelioid appearance. Cartilage can occasionally form up to 75% of the tumor but may be present only in minute amounts. Calcifications, cyst formation and areas of hemorrhage may sometimes be seen (Fig 28.12).

Findings that may add to the impression of malignancy are pleomorphic cells with large hyperchromatic nuclei or that are binucleate, and osteoclast-like giant cells, which are sometimes numerous. However, mitoses are scarce. Features helping to distinguish this tumor from a chondrosarcoma are an earlier age of onset, its sclerotic margins, and frequent lack of calcifications, or calcifications of a different type from those seen in chondrosarcomas.

BEHAVIOR AND MANAGEMENT

Differentiation from chondrosarcoma by adequate biopsy is essential. Excision of chondromyxoid fibroma with as wide as

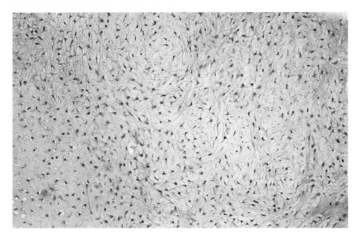

Fig. 28.12 Chondromyxoid fibroma. Stellate cells in a myxoid stroma and an ill-defined area of hyaline chondroid tissue in one corner are present.

possible a margin of normal tissue, followed by grafting if necessary, has frequently been recommended. However, of 12 cases treated by enucleation or curettage only two are known to have recurred within periods of follow-up ranging from 5 months to 18 years. Like other chondroid tumors, chondromyxoid fibroma can grow in the soft tissues as a result of seeding of tumor cells at operation. However it is doubtful whether sarcomatous change has been authenticated unless radiotherapy has been used.

Chondroblastoma

Chondroblastoma is a benign tumor that involves the maxillofacial region even more rarely than chondromyxoid fibroma. Out of 495 cases reviewed by Kurt et al,[14] only seven were in the mandible.

CLINICAL FEATURES

The median age of presentation of these tumors in the head and neck region is approximately 40 years; males have been affected twice as frequently as females.

RADIOGRAPHY

Characteristic radiographic appearances in the long bones are a rounded area of radiolucency with a thin sclerotic border, which may sometimes appear scalloped, and varying amounts of calcification. These appearances may be less well defined in the jaws.

MICROSCOPY

Chondroblastoma is highly cellular. Rounded cells, with well-defined outlines, eosinophilic or amphophilic cytoplasm, and an epithelioid appearance are the main components. Multinucleate giant cells are common, and range from those with only two or three nuclei, to large osteoclast-like cells. They are usually associated with areas of hemorrhage or necrosis, and secondary aneurysmal bone cyst formation has been seen in up to 25% of cases. The frequency of giant cells in these tumors is emphasized by its earlier names of 'calcifying giant cell tumor' and 'epiphyseal chondromatous giant cell tumor'.

Chondroid areas can be sharply defined or merge imperceptibly into the epithelioid areas. A net-like pattern of calcification extending between the cells or punctate calcifications are characteristic. Calcification in the cartilaginous areas may be seen, but ossification is rare and myxoid areas are absent.

BEHAVIOR AND MANAGEMENT

As indicated earlier, information about chondroblastomas of the jaws is scanty. Curettage, followed if necessary by bone grafting, has frequently been successful, but up to 30% of cases may recur. If aneurysmal bone cyst is associated, curettage alone is inadequate and combination treatment with cryosurgery is probably more effective. There is, in either case, a good response to radiotherapy for otherwise uncontrollable or surgically inaccessible lesions.

REFERENCES

1. Batsakis JG, Solomon AR, Rice DH 1980 The pathology of head and neck tumors: neoplasms of cartilage, bone and the notochord. Part 7. Head Neck Surg 3: 43–57
2. Garrington GE, Collett WK 1988 Chondrosarcoma. 1. A selected literature review. J Oral Pathol 17: 1–11
3. Lichtenstein L, Jaffe HL 1943 Chondrosarcoma of bone. Am J Pathol 19: 553–589
4. Garrington GE, Collett WK 1988 Chondrosarcoma. II. Chondrosarcoma of the jaws: analysis of 37 cases. J Oral Pathol 17: 12–20
5. Hackney FL, Aragon SB, Aufdemorte TB, Holt RG, Sickels JEV 1991 Chondrosarcoma of the jaws: clinical findings, histopathology and treatment. Oral Surg Oral Pathol Oral Med 71: 139–143
6. Ormiston IW, Piette E, Tideman H, Wu PC 1994 Chondrosarcoma of the mandible presenting as periodontal lesions: report of 2 cases. J Cranio-Maxillo-Fac Surg 22: 231–235
7. Slootweg PJ 1980 Clear-cell chondrosarcoma of the maxilla. Report of a case. Oral Surg Oral Med Oral Pathol 50: 233–237
8. Unni KK, Dahlin DC, Beabaut JW, Sim FH 1976 Chondrosarcoma; clear cell variant: a report of sixteen cases. J Bone Joint Surg 58A: 676–683
9. Le Charpentier Y, Forest M, Postel M, Tomeno B, Abelnet R 1979 Clear cell chondrosarcoma. A report of five cases including ultrastructural study. Cancer 44: 622–629
10. Lustman J, Gazit D, Ulmansky M, Lewin-Epstein J 1986 Chondromyxoid fibroma of the jaws: a clinicopathological study. J Oral Pathol Med 15: 343–346
11. Damm DD, White DK, Geissler RH, Drummond JK, Gonty AA 1985 Chondromyxoid fibroma of the maxilla. Electron microscopic findings and review of the literature. Oral Surg Oral Med Oral Pathol 59: 176–183
12. Zillman DA, Dorfman HD 1989 Chondromyxoid fibroma of bone: thirty-six cases with clinicopathologic correlation. Hum Pathol 20: 952–964
13. Lingen MW, Polverini PJ 1993 Unusual presentation of chondromyxoid fibroma of the mandible. Report of a case and review of the literature. Oral Surg Oral Med Oral Pathol 75: 615–621
14. Kurt A-M, Unni KK, Sim FH, McLeod RA 1989 Chondroblastoma of bone. Hum Pathol 20: 965–978

Multiple myeloma, solitary plasmacytoma, and oropharyngeal plasmacytosis

29

Multiple myeloma

Multiple myeloma, a neoplasm of plasma cells, causes multifocal bone-destructive lesions which are usually painful and tender. A jaw lesion occasionally gives rise to the first symptoms. A review of the literature by Epstein et al[1] suggested that there had then been reports of 783 cases of some manifestation of multiple myeloma in the mouth or jaws and that, overall, 14% of multiple myelomas had previously had oral manifestations. Of 41 patients in whom oral lesions were the initial manifestation of multiple myeloma, most were tumors in the jaws, but three cases were of amyloid deposits. Of the 59 patients studied by Bruce & Royer,[2]

12% had oral manifestations as the first sign or symptom of multiple myeloma. These figures may seem high but, as Cataldo & Meyer[3] have pointed out, painless, unsuspected jaw lesions can more frequently be found if appropriate radiographs are taken.

Amyloid deposition in the oral tissues is usually a late complication but, rarely, macroglossia due to this cause is the first sign.[4]

Skeletal radiographs typically show multiple punched-out areas of radiolucency, particularly in the vault of the skull. These areas are typically 1–5 cm in diameter and lack a sclerotic margin (Figs 29.1 and 29.2).

As a result of the proliferation of myeloma cells in the marrow, there is frequently anemia and sometimes thrombocytopenia. Abnormal susceptibility to infection may result from depressed production of normal immunoglobulins.

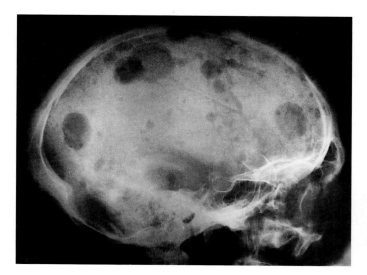

Fig. 29.1 Multiple myeloma. The radiograph shows the typical punched-out areas of radiolucency in the calvarium.

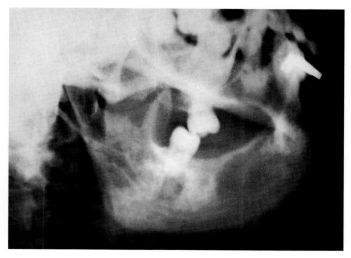

Fig. 29.2 Multiple myeloma. These deposits in the mandible have a less well-circumscribed appearance than those in the skull.

The picture just described is that of established disease. Myeloma may be suspected in its asymptomatic phase by the chance finding in a routine blood examination, of a greatly raised ESR or even rouleaux formation in the blood sample as a result of the overproduction of immunoglobulin. The diagnosis is confirmed by electrophoresis showing a monoclonal immunoglobulin or fragment spike, and histopathology.

MICROSCOPY

Myeloma appears as sheets of plasma cells which, when well-differentiated, have an eccentric nucleus with peripheral clumping of the chromatin, giving a so-called cartwheel appearance and a perinuclear halo (Figs 29.3 and 29.4). The area of cytoplasm is relatively large and baso- or amphophilic. However, as Fechner & Mills[5] point out, even in well-differentiated myeloma some of the cells may be more polygonal in shape. Some lack a perinuclear halo, the chromatin pattern may be irregularly dispersed, and occasional binucleate or trinucleate forms may be seen. With

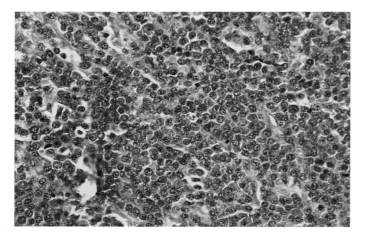

Fig. 29.3 Multiple myeloma. Medium-power view shows atypical plasma cells and a few that are well differentiated.

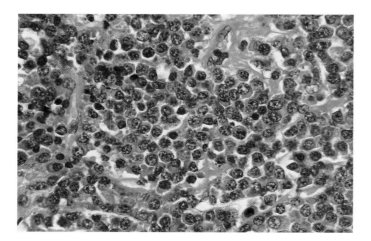

Fig. 29.4 Multiple myeloma. Higher power view shows moderately well-differentiated but slightly pleomorphic plasma cells.

loss of differentiation, the nuclei become larger and lose their characteristic chromatin pattern, but show coarse irregular clumping, and the cytoplasm may form no more than a rim around the nucleus. Multiple nuclei and mitoses may be seen. Amyloid is occasionally seen and may, rarely, be so abundant as to obscure the tumor cells, and in a neglected tumor the amyloid may calcify to give radioopacities in a radiograph.

Myeloma cells are monoclonal and show κ- or λ-light-chain restriction. Fechner & Mills[5] state that if the ratio of one or the other is greater than 16 : 1, the diagnosis is assured and distinguishes the tumor from reactive plasmacytic proliferation.

Histological differentiation between poorly differentiated myeloma and B-cell immunoblastic lymphoma may be difficult, but the latter typically also involves lymph nodes.

BEHAVIOR AND MANAGEMENT

Bone marrow biopsy is usually diagnostic, but recognition, by microscopy alone, of poorly differentiated myeloma may be difficult. Confirmation depends on the electrophoretic findings as well as the clinical features. Serological findings in multiple myeloma are a greatly raised ESR, rouleaux formation of red cells in a blood sample, and raised plasma protein levels, all of which result from immunoglobulin (Ig) overproduction. Serum electrophoresis shows a monoclonal spike of IgG and light-chain restriction in the majority of cases. IgA-producing myeloma is less common.

Immunocytochemical demonstration of monoclonal production of immunoglobulin or immunoglobulin fragments provides substantiation. Light-chain overproduction is common and leads to Bence–Jones proteinuria.

There is frequently an initial response to treatment with combination chemotherapy, but the median survival for multiple myeloma is about 2–3 years. Fewer than 20% of patients survive for 5 years or more.

Complications include anemia, hemorrhagic tendencies, abnormal susceptibility to infection, and amyloidosis.

SOLITARY PLASMACYTOMA OF BONE

This tumor comprises approximately 24% of cases of myeloma. It has a significantly better prognosis than soft tissue plasmacytoma, as discussed below. The diagnosis can only be made if a skeletal survey shows absence of other myelomatous lesions. The majority of patients are over 50 years of age. Clinically, bone pain, tenderness or a swelling, and a sharply defined area of radiolucency or, rarely, a soap-bubble appearance are typical features.

Microscopically, the cellular features are the same as those of multiple myeloma, which should be excluded as described earlier. A small rise in serum or urine monoclonal immunoglobulin is detectable in 50–77% of patients with solitary endosteal plasmacytoma. The monoclonal peak in the serum should disappear with treatment, but persistence indicates that treatment has been inadequate or that the disease has disseminated.

Treatment is by localized radiotherapy. Up to 55% of patients survive for 10 years or more, but the majority develop multiple myeloma, sometimes within a few months but occasionally even after several decades.

SOLITARY, SOFT TISSUE (EXTRAMEDULLARY) PLASMACYTOMA

These are rare tumors, but approximately 80% of them form in the head and neck, usually in the nasal cavity or nasopharynx rather than the mouth. Involvement of the antrum may, however, give rise to a maxillary tumor.

Microscopically, extramedullary plasmacytoma does not differ from multiple myeloma, and can be shown to be monoclonal by immunocytochemistry. Solitary extramedullary plasmacytoma is not associated with a monoclonal peak in the serum.

Irradiation is highly effective, but multiple myeloma develops in up to 50% of patients, usually within 2 years.

MULTIPLE MYELOMA AFFECTING THE JAWS

As noted earlier, osteolytic jaw lesions are occasionally the presenting symptom of multiple myeloma. Lambertenghi-Delilliers et al[6] found, among 193 cases, jaw lesions in 10 patients whose ages ranged from 47 to 83 years. All except one had multiple lytic deposits, but these caused no symptoms in eight of them. In five cases the deposits were detected at the time of diagnosis of multiple myeloma and the remainder developed 6 months to 3 years afterwards. In those with jaw lesions, IgG-secreting tumors accounted for 53%.

González et al[7] reported two cases of multiple myeloma with painful deposits in the mandibular condyle. They reviewed the findings in 18 other cases, of which oral or maxillofacial lesions were the first sign of myeloma in 72%. Ten lesions involved the mandible and eight involved the maxilla.

Furutani et al[8] noted jaw lesions in five of 38 patients with multiple myeloma. Their ages ranged from 58 to 83 years. The jaw lesions caused no symptoms except in one patient who sustained a pathologic fracture due to multilocular lytic lesions. In this patient and one other, oral radiographs led to the diagnosis of multiple myeloma. The duration of survival after recognition of deposits in the jaws ranged from 11 to 28 months. Furutani et al[8] noted seven other reports, apart from those already quoted, of jaw involvement by multiple myeloma.

These reports show that deposits of multiple myeloma in the jaws have variable radiographic appearances, from multiple osteolytic areas with ill-defined margins to a single well-circumscribed round area of radiolucency.

SOLITARY PLASMACYTOMA OF THE MANDIBLE

Although solitary plasmacytoma of bone forms only 3–5% of all plasma cell malignancies, there appear to be at least as many reports of solitary plasmacytoma of the jaws as involvement of these bones by multiple myeloma. Loh[9] was able to find reports of 23 cases between 1948 and 1982, and added another. Multiple myeloma failed to develop after periods of follow-up ranging from 4 months to 16 years in the 16 patients for whom such data were available. Kanazawa et al[10] reported on a 49-year-old woman with a painless gingival swelling due to extension of a bony deposit of solitary plasmacytoma in the mandible. Both the jaw deposit and serum showed monoclonal IgG production with λ-light-chain restriction. Multiple myeloma failed to develop within a year. Kanazawa et al[10] were able to retrieve 12 additional reports of solitary plasmacytoma of the mandible. Review of these cases showed that the radiographic appearances varied from well-circumscribed, cyst-like areas of radiolucency, multilocular radiolucency mimicking an ameloblastoma, multiple or irregular areas of radiolucency, or a soap-bubble appearance, to a cyst-like unilocular area in the right mandible and an irregular osteolytic area in the left mandible. In 10 cases for which follow-up data were available, there was no evidence of disseminated disease after periods ranging from 4 to 151 months. Of these, five patients showed no evidence of disease for 5–12.5 years. Two patients developed multiple myeloma after 9 and 12 months. Most of these patients had received local radiotherapy, either alone or with surgery.

PLASMACYTOMA OF THE ORAL SOFT TISSUES

Solitary plasmacytoma of the oral soft tissues is considerably more uncommon than similar tumors in the jaws. Kapadia et al[11] noted a single case involving the gingiva and one of the nasopharynx that had extended into the soft tissues of the palate, among 20 examples of extramedullary plasmacytoma of the head and neck. In 16 cases (80%), the extramedullary plasmacytoma was the primary tumor, and in the remainder it was associated with multiple myeloma. Wiltshaw[12] noted a single case of tongue involvement in extramedullary plasmacytomas of the head and neck. Layton et al[13] have reported an unusual case characterized by diffuse, sumucosal aggregates of monotypic IgG-producing λ- and κ-light-chain restricted plasma cells associated with ulcerative stomatitis. An immunoglobulin screen showed a monoclonal IgG κ with integrated paraprotein of 3.1 g/l. Although the relationship between the ulcerative stomatitis and the plasma cell dyscrasia is unclear, Bowden et al[14] have also reported oral bullous lichenoid lesions associated with multiple myeloma. The lichenoid lesions resolved when the multiple myeloma was treated with cyclophosphamide.

AMYLOIDOSIS

Amyloidosis is the deposition in the tissues of an abnormal protein. It has characteristic staining properties and electron-microscopic appearances. It can be systemic or localized, and is classified according to the nature of the amyloid fibril and of the related serum protein. A fibrillary protein forms the essential structural element, but a nonfibrillary glycoprotein (amyloid P component (AP)) is present in virtually all types. In the case of myeloma and monoclonal gammopathies, amyloidosis results from overproduction of immunoglobulin light chains.

The relevance of oral amyloidosis in the present context is that it may rarely provide the first sign of multiple myeloma or of other monoclonal gammopathies. Moreover, it is a highly unfavorable prognostic sign.

Amyloid deposition in the mouth, particularly the tongue, is most commonly a manifestation of a monoclonal gammopathy (non-neoplastic, plasma cell dyscrasias with overproduction of immunoglobulin) or of myeloma. In a survey of 225 patients, Kyle & Greip[15] found macroglossia in 32% of cases of amyloidosis due to myeloma and in 19% of patients with monoclonal gammopathy. Reinish et al[16] found reports of 54 cases of oral amyloidosis secondary to multiple myeloma. The tongue was involved in all these cases, but in some, other oral sites or salivary glands were affected. Although in the past it was believed that gingival biopsy was a valuable aid to the diagnosis of amyloidosis, it may be noted that only a single case of gingival involvement was recorded among these 54 cases. In three of the five patients with oral amyloidosis reported by van der Wal et al,[17] it was the first and main symptom of multiple myeloma.

Reactionary (secondary) amyloidosis resulting from rheumatoid arthritis or chronic infections is more common overall, but rarely affects the mouth.

CLINICAL FEATURES

Clinically, deposits of amyloid can cause macroglossia, or soft-tissue tags or swellings, sometimes on the gingivae. An enlarged tongue due to amyloid is frequently lobulated, particularly along the margins, and can be so large as to protrude from the mouth. Purpura and anemia may be associated and give the tongue a pale or purplish color, or cause ecchymoses in the surrounding tissues.

Gertz et al[18] have reported jaw pain on mastication (misnamed 'jaw claudication' – claudication is, literally, 'limping') in 9% of 237 patients with primary amyloidosis, and was the only cause of symptoms in four cases of myeloma-associated amyloidosis.

Amyloidosis of salivary glands is a rare cause of xerostomia.

MICROSCOPY

Amyloid appears as weakly eosinophilic, hyaline homogeneous material, which is often perivascular. It stains positively with Congo red, which also shows a characteristic apple-green birefringence under polarized light. There is also positive fluorescence with thioflavine T and a characteristic fibrillary structure is seen on electron microscopy.

If the underlying disease has not already been identified, a blood picture and plasma protein electrophoresis should be followed, if positive, by marrow biopsy and skeletal radiographs.

BEHAVIOR AND MANAGEMENT

The prognosis of myeloma-associated amyloidosis is poor, either from the tumor itself or from widespread amyloid deposition and, in particular, renal damage. So-called *benign monoclonal gammopathy* has a poor prognosis ultimately, either as a result of eventual development of myeloma or of widespread amyloid deposition and renal failure. Although progress of the disease may be delayed by chemotherapy with melphelan and prednisolone, Kyle & Greip[15] noted that the median duration of survival of 229 patients with amyloidosis (with or without myeloma) was 12 months, and fewer than 25% of patients were alive after 3 years. Hawkins[19] quotes a median duration of survival of 12–15 months for this type (AL) of amyloidosis.

Oral amyloidosis as a late manifestation of multiple myeloma is also an unfavorable prognostic finding. Salisbury & Jacoway[20] described a patient with a 6-year history of multiple myeloma, who died 4 months after nodular deposits of amyloid developed in the oral soft tissues.

Tongue reduction for macroglossia due to amyloidosis, though desirable, should be avoided if possible, as the tissue is friable, bleeding can be difficult to control, and any benefit is often only temporary.

Oropharyngeal plasmacytosis

Intense, aerodigestive tract, submucosal plasmacytic proliferation, which had been mistaken for extramedullary plasmacytoma, has been described by White et al,[21] Timms & Sloan,[22] and Ferriero et al.[23] Nineteen cases of gingival plasmacytosis were reported by Perry et al.[24] This condition was thought to have been caused by a component of toothpaste, as suggested by its virtual disappearance a few years later.[25]

Unlike these cases of plasma cell gingivitis, plasmacytosis can involve the upper aerodigestive tract more widely. In the three patients reported by Timms & Sloan[22] there was supraglottic erythematous swelling due to intense plasmacytic proliferation. In the nine cases reported by Ferreiro et al,[23] four involved the lips, tongue, or palate, or multiple sites including the naso-pharynx, larynx, and trachea. Clinically, the oral lesions consisted of warty or cobblestone thickening, sometimes with fissuring of the mucosa, ulceration, and soreness. Three of these patients were male and one female, and their ages ranged from 56 to 67 years. No risk factors were identifiable.

MICROSCOPY

In the cases reported by Timms & Sloan[22] the lesions showed pseudoepitheliomatous hyperplasia of the epithelium. All the lesions reported by Ferreiro et al[23] showed psoriasiform epithelial changes, with parakeratosis, elongation of the rete ridges, and suprapapillary epithelial thinning. Aggregation of neutrophils with Monro-abscess-like formation was sometimes seen, but deep cell keratinization was present in all cases.

Submucosally there was intense infiltration by plasma cells which, because of its density and uniformity, had been mistaken for an extramedullary plasmacytoma in many cases. However, the plasma cells showed no loss of differentiation or prominent nucleoli and were polyclonal for κ and λ light chains. In one of the cases reported by Ferreiro et al,[23] where molecular genetic probes for immunoglobulin-encoding genes were used, no gene rearrangement was detectable.

BEHAVIOR AND MANAGEMENT

The lesions reported by Timms & Sloan[22] responded to corticosteroid therapy, but no prolonged follow-up was mentioned. None of the cases reported by Ferreiro et al[23] responded to antimicrobial treatment. One case responded temporarily to administration of corticosteroids, but then progressed. None of the lesions regressed spontaneously, and most progressed. Surgery was required for lesions that led to airways obstruction. There were no other complications, and none of the patients developed malignant disease in periods of follow-up ranging from 1 to 16 years.

This condition, apart from the risk of airways obstruction, therefore appears to be benign. Its importance lies in the need to distinguish it from a plasmacytoma and to avoid cytotoxic chemotherapy. However, prolonged follow-up is required.

REFERENCES

1. Epstein JB, Voss NJS, Stevenson-Moore P 1984 Maxillofacial manifestations of multiple myeloma. An unusual case and review of the literature. Oral Surg Oral Med Oral Pathol 57: 267–271

2. Bruce KW, Royer RQ 1953 Multiple myeloma occurring in the jaws: a study of 17 cases. Oral Surg Oral Med Oral Pathol 6: 729–744

3. Cataldo E, Meyer I 1966 Solitary and multiple plasma cell tumor of the jaws and oral cavity. Oral Surg Oral Med Oral Pathol 22: 628–639

4. Flick WG, Lawrence FR 1980 Oral amyloidosis as initial symptom of multiple myeloma. Oral Surg Oral Med Oral Pathol 49: 18–20

5. Fechner RE, Mills SE 1992 Tumors of the bones and joints. Atlas of tumor pathology. Armed Forces Institute of Pathology, Washington, DC, third series, fascicle 8

6. Lambertenghi-Delilliers G, Bruno E, Cortelezzi A, Fumagalli L, Morosini A 1988 Incidence of jaw lesions in 193 patients with multiple myeloma. Oral Surg Oral Med Oral Pathol 65: 533–537

7. González J, Elizondo J, Trull JM, De Torres I 1991 Plasma-cell tumours of the condyle. Br J Oral Maxillofac Surg 29: 274–276

8. Furutani M, Ohnishi M, Tanaka Y 1994 Mandibular involvement in patients with multiple myeloma. J Oral Maxillofac Surg 52: 23–25

9. Loh HS 1984 A retrospective evaluation of 23 reported cases of solitary plasmacytoma of the mandible, with an additional case report. Br J Oral Maxillofac Surg 22: 216–224

10. Kanazawa H, Shoji A, Yokoe H, Midorikawa S, Takamiya Y 1993 Solitary plasmacytoma of the mandible. Case report and review of the literature. J Cranio-Maxillo-Fac Surg 21: 202–206

11. Kapadia SB, Desai U, Cheng VS 1982 Extramedullary plasmacytoma of the head and neck. A clinicopathologic study of 20 cases. Medicine 61: 317–329

12. Wiltshaw E 1976 The natural history of extramedullary plasmacytoma and its relationship to solitary myeloma of bone and myelomatosis. Medicine 55: 217–238

13. Layton SA, Cook JN, Henry JA 1993 Monoclonal plasmacytic ulcerative stomatitis. A plasma cell dyscrasia? Oral Surg Oral Med Oral Pathol 75: 483–487

14. Bowden JR, Scully C, Eveson JW, Flint S, Harman RRM, Jones SK 1990 Multiple myeloma and bullous lichenoid lesions: and unusual association. Oral Surg Oral Med Oral Pathol 70: 587–589

15. Kyle RA, Greipp PR 1983 Subject review, amyloidosis (AL): clinical and laboratory features in 229 cases. Proc Mayo Clin 58: 665–683

16. Reinish EI, Raviv M, Srolovitz, Gornitsky M 1994 Tongue, primary amyloidosis and multiple myeloma. Oral Surg Oral Med Oral Pathol 77: 121–125

17. Van der Wal N, Henzen-Logmans S, van der Kwast WAM, van der Waal I 1984 Amyloidosis of the tongue: a clinical and postmortem study. J Oral Pathol 13: 632–639

18. Gertz MA, Kyle RA, Griffing WL. Hunder GG 1986 Jaw claudication in primary systemic amyloidosis. Medicine 65: 173–179

19. Hawkins PN 1994 Amyloidosis. Med Intl 22: 76–82

20. Salisbury PL, Jacoway JR 1983 Oral amyloidosis: a late complication of multiple myeloma. Oral Surg 56: 48–50

21. White JW, Olsen KD, Banks PM 1986 Plasma cell orificial mucositis: report of a case and review of the literature. Arch Dermatol 122: 1321–1324

22. Timms MS, Sloan P 1991 Association of supraglottic and gingival idiopathic plasmacytosis. Oral Surg Oral Med Oral Pathol 71: 451–453

23. Ferreiro JA, Egorshin EV, Olsen KD, Banks PM, Weiland LH 1994 Mucous membrane plasmacytosis of the upper aerodigestive tract. A clinicopathologic study. Am J Surg Pathol 18: 1048–1053

24. Perry HO, Deffner NF, Sheridan PJ 1973 Atypical gingivostomatitis: nineteen cases. Arch Dermatol 107: 872–878

25. Silverman S, Lazada F 1977 An epilogue to plasma-cell gingivitis. Oral Surg Oral Med Oral Pathol 38: 211–217

Langerhans cell histiocytosis and eosinophilic granuloma **30**

Langerhans cell histiocytosis

This uncommon, predominantly osteolytic, tumor-like disease, also known as *histiocytosis X* is due to proliferation of Langerhans cells. The latter are predominantly cutaneous, antigen-presenting cells. They resemble histiocytes histologically, but have characteristic surface markers and contain Birbeck granules. Although there has been doubt whether this disease is a true neoplasm, Willman et al[1] have shown, by use of X-linked polymorphic DNA probes, that the proliferating Langerhans cells were monoclonal in nine out of 10 cases in females with all types of the disease. However, as discussed later, solitary bone lesions in particular sometimes undergo spontaneous resolution.

Langerhans cell histiocytosis, whatever its nature, has highly variable manifestions and behavior, ranging from solitary bone lesions to disseminated, potentially fatal disease. It may therefore be a group of diseases with certain common features.[2] Clinical manifestations, diagnosis, treatment, and possible etiology of Langerhans cell histiocytosis have been reviewed by Egeler & D'Angio.[3]

Three main forms, in order of severity, are usually recognized:

- solitary eosinophilic granuloma
- multifocal eosinophilic granuloma (including Hand–Schuller–Christian disease)
- Letterer Siwe disease.

In a review of 1120 cases, Hartman[4] found that there was oral involvement in 114 and that the mandible was affected in 73%, either alone or in polyostotic disease. Kilpatrick et al[5] found that the jaws were involved in 11% of 263 children and adults. Other perioral sites of involvement are the cervical lymph nodes, which can become enlarged either in isolation, in association with restricted bone lesions or, more frequently, with multisystem disease. Cervical lymphadenopathy can sometimes be massive.

SOLITARY EOSINOPHILIC GRANULOMA

INCIDENCE

Solitary eosinophilic granuloma of bone affects adults slightly more frequently than children. Jaw lesions more frequently involve the mandible to cause a localized area of bone destruction.

CLINICAL FEATURES

Pain is the most common symptom, and swelling.

RADIOGRAPHY

Radiographically, a typical appearance is a rounded area of radiolucency, frequently extending into the alveolar ridge. Dagenais et al,[6] reviewing the radiographic findings in 29 cases, noted solitary intraosseous lesions, multiple lesions of the alveolar ridge, saucerization or scooped out lesions of the alveolar ridge, periosteal new bone formation and, in 10 of 15 cases, root resorption. The radiolucent areas were well defined, but only those involving the alveolar ridge showed marginal sclerosis. The mandible alone was involved in 20 of the 29 cases, and together with the maxilla was involved in eight more. The maxilla was the sole site in only one case.

Occasionally, gross periodontal destruction with exposure of the roots of the teeth is a feature. Teeth that appear on radiographs to be floating in air is typical, and Kilpatrick et al[5] noted that 9% of children and 13% of adults with biopsy-proven Langerhans cell histiocytosis had loosened teeth. Oral ulcers were present in 3% of children and 7% of adults.

MICROSCOPY

Langerhans cells are associated with eosinophils; other types of granulocytes are often present in variable numbers. The

Langerhans cells have pale, vesiculated, weakly eosinophilic cytoplasm and nuclei, which are folded or lobulated. Mitotic activity is typically absent. Eosinophils may be scattered among the Langerhans cells, or be arranged in conspicuous clusters. The matrix consists of unremarkable poorly fibrillar or granular material. These appearances may vary with the stage of the disease, with a high proportion of eosinophils at first, then growing numbers of histiocytes and, finally, in resolving cases, increasing fibrosis (Figs 30.1–30.3).

Electron microscopy shows Birbeck granules in the Langerhans cells. The granules appear as lamellar plates with a central striated line. They occasionally have a terminal vesicular dilatation, giving them a racquet shape.

Diagnostic criteria are summarized in Table 30.1. Fartasch et al[8] have reported that positive staining of Langerhans cells for S-100 protein and peanut agglutinin is as reliable as electron microscopy. Emile et al[9] have described the use of a mouse monoclonal CD1a antibody (mAb O10) that recognizes a formalin-resistant epitope of CD1a. In paraffin-embedded

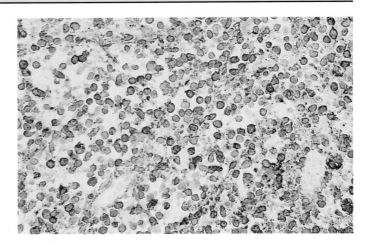

Fig. 30.3 Langerhans cell histiocytosis. Positive S-100 staining of Langerhans cells.

Table 30.1 Confidence levels for the diagnosis of Langerhans cell histiocytosis[7]

1. Presumptive diagnosis: light morphological characteristics
2. Designated diagnosis
   (a) Light morphological features
      plus
   (b) Two or more supplemental positive stains for
      – adenosinetriphosphatase
      – S-100 protein
      – α-d-mannosidase
      – peanut lectin
3. Definitive diagnosis
   (a) Light morphological features
      plus
   (b) Birbeck granules in the lesional cell by electron microscopy
      and/or
   (c) Positive staining for CD1 antigen (T6) on the lesional cell

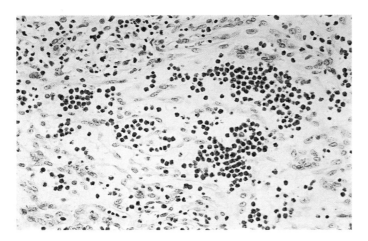

Fig. 30.1 Langerhans cell histiocytosis. In this field clusters of eosinophils are prominent.

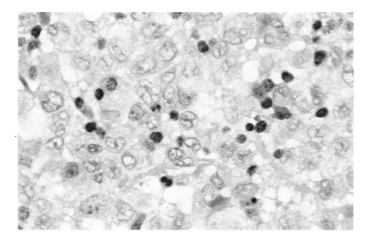

Fig. 30.2 Langerhans cell histiocytosis. Higher power view shows the lobed nuclei of the Langerhans cells.

sections, they found the histiocytes to stain positively for mAb O10 in all but one, although this specimen was strongly CD1a positive in frozen sections. mAb O10 staining closely corresponded with S-100 positivity, but was negative in nevi, melanomas and neurofibromas, and non-Langerhans cell histiocytoses used for controls. The phenotypic and functional features of Langerhans cells have been reviewed by Barratt et al,[10] who tabulate the adhesion and other molecules that are constitutively or transiently expressed by oral Langerhans cells.

MULTIFOCAL EOSINOPHILIC GRANULOMA

As well as the mandible, other sites of predilection are the skull, axial skeleton, and femora. Almost any of the viscera (particularly hepatosplenomegaly) or the skin (seborrheic dermatitis) may be involved in multifocal disease, but rarely without osseous lesions. Such disease may be termed *Hand–Schuller–Christian disease*, but the classical triad of exophthalmos, diabetes insipidus, and lytic skull lesions is present only in a minority of cases.

LETTERER-SIWE DISEASE

Letterer-Siwe disease differs from other types of Langerhans cell histiocytosis in that infants or young children are affected. It can be rapidly fatal. Although it was believed that Letterer-Siwe disease was a separate entity, Birbeck granules can be found and the microscopic appearances may not be distinguishable from those seen in other forms of the disease. As Willman et al[1] have also shown, this type of disease shows a similar pattern of clonality to other forms of Langerhans cell histiocytosis.

CLINICAL FEATURES

Both soft tissues and bone are commonly involved, and rashes may be the earliest manifestation. Other features can include lymphadenopathy and splenomegaly, fever, anemia and thrombocytopenia, and infections such as otitis media. Many organs can become involved and become enlarged as a result of histiocytic infiltration.

RADIOGRAPHY

Radiographically, the bone lesions do not differ from those in other types of Langerhans cell histiocytosis.

BEHAVIOR AND MANAGEMENT

The natural history ranges from isolated lesions with spontaneous regression, to widespread disease and a rapidly fatal outcome, despite treatment. Although the behavior is unpredictable, the very young have the worst prognosis, and have a mortality rate of 50% or more. In those aged over 2 years, the mortality has been considered to be about 15%. However, in the large series reported by Kilpatrick et al,[5] no patients without extraskeletal complications died. In general, the greater the number of organ systems affected, the poorer the prognosis. Monocytosis or thrombocytopenia are also associated with a high mortality.

In addition to biopsy of oral lesions, physical examination, skeletal survey, and blood picture will give an indication of any dissemination and its degree.

Isolated jaw lesions tend to regress spontaneously over a period of months to years, but usually a more rapid solution is required or intervention is necessary because of pain, pathological fracture, or loss of teeth. Curettage usually suffices or, as Egeler & D'Angio[3] have suggested, biopsy alone may initiate healing. Intralesional injection of corticosteroids may be given as adjunctive treatment or, as McLelland et al[11] have reported, may be a safe and effective primary treatment for monostotic disease. Irradiation (150 cGy/day for 4 days) may be given if other measures fail. Prolonged careful follow-up is desirable, and sometimes further treatment is required. However, a single skeletal radiographic survey 6 months after treatment may be adequate for monostotic disease.[12]

For multisystem disease, a combination of cytotoxic agents (often vinca alkaloids), corticosteroids, and irradiation of active bone lesions is required. Nevertheless, some cases, particularly those in young children, are refractory to currently available treatments, so that such treatments as marrow transplantation, gene transfer therapy, and monoclonal antibodies against the CD1a antigen are under trial, as reviewed by Arceci.[13] Rarely, the soft-tissue lesion, eosinophilic ulcer has been mistaken for Langerhans cell histiocytosis.

Eosinophilic ulcer (atypical or traumatic eosinophilic granuloma)

Tumor-like, often ulcerated lesions with a microscopic picture that may resemble that of Langerhans cell histiocytosis may sometimes be seen in the oral soft tissues. The tongue is most frequently affected.

Elzay,[14] in giving the background to this lesion, relates it to Riga–Fede's disease. The latter refers to traumatic ulceration of the frenulum of the tongue caused by trauma from the lower incisor teeth, and is typically a result of whooping cough. Ten of the 47 cases reviewed by Elzay were in infants aged between 1 week and 11 months.

Experimentally, crush injury to tongue muscle can induce a proliferative response, with tissue eosinophilia.[15] However, Doyle et al[16] found trauma to be a possible cause in only five of 15 cases. Of five new cases in patients aged 8–46 years reported by Movassaghi et al,[17] only two gave a history of injury.

CLINICAL FEATURES

Clinically, the ulcerated mass may be mistaken for a carcinoma. Almost any age can be affected; the 38 patients reported by El Mofty et al[18] ranged in age from 6 to 88 years (average 56.6 years). Twenty-two of their patients were females. The two most frequent sites were the tongue (16 cases) and the buccal mucosa or fold (15 cases). Nineteen of the lesions were ulcerated and 16 were raised and indurated. A history of trauma was elicited in only seven cases, but unnoticed trauma could have been inflicted during mastication. Mezei et al[19] reported three new cases and reviewed reports of 134 more. Males and females were virtually equally frequently affected, and the average age was 52 years (range 6 months to 92 years). The duration before treatment averaged 41 days, but ranged from 3 days to 1 year. A history of trauma was recorded in 57% of 68 cases. The most frequent sites were the tongue (60%), buccal mucosa (18%), lip (6%), palate or floor of mouth (5%), vestibule (5%), and frenum (1%).

MICROSCOPY

The picture is variable, but typically there is a dense polymorphic inflammatory infiltrate with many eosinophils and large mononuclear histiocyte-like cells with pale ovoid nuclei with small nucleoli and indistinct cell membranes. These histiocyte-like cells lack the surface markers and ultrastructural features of Langerhans cells, but occasionally are pleomorphic and show prominent nucleoli and mitotic activity.

The cellular infiltrate typically spreads between muscle fibers and may extend into the epithelium. Degeneration and death of muscle fibers is consistently found. El Mofty et al[18] also noted that mast cells were prominent in the connective tissue deep to the lesion, but not at its centre.

The differential diagnosis is from Langerhans cell histiocytosis, lymphoma or pseudolymphoma, and angiolymphoid hyperplasia with eosinophils. Langerhans cell histiocytosis can be excluded by means of the investigations suggested earlier. Eosinophilic ulcer differs from lymphoma and pseudolymphoma in its polymorphic infiltrate. El Mofty et al[18] found that the cell populations varied from specimen to specimen, but that overall there was an inverse relationship between the numbers of large mononuclear and inflammatory cells, and that T lymphocytes predominated over B lymphocytes. Regezi et al[20] noted that there were separate populations of large mononuclear cells, which were CD68-positive macrophages, and factor-XIIIa-positive dendrocytes. CD3-positive T lymphocytes were also abundant. However, El Mofty et al[18] found that the large mononuclear cells stained only with vimentin, and suggested that these cells might be related to myofibroblasts involved in reparative processes.

Mezei et al,[19] who reviewed the histologic findings in a very large number of reported cases, also noted the similarities between eosinophilic granuloma and angiolymphoid hyperplasia with eosinophils. Both they and El Mofty et al[18] noted occasional cases with plump endothelial cells resembling those seen in angiolymphoid hyperplasia with eosinophils. However, unlike the latter, eosinophilic ulcer typically resolves spontaneously.

BEHAVIOR AND MANAGEMENT

Spontaneous resolution, usually within 3–8 weeks, is to be expected, and with an isolated soft tissue mass having the characteristics described earlier, an expectant policy is usually justified.

REFERENCES

1. Willman CL, Busque L, Griffith BB et al 1994 Langerhans-cell histiocytosis (histiocytosis X) – a clonal proliferative disease. New Engl J Med 331 154–160
2. Favara BE, Jaffe R 1994 The histopathology of Langerhans cell histiocytosis. Br J Cancer 70(Suppl 23): S17–S23
3. Egeler RM, D'Angio GJ 1995 Langerhans cell histiocytosis. J Pediat 127: 1–11
4. Hartman KS 1980 Histiocytosis X. A review of 114 cases with oral involvement. Oral Surg Oral Med Oral Pathol 49: 38–54
5. Kilpatrick SE, Wenger DE, Gilchrist GS, Shives TC, Woolan PC 1995 Langerhans cell histiocytosis (histiocytosis X) of bone. A clinicopathologic analysis of 263 pediatric and adult cases. Cancer 76: 2471–2484
6. Dagenais M, Pharoah MJ, Sikorski PA 1992 The radiographic characteristics of histiocytosis X. A study of 29 cases that involve the jaws. Oral Surg Oral Med Oral Pathol 74: 230–236
7. Writing Group of the Histiocytic Society 1987 Histiocytic syndromes in children (Chu T, D'Angio GJ, Favara B, Ladisch S, Nesbit M, Pritchard J) 1987 Lancet i: 208–209
8. Fartasch M, Vigneswaran N, Diepgen TL, Hornstein OP 1990 Immunohistochemical and ultrastructural study of histiocytosis X and non-X histiocytoses. J Am Acad Dermatol 23: 885–892
9. Emile J-F, Wechsler J, Brousse N et al 1995 Langerhans cell histiocytosis. Definitive diagnosis with the use of monoclonal antibody 010 on routinely paraffin-embedded samples. Am J Surg Pathol 19: 636–641
10. Barrett AW, Cruchley AT, Williams DM 1996 Oral mucosal Langerhans cells. Crit Rev Biol Med 1: 36–58
11. McLelland J, Broadbent V, Yeomans E, Malone M, Pritchard J 1990 Langerhans cell histiocytosis: the case for conservative treatment. Arch Dis Child 65: 301–303
12. Clinical Writing Group of the Histiocyte Society (Broadbent V, Gander H, Komp DM, Ladisch S) 1989 Histiocytoses syndromes in children: II. Approach to the clinical and laboratory evaluation of children with Langerhans cell histiocytosis. Med Pediatr Oncol 17: 492–495
13. Arceci RJ 1994 Treatment options – commentary. Br J Cancer 23: S58–S60
14. Elzay RP 1983 Traumatic ulcerative granuloma with stromal eosinophilia (Riga–Fede's disease and traumatic eosinophilic granuloma). Oral Surg 55: 497–506
15. Bhaskar SN, Lilly GE 1964 Traumatic granuloma of the tongue (human and experimental). Oral Surg Oral Med Oral Pathol 18: 206–218
16. Doyle JL, Geary W, Baden E 1989 Eosinophilic ulcer. J Oral Maxillofac Surg 47: 349–352
17. Movassaghi K, Goodman ML, Keith D 1996 Ulcerative eosinophilic granuloma: a report of five new cases. Br J Oral Maxillofac Surg 34: 115–117
18. El Mofty SK, Swanson PE, Wick MR, Miller AS 1993 Eosinophilic ulcer of the oral mucosa. Report of 38 new cases with immunohistochemical observations. Oral Surg Oral Med Oral Pathol 75: 716–722
19. Mezei MM, Tron VA, Stewart WD, Rivers JK 1995 Eosinophilic ulcer of the oral mucosa. J Am Acad Dermatol 33: 734–740
20. Regezi HA, Zarbo RJ, Daniels TE, Greenspan JS 1993 Oral traumatic granuloma. Characterisation of the cellular infiltrate. Oral Surg Oral Med Oral Pathol 75: 723–727

Tumors of the oral epithelium

Benign epithelial tumors 31

Papilloma

Squamous cell papillomas are relatively common. They are usually clinically recognizable by their warty surfaces or long, papillary, finger-like processes. They are white when keratinized or pink if not. Abbey et al,[1] in an analysis of 464 oral squamous cell papillomas, found that these tumors comprised 2.4% of all oral biopsies and affected ages ranged from 2 to 91 years, the average age being 31.4 years. The tumors were found slightly more frequently (53.8%) in men and located most frequently on the palate (34.4%), tongue (23.5%), and lips or gingivae (11.5% each). Nearly 70% were described as being white in color.

Human papilloma virus (particularly HPV 6 or 11) DNA can be detected in papillomas by in situ hybridization. However, unlike infective warts, evidence of viral proliferation is not seen by light microscopy. Also, simple papillomas are not infective and have no tendency to spread by autoinoculation to other sites.

MICROSCOPY

Papillomas have a branching structure consisting of a vascular connective tissue core, supporting a thick hyperplastic epithelium, which is often heavily keratinized (Fig. 31.1). According to Abbey et al,[1] 72% of papillomas judged to be hyperkeratotic showed parakeratinization only. They also recorded one or more features of atypia in the epithelium in 30% of 176 papillomas. However, malignant change in oral papillomas is virtually unknown.

BEHAVIOR AND MANAGEMENT

Clinically, papillomas may be mistaken for infective warts, fibrous polyps, pyogenic granulomas or, exceptionally rarely, sialadenoma papilliferum (see Ch. 51). Confirmation of diagnosis therefore depends on microscopy. Excision should be curative and recurrence is rare. Cryotherapy is effective, but may be followed by severe postoperative edema.

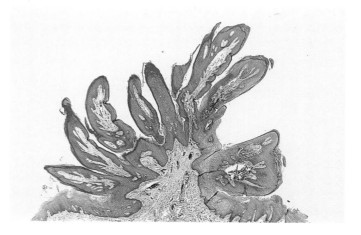

Fig. 31.1 Squamous cell papilloma. The branching finger-like process have a fibrovascular core and are keratinized in this example.

Verruca vulgaris

Infective warts occasionally affect the oral mucosa, particularly in children with warts of the fingers. Clinically, oral warts are pink or white and similar in appearance to papillomas. HPV 2a–e can be found in common warts and HPV 6a–f can be found in oral warts.

MICROSCOPY

Warts are similar to papillomas, but are distinguishable by the presence of intranuclear inclusion bodies (Fig. 31.2).

Excision is the treatment of choice, but further lesions may develop as a result of repeated autoinoculation.

Florid oral papillomatosis

This rare condition of widespread oral papilloma formation may

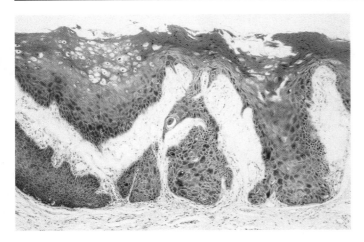

Fig. 31.2 Viral wart. The viral-induced nuclear changes have a striking resemblance to atypia. In situ hybridization showed Epstein–Barr virus DNA in the nuclei.

involve the whole of the buccal mucosa, lip, or other sites, which become pebbly in character. It has been reported in Down's syndrome[2] and massive oropharyngeal papillomatosis causing obstructive sleep apnea in a child has been reported by Brodsky et al.[3] Multiple papilloma-like lesions in 110 Guatemalans, mainly children and adolescents, with multifocal papilloma virus hyperplasia (focal epithelial hyperplasia) were described by Carlos & Sedano,[4] who reviewed earlier reports. The latter condition, unlike oropharyngeal papillomatosis, typically spares the palate.

Oral papillomatosis is also a feature of Cowden's syndrome, as described below. Papillomatosis should be differentiated particularly from naevus unius lateris.

Clinically, multiple oral papillomatosis causes the mucosa to acquire a cobblestone appearance.

Surgical excision may be justified, particularly for cosmetic reasons when the lips are affected, but the condition is otherwise benign.

Focal epithelial hyperplasia (Heck's disease)

Focal epithelial hyperplasia is an HPV-associated disease, but is probably dependent on a genetic predisposition. It was first noted among American Indians and an Eskimo boy. The reported incidence in various racial groups was reviewed by Praetorius-Clausen,[5] who showed that it may be seen in up to 20% of Greenlandic Eskimos and nearly 34% of Venezuelan Indians. It is rare in Britain, but isolated cases have been reported from many parts of the world, including Africa. HPV 13 and 32 appear to be virtually specific to this disease.

CLINICAL FEATURES

Focal epithelial hyperplasia appears as creamy, slightly elevated,

nodular, soft masses that are usually about 6–7 mm across. They are asymptomatic and are frequently noticed by chance. The labial and buccal mucosa are typical sites, but the palate appears to be spared. Almost any age and either sex may be affected, but among Guatemalans, Carlos & Sedano[4] found multifocal lesions mainly in children and adolescents, and males to be twice as frequently affected as females.

MICROSCOPY

The epithelium is hyperplastic, mildly parakeratotic, and has vacuolated, koilocyte cells with pyknotic nuclei just below the surface (Figs 31.3 and 31.4). The rete ridges are broad and often confluent. Carlos & Sedano[4] describe mitosoid abnormalities of keratinocyte nuclei as pathognomonic of the condition, but note that serial sections may be needed to find them. Virus-like particles can be identified by electron microscopy and viral DNA can be detected by in situ DNA hybridization.

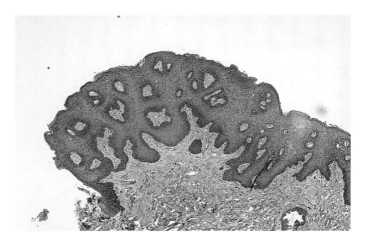

Fig. 31.3 Focal epithelial hyperplasia. Low-power view.

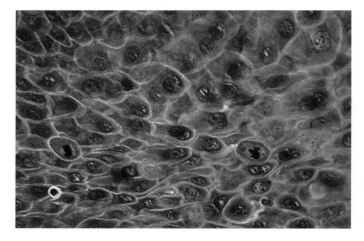

Fig. 31.4 Focal epithelial hyperplasia. The mitosoid cells in the epithelium are typical.

BEHAVIOR AND MANAGEMENT

The diagnosis is confirmed by biopsy. Treatment is not normally required and may be impractical if lesions are widespread. Spontaneous resolution has also been seen.

Condyloma acuminatum

Condyloma acuminatum is a sexually transmitted lesion seen mainly in the anogenital region. It is rare in the mouth but it is increasingly frequently seen in patients with human immuno-deficiency virus (HIV) infection as an opportunistic infection probably transmitted by orogenital contact. HPV 6 and 11 DNA has been identified in 85% of condylomata acuminata by in situ hybridization, although HPV 11 may be found in all types of papilliferous lesions.

CLINICAL FEATURES

Condyloma acuminatum appears as a white or pink nodule with prominent papillary processes, which are larger and broader than those of papillomas. It is usually sessile and may be single or multiple.

MICROSCOPY

The epithelium is thrown up into folds or broad papilla, giving a clefted appearance (Fig. 31.5). It is supported by a vascular stroma with a thin chronic inflammatory infiltrate. There is para-keratosis with a clear zone in the upper levels of the epithelium due to vacuolated koilocytic cells with pyknotic nuclei. Acanthosis is characterized by broad, long rete ridges. Never-theless, there are no reliable histological criteria for distin-guishing condyloma acuminatum from infective warts.

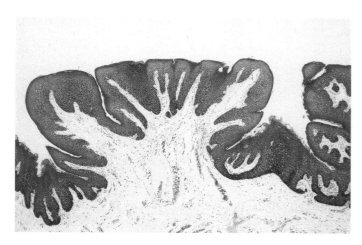

Fig. 31.5 Condyloma acuminatum. Low-power view.

Molluscum contagiosum

The molluscum contagiosum virus, a member of the poxvirus family, spreads by contact. It causes pearly umbilicated nodules on the skin, particularly of the neck, limbs, and trunk. The nodules can reach 1 cm in diameter. They are exceedingly rare in the mouth,[6] but may be seen in the perioral region in those with HIV infection.

MICROSCOPY

Molluscum contagiosum consists of a goblet-shaped mass. The proliferating epithelium forms compressed papillae pushing down into the corium and surrounding a central cavity open to the surface (Fig. 31.6). The superficial epithelial cells are distended by molluscum bodies, which are large, hyaline, eosinophilic inclusion bodies containing enormous numbers of the virus (Fig. 31.7). The central cavity is filled mainly with desquamated keratin-containing molluscum bodies.

Papillary hyperplasia of the palate

Palatal papillary hyperplasia consists of multiple soft-tissue nodules giving a coarsely granular or cobblestone texture to the vault of the palate. It is frequently regarded as a response to trauma from or infection under a denture. However, it may occasionally be seen in the absence of a denture, but the latter certainly aggravates the condition, particularly when harboring *Candida albicans*. The papillae are then red and edematous.

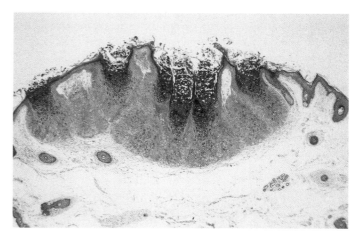

Fig. 31.6 Molluscum contagiosum. Low-power view showing epithelial hyperplasia and clefting.

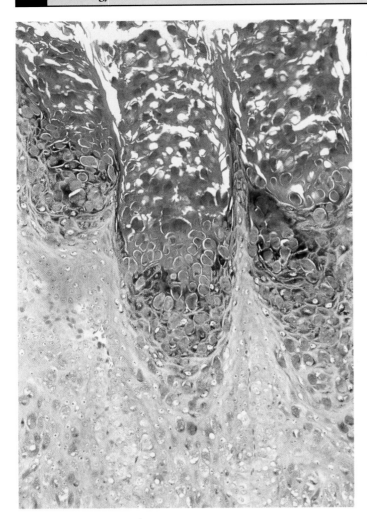

Fig. 31.7 Molluscum contagiosum. Higher power view showing striking viral inclusions.

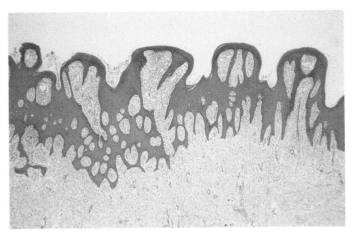

Fig. 31.8 Papillary hyperplasia of the palate. Low-power view shows multiple nodular projections of fibrous tissue with epithelial covering.

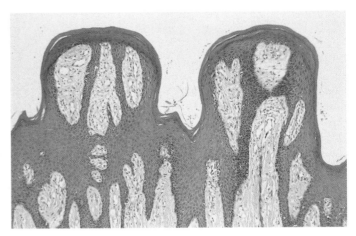

Fig. 31.9 Papillary hyperplasia of the palate. Higher power view showing the fibrovascular core to the nodules and hyperkeratosis of the epithelium.

MICROSCOPY

Papillary hyperplasia consists of multiple, closely set, rounded nodules of connective tissue covered by hyperplastic epithelium and infiltrated by varying numbers of inflammatory cells (Figs 31.8 and 31.9).

BEHAVIOR AND MANAGEMENT

If a denture is worn, the main requirement is to correct any defects and to treat any candidal infection with a topical antifungal drug. There is little or no justification for surgical intervention.

Cowden's (multiple hamartoma) syndrome

Cowden's syndrome is a rare autosomal dominant, genetic disorder characterized by hamartomas at almost any site and, later, by malignant neoplasms. The mouth, skin, thyroid, breast, gastrointestinal tract, and reproductive system are most frequently involved, and papular facial lesions may bring the patient to seek attention.

CLINICAL FEATURES

Cowden's syndrome often remains unrecognized until middle age, although the patient may have had treatment for what seemed to be disparate conditions for several years. Skin lesions are concentrated round the center of the face and consist of fine, hyperkeratotic papular lesions which can give a toad-skin appearance. Oral lesions are present in most patients and consist of multiple, often almost confluent, small papules on the lips, buccal mucosa, gingivae tongue, or uvula, resembling florid oral papillomatosis. The tongue may also be scrotal. The papules are initially painless, but may be so numerous as to interfere with mastication and, if abraded, become sore. Due to incomplete penetrance, relatives may have minor manifestations such as telangiectasia. The oral and systemic manifestations have been reviewed by Porter et al.[7] The oral abnormalities may be regarded as markers for possible internal malignancy.

MICROSCOPY

The oral papules consist of a fibrous core, which may be highly vascular, and are covered by acanthotic epithelium.

BEHAVIOR AND MANAGEMENT

Diagnosis depends on the clinical orofacial features and usually also a history of removal of multiple, initially benign, tumors, particularly in the sites mentioned earlier. Oral lesions require no treatment unless they trouble the patient. If so, they can be excised, but Devlin et al[8] reported persistent bleeding as a complication. Continued observation is required to enable internal cancers to be recognized and treated as early as possible.

Verruciform xanthoma

This uncommon lesion can appear as a papilloma-like warty swelling with a whitish surface, but is more frequently plaque-like. It is readily recognizable microscopically by the large subepithelial xanthoma cells.

Adenomas and adenocarcinomas

These tumors arise from minor intraoral salivary glands and can therefore appear in the oral mucosa as submucosal nodules or swellings, most commonly on the palate, in the lip, or buccal mucosa. Only sialadenoma papilliferum mimics a papilloma clinically.

REFERENCES

1. Abbey LM, Page DG, Sawyer DR 1980 The clinical and histopathologic features of a series of 464 oral squamous cell papillomas. Oral Surg 49: 419–427
2. Eversole LR, Sorenson HW 1974 Oral florid papillomatosis in Down's syndrome. Oral Surg Oral Med Oral Pathol 37: 202–207
3. Brodsky L, Siddiqui SY, Stanievich JF 1987 Massive oropharyngeal papillomatosis causing obstructive sleep apnea in a child. Arch Otolaryngol Head Neck Surg 113: 882–884
4. Carlos R, Sedano HO 1994 Multifocal papilloma virus epithelial hyperplasia. Oral Surg Oral Med Oral Pathol 77: 631–635
5. Praetorius-Clausen F 1973 Geographical aspects of oral focal epithelial hyperplasia. Pathol Microbiol 39: 204–213
6. Barsh LI 1966 Molluscum contagiosum of the oral mucosa. Oral Surg Oral Med Oral Pathol 22: 42–46
7. Porter S, Cawson R, Scully C, Eveson J 1996 Multiple harmatoma syndrome presenting with oral lesions. Oral Surg Oral Med Oral Pathol Oral Radiol Endod 82: 295–301
8. Devlin MF, Barrie R, Ward-Booth RP 1992 Cowden's disease: a rare but important manifestation of oral papillomatosis. Br J Oral Maxillofac Surg 30: 335–336

32

Chronic oral mucosal white lesions

The appearance of most mucosal white lesions is due to hyperkeratosis. Apart from the lingual filiform papillae, visible keratinization of any significant degree is abnormal in the mouth. Any excess keratin, becoming sodden with saliva, appears white.

Leukoplakia literally means no more than a white plaque, but in the past was widely, but mistakenly, regarded as virtually synonymous with premalignancy. The term 'leukoplakia' should therefore be used only as defined by a World Health Organization (WHO) committee[1] as 'a white patch or plaque which cannot be characterized clinically or pathologically as any other condition,' or avoided altogether. However, this is a diagnosis by exclusion and the WHO definition is ignored in some conditions such as hairy leukoplakia. Concern about the clinical diagnosis of precancerous lesions has led Axell et al[2] to devise more precise definitions, in particular in order to provide more reliable results from epidemiological studies.

Only a few white lesions undergo malignant change, and hyperkeratosis per se is of no premalignant significance, except when associated with epithelial dysplasia. Also, as discussed later, erythroplastic (red) lesions are more frequently dysplastic than white lesions.

In an attempt to ease the difficult problem of deciding the probable behavior of a chronic white lesion, those with little or no malignant potential are discussed first.

Chronic white lesions with little or no malignant potential

WHITE SPONGE NAEVUS

White sponge naevus is a developmental anomaly inherited as an autosomal dominant trait, and occasionally other affected members of a family may be seen.

CLINICAL FEATURES

The appearance is distinctive. The affected mucosa is white, soft,

and irregularly thickened. Unlike other white lesions, this change can cross the midline and involves the whole oral mucosa. It lacks well-defined borders and its edges fade imperceptibly into normal tissue. It can involve the esophagus,[3] anus, and vagina.[4]

MICROSCOPY

The epithelium is hyperplastic with uniform thickening, and the rete ridges extend to a uniform depth. Shaggy hyperparakeratosis and intracellular edema with abnormally prominent cell membranes produces a so-called basketweave appearance. There is no dysplasia, and inflammatory infiltration in the corium is typically absent (Figs 32.1 and 32.2).

BEHAVIOR AND MANAGEMENT

The appearance is readily recognized, particularly when there is widespread mucosal involvement. A positive family history is virtually confirmatory. If there is any doubt, a biopsy will confirm the diagnosis. Occasionally, patients claim that antibiotic treatment has caused the whiteness to disappear, but any such response is unreliable. The main requirement is to reassure the patient of the benign nature of the condition.

PACHYONYCHIA CONGENITA

Pachyonychia congenita is an uncommon congenital disorder, characterized by hypertrophy of the nail beds, skin lesions (particularly hyperkeratosis of the palms and soles), and oral white lesions. Premature eruption, including natal teeth, may be an associated feature.

CLINICAL FEATURES

The oral lesions typically consist of widespread, translucent thickening of the mucosal surface (leukokeratosis), sometimes with localized soft white plaques. Leukokeratosis may be present

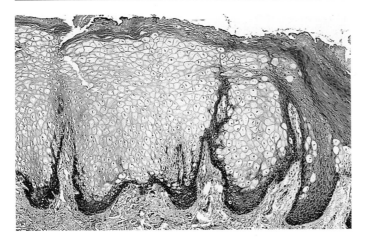

Fig. 32.1 White sponge naevus. Low-power view shows the hyperplastic epithelium with the vacuolated superficial cells.

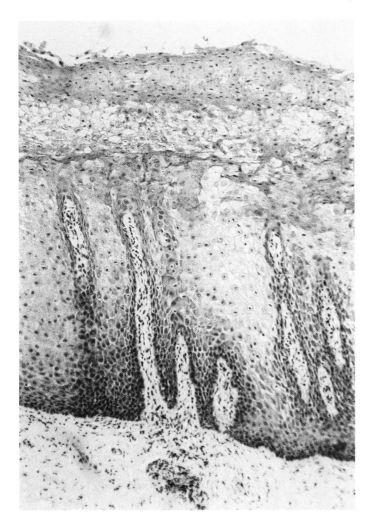

Fig. 32.2 White sponge naevus. Higher power view shows a variation on the possible appearances. The basketweave appearance of the superficial epithelial cells due to their clear cytoplasm and cell membranes is unusually well defined.

in infancy, but becomes prominent, especially in areas subject to trauma, over the course of years. White sponge naevus, by contrast, produces considerably more diffuse and widespread white mucosal thickening and lacks ungual or cutaneous abnormalities.

MICROSCOPY

The oral plaques show acanthosis and widespread hyperparakeratosis. The epithelial cells show intracellular vacuolation, somewhat like those of white sponge naevus, but in a more limited zone in the spinous cell layer and surrounded by normal cells. No treatment other than reassurance is required.

FORDYCE'S GRANULES

Sebaceous glands are present in the oral mucosa in at least 80% of adults. They appear in the oral mucosa as creamy white spots a few millimeters in diameter. They are soft, symmetrically distributed and, as they increase in size with age as a consequence of androgen dependence, may become conspicuous. The buccal mucosa is the main site, but sometimes the lips, and rarely even the tongue, palate, or gingivae are involved.

If these glands are mistaken for disease, patients can be reassured, but if a biopsy is carried out it shows a normal sebaceous gland with two or three lobules (Fig. 32.3).

SEBACEOUS GLAND HYPERPLASIA

Sebaceous gland hyperplasia has been defined by Daley[5] as a clinically distinct lesion that requires biopsy for definitive diagnosis. The condition has been reviewed by Dent et al,[6] who presented a case.

Intraoral sebaceous gland hyperplasia is uncommon. It appears clinically as an asymptomatic slightly raised submucosal mass typically of approximately 0.5 cm diameter and giving the mucosa a yellowish tint.

Histologically, sebaceous gland hyperplasia consists of sebaceous tissue with 15 or more lobules per gland and distended ducts, which may contain sebum-like material.

Treatment beyond confirmation of the histological diagnosis is not required.

FRICTIONAL KERATOSIS AND CHEEK BITING

Abrasion of the mucous membrane can be caused by such irritants as a sharp tooth, cheek biting, or dentures.

CLINICAL FEATURES

In the early stages, the patches are pale and translucent, but later

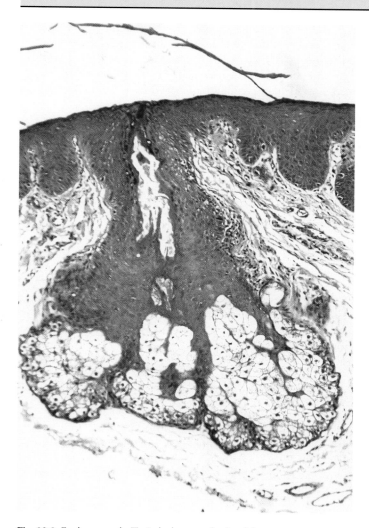

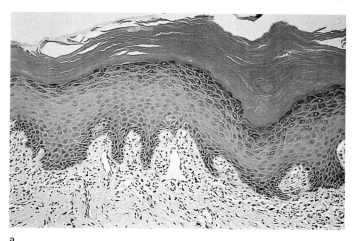

a

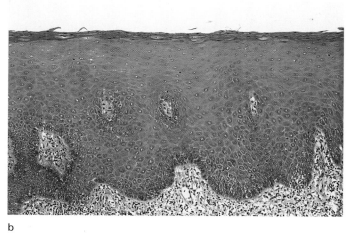

b

Fig. 32.3 Fordyce granule. Typical sebaceous gland and duct.

Fig. 32.4 Frictional keratosis. **a** The simple hyperorthokeratosis is nonspecific in appearance. **b** In this area the epithelium is parakeratinized.

become dense and white, sometimes with a rough surface. Habitual cheek biting causes an area of buccal mucosa to appear patchily red and white with a rough surface.

MICROSCOPY

The epithelium is moderately hyperplastic with a prominent granular cell layer and thick hyperkeratosis, but no dysplasia (Fig. 32.4). There are often scattered chronic inflammatory cells in the corium.

BEHAVIOR AND MANAGEMENT

Removal of the irritant causes the patch to disappear quickly and should make biopsy unnecessary. Frictional keratosis is completely benign, and there is no evidence that continued minor trauma alone has any carcinogenic potential.

PIPE-SMOKER'S KERATOSIS ('NICOTINIC STOMATITIS')

Smoker's keratosis is seen among heavy, long-term pipe smokers and some cigar smokers. By contrast, there is no specific lesion associated with the far more common habit of cigarette smoking.

CLINICAL FEATURES

The appearances are distinctive in that the palate is affected, but any part protected by a denture is spared. Changes are then seen behind the posterior border of the denture, mainly on the soft palate.

The lesion has two components: hyperkeratosis and inflammatory swelling of minor mucous glands. Either may predominate but, typically, white thickening of the palatal mucosa is associated with small umbilicated swellings with red centers. The white plaque is sometimes distinctly tesselated (Fig. 32.5).

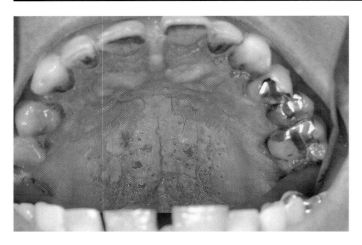

Fig. 32.5 Pipe-smoker's keratosis. The clinical appearance and history are more specific than the histological findings.

MICROSCOPY

The white areas show hyperorthokeratosis and acanthosis with a variable inflammatory infiltrate beneath. The diagnostic feature is the swollen, inflamed mucous glands with hyperkeratosis extending up to the margins of the duct orifice (Fig. 32.6).

BEHAVIOR AND MANAGEMENT

The clinical appearances and history are so distinctive that biopsy should not be necessary. Moreover, if the patient stops smoking the lesion resolves rapidly.

Epidemiological evidence suggests that pipe smoking raises the risk of cancer, but when oral cancer develops in association with pipe-smokers' keratosis, it typically appears *not* in the keratotic area on the palate (one of the least common sites for cancer), but low down in the mouth, often in the lingual retromolar region. This may be the result of carcinogens pooling and having their

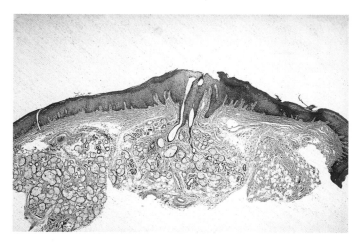

Fig. 32.6 Pipe-smoker's keratosis. Simple hyperorthokeratosis and an inflamed mucous gland with swelling round the duct orifice.

maximal effect in drainage areas of the mouth. It also suggests that there are different causes for the hyperkeratosis and any carcinomatous change.

It is noteworthy, therefore, that although tobacco is frequently incriminated in the etiology of oral cancer, the hyperkeratotic palatal lesion of pipe smokers is benign.

By contrast the palatal lesion caused by reverse smoking has a strong malignant potential. In this habit, which is practised in, for example, the Philippines and some parts of India[7] and South America, the lighted end of the cigar or cigarette is held in the mouth.

HIV-ASSOCIATED HAIRY LEUKOPLAKIA

Patients with HIV infection may develop a clinically and histologically distinctive type of white lesion, which was first described by Greenspan et al.[8] Hairy leukoplakia is an important manifestation of HIV infection and, although not entirely unique to it, is otherwise exceedingly rare. Hairy leukoplakia also has important prognostic significance.

CLINICAL FEATURES

Male homosexuals are predominantly affected; all 155 patients with hairy leukoplakia reported by Greenspan et al[9] were in this group. The lateral margins of the tongue are usually affected, and the plaque is soft, white, and usually asymptomatic. The surface is vertically corrugated, but only rarely has hair-like filamentous projections of keratin. Hairy leukoplakia has been reported in children, but to date there have been only three reported cases. Laskaris et al[10] reviewed the two earlier reports and described a case in a 9-year-old boy with a CD4 count of 95/μl. The condition resolved completely after treatment with aciclovir (600 mg/day for 1 month).

MICROSCOPY

Hairy leukoplakia shows hyperkeratosis, parakeratosis, or both, with a ridged or shaggy surface or, rarely, hair-like extensions of keratin. Secondary invasion of the surface by candidal hyphae is relatively common, but microscopic features of candidosis are lacking (Fig. 32.7). More important is the presence of *koilocytes*, which are vacuolated and ballooned prickle cells with pyknotic nuclei surrounded by a clear halo (Fig. 32.8). There is little or no inflammatory infiltrate in the corium (Fig. 32.9).

Epstein–Barr virus (EBV) capsid antigen can be identified by in situ hybridization in the epithelial cell nuclei (Fig. 32.10). Viral particles resembling EBV can also be seen by electron microscopy. This finding appears to be unique to hairy leukoplakia, and the likelihood that the EBV is the etiological agent is also suggested by the report by Resnick et al,[11] among others, that hairy leukoplakia responds to treatment with aciclovir or its analogs. Langerhans

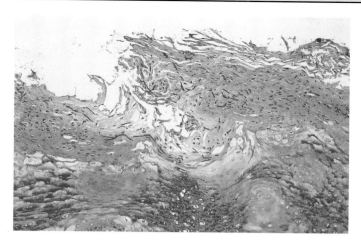

Fig. 32.7 Candidosis in HIV infection. Superimposed candidal infection without intraepithelial inflammatory response in hairy leukoplakia.

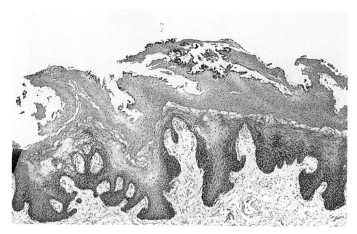

Fig. 32.9 Hairy leukoplakia. The parakeratotic layer shows hair-like extensions. The zone of clear, koilocyte-like cells is clearly defined and there is a notable absence of inflammatory infiltration in the lamina propria.

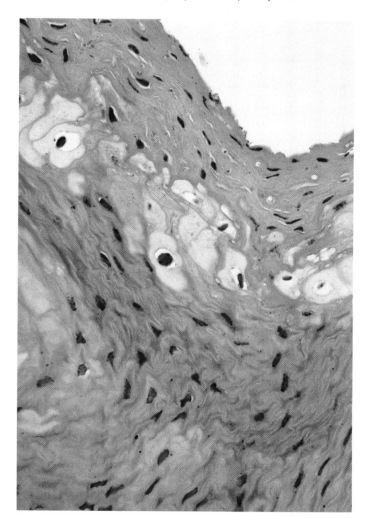

Fig. 32.8 Hairy leukoplakia. Cowdray type A inclusion body.

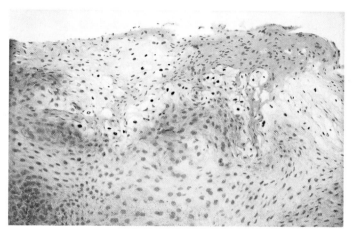

Fig. 32.10 Hairy leukoplakia. In situ hybridization to show intranuclear Epstein–Barr virus DNA.

Up to 70% of patients with HIV-associated hairy leukoplakia develop the full acquired immune deficiency syndrome within less than 5 years. Because of this poor prognosis, confirmation of the diagnosis is important.

Incisional biopsy (with all the disadvantages of an invasive procedure in an HIV-positive patient) may be avoided by using exfoliative cytology as reported by Epstein et al.[12] Their criterion of diagnosis was margination (beading) of the nuclear chromatin in the superficial cells. This change was confirmed by electron microscopy, which also showed the nuclei to be packed with viral particles.

Hairy leukoplakia is not premalignant and the incidence of intraoral cancer is no higher in HIV-positive persons than in the rest of the population. It has a remittant course and can regress spontaneously. However, as mentioned earlier, it is an important indicator of progression to AIDS.

cells may be few or absent, so that a defect of local immunity may contribute to the development of this lesion. Human papilloma virus can frequently also be detected, but appears to play no part in the pathogenesis.

HAIRY LEUKOPLAKIA IN THE ABSENCE OF HIV INFECTION

Hairy leukoplakia is not completely unique to HIV infection. It has been reported in both immunocompetent and immuno-deficient patients, but this is rare in comparison with the incidence in those with HIV infection. Eisenberg et al[13] described two immunocompetent patients in whom unexplained hairy leukoplakia developed and in which EBV DNA was detected by in situ hybridization. Epstein et al[14] have described it in 10 patients after bone marrow transplantation. In both the immunocompetent and immunosuppressed patients the lesion resolved spontaneously.

ORAL KERATOSIS OF RENAL FAILURE

White oral lesions are an occasional and unexplained complication of long-standing renal failure.

CLINICAL FEATURES

Clinically, the plaques are soft, have a crenated surface and are typically symmetrically distributed. Effective dialysis or renal transplantation bring resolution. No local treatment is necessary or likely to be effective.

MICROSCOPY

The features do not appear to be sufficiently distinctive to enable a diagnosis to be made without knowledge of the underlying disease. There is irregular acanthosis, with mild atypia of the epithelial cells and moderate parakeratosis. The appearances are somewhat similar to those of hairy leukoplakia (Fig. 32.11). Biopsy may be useful also to distinguish these lesions from adherent bacterial plaques, which may also develop in patients with renal failure.

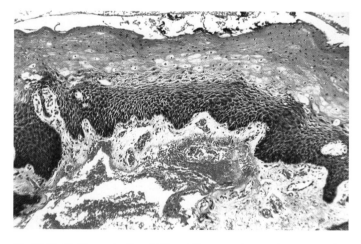

Fig. 32.11 Oral keratosis of renal failure. Microscopy shows a picture suggestive of hairy leukoplakia but in situ hybridization for EBV was negative.

PSORIASIS

Psoriasis is a common skin disease estimated to affect 2% of the population. Oral psoriatic plaques are rare, but a significant association has been noted between both benign migratory glossitis (geographical tongue) and stomatitis areata migrans (its counterpart on other parts of the oral mucosa) and cutaneous psoriasis, which these lesions closely resemble histologically.

CLINICAL FEATURES

Oral psoriatic plaques are typically associated with severe pustular psoriasis, but occasionally with psoriasis vulgaris. The appearance of oral lesions is variable.[15,16] Whitish translucent plaques are most characteristic or there may be the circinate white lesions of migratory glossitis or stomatitis areata migrans. Macules, diffuse erythema, and pustules may occasionally be seen. Oral lesions are frequently asymptomatic and may not be noticed.

MICROSCOPY

Oral and cutaneous lesions have essentially the same histologic appearances. There is parakeratosis, superficial spongiosis, and an inflammatory infiltrate which can form Monro microabscesses superficially in the epithelium (Fig. 32.12). There may also be the characteristic pattern of acanthosis, with long, slender, square-tipped or club-shaped epithelial downgrowths (Fig. 32.13). The inflammatory infiltrate in the corium is usually sparse.

Migratory glossitis, chronic candidosis, and Reiter's disease can also have a psoriasiform microscopic appearance. The diagnosis of oral psoriasis should only, therefore, be made when it has the characteristic microscopic features and is associated with cutaneous psoriasis.

VERRUCIFORM XANTHOMA

Verruciform xanthoma is a rare proliferative lesion, which can have a white, hyperkeratotic surface.

CLINICAL FEATURES

Clinically, verruciform xanthoma is most common in the fifth to seventh decades. It is usually found on the gingiva, but can form in almost any site in the mouth. It can be white or red in color, be sessile or pedunculated, have a warty surface, and range in size from one to several centimeters across. It may be mistaken for a papilloma, leukoplakia, or carcinoma clinically, but is readily recognizable histologically. Verruciform xanthoma is benign and has no known relationship with diseases, such as hyperlipidemia or diabetes mellitus, that are associated with cutaneous xanthoma formation. Simple surgical excision is curative. Nowparast et al[17] have reviewed the clinicopathologic findings in 54 cases.

MICROSCOPY

The warty surface is due to the much infolded epithelium which,

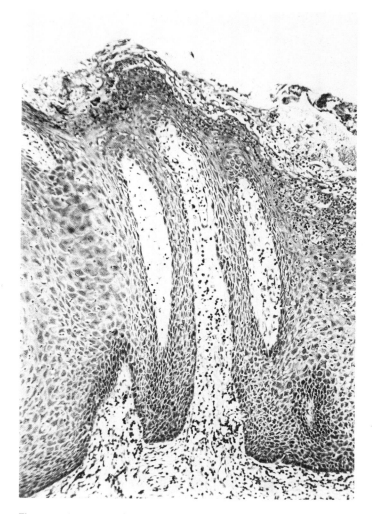

Fig. 32.12 Psoriasis. In this area the spongiotic changes and inflammatory infiltration of the superficial epithelium is prominent.

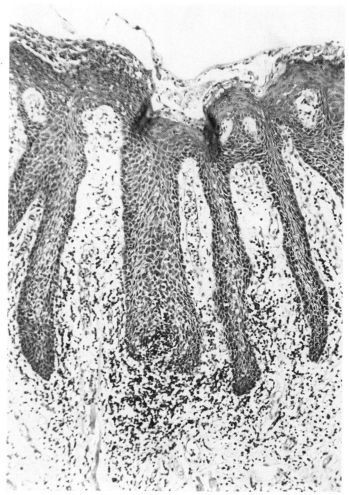

Fig. 32.13 Psoriasis. The rete ridges show the typical slender, club shape.

in white variants, is hyperkeratinized or, sometimes, parakeratinized. In hematoxylin and eosin (H&E) stained sections, the parakeratin layer stains a distinctive orange color (Fig. 32.14). The elongated rete ridges are uniformly elongated and extend to a straight, well-defined lower border.

The diagnostic feature is the large, foamy, xanthoma cells that fill the connective tissue papillae but extend only to the lower border of the lesion (Figs 32.15 and 32.16). These cells contain lipid and periodic acid Schiff (PAS) positive granules, and are positive for macrophage markers (Fig. 32.17).

Chronic white lesions with possible or recognized malignant potential

CANDIDOSIS

Candidosis can cause acute lesions (thrush), chronic white plaques (chronic hyperplastic candidosis), and also red lesions such as denture stomatitis.

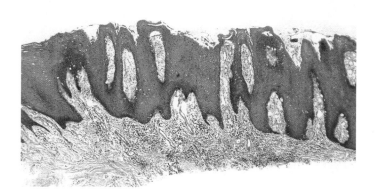

Fig. 32.14 Verruciform xanthoma. Low-power view showing the hyperplastic epithelium and the orange coloration that is frequently seen in H&E stained specimens.

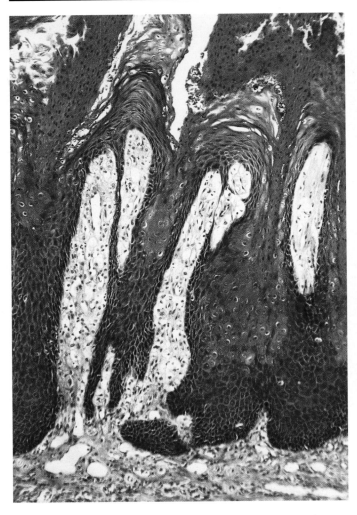

Fig. 32.15 Verruciform xanthoma. Higher power view showing prominent acanthosis, parakeratosis, and foam cells.

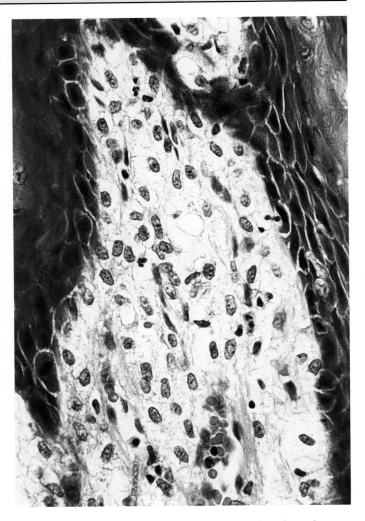

Fig. 32.16 Verruciform xanthoma. Higher power view to show the xanthoma cells in more detail.

CHRONIC HYPERPLASTIC CANDIDOSIS (CANDIDAL LEUKOPLAKIA)

Adults, typically males of middle age or over, are affected. The usual sites are the dorsum of the tongue and the postcommissural buccal mucosa. The plaque is tough and adherent, and distinguishable only by biopsy from other chronic white lesions. It is variable in thickness and often rough or irregular in texture, or nodular with an erythematous background, giving it a speckled appearance. Angular stomatitis may be associated, is sometimes continuous with intraoral plaques and suggests the candidal nature of the lesion.

Microscopy

Unlike thrush, the plaque cannot be wiped off, but fragments can be detached by firm scraping. Gram-staining then shows candidal hyphae embedded in clumps of detached epithelial cells.

The rete ridges are typically grossly enlarged and bulbous

(Fig. 32.18). Like thrush, the plaque of chronic candidosis is parakeratotic, but it is more coherent, containing only beads of inflammatory exudate which give it a psoriasiform appearance. In H&E stained sections, hyphae appear as no more than clear or faintly basophilic tracks through the epithelium (Fig. 32.19). PAS stain clearly shows the hyphae growing (as in thrush) through the full thickness of the plaque to the glycogen-rich zone, where the inflammatory exudate tends to be more concentrated and can form microabscesses (Fig. 32.20).

Electron microscopy shows *C. albicans* to be an intracellular parasite growing within the epithelial cytoplasm.[18] The hyphae, therefore, grow in relatively straight lines and do not follow a tortuous path along the intercellular spaces (Fig. 32.21).

Acanthosis of the epithelium can sometimes be extensive, with rounded downgrowths, and there may be dysplasia. Induction of epithelial proliferation by *C. albicans* infection has been demonstrated experimentally.[19]

The chronic inflammatory infiltrate in the corium is variable in density but may not break into the deeper epithelium. The

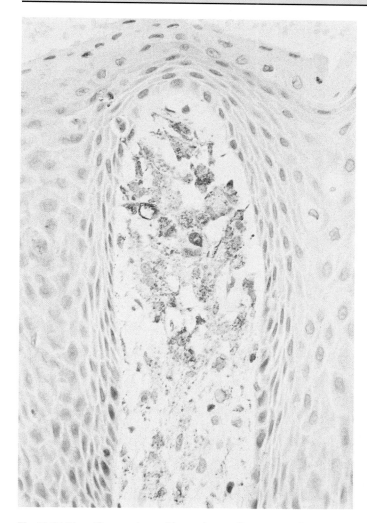

Fig. 32.17 Verruciform xanthoma. The xanthoma cells are positive for the macrophage marker CD68.

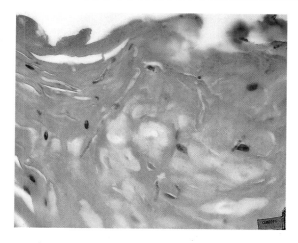

Fig. 32.19 Chronic hyperplastic candidosis. With H&E staining, hyphae (if visible at all) appear as clear or faintly basophilic tracts through the epithelium.

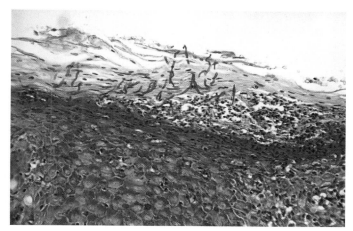

Fig. 32.20 Chronic hyperplastic candidosis. PAS staining shows hyphae in the plaque and intraepithelial abscess formation

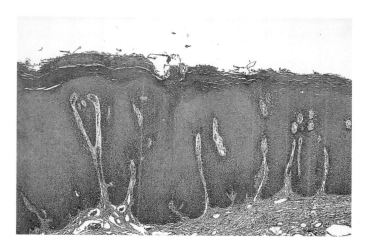

Fig. 32.18 Chronic hyperplastic candidosis. Low-power view showing the parakeratotic plaque and grossly enlarged, bulbous rete ridges.

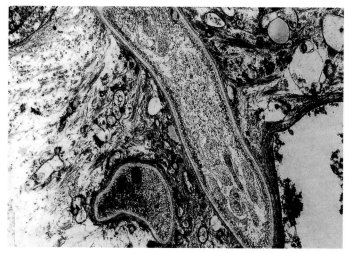

Fig. 32.21 Chronic hyperplastic candidosis. Electron micrograph of candidal hypha migrating through an epithelial cell.

basement membrane then remains intact and may appear to be thickened. This unusual feature in an oral keratotic lesion is typical of chronic candidosis.

Behavior and management

After confirmation of the diagnosis by biopsy, treatment should be with a systemically acting antifungal agent such as fluconazole, but this may have to be continued for several months. Other factors likely to perpetuate candidal infection should be controlled. Stopping the patient from smoking and elimination of a reservoir of candidal infection from under an upper denture are important. Any iron deficiency should also be treated.

Excision of candidal plaque alone is of little value, as the infection can recur in the same site even after skin grafting. Vigorous antifungal therapy is therefore essential, but sometimes some residual (uninfected) plaque may persist after treatment, and probably once the process has been initiated it may become (as in syphilitic leukoplakia) autonomous.

Chronic mucosal candidal infection can undoubtedly cause hyperplastic white lesions in which dysplasia is sometimes present.[20] Occasional cases of malignant change in chronic hyperplastic candidosis have also been described and, although the malignant potential of chronic candidosis remains controversial, the risk has been assessed by Cawson & Binnie,[21] Field et al,[22] and O'Grady & Reade.[23]

CHRONIC MUCOCUTANEOUS CANDIDOSIS SYNDROMES

These syndromes are all rare, but are difficult to manage. However, unlike isolated chronic hyperplastic candidosis, these syndromes do not appear to have any malignant potential.

The following classification is mainly based on that of Higgs & Wells:[24]

- familial (limited) type
- diffuse type (*Candida* 'granuloma')
- endocrine candidosis syndrome
- late onset (thymoma syndrome).

HIV-ASSOCIATED CANDIDOSIS

Any form of candidosis can be seen in HIV-positive patients. Thrush is most common as an early manifestion of the immune deficiency, but various forms of erythematous candidosis, angular stomatitis or, occasionally, chronic hyperplastic candidosis may be seen. HIV-related oral candidosis is associated with a low CD4 count (less than 200 cells/mm³) and is indicative of a poor prognosis. In a series of 1172 HIV-positive, hospitalized patients the mean survival time of those with oral candidosis was only 662 days.[25]

There is no evidence that HIV-associated candidosis has any malignant potential.

DYSKERATOSIS CONGENITA

Dyskeratosis congenita is heritable as a rare recessive or dominant trait. Dysplastic lesions of the oral mucosa, dermal pigmentation, dystrophies of the nails, and hemopoietic defects are the main features.

CLINICAL FEATURES

Oral white patches are seen in over 80% of patients, or there may be inconspicuous erythematous areas. Dental defects may be associated.[26] The cutaneous pigmentation is grayish brown, reticulate, and predominantly affects the neck, arms, and upper chest. The nails become dystrophic early and, by adolescence, may be completely destroyed. Alopecia is present in over 30% and hematological abnormalities are seen in 51% of patients. Many patients also appear to be immunodeficient or have other abnormalities: the findings in 104 cases of the disease have been reviewed by Davidson & Connor.[27]

MICROSCOPY

However slight the symptoms and however innocent the oral lesions appear clinically, they frequently show cytological atypia microscopically and the risk of carcinomatous change is high (Fig. 32.22). Multiple oral carcinomas can result, and the life expectancy is poor. Close observation and repeated biopsies should be prompted by the slightest symptoms so that each tumor can be treated as early as possible.

BEHAVIOR AND MANAGEMENT

The management is the same as for other dysplastic epithelial lesions (as discussed later) but, overall, the prognosis is poor. The

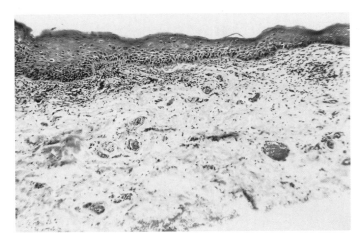

Fig. 32.22 Dyskeratosis congenita. An atrophic epithelium with mild dyskeratosis.

mean life expectancy is less than 25 years. Causes of death include cancers of the mouth or other sites, bleeding (gastrointestinal or cerebral), and aplastic anemia, but in 50% of cases death is due to infection, which is frequently opportunistic.

SNUFF-DIPPERS' KERATOSIS AND OTHER SMOKELESS TOBACCO LESIONS

Tobacco chewing or snuff dipping (holding flavored tobacco powder in an oral sulcus) causes a white hyperkeratotic lesion. Oral snuff appears to cause more severe changes than does tobacco chewing.[28]

CLINICAL FEATURES

The habit of snuff dipping may be maintained for decades, and gives rise to keratoses in the buccal or labial sulcus, where the tobacco is held. Early changes are erythema and mild, whitish thickening. Long-term snuff use gives rise to extensive white thickening and wrinkling of the buccal mucosa.

MICROSCOPY

The main changes are thickening of the epithelium, with plump or squared-off rete ridges. There are varying degrees of hyper-orthokeratosis or parakeratosis. Chevron keratosis is sometimes regarded as characteristic, but was seen in only 17% of 132 biopsies examined by Daniels et al[28] (Fig. 32.23). Hyalinization is seen deep to the lamina propria (Fig. 32.24). Dysplasia may eventually be seen and, occasionally, malignant change can follow, but only after several decades of use. A high proportion of these carcinomas are verrucous.

The heaviest users of oral snuff in the Western World are in Sweden, but in an extensive study Larsson et al[29] found no carcinomas among users and stated that they had never seen such a carcinoma in the great number of biopsies from all parts of Sweden over many years. The prevalence of oral lesions in smokeless tobacco users in the USA and the risk factors involved have been reviewed by Kaugars et al.[30]

BEHAVIOR AND MANAGEMENT

Diagnosis is based on the history of snuff use and the white lesion in the area where the tobacco is held. Biopsy is required to exclude dysplasia or early malignant change.

Larsson et al[29] have shown that snuff-dippers' lesions will resolve on stopping the habit, even after 25 years of use. This, therefore, is the main measure. If this fails, regular follow-up and biopsies are required.

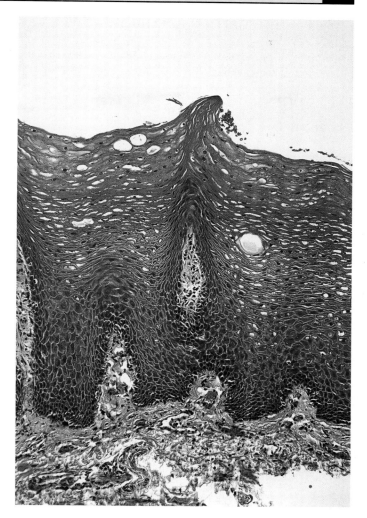

Fig. 32.23 Snuff-dipper's keratosis. 'Chevron' keratosis is a typical appearance.

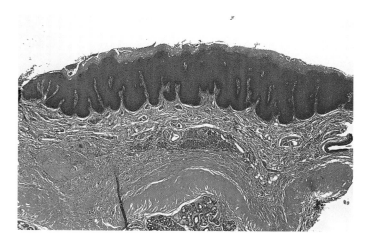

Fig. 32.24 Snuff-dipper's keratosis. Hyalinization deep to the lamina propria is prominent.

SYPHILITIC LEUKOPLAKIA

Leukoplakia of the dorsum of the tongue is a characteristic complication of tertiary syphilis, but is of little more than historical interest.

CLINICAL FEATURES

Syphilitic leukoplakia has no distinctive features, but typically affects the dorsum of the tongue and spares the margins (Fig. 32.25). The plaque has an irregular outline and surface. It is usually regarded as having a high risk of malignant change. Surface cracks, small erosions, or nodules may prove to be foci of invasive carcinoma. Carcinoma developing near the center of the dorsum of the tongue is typically a sequel to syphilitic leukoplakia and, as a consequence of the great decline in the incidence late-stage syphilis, is exceedingly rare in this site now.

MICROSCOPY

In addition to hyperkeratosis and acanthosis, often with dysplasia, the characteristic late syphilitic chronic inflammatory changes, with plasma cells predominating, may be seen in the connective tissue. Giant cells and, rarely, granulomas may be present. Endarteritis of small arteries is particularly characteristic. However, any distinctive features of a syphilitic inflammatory reaction may be totally lacking.

BEHAVIOR AND MANAGEMENT

The diagnosis is confirmed mainly by the serological findings. However, even if positive, biopsy is still essential, as minute areas of malignant change may be found, and the management is affected accordingly. In particular, the presence of syphilitic endarteritis, may be a contraindication to radiotherapy.

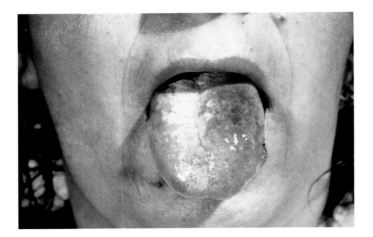

Fig. 32.25 Syphilis. This clinical picture of a now rare lesion shows a carcinoma of the dorsum of the tongue in syphilitic leukoplakia.

Antibiotic treatment of syphilis does not cure the leukoplakia, which persists and can undergo malignant change even after serology has become negative.

LICHEN PLANUS

Lichen planus, a common chronic inflammatory mucocutaneous disease, can give rise to mucosal white lesions, atrophic areas, or erosions.

ETIOLOGY AND PATHOGENESIS

Despite histological changes which can be highly characteristic and specific, the etiology of lichen planus remains unclear. The predominantly T-lymphocyte infiltrate suggests cell-mediated immunological damage to the epithelium and although it is inappropriate to discuss them here in detail, there is a plethora of reported immunological abnormalities. Tests of cellular immune responses to extracts of skin lesions of lichen planus have produced inconclusive results, and it has not yet been possible to demonstrate humoral or lymphocytotoxic mechanisms. However, the inflammatory infiltrate consists mainly of CD4 and CD8 T lymphocytes. CD8 T cells are more numerous in relation to the epithelium, and their numbers rise with disease. Which of the numerous reported phenomena are responsible for promoting accumulation of lymphocytes in the lesions and the precise trigger mechanisms remain unclear, but lichen planus undoubtedly appears to be a T-lymphocyte-mediated disorder.

The fact that a disease indistinguishable from lichen planus can be induced by various drugs also suggests an immuno-pathogenesis. Lichen planus is also a characteristic feature of graft-versus-host disease. Nevertheless it is not regularly associated with any of the recognized autoimmune diseases. Lichen planus responds well to immunosuppressive drugs (though not when associated with graft-versus-host disease), but the nature of any immunological mechanism remains unclear.

The belief that lichen planus may be associated with an unusually high incidence of glucose intolerance or diabetes mellitus or, alternatively, with rheumatoid arthritis has not been confirmed. The so-called *Grinspan syndrome* of lichen planus, diabetes mellitus, and hypertension appears to be no more than a chance association of common disorders or related to the drugs used. An association between lichen planus and hepatitis C virus infection has also been noted, particularly in Italy, but Cribier et al[31] found no higher frequency of hepatitis C antibody carriage in 52 patients with lichen planus than in controls.

The traditional view that lichen planus is associated with emotional stress is difficult to evaluate or substantiate.

CLINICAL FEATURES

White lesions are frequently asymptomatic. By contrast, lichen planus is probably the only disease which, if untreated, can cause unrelieved soreness of the mouth for 10 or more years. The middle-aged or older are predominantly affected, and the disease is rarely seen before the age of 30 years. Women account for at least 65% of patients.

The lesions have characteristic clinical appearances and distribution. The buccal mucosae are most frequently affected and the next most common site is the tongue. The gingivae are occasionally involved but the lips or palate are rarely so. Lesions are frequently symmetrical, sometimes strikingly so, but may be more prominent on one side than another.

Striae are sharply defined, bluish white, and form lacy, starry, or annular patterns. They may occasionally be interspersed with minute, white papules: rarely, papules may predominate. Striae may be impalpable or felt to have a stringy texture. *Atrophic areas* with redness and thinning, but not ulceration of the mucosa, are often combined with striae.

Erosions are shallow, irregular, and sometimes extensive areas of epithelial destruction. The margins may become slightly sunken due to fibrosis and gradual healing at the periphery. Striae radiating from the margins may also be seen. Erosions are sometimes covered by a raised yellowish layer of fibrin. This appearance often gives rise to the idea that they are intact or recently ruptured bullae. However, oral bullous lichen planus is a rarity that is hardly ever authenticated.

The three main types of lesion have corresponding microscopic features, as discussed below. Lichen planus occasionally also causes plaque-like lesions, particularly on the dorsum of the tongue and in long-standing disease. The plaques may be thick, are characteristically snowy white, and may have ill-defined margins giving them a fluffy or cotton-wool outline. However, it does not appear that the risk of malignant change is greater in plaque-like lichen planus.

Skin lesions

Lichen planus is a common skin disease, and 25–35% of patients with oral lichen planus may also have skin involvement. The skin lesions characteristically form purplish papules 2–3 mm in size. They have a glistening surface marked by fine (Wickham's) striae which, unlike those in the mouth, may only be visible with a magnifying glass. The rash is usually irritating and its appearance may be changed by scratching. Skin lesions should be looked for on the flexor surface of the forearms, especially on the wrists.

MICROSCOPY

The classical features of lichen planus are:

- a saw-tooth profile of the rete ridges (uncommon in oral lesions)
- liquefaction degeneration of the basal cell layer
- a band-like lymphocytic infiltrate which hugs the epitheliomesenchymal junction.

Striae show parakeratosis or hyperorthokeratosis, sometimes

with a prominent granular cell layer. The rete ridges tend to be pointed and are sometimes saw-tooth in shape (Fig. 32.26). Along the junction between the epithelium and connective tissue, there may be degeneration and liquefaction, with beads of fluid accumulating along the basement membrane (Fig. 32.27). The basal cell layer is not usually identifiable, but colloid (Civatte) bodies (apoptotic bodies) may be present in the depths of the epithelium or extruded into the immediately underlying connective tissue (Fig. 32.28). Fibrillar fibrinogen deposition along the basement membrane zone may be conspicuous, and there is often pigmentary incontinence. Antibodies are not found, but there may be nonspecific immunoglobulin deposits.

In the corium, the infiltrate consists mainly of T lymphocytes, packed beneath the epithelium in a band-like distribution. These inflammatory cells form a compact zone, which hugs and may cross the epitheliomesenchymal junction, but has a well-defined deep border.

Atrophic lesions show severe thinning and flattening of the

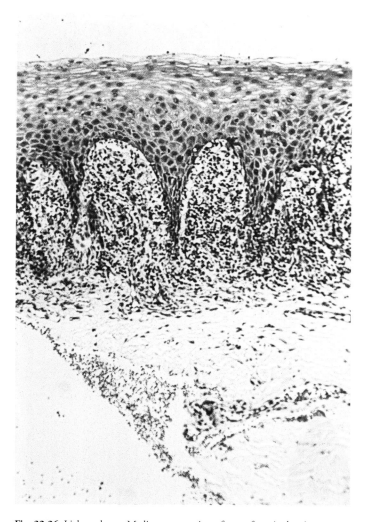

Fig. 32.26 Lichen planus. Medium-power view of part of a stria showing parakeratosis, 'classical' saw-tooth rete ridges, and band-like distribution of the inflammatory infiltrate.

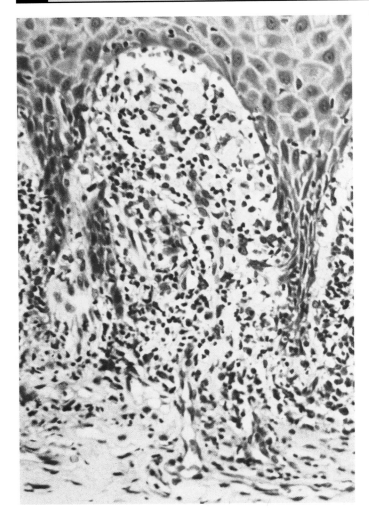

Fig. 32.27 Lichen planus. Higher power view showing the tips of the rete ridges, liquefaction degeneration of the basal cell layer, and the mixed chronic inflammatory infiltrate.

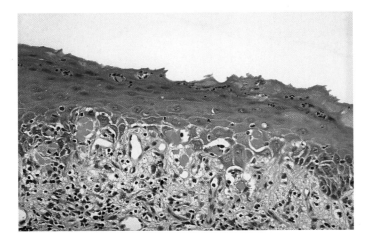

Fig. 32.28 Lichen planus. Higher power view showing liquefaction degeneration, loss of a defined basal cell layer, and eosinophilic colloid (Civatte) bodies.

epithelium, but the inflammatory infiltrate often retains its characteristic distribution and may be more dense.

In erosions, destruction of the epithelium leaves only a granulating connective tissue floor, so that the appearances are nonspecific. The diagnosis must be confirmed by finding typical lesions elsewhere in the mouth or skin.

In many cases the microscopic features are not absolutely distinctive and no more than 'consistent with' lichen planus or difficult to distinguish from lupus erythematosus. There are no reliable criteria to distinguish spontaneous lichen planus from drug-associated disease. The diagnosis must then be made in conjunction with the clinical features and laboratory investigation in order to exclude lupus erythematosus.

DRUG-ASSOCIATED LICHEN PLANUS

A great variety of drugs, notably methyldopa, gold and anti-malarial agents, but many others also, have been reported to cause disease ('lichenoid' lesions) indistinguishable from lichen planus. The treatment is, wherever possible, to change the drug for an appropriate alternative.

REACTIONS TO AMALGAM RESTORATIONS

The possibility that amalgam restorations can induce lichenoid lesions has been explored extensively. Overall, the findings have have been inconclusive.[32,33]

POTENTIAL OF ORAL LICHEN PLANUS FOR MALIGNANT CHANGE

This point has long been controversial. A study by Holmstrup et al[34] involved 611 patients followed for a mean period of 7.5 years, and in this group malignant change developed in 1.5%. All but one of the latter were women, and malignant change followed the initial diagnosis after a mean period of 10 years (range 5–24 years). Compared with the estimated cancer risk in the population of Denmark, lichen planus would thus appear to increase it approximately 50-fold. By contrast, in their follow-up study of 113 patients, Voute et al[35] concluded that the three cases of oral cancer found after an average period of 7 years provided 'some but not very strong support' for the belief that lichen planus is premalignant, because of doubt about the original diagnosis.

Also apparently anomalous findings are those of Murti et al,[36] who concluded from a study of 722 patients in India, where susceptibility to oral cancer is strong, that the 0.3% incidence of malignant change in oral lichen planus could not confirm its precancerous nature. Sigurgeirsson & Lindelöf,[37] in a study from a dermatology department of 2071 patients with lichen planus, followed for an average of 9.9 years, found an incidence of oral cancer of 0.4%. However, they could not specify how many of the patients had oral lichen planus, and it seems likely that many of their patients had cutaneous disease. They also reviewed reports of skin cancer developing in cutaneous lichen planus, but could only find 36 cases between the years 1903 and 1989. However the findings of these workers are interpreted, it appears that the malignant potential of oral lichen planus is far higher than that of the cutaneous form.

On the basis of five previous studies reported since 1985, Holmstrup[38] felt that there was no longer any doubt about this risk and that its magnitude was between 0.5% and 2.5%, but he was unable to identify any predictive factors. Barnard et al[39] examined retrospectively the records of a further 241 patients, in 3.7% of whom carcinoma or carcinoma in situ developed. They also reviewed 22 earlier reports including those mentioned, and in those where more than 100 patients had been followed-up the rate of malignant change ranged from 0.4% to 2.7%.

Under such circumstances it seems strange that the risk of malignant change in oral lichen planus has for so long remained controversial. It may be noted that such figures refer to cases of lichen planus referred to hospital but, as the disease can be asymptomatic, there are probably many more cases in the general population and the risk of malignant change is therefore lower than the quoted figures suggest.

BEHAVIOR AND MANAGEMENT

The diagnosis of lichen planus can usually be made from the history, appearance, and distribution of the lesions. If there is any doubt, a biopsy should be taken, particularly when striae are ill-defined or carcinoma is suspected by changes in the appearance of the lesion. A streaky whitish appearance is occasionally due to dysplastic disease. The main management considerations are first to relieve symptoms, and second to follow up the patient for possible malignant change.

Corticosteroids are frequently effective. Eisen et al[40] reported cyclosporin mouth rinses to be effective in a small group of patients, but this has not been widely confirmed. Systemic cyclosporin treatment has been reported to be effective for otherwise intractable lichen planus.[41]

Baudet-Pommel et al[42] have reported the effects of treatment with tretinoin and etretinate, but these drugs have significant toxic effects and are of known teratogenicity. Whether the risk of malignant change is affected by early treatment or the type of lesion is unknown.

LUPUS ERYTHEMATOSUS

Lupus erythematosus is an uncommon connective tissue disease which may be systemic or discoid. Either can give rise to oral lesions that may resemble to some degree those of oral lichen planus. Systemic lupus erythematosus has protean effects. Arthralgias and rashes are most common, but virtually any organ system or serous surface can be affected. The most serious consequences are from renal or cerebral involvement. A great variety of auto-

antibodies is produced and, of these, antinuclear antibodies are the most characteristic and regularly detectable.

Discoid lupus is essentially a skin disease with mucocutaneous lesions indistinguishable clinically from those of systemic lupus. These may be associated with arthralgias or, rarely, with significant autoantibody production.

CLINICAL FEATURES

Oral lesions are seen in about 20% of cases of systemic lupus, in an unknown number of patients with discoid disease and, rarely, can be presenting signs of this disease.[43] Typical lesions are white, often striate areas with irregular atrophic areas or shallow erosions, but the patterns, particularly those of the striae, are typically far less sharply defined than in lichen planus. They may involve only a small area of one side of the mouth and may be in the vault of the palate, which is an unusual site for lichen planus.

Lesions can be widespread and form variable patterns of white and red areas. There may also be small slit-like ulcers just short of the gingival margins. In about 30%, Sjögren's syndrome develops. Rarely, cervical lymphadenopathy is the first clinical sign.

MICROSCOPY

Oral lesions of discoid and systemic lupus show an irregular pattern of epithelial atrophy and acanthosis. The downgrowths of the latter may be flame-like in contour, or long and slender extending deeply into the lamina propria (Fig. 32.29). There may be surface keratinization, which may rarely appear to be invaginating the epithelium (keratotic plugging), liquefaction degeneration of the basal cell layer, and thickening of the basement membrane zone by deposition of antigen–antibody complexes, which also appear in blood vessel walls, as shown by PAS staining (Figs 32.30 and 32.31). In the lamina propria there

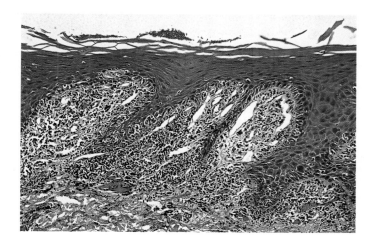

Fig. 32.29 Lupus erythematosus. The acanthosis has a more ragged profile than that of lichen planus, and the inflammatory infiltrate is more scattered.

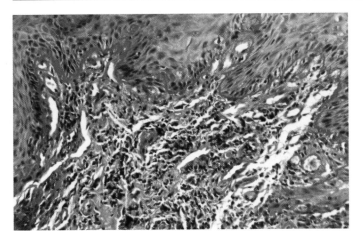

Fig. 32.30 Lupus erythematosus. Thickening of the basement membrane zone due to deposition of immune complexes demonstrated by PAS staining.

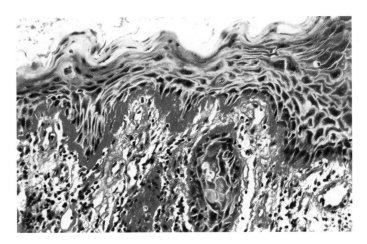

Fig. 32.31 Lupus erythematosus. Higher power view of thickening of the basement membrane zone due to deposition of immune complexes, as demonstrated by PAS staining.

is edema and often a hyaline appearance. The inflammatory infiltrate is highly variable in density, typically extends deeply into the connective tissue, and may have a perivascular distribution, but it is frequently scanty in the lamina propria.

Though the appearances can sometimes suggest either lichen planus or lupus erythematosus, the latter is unlikely to show the regular patterns of acanthosis or, more particularly, the band-like distribution of lymphocytes in the papillary corium.

In a statistical analysis of a range of microscopic features seen in lichen planus and lupus erythematosus, Karjalainen & Tomich[44] found that distinguishing features of the latter were vacuolization of keratinocytes, thick patchy PAS-positive subepithelial deposits, edema of the upper lamina propria, PAS-positive thickening of blood vessel walls, and dense, deep, or perivascular inflammatory infiltrate.

Using frozen sections, a band of immunoglobulins and complement (C3) with a granular texture deposited along the line of the basement membrane may be shown by immunofluorescence. This deposit underlies the lesions alone in discoid disease, but also underlies normal epithelium in systemic disease. In paraffin sections, immunoglobulin deposits may be detectable using immunoperoxidase staining. The only other feature that distinguishes systemic from discoid lupus microscopically is the characteristic, but rare, finding of frank vasculitis.

Diagnosis of discoid lupus depends on the clinical features and, in particular on the presence of rashes, often of a photosensitivity type. The autoantibody findings in discoid disease are important mainly to distinguish it from systemic lupus.

Mild systemic lupus can be difficult to distinguish clinically from discoid disease and, rarely, there can be transition from discoid to systemic disease. However, systemic lupus should be recognizable by the pattern of multiple autoantibody production. The most specific is that to double-stranded (native) DNA (dsDNA, nDNA).

Hematologic findings in active systemic lupus erythamatosus include a raised ESR, anemia and, often, leukopenia or thrombocytopenia. Renal involvement is indicated by hematuria, proteinuria, and red and white cell casts.

Oral lesions of discoid and systemic lupus respond in some degree to topical corticosteroids. Mild systemic lupus may be treated with anti-inflammatory agents alone, but more severe disease requires systemic corticosteroid or other immunosuppressive treatment. However, oral lesions frequently do not respond to doses of corticosteroids adequate to control systemic effects of the disease. Under such circumstances, palliative treatment is needed until disease activity abates.

PROGNOSIS

Sjögren's syndrome is associated in up to 30% of patients. As with other connective tissue diseases, there is a raised risk of cancer, especially lymphomas. There is also a small risk of malignant change in cutaneous lupus, particularly that of the lip.

SUBLINGUAL KERATOSIS

A white soft plaque with a wrinkled surface, with an irregular but well-defined outline, and sometimes with a butterfly shape may appear in the sublingual region (Fig. 32.32). The plaque typically extends from the anterior floor of the mouth to the undersurface of the tongue.

MICROSCOPY

Sublingual keratosis may show atypia, but the appearances are not distinctive (Fig. 32.33). Malignant change was associated in 24% of 29 cases reported by Kramer et al.[45] Such a high risk of malignant change has not been widely confirmed, and it is puzzling that more than 20 years should elapse between the

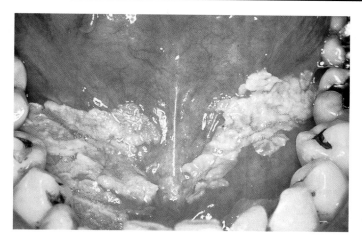

Fig. 32.32 Sublingual keratosis. Typical clinical appearance.

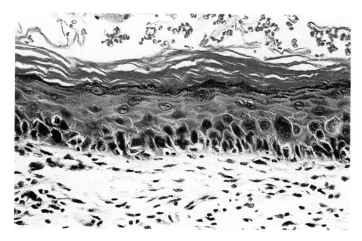

Fig. 32.33 Sublingual keratosis. Higher power view shows an atrophic epithelium, with moderate atypia and hyperorthokeratosis.

reporting of this potential and the description of sublingual keratosis as a harmless naevus by Cooke.[46] Moreover, malignant change has not apparently been seen in any of the patients that Cooke[46] reported.

ORAL SUBMUCOUS FIBROSIS

Oral submucous fibrosis is a disease that causes changes similar to those of systemic sclerosis (scleroderma) but limited to the oral tissues. The disease is seen in those from the Indian sub-continent and from many parts of South-East Asia such as Taiwan.

In their review, Pillai et al[47] conclude that the etiology is unknown but is probably multifactorial. Despite the histologic similarities, there are no immunologic abnormalities to suggest any relationship between oral submucous fibrosis and systemic sclerosis.

The main contributor is thought by Jayanthi et al[48] to be the use of *pan*, which typically consists of areca nut, tobacco, and

lime wrapped in betel leaf. Experimentally, an alkaloid component of the areca nut, arecoline, can induce fibroblast proliferation and collagen synthesis and may penetrate the oral mucosa to cause progressive cross-linking of collagen fibers.[49] Susceptibility to submucous fibrosis also appears to be related to specific HLA types. This also suggests a genetic factor. It is probably the tobacco content of the betel quid, rather than an areca nut, that induces epithelial atypia. While tobacco may possibly contribute to the malignant potential of this disease, it does not contribute to the fibrosis, which is not seen in the oral mucosa after long-term use of oral tobacco in other countries.

CLINICAL FEATURES

Clinically, affected areas of the oral mucosa, such as the palate or buccal mucosa, appear almost white. This is not a white plaque. The mucosa is typically smooth, thin and atrophic, and the pallor is due to the underlying fibrosis and ischemia. However, leukoplakia or a vesiculating stomatitis may be associated. Fibrosis is symmetrically distributed and also causes the affected area to become so hard that it cannot be indented with the finger. Ultimately, opening the mouth may become so limited that eating and dental treatment become increasingly difficult, and tube feeding may become necessary.

MICROSCOPY

The subepithelial connective tissue becomes thickened, hyaline, and avascular, and there may be infiltration by modest numbers of chronic inflammatory cells. The epithelium usually becomes thinned and may show atypia. Underlying muscle fibers undergo progressive atrophy (Fig. 32.34).

BEHAVIOR AND MANAGEMENT

In patients from Asia with these lesions, and especially with the characteristic histological changes on biopsy, the diagnosis can rarely be in doubt. Scleroderma should be readily differentiated by cutaneous and visceral involvement, the different character of any oral changes, and the immunological abnormalities. Murti et al[50] reported the development of oral carcinoma in 7.6% of 66 patients with submucous fibrosis who were followed up for a median period of 10 years.

Treatment is unsatisfactory. Patients must stop the habit of betel chewing. Intralesional injections of corticosteroids may be tried in association with muscle stretching exercises to prevent further limitation of opening, but the benefit is not great. Wide surgical excision of the affected tissues, including the underlying buccinator muscle, together with skin grafting can be carried out, but is likely to be followed by relapse. Borle & Borle,[51] in comparing treatments in 326 patients, concluded that injections could be hazardous, and conservative treatment by topical applications of

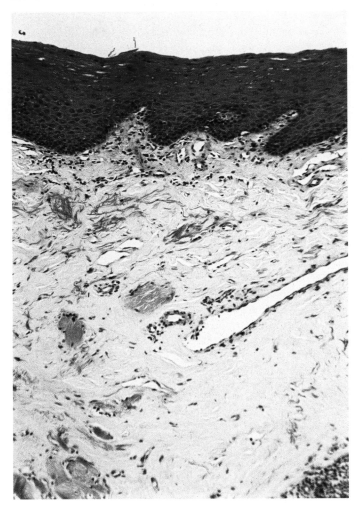

Fig. 32.34 Oral submucous fibrosis. Deeply extending, poorly cellular fibrous tissue has replaced the muscle, a few remnants of which are still present.

The most extensive follow-up studies suggest that this idiopathic group now has the highest risk of developing cancer. In most lesions of definable cause, the risk of malignant change is low, especially now that late-stage syphilis forms a negligibly small group.

The definition of premalignancy is difficult. In practice, lesions can only be termed precancerous *after* malignant change has developed, since there is, as yet, no means of predicting with certainty the risk of cancerous transformation. Microscopy is the best available guide, but even severely dysplastic lesions can undergo spontaneous regression. The histological findings therefore indicate no more than that a lesion has a malignant potential, but cannot be used for confident prediction of malignant change.

Clinically, the main lesions with malignant potential are idiopathic white lesions, speckled leukoplakias, and erythroplasias. Microscopically, the main feature suggesting premalignancy is epithelial dysplasia. Although there is no doubt about the malignant potential of some white lesions, the level of risk cannot be accurately assessed from the histopathology.

The most extensive clinical study was carried out by Einhorn & Wersall[52] and was based on 782 cases of histologically unspecified oral white lesions followed for an average of 12 years. Of these, 2.4% underwent malignant change in 10 years and fewer than 5% did so after 20 years. However, even this low rate represents a risk of malignant change 50–100 times that in the normal mouth. It was also conspicuous that in this very large study the rate of malignant change in oral leukoplakias was 10 times higher in nonsmokers than in smokers. Silverman et al[53] reported transformation rates of 0.12% in India and 6% in the USA. By contrast, in a study of 257 patients with leukoplakia who had been followed for an average of 8 years, Silverman et al[54] found malignant transformation in 17.5%. However, malignant change was also more frequent among nonsmokers. Other, smaller, series have suggested transformation rates of 30% or more, although in many cases no time scale was indicated. The wide variation in the rate of malignant change in these different series suggests that the findings have been significantly affected by selection of cases.

It must be emphasized that these large-scale studies have been done on histologically unspecified oral keratoses. Because of the rarity of dysplastic oral lesions there are very few studies, and none on a large scale, that have followed their progress for adequate periods. In the study by Mincer et al,[55] 45 patients with oral dysplastic lesions were followed for up to 8 years. Only 11% of lesions underwent malignant change in this period, and up to 30% regressed or even ultimately disappeared spontaneously. Eveson,[56] in a review of published surveys, found that dysplastic lesions appeared to regress more frequently than to undergo malignant change. As a consequence, it is not possible to prognosticate solely on the basis of the histologic changes. An additional problem is that, apart from the subjective nature of the assessment, if part is taken for biopsy purposes, there is no certainty that it is representative of the whole. The etiologies of cancer and of precancerous lesions overlap at many points, and they are therefore discussed in the next chapter.

such preparations as corticosteroids or vitamin A derivatives, and oral iron were as effective. However, no form of treatment is more than palliative, and in some cases operative treatment may become unavoidable. Jayanthi et al[48] (1992) suggest that the most important measure is prevention, and that use of pan should be forbidden in patients. This may be initially effective, but fibrosis often recurs even though the patient complies. Regular follow-up is important because of the malignant potential of this disease, but whether this is affected by early treatment is unknown.

IDIOPATHIC (INCLUDING DYSPLASTIC) LEUKOPLAKIA

For the majority of persistent white plaques, no etiologic factor can be identified. The histopathology is also highly variable, ranging from hyperkeratosis and hyperplasia to severe dysplasia.

CLINICAL FEATURES

Idiopathic leukoplakias and dysplastic lesions do not have any specific clinical appearance. Small and innocent-looking white patches are as likely to show epithelial dysplasia as are large and irregular ones. However, red (erythroplastic) lesions or erythroplasia in leukoplakias (speckled leukoplakia) are usually dysplastic or frank carcinomas.

MICROSCOPY

The epithelium may or may not be hyperplastic and is often thinner than normal. The plaque may show hyperorthokeratosis and parakeratosis in different parts, and the two may alternate along the length of the specimen. The epithelium is characterized by any of the cytologic changes of dysplasia (Figs 32.35–32.38):

- *Nuclear hyperchromatism.* The nuclei stain more densely due to greater nucleic acid content.
- *Nuclear pleomorphism and altered nuclear/cytoplasmic ratio.* The nuclei are variable in size, out of proportion to that of the cell; there may then be little cytoplasm surrounding the nucleus.
- *Mitoses.* These may be frequent and at superficial levels.
- *Loss of polarity.* The basal cells in particular may lie in a disordered fashion at angles to one another.
- *Deep-cell keratinization.* Individual cells may start to degenerate long before the surface is reached and show eosinophilic change deeply within the epithelium. The term 'dyskeratosis' applies only to this particular cellular change.
- *Differentiation.* The organization of the individual cell layers becomes lost and no clearly differentiated basal and spinous cell layers can be identified. Drop-shaped rete ridges are regarded as a particularly adverse feature.
- *Loss of intercellular adherence.* The boundaries of the cells may become separated.

A lymphoplasmacytic infiltrate of highly variable intensity is usually present in the lamina propria.

The histologic assessment of oral epithelial dysplasia is notoriously unreliable. Abbey et al[57] tested six board-certified oral pathologists for their consistency of histologic diagnosis of 120 oral biopsies, which ranged from simple hyperkeratosis to severe dysplasia. Exact agreement ('mild' or 'moderate' dysplasia) with the sign-out diagnosis was achieved in only 50.5%. Moreover, examiners agreed with their own first assessment on a second showing on only 50.8% of occasions. Agreement with the original diagnosis of the presence or absence of dysplasia was 81.5% and agreement by pathologists with their own diagnoses of dysplasia was 80.3%. Thus in nearly 20% of cases expert pathologists could not even confirm their own earlier diagnoses of dysplasia or its absence.

CARCINOMA IN SITU

'Carcinoma in situ' is a controversial term used for severe dysplasia where the abnormalities extend throughout the thickness of the

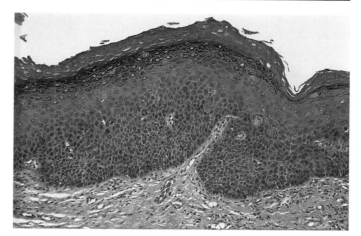

a

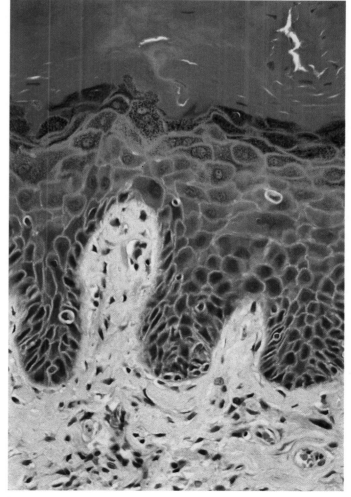

b

Fig. 32.35 a, b Mild epithelial dysplasia and hyperorthokeratosis.

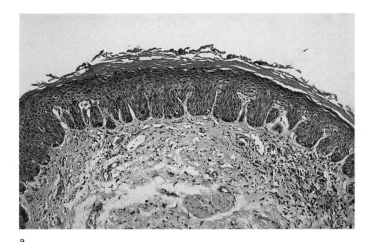

a

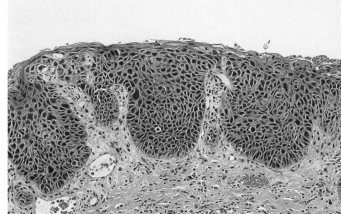

Fig. 32.37 Severe, full-thickness dysplasia (top-to-bottom change).

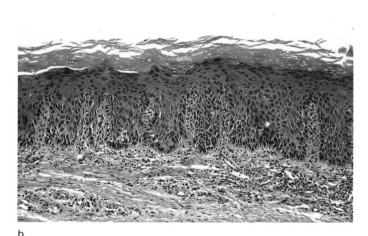

b

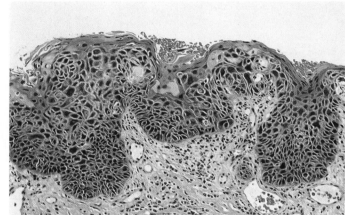

Fig. 32.38 Severe, full-thickness dysplasia. This view shows virtually all the possible nuclear and cytoplasmic abnormalities described in the text.

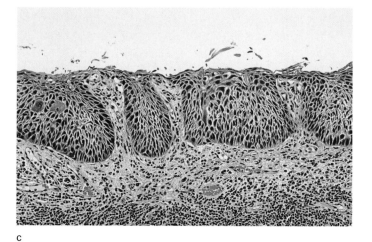

c

Fig. 32.36 a–c Moderate to severe epithelial dysplasia with nuclear pleomorphism and hyperchromatism.

epithelium – a state sometimes graphically called 'top-to-bottom change.' All the cellular abnormalities characteristic of malignancy may be present; only invasion of the underlying connective tissue is absent.

Top-to-bottom epithelial dysplasia, like other dysplastic lesions, has no characteristic clinical appearance. However, as discussed below, erythroplasia often proves to be carcinoma in situ or early invasive carcinoma (Figs 32.39 and 32.40).

MANAGEMENT OF DYSPLASTIC LESIONS

The management of dysplastic oral lesions remains controversial, as their relative rarity has made it impossible as yet to accumulate enough data to make reliable predictions. It is frequently also assumed that dysplasia is no more than an early stage in the development of carcinoma, which will subsequently behave like any other carcinoma. This leads to the assumption that treatment

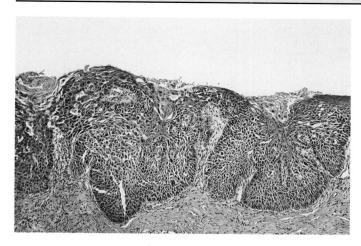

Fig. 32.39 Gross, full-thickness dysplasia, which could be graded as carcinoma in situ.

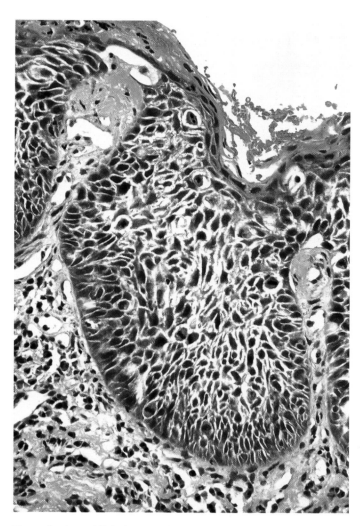

Fig. 32.40 Gross, full-thickness dysplasia. Higher power view of the same specimen as shown in Figure 32.39.

of a dysplastic lesion provides an opportunity to treat carcinoma at an exceptionally early, and potentially curative, preinvasive stage.

In contrast to an optimistic viewpoint of this sort, is the finding (discussed earlier) from the large survey by Einhorn & Wersall[52] that, after prolonged follow-up, lesions that had been treated by surgery more frequently became frankly malignant than did lesions that had not been so treated. Although the selection of patients may have biased these results, the latter certainly do not endorse the value of surgery.

From the histologic viewpoint it is also noticeable that the degree of atypia in many dysplastic lesions is considerably more severe than that seen in many frank carcinomas of the mouth. This may possibly be an indicator (on the assumption that the degree of differentiation of carcinomas is a guide to prognosis) of particularly aggressive behavior.

Furthermore, small dysplastic lesions, despite excision, can be followed by multiple carcinomas and a fatal outcome, as confirmed by the report by Shibuya et al[58] of 522 cases of carcinoma or carcinoma in situ of the tongue. They found that the risk of multiple carcinomas was five times greater in patients with carcinoma preceded by leukoplakia than in those carcinomas that had no such precursor. This large study, therefore, appears to confirm the possibility that some dysplastic leukoplakias may have a worse prognosis than isolated carcinomas without leukoplakia. Although such phenomena may be described as 'field change,' this is of little help to either the patient or surgeon.

By contrast, there is the evidence, discussed earlier, that many dysplastic lesions can regress spontaneously. It is clear, therefore, that the behavior of dysplastic lesions is unpredictable and that there is no reliable protocol of management. If they are of manageable size, it is tempting to excise them – this may do no harm, but it is essentially a treatment of hope rather than certainty. Prolonged, close follow-up is therefore essential. Even then, the prognosis may be poor. An alternative policy is to avoid surgical interference unless there are signs of progression and deterioration.

Another approach is cryotherapy ablation. In the short term the area usually heals rapidly to leave an apparently normal mucosa. However, there is some uncertainty about the risk of invasive carcinomas subsequently arising in sites previously treated by cryotherapy. Carbon dioxide laser ablation has also been advocated, but the same objections may apply.

Treatment with systemic or topical retinoids has also been tried. Topical retinoids are largely ineffective and, although a proportion of white lesions resolve with systemic treatment, the toxic effects are usually unacceptable. Furthermore, lesions that resolve with treatment recur on withdrawal of the drugs. Lippman et al[59] have reported that high-dose induction followed by low-dose systemic isotretinoin did not cause unacceptable toxicity, stabilized the majority of lesions, and was more effective than β-carotene in preventing malignant change. This seems an approach worth considering for lesions that are accessible for clinical and pathological assessment of progress.

With regard to possible predictors of malignant change in leukoplakias, there is good evidence that such change is more common in women. This also appears to apply to malignant change in lichen planus, as discussed earlier.

In summary, assessment of the severity of epithelial dysplasia is unreliable. As to treatment, excision may be considered, but frequent clinical observation, preferably with photographic records, and immediate biopsy of any areas that are suspicious or change in appearance, is an option that may be justified in view of the unpredictable behavior of dysplastic lesions.

SPECKLED (NONHOMOGENEOUS) LEUKOPLAKIA

This term applies to lesions consisting of white flecks or fine nodules on an atrophic erythematous base. They can be regarded as a combination of or transition between leukoplakia and erythroplasia. Speckled leukoplakia also more frequently shows dysplasia than lesions with a homogeneous surface. The histological characteristics are usually, therefore, intermediate between leukoplakia and erythroplasia.

Many cases of chronic candidosis have this appearance.

ERYTHROPLASIA ('ERYTHROPLAKIA')

In contrast to the foregoing lesions, erythroplasias are red. The surface is frequently velvety in texture and the margin may be sharply defined. Lesions of this type typically do not form plaques (hence the term 'erythroplakia' is inappropriate); instead, their surface is often depressed below the level of the surrounding mucosa.

Erythroplasia is uncommon in the mouth.

MICROSCOPY

Erythroplastic lesions usually show epithelial dysplasia, which may be severe, or there may be microinvasive or frankly invasive carcinoma. The risk of development of cancer is, therefore, highest in these lesions if they are not already carcinomas.

EARLY SQUAMOUS CELL CARCINOMA

Occasionally, early carcinomas produce sufficient surface keratin to appear as white plaques. These should not be confused with carcinomatous change in pre-existing leukoplakia. The carcinomas are always small (5–7 mm across), as further progress produces a more typical mass or ulcer.

REFERENCES

1. World Health Organization Collaborating Centre for Oral Precancerous Lesions 1978 Definition of leukoplakia and related lesions: an aid to studies on oral precancer. Oral Surg Oral Med Oral Pathol 46: 518–539
2. Axell T, Pindborg JJ, Smith CJ, van der Waal I, International Collaborative Group on Oral White Lesions 1996 Oral white lesions with special reference to precancerous and tobacco-related lesions: conclusions of an international symposium held in Uppsala, Sweden, May 18–21 1994. J Oral Pathol Med 25: 49–54
3. Krajewska IA, Moore L, Brown JH 1992 White sponge nevus presenting in the esophagus – case report and literature review. Pathology 24: 112–115
4. Nichols GE et al 1990 White sponge nevus. Obstet Gynecol 76: 545–548
5. Daley TD 1993 Intraoral sebaceous gland hyperplasia. Diagnostic criteria. Oral Surg Oral Med Oral Pathol 75: 343–346
6. Dent CD, Hunter WE, Svirsky JA 1995 Sebaceous gland hyperplasia: case report and literature review. J Oral Maxillofac Surg 53: 936–938
7. Reddy CRR, Kameswari VR, Chandramouli KB et al 1975 Evaluation of oral, pharyngeal, laryngeal and esophageal cancer risk of reverse smoking of chuttas. Int Surg 60: 266–269
8. Greenspan D, Greenspan JS, Conant M, Petersn V, Silverman S, DeSouza 1984 Oral 'hairy' leukoplakia in male homosexuals: evidence of an association with both papillomavirus and a herpes group virus. Lancet ii: 831–834
9. Greenspan D, Greenspan JS, Hearst NG et al 1987 Relation of oral hairy leukoplakia to infection with the human immunodeficiency virus and the risk of developing AIDS. J Infect Dis 155: 475–481
10. Laskaris G, Laskaris M, Theodoridou M 1995 Oral leukoplakia in a child with AIDS. Oral Surg Oral Med Oral Pathol 79: 570–571
11. Resnick L, Herbst JS, Ablashi DV et al 1988 Regression of oral hairy leukoplakia after orally administered acyclovir therapy. JAMA 259: 384–388
12. Epstein JB, Fatahzadeh M, Matisic J, Anderson G 1995 Exfoliative cytology and electron microscopy in the diagnosis of hairy leukoplakia. Oral Surg Oral Med Oral Pathol 79: 564–569
13. Eisenberg E, Krutchkoff D, Yamase H 1992 Incidental oral hairy leukoplakia in immunocompetent persons. A report of two cases. Oral Surg Oral Med Oral Pathol 74: 332–333
14. Epstein JB, Sherlock CH, Wolber RA 1993 Hairy leukoplakia after bone marrow transplantation. Oral Surg Oral Med Oral Pathol 75: 690–696
15. Morris LF, Phillips CM, Binnie WH et al 1992 Oral lesions in patients with psoriasis. Cutis 49: 339–334
16. Sklavounou A, Laskaris G 1990 Oral psoriasis: report of a case and review of the literature. Dermatologica 180: 157–159
17. Nowparast B, Howell FV, Rick GM 1981 Verruciform xanthoma: a clinicopathologic review and report of fifty-four cases. Oral Surg Oral Med Oral Pathol 51: 619–625
18. Cawson RA, Rajasingham KC 1971 Ultrastructural features of the invasive phase of Candida albicans. Br J Dermatol 87: 435–438
19. Cawson RA 1973 Induction of epithelial hyperplasia by Candida albicans. Br J Dermatol 89: 497–483
20. Cawson RA 1966 Chronic oral candidiasis and leukoplakia. Oral Surg Oral Med Oral Pathol 22: 582–584
21. Cawson RA, Binnie WH 1980 Candida leukoplakia and carcinoma: a possible relationship. In: Mackenzie IC, Dabelsteen E, Squier CA (eds). Oral premalignancy. Proceedings of the First Dow Symposium. Iowa: University Iowa, p 59–66
22. Field EA, Field JK, Martin MV 1989 Does Candida have a role in epithelial neoplasia? J Med Vet Mycol 27: 277–294
23. O'Grady JF, Reade PC 1992 Candia albicans as a promoter of oral neoplasia. Carcinogenesis 13: 783–786
24. Higgs JM, Wells RS 1974 Classification of chronic muco-cutaneous candidosis. Clinical data and therapy. Hautartz 25: 159–165
25. Lin RY, Goodhart P 1993 The role of oral candidiasis in survival and hospitalization patterns: analysis of an inner city hospital human immunodeficiency virus/acquired immune deficiency registry. Am J Med Sci 305: 345–353
26. Yavalzilmaz E, Yamalik N, Yetgin S, Kansu O 1992 Oral-dental findings in dyskeratosis congenita. J Oral Pathol Med 21: 280–284
27. Davidson HR, Connor JM 1988 Dykeratosis congenita. J Med Genet 25: 843–846
28. Daniels TE, Hansen LS, Greenspan JS et al 1992 Histopathology of smokeless tobacco lesions in professional baseball players. Associations with different types of tobacco. Oral Surg Oral Med Oral Pathol 73: 720–725
29. Larsson A, Axéll T, Andersson G 1991 Reversibility of snuff dippers' lesions in Swedish moist snuff users: a clinical and histologic follow-up study. J Oral Pathol Med 20: 258–264
30. Kaugars GE, Riley WT, Brandt RB et al 1992 The prevalence of oral lesions in smokeless tobacco users and an evaluation of risk factors. Cancer 70: 2579–2585
31. Cribier B, Garnier C, Lausriat D, Heid E 1994 Lichen planus and hepatitis C virus infection: an epidemiologic study. J Am Acad Dermatol 31: 1070–1072
32. Hietanen J, Pihlman K, Linder E, Reunala T 1987 No evidence of hypersensitivity to dental restorative materials in oral lichen planus. Scand J Dent Res 95: 320–327
33. Laine J, Kalimo K, Forssell H, Happonen R-P 1992 Resolution of oral lichenoid lesions in patients allergic to mercury compounds. Br J Dermatol 126: 10–15
34. Holmstrup P, Thorn JJ, Rindum J, Pindborg JJ 1988 Malignant development of lichen planus-affected oral mucosa. J Oral Pathol Med 17: 219–225
35. Voute ABE, de Jong WFB, Schulten EAJM, Snow GB, van der Waal I 1992 Possible premalignant character of oral lichen planus; the Amsterdam experience. J Oral Pathol Med 21: 326–329
36. Murti PR, Daftary DK, Bhonsle RB, Gupta PC, Mahta FS, Pindborg JJ 1986 Malignant potential of oral lichen planus: observations in 722 patients from India. J Oral Pathol 15: 71–77
37. Sigurgeirsson B, Lindel öf B 1991 Lichen planus and malignancy. An epidemiologic study of 2071 patients and a review of the literature. Arch Dermatol 127: 1684–1688
38. Holmstrup P 1992 The controversy of a premalignant potential of oral lichen planus is over. Oral Surg Oral Med Oral Pathol 73: 704–706

39. Barnard NA, Scully C, Eveson JW, Cunningham S, Porter SR 1993 Oral cancer development in patients with oral lichen planus. Oral Pathol Med 22: 421–424

40. Eisen D, Ellis CN, Duell EA, Griffiths CEM, Voorhees JJ 1990 Effect of topical cyclosporine rinses on oral lichen planus. A double blind analysis. N Engl J Med 323: 290–294

41. Ho VC, Gupta AK, Ellis CN, Nickoloff BJ, Vorrhees JJ 1990 Treatment of severe lichen planus with cyclosporine. J Am Acad Dermatol 22: 64–68

42. Baudet-Pommel M, Janin-Mercier A, Souteyrand P 1991 Sequential immunopathologic study of oral lichen planus treated with tretinoin and etretinate. Oral Surg Oral Med Oral Pathol 71: 197–202

43. Rhodus NL, Johnson DK 1990 The prevalence of oral manifestations of lupus erythematosus. Quintessence Int 21: 461–465

44. Karjalainen TK, Tomich CE 1989 A histopathologic study of oral mucosal lupus erythematosus. Oral Surg Oral Med Oral Pathol 67: 547–554

45. Kramer IRH, El-Labban N, Lee KW 1978 The clinical features and risk of malignant transformation in sublingual keratosis. Br Dent J 144: 171–176

46. Cooke BED 1956 Leukoplakia buccalis and oral epithelial naevi. Br J Dermatol 68: 151–174

47. Pillai R, Balaram P, Reddiar KS 1992 Pathogenesis of oral submucous fibrosis. Relationship to risk factors associated with oral cancer. Cancer 69: 2011–2020

48. Janthi V, Probert CSJ, Sher KS, Mayberry JF 1992 Oral submucosal fibrosis – a preventable disease. Gut 33: 4–6

49. Maher R, Lee AJ, Warnakulasuriya KAAS et al 1994 Role of areca nut in the causation of oral submucous fibrosis: a case-control study in Pakistan. J Oral Pathol Med 23: 65–69

50. Murti PR, Bhonsle RB, Pindborg JJ, Daftary DK, Gupta PC, Mehta FS 1985 Malignant transformation rate in oral submucous fibrosis over a 17-year period. Community Dent Oral Epidemiol 13: 340–341

51. Borle RM, Borle SR 1991 Management of oral submucous fibrosis: a conservative approach. J Oral Maxillofacial Surg 49: 788–791

52. Einhorn J, Wersall J 1967 Incidence of oral carcinoma in patients with leukoplakia of the oral mucosa. Cancer 20: 2184–2193

53. Silverman S, Bhargava R, Mani NJ, Smith LW, Malaowalla AM 1976 Malignant transformation and natural history of oral leukoplakia in 57 518 industrial workers in Gujerat, India. Cancer 38: 1790–1795

54. Silverman S, Gorsky M, Lozada F 1984 Oral leukoplakia and malignant transformation. A follow-up study of 257 patients. Cancer 53: 563–568

55. Mincer, HH, Coleman, SA, Hopkins, KP 1972 Observations on the clinical characteristics of oral lesions showing histologic epithelial dysplasia. Oral Surg 33: 389–399

56. Eveson JW 1983 Oral premalignancy. Cancer Surv 2:403–424

57. Abbey LM, Kaugars GE, Gunsolley JC et al 1995 Interexaminer and intraexaminer reliability in the diagnosis of oral epithelial dysplasia. Oral Surg Oral Med Oral Pathol Oral Radiol Endod 80: 188–191

58. Shibuya H, Amagasa T Seto K-I et al 1986 Leukoplakia-associated multiple carcinomas in patients with tongue carcinoma. Cancer 843–846

59. Lippman SM, Batsakis JG, Toth BT et al 1993 Comparison of low-dose isotretinoin with β-carotene to prevent oral carcinogenesis. N Engl J Med 328: 15–20

Carcinoma of the oral mucosa

33

Squamous cell carcinoma is by far the most common oral mucosal malignant tumor.

EPIDEMIOLOGICAL ASPECTS

Oral cancer is a disease of the elderly, having a peak incidence in the sixth or seventh decades. Overall, mouth cancer is uncommon in the UK compared with other countries. Although there are regional variations, oral cancer is also uncommon in most parts of the world where reliable data are available. The main exception is the Indian subcontinent, where the incidence reaches 40% in some areas, and the mouth is one of the most frequent sites of cancer in any part of the body.

INCIDENCE

In England and Wales, the number of registrations in 1989 (latest available figures) for intraoral cancer was 1494 (or 1843 if oropharyngeal cancer is included) and for cancer of the lip was 237. Together these accounted for less than 1% of all malignant neoplasms.

Incidence rates expressed as annual age-adjusted rates per 100 000 population provide a better basis for comparisons. Where reliable national cancer registries exist, these figures may be used for international comparisons. However, in India, where oral cancer has been reported to account for 40% of all cancers, this does not apply to all areas, and figures for the country as a whole may not be reliable. Within Europe, the incidence varies from approximately 6 per 100 000 in England and Wales to 16.5 per 100 000 in Malta where there is an unusually high incidence of lip cancer, probably due to the strong sunlight. The different incidence rates for rural and metropolitan Poland and Spain are probably similarly explained by exposure of rural workers to sunlight. Binnie et al[1] remarked on the exceptionally high mortality from oral cancer in France, where there appeared to be an association between oral cancer, cirrhosis, and consumption of immature pot-still spirits containing toxic byproducts.

In North America and Canada there appear to be even greater variations in incidence than in Europe. Newfoundland has the highest rate for oral cancer in the Western world. This high incidence may also be due to the high rate of lip cancer amongst fishermen. The chances of a fisherman in Newfoundland developing lip cancer is 4.4 times higher than that for a comparable male in other occupations. In the USA, the incidence of oral cancer varies considerably between states and between whites and blacks. The low incidence of lip cancer amongst blacks may contribute to these differences.

As previously mentioned, figures for Asia are also less reliable due to the absence of national cancer registries. Waterhouse et al[2] quote an incidence of 19.6 per 100 000 for Bombay, but this figure is considerably lower than that quoted in other studies undertaken in different areas of India, such as 33 per 100 000 in Ernakulam. Conspicuous differences in incidence are seen between the various races in Singapore, with the highest rate being in Indians. Although this may be due to tobacco and betel chewing, or submucous fibrosis (see Ch. 32), a genetic factor cannot be excluded.

Age distribution

Oral cancer is largely a disease of the elderly and the incidence rises sharply with age. Seventy-seven per cent of all oral cancers develop between the ages of 55 and 77 years. In Britain the mean age for oral cancer is 64 years for males and 61 years for females.

Gender distribution

Cancer of the mouth is traditionally regarded as a disease predominantly of males. The Registrar General's figures for 1921, for example, showed that the male/female ratio for deaths from mouth cancer was 13:1 in England and Wales. The magnitude of this difference is all the more remarkable if account is taken of the heavy predominance of females in the population as a whole at that time, as a result of the deaths in the 1914–1918 war. However, the 1989 figures for England and Wales show a male/female ratio for cancer of the tongue of no more than 1.7 : 1. Moreover, for most sites within the mouth this ratio is even smaller, but for cancer of the floor of the mouth the male/female ratio is 3 : 1. This change is due to a fall in the incidence of mouth cancer in males since (approximately) 1916–1920, while the incidence in females has declined considerably more slowly.

Evidence for a rising incidence of oral cancer has been produced for several countries, including Britain,[3,4] and the USA.[5] However, Goldberg et al[6] found a fall in the mortality from oral and pharyngeal cancer of no less than 19% in the 15-year period 1973–1987 in the USA as a whole. They considered that improvements in treatment were the probable explanation, as the Surveillance, Epidemiology and End Results Survey (SEER) program had found no change in incidence over this period. However, the SEER program only covered 10% of the population and, unexpectedly, the National Cancer Institute[7] found that the overall survival rates for oral and pharyngeal cancer (unlike cancers in other sites) had not improved for whites and had actually deteriorated for blacks during this period. Goldberg et al[6] in fact concede that the SEER program might have failed to detect a decline in incidence.

Hindle et al[8] noted that the rise in incidence of oral cancer in younger males in Britain was cohort related and affected those born after 1911–1912. The postulated cause was greater alcohol consumption, as tobacco consumption has declined.

The many quoted figures and apparent contradictions are therefore difficult to interpret because of such factors as variation in the area of residence and the precision with which the anatomic subsite is defined. While, for unexplained reasons, there may be a rising incidence of cancer in one particular part of the mouth it may be declining in another. The relative frequency with which these sites are affected then determines the overall effect.

Nevertheless, the lengthening life expectancy, leading to an aging population in many Western countries, must lead to a growing incidence of mouth and other cancers, as these are largely age-related phenomena.

Site distribution

The floor of the mouth, bounded by the lateral and ventral aspects of the tongue and the mandibular alveolar ridge, forms a horseshoe-shaped sump into which any soluble carcinogens could pool. Although this area comprises only 30% of the surface area of the oral cavity, it accounts for 70% of carcinomas.[9] This fact suggests that exogenous carcinogens may operate.

By contrast, cancer is so rare in the center of the dorsum of the tongue and the vault of the palate for cases to be clinical curiosities. Cancer of the center of the dorsum of the tongue is so rare that a retrospective survey of the microscopy of six such cases[10] showed that the histological diagnosis had been incorrect in all of them. Several were granular cell tumors with pseudoepitheliomatous hyperplasia.

Though squamous cell carcinoma of the mouth does not show any significant variation in its histological features in different areas of the mouth, there are differences in behavior and in prognosis according to site. Therefore, the following sites are usually identified:

- lip (vermilion border, ICD 140)
- tongue (ICD 141)
- alveolar ridge or gingival margin (ICD 143)
- floor of the mouth (ICD 144)
- buccal mucosa
- palate.

Table 33.1 Newly registered cases of cancer in England and Wales, 1989*

Cancer type	Sex	No. of cases
All malignant neoplasms	M	117 560
	F	119 669
Malignant neoplasm of lip	M	175
	F	62
Malignant neoplasm of tongue	M	413
	F	247
Malignant neoplasm of major salivary glands	M	171
	F	158
Malignant neoplasm of gum	M	51
	F	58
Malignant neoplasm of floor of mouth	M	216
	F	85
Malignant neoplasm of other and unspecified parts of mouth	M	238
	F	186

*From the Office of Population Censuses and Surveys 1994 Cancer in England & Wales OPCS cancer statistics, registrations 1989. Series MB1, No 22. HMSO, London.

For cancer registration and data collected on a national or international scale, the International Classification of Diseases (ICD) is used, and in Britain at least, only the first four of these sites are considered in terms of incidence and survival. The remaining two sites are categorized as 'Other and unspecified' (ICD 145).

Frequency in different sites

Figures for England and Wales for 1989 registrations are summarized in Table 33.1. It can seen that the tongue is the single most frequently affected site. In women, the lip is one of the least frequently affected sites. The reason for the considerable and persistent difference between men and women in the incidence of cancer of the floor of the mouth is unknown.

Of 589 mouth cancers registered in 1 year at the South Thames Cancer Registry area (covering a population of approximately 6.5 million), 83% of the tongue tumors were squamous cell carcinomas, while for the gum and floor of the mouth and other unspecified sites the figures were 78%, 83%, and 60%, respectively. These figures are slightly low because not all diagnoses were verified histologically.

ETIOLOGY

Much has been written, but relatively little is known for certain, about the etiology of cancer of the mouth or of precancerous conditions. Although the two are discussed together here, it must be emphasized that oral carcinoma developing in an identifiable precancerous lesion is found in only a minority of cases. In a study of the association between leukoplakia and cancer in 77 patients over the period 1935–1948, Bouquot et al[11] found leukoplakia juxtaposed to intraoral carcinoma in 1–9% of cases according to the site, although they found juxtaposition to be more frequent (66%) on the vermilion border of the lip. More puzzling is that, in a study of 212 patients with oral cancer, Hogewind et al[12] found that 48% of them had *separate* white lesions.

Conditions or factors related to or thought to be involved in the etiology of cancer of the mouth include the following:

- tobacco
- alcohol
- areca ('betel') nut
- experimental carcinogens
- industrial hazards:
  – woollen textile work
  – some chemical industries
- infections (possibly with co-carcinogens):
  – syphilis
  – candidosis
  – viruses
- Genetic (specific syndromes):
  – dyskeratosis congenita
  – Fanconi's anemia
  – Bloom's syndrome
- Mucosal or mucocutaneous diseases:
  – iron deficiency (Paterson Kelly syndrome)
  – lichen planus
  – lupus erythematosus
  – oral submucous fibrosis
  – Dysplastic leukoplakias and erythroplakias
- Physical factors:
  – sunlight (lip cancer only).

Race and actinic radiation

Dark-skinned ethnic groups have very low lip cancer rates in comparison with fair-skinned people living in the same areas. Anderson[13] has shown that melanin acts as a protector, either as a physical barrier that blocks the passage of ultraviolet rays, or by the chemical absorption of carcinogens released by ultraviolet radiation. This protective influence of melanin is not confined to blacks. Belamarie[14] reported that among the Chinese in Hong Kong the incidence of lip cancer was only 4% of mouth cancers, in contrast to a figure of 25–30% reported for the Western World.

Dorn & Cutler[15] also showed that the incidence of lip cancer in the USA rose from the north-eastern states to the south-western states in line with the sunnier weather. This finding has been generally confirmed in countries such as America and Australia where immigrant populations with fair complexions are exposed to stronger sunlight than in their country of origin. The protective function of skin pigmentation is suggested by the lower incidence of lip and skin cancer in such countries among the indigenous populations.

In Britain, lip cancer has a higher incidence in Scotland than in England and Wales, and this too may possibly be explained by the higher proportion of fair- and red-haired Scots than English or Welsh. The amount of exposure to sunshine or the degree of

protection from it among outdoor workers is nevertheless difficult to assess. For example, there are many fewer hours of strong sunshine during the year in Britain than in Texas, but in Texas the wearing of an unusually broad brimmed ('ten gallon') hat is traditional. By contrast, Lindquist & Teppo[16] have reported an inverse relationship between the mean annual amount of solar radiation and lip cancer incidence in Finland, but this result is exceptional and unexplained.

In general, therefore, the incidence of lip cancer is greater in rural than in urban populations living in the same geographical area, and outdoor occupations carry a higher risk of developing lip cancer. Sunlight is usually implicated as the causative factor and, microscopically, cancer of the lip is typically associated with a wider area of actinic damage (solar elastosis, cholastic change).

Though genetically determined racial skin pigmentation protects against lip and skin cancer in tropical climates, a genetic factor in some races may confer susceptibility to intraoral cancer. This is suggested by the exceptionally high incidence of oral cancer in the Indian subcontinent. Oral submucous fibrosis contributes to this high incidence to some extent, and a genetic influence is suggested by the high frequency of HLA10, DR3, and DR7.[17] Murti et al[18] reported a malignant transformation rate of 7.6% in 66 patients with oral submucous fibrosis (a disease almost restricted to that subcontinent) observed over a median period of 10 years.

Tobacco use

Pipe smoking Historically, it has been claimed that there is a link between clay pipe smoking and lip cancer. For example, the decline in pipe smoking in Britain has been associated with a steady decline in mouth cancer in males. However, as this habit is now rare in most countries, evidence is lacking to prove or refute this claim. A high incidence of lip cancer in one region of Czechoslovakia has been attributed to a combination of actinic radiation, spicy food, and the use of the tschibuk, a short-stemmed clay pipe.

In Gujarat, India, the hookli, a short-stemmed clay pipe is widely used. Mehta et al[19] noted that 7% of hookli smokers developed labial leukoplakia.

Conventional pipe smoking can also cause a characteristic leukoplakia of the palate but, as discussed earlier (see Ch. 32), any associated carcinoma develops in another part of the mouth.

Cigarette smoking

Unfortunately, few workers have attempted to distinguish between the effects of cigarette smoking and other tobacco habits in the etiology of mouth cancer. Wynder et al[20] and Keller[21] both demonstrated a relationship between cancer of the tongue and of the floor of the mouth cancer and total tobacco smoked. Martinez[22] estimated that, in Puerto Rico, the risk of developing oral cancer was 2.5 to 5 times higher for heavy smokers than for nonsmokers, but no distinction was made between different smoking habits. Graham et al,[23] in the USA, have shown that heavy smokers (more than 20 cigarettes or five cigars daily) are six times more likely to develop oral cancer than are those who do not smoke.

Although cigarette smoking is widely believed to play a major role in the onset of oral cancer, its influence must be limited. In several countries the incidence of oral cancer was declining during the same period that cigarette consumption was rising. In Britain in particular, where detailed and accurate national data are available, the steady increase in cigarette smoking since the beginning of the century was associated with a steady decline in the incidence of mouth cancer in males and no increase in this disease in females, despite the steady increase in cigarette consumption, in the latter.

Moreover, unlike pipe smoking, there is no recognized or consistently found lesion caused by long-term cigarette smoking. Detailed follow-up studies have also shown that malignant change in leukoplakias is more common in nonsmokers than in smokers.

Other smoking habits

Wynder et al[20] have also presented some evidence to link pipe and cigar smoking with oral cancer. Cheroot smoking is a common habit among Danish females, and Pindborg et al[24] have shown that leukoplakia of the floor of the mouth is associated with cheroot smoking.

Reverse smoking, in which cigarettes are smoked with the burning end in the oral cavity, is practised in parts of the Caribbean, South and Central America, India, and Sardinia. In the Indian subcontinent, cancer of the hard palate is common, and this has been linked with the reverse smoking of chuttas. However, in the Caribbean, where a similar habit is practised, there is no link with oral cancer. These differences may be due to variations in the composition or curing method of the tobacco product used.

Bidi smoking, as practised in India, is related to oropharyngeal cancer. A bidi consists of a small amount of Nipani tobacco rolled up in a dried temburni leaf. Hoffman et al[25] have shown that bidi smoke has a higher content of carbon monoxide, ammonia, hydrogen cyanide, phenol, and carcinogenic hydrocarbons than cigarette smoke. Pindborg et al[26] have shown a high incidence of commissural leukoplakia with bidi smoking, and that 16% of bidi smokers had leukoplakia.

Snuff dipping and use of smokeless tobacco

Link et al[27] compared the frequency of oral carcinomas in smokeless tobacco users with those in nonusers. Of 874 patients with squamous cell carcinomas, 1.4% used smokeless tobacco, while of 129 patients with verrucous carcinomas 7.7% were smokeless tobacco users. The numbers at risk from smokeless tobacco use are unknown, but it is noticeable that, as Link et al have confirmed, both squamous cell and verrucous carcinomas far more frequently affect the buccal mucosa, the area in which smokeless tobacco is held. More remarkably, they found that cancers developed later in users than in nonusers. The mean age of smokeless tobacco users developing either type of carcinoma was 70.5 years and of nonusers was 64.2 years. Moreover, the

squamous cell carcinomas in users were, overall, better differentiated than those in nonusers. Any carcinogenic potential for smokeless tobacco therefore appears to be low. Indeed, in Sweden where the use of smokeless tobacco is reputedly heaviest, Larsson et al[28] in reporting the findings from no fewer than 252 biopsies from regular snuff dippers emphasized that over a period of many years they had never seen a carcinoma develop in a pre-existing snuff-dipper's lesion. In short, despite the fact that tobacco-specific carcinogens can be identified, a relatively low proportion of long-term snuff users develop carcinomas. If malignant change develops it is only likely to follow several decades of use.

In the south-eastern states of the USA, lower gingival and alveolar ridge carcinoma is common, and women account for 45% of such cases.[29] This has been linked with the widespread habit among women of snuff dipping over many years. Relatively recently, Skoal Bandits (small permeable paper bags, resembling teabags but containing tobacco) have been introduced.

Betel chewing

There is a high prevalence of oral cancer in India, where betel quid (pan) chewing is widespread, and attempts have been made to link these observations. Support for this hypothesis arises from the greater prevalence of oral cancer:

- among individuals who chew betel quid compared with those who do not
- in the site where betel quid is habitually held[30]
- among individuals who used betel for prolonged periods or particularly frequently.

The composition of the betel quid varies from district to district, but usually contains tobacco, slaked lime, catachu, and areca nut wrapped in a betel leaf. Recent epidemiological surveys have shown that it is only in those areas where tobacco is present in the quid that oral cancer is associated with the habit, although potential carcinogens such as arecoline have been identified in areca nuts.

Jaftarrey & Zaidi[31] have shown that in Pakistan the combination of betel chewing (with tobacco) and smoking enhances the risk of developing oral cancer by 23 times in men and 35 times in women.

Alcohol

Mortality statistics in the UK showed an association between death from oral cancer and occupations in the liquor trade. Others have confirmed the association of excessive alcohol consumption and oral cancer. Wynder et al[32] calculated that heavy drinkers (more than six ounces daily of spirits or equivalent) had a 10 times higher risk of developing oral cancer than occasional drinkers. However, it should be realized that many heavy drinkers are also heavy smokers. It is difficult to separate these risks, and Lemon et al[33] found a low mortality from oral cancer among Seventh Day Adventists, a group who abstain from both alcohol and tobacco. By contrast, Binnie et al[34] noted, in a national survey, that there was a negative association in Britain between overall alcohol consumption and the incidence of oral cancer. Both alcohol and tobacco consumption had grown considerably during the previous 40 years, but during this time the incidence of oral cancer had progressively fallen in Britain. Binnie[35] also noted that any association between alcohol consumption and oral cancer in the USA and France could be related to consumption of un-matured pot-stilled spirits containing toxic byproducts.

Other authors have found an association between cirrhosis and oral cancer. They have suggested that alcohol-induced liver damage helps to initiate or accelerate malignant changes in the oral mucosa. Protzel et al[36] have shown in animal experiments that alcohol may be an etiological factor in oral cancer through a systemic effect, and that other substances which damage the liver can potentiate the action of carcinogens on the oral mucosa.

Infection and immunological factors

Syphilitic leukoplakia holds pride of place as a precancerous disease, in that the suggested rate of malignant change is between 30% and 100%. However, the condition has become so rare that investigation of possible mechanisms has now become impossible.

The role of chronic candidosis is also obscure. The evidence rests on the following facts. (a) *Candida albicans* is an intracellular parasite[37] and that candidal infection induces epithelial hyperplasia experimentally.[38] (b) Chronic candidosis (candidal leukoplakia) is frequently speckled in character clinically, and dysplasia is frequently associated. (c) Cawson[39] found that in randomly selected leukoplakias, in which the microscopic features of chronic candidosis were later found, the incidence of malignant change had been exceptionally high. Finally, (d) cancer developing in cases of chronic candidosis have been reported. The possible role of candidosis in the etiology of oral cancer has been summarized by Cawson & Binnie,[40] but even if chronic candidosis does promote malignant change, it accounts for relatively few cases.

Currently there is active consideration of the oncogenic potential of viruses, and some evidence has been produced to suggest the herpes virus genome or, more recently, human papilloma virus (particularly HPV 16) genomes can be found, incorporated into mouth cancer cells. The importance of this finding is as yet unclear, especially as HPV is found equally frequently in normal mucosa.

There is no evidence of any increased susceptibility to intraoral cancer among patients who are deeply immunosuppressed or who have the acquired immune deficiency syndrome (AIDS). However, the former have high rates of lip cancer if exposed to strong sunshine.

Various immunological abnormalities have been described among 'head and neck cancer' patients, but again their significance is as yet uncertain.

Genetic syndromes and oncogenes

The susceptibility to mouth cancer is significantly increased in dyskeratosis congenita (see Ch. 32). Oral cancer is also a complication of Fanconi's anemia, as discussed below, and is occasionally seen in Bloom's syndrome (telangiectatic erythema with growth retardation). A strain of rat with a high genetic susceptibility to cancer has also been described. However, the low incidence of mouth cancer in the population at large suggests that any genetic component in the etiology is insignificant, although the possibility that it may contribute to the high incidence of the disease in the Indian subcontinent cannot be discounted.

Fanconi's anemia. This is a rare genetic chromosomal defect typically complicated by leukemia in approximately 10% or myelodysplastic syndromes in approximately 5% of cases. Aplastic anemia is another possibility. There is also susceptibility to solid tumors. Oral squamous cell carcinomas developed in 57% of 14 cases of reviewed by Kennedy & Hart.[41] However, in an analysis of more than 950 reported cases, Alter[42] found that solid tumors developed in approximately 5% and that 13 (24%±) of these, 55 neoplasms were in the oral cavity or mandible.

Bone marrow failure usually starts to become apparent before the age of 10 years and most patients die of anemia or leukemia within the next 10 years. In those where the marrow failure is less rapidly progressive, carcinomas appear in the teens and usually before the age of 30 years, but the risk steadily rises with age. Overall, however, tumors develop far earlier in Fanconi's anemia patients than in those without this genetic defect. Females are more frequently affected, in a ratio of 3:1.

Treatment of the oral carcinomas is according to accepted protocols but the life expectancy is short.

Oncogenes and anti-oncogenes

The p53 tumor-suppressor gene may undergo mutation to contribute to the development of cancer. Mutant p53 proteins are stable and their concentration in cancer cells is considerably higher than that of normal p53 protein in non-neoplastic cells. Ogden et al[43] reported that 54% of 20 oral cancers expressed the stable p53 protein, but they failed to identify it in what they termed 'normal', 'benign,' or 'premalignant' mucosa.

Currently there is controversy concerning the detection of p53 protein and its role in carcinogenesis. Thus Piffko et al[44] used a panel of no fewer than four anti-p53 antibodies and assessed the effect on antigen retrieval of pretreatment of sections by micro-waving or wet autoclaving. Without pretreatment none of 22 oral cancers stained positively with Pab 240 and only two stained positively with CM-1, Pab 1801 or DO7. The best results were obtained after wet autoclaving, but even then p53 protein was detected in a maximum of nine of the 22 specimens. It appears, therefore, that the rate of detection of p53 protein overexpression is heavily dependent on technique.

Dental factors

Poor oral hygiene, rough restorations, sharp edges of teeth, and ill-fitting dentures have often been implicated in the etiology of oral cancer, particularly in the past. Indeed, it is uncommon to find a patient with oral cancer with a well-preserved dentition.

However, the incidence of these dental irritants is so high that it is difficult to prove a causal relationship with oral cancer.

Renstrup et al[45] have demonstrated that chronic irritation enhances oral carcinogenesis in experimental animals. Graham et al[46] attempted to assess dental status using a 'dentition index,' and found that a low dental status was associated with a greater risk of oral cancer. They found that men who smoked heavily, drank large quantities of alcohol, and had a poor dentition had an eight-fold higher risk than matched controls.

The well-established improvement in dental health over the years in Britain has also been associated with an overall decline in oral cancer, although, strangely, not in women, who have a record of better dental attendance than men. Also, the lowest socioeconomic groups, who have the lowest standards of dental health, are at highest risk for oral cancer. However, like so much of the data already discussed, any evidence for the role of oral sepsis in the etiology of mouth cancer is circumstantial.

Mucosal disease

The precancerous potential of various mucosal diseases has been discussed in Chapter 32. Of these diseases the only common condition with a small but significant risk of malignant change is lichen planus. There is also a risk of malignant change in the less frequently seen lupus erythematosus and epidermolysis bullosa, but the overall contribution of such diseases to oral cancer must be small. Of other diseases listed, Paterson Kelly syndrome appears to have strong precancerous potential, both in the mouth and the esophagus, but the importance of iron or other hematinic deficiency in this process is unclear. Moreover, the condition has become rare both in Britain and Sweden, and both this and other mucosal diseases, insofar as they may be premalignant, contribute little to the incidence of mouth cancer overall.

MICROSCOPY

Approximately 90% of cancers of the mouth are squamous cell carcinomas, and are usually well differentiated. Characteristic features are the retention of an obvious epidermoid character (sheets of polygonal cells with intercellular bridges) by all but the most peripheral cells of the tumor processes, loss of definition or disappearance of the basal lamina, nuclear pleomorphism and hyperchromatism, deep-cell keratinization, and invasion of normal structures in the path, of the tumor. There is almost invariably an inflammatory reaction (predominantly lympho-plasmacytic) around the tumor margins, and many believe that this represents an immunological response to the disease.

Abnormal keratinization frequently leads to the formation of whorls of keratin (cell nests) within the tumor processes. In addition to deep keratinization, these tumors, in their earlier stages at least, occasionally produce significant amounts of surface keratin, and this can cause them to be mistaken clinically for leukoplakia.

As tissue destruction progresses, the surface usually ulcerates, and the ulcer typically has thickened margins infiltrated by tumor.

In less well-differentiated neoplasms, cell nests are absent, prickle cells become less obvious, and there is increasing atypia. The most obvious features of the latter are the increased nuclear cytoplasmic ratio, so that the tumor may consist largely of closely packed, hyperchromatic nuclei of variable shape and size. However, there is frequently variation in the degree of differentiation from one area of the tumor to another, and this inevitably makes grading (a subjective assessment at best) even more difficult, as discussed later.

Anaplastic carcinomas are rare in the mouth and, by definition, lack features indicative of their epidermoid origin, and prickle cells cannot be identified. These tumors can therefore be difficult to distinguish by light microscopy, from metastases, or even from lymphomas. However, with the use of immunocytochemistry and of epithelial markers, particularly cytokeratins, it is possible to identify epithelial tumors with more certainty.

Examples of these variations in microscopic differentiation are more satisfactorily illustrated than described (Figs 33.1–33.7).

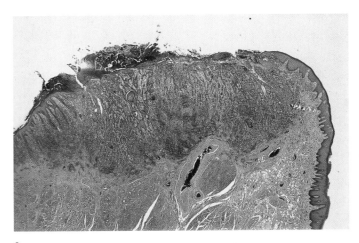

a

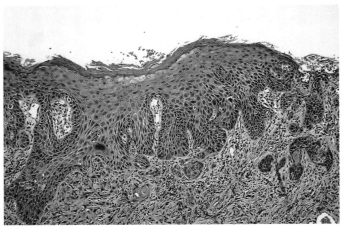

b

Fig. 33.1 a Early, well-differentiated squamous cell carcinoma of the lip. Note, in particular, cell-nest formation and dense inflammatory infiltrate. **b** Higher power view of the same lesion.

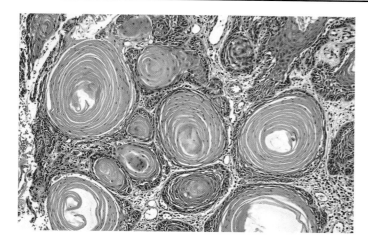

Fig. 33.2 Squamous cell carcinoma. Higher power view to show the formation of cell nests by intraepithelial keratin production.

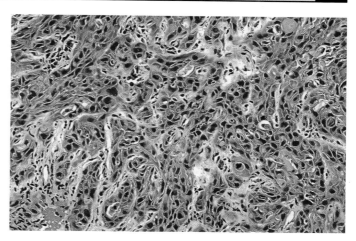

Fig. 33.5 Squamous cell carcinoma. Moderate to poorly differentiated tumor showing widespread nuclear pleomorphism and hyperchromatism, and aberrant mitotic figures.

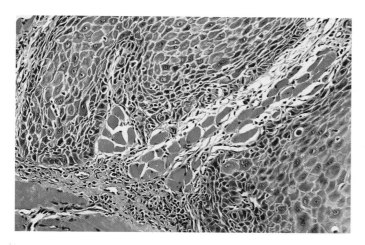

Fig. 33.3 Squamous cell carcinoma. Muscle destruction

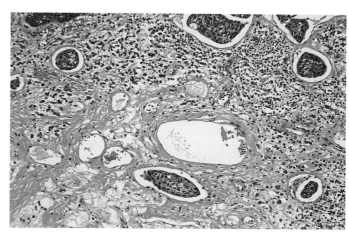

Fig. 33.6 Squamous cell carcinoma. Lymphatic permeation.

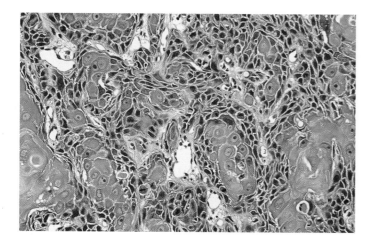

Fig. 33.4 Squamous cell carcinoma. A moderately well-differentiated tumor showing nuclear pleomorphism, mitotic activity, and deep-cell keratinization.

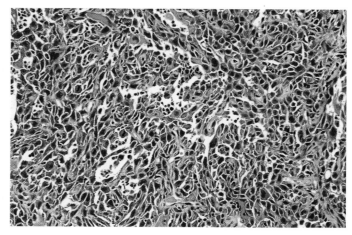

Fig. 33.7 Squamous cell carcinoma. A poorly differentiated tumor with nuclear and cellular pleomorphism, but still retaining obvious squamous characteristics.

SPREAD OF CARCINOMA OF THE MOUTH

The critical feature of carcinomas is their capacity to invade local structures and to spread into the neck through the lymphatics and beyond. Control of the disease in the mouth and neck dominates all aspects of management.

Knowledge of patterns of spread of oral cancer is clearly important if excision is to be complete but within practical limits. Nevertheless, there are obvious difficulties in adequately defining such patterns. It must therefore be appreciated that, despite all the research carried out so far, the following account should be regarded only as a general guide and that cancers can behave unpredictably. It is essential, as described below, to check that resection margins are clear of tumor.

Local spread

Invasion of soft tissues

Mouth cancers often infiltrate widely into adjacent connective tissues. Particularly in the tongue, extensive infiltration beneath intact mucosa is common and very difficult to detect preoperatively. The risk is therefore of encroachment of tumor into resection margins which, of necessity, are often very narrow in the oral cavity. Meticulous frozen section control of all soft tissue margins is therefore essential during resections and, when radiotherapy is used, any such local extension must be taken into consideration when determining the volume of tissue to be treated.

Carcinomas penetrate deeply between and occasionally within the intrinsic muscle bundles of the tongue, but extension through the mylohyoid and hyoglossus muscles in the floor of the mouth is uncommon. In the tongue, infiltration is usually more extensive posteriorly than anteriorly. Tumors arising more posteriorly in the region of the linguotonsillar groove may, however, spread behind the mylohyoid and enter the submandibular space.

These natural soft tissue barriers and pathways become obliterated by previous surgery and/or irradiation, due to progressive fibrosis. Under such circumstances, the extent and direction of local spread becomes unpredictable.

Invasion of perineural spaces

Perineural spread in the head and neck region is particularly characteristic of adenoid cystic carcinomas, but may also be seen with squamous cell carcinomas. Once within perineural spaces, tumor cells can track long distances both distally and proximally. Such centripetal infiltration of tumor along branches of the mandibular nerve (inferior dental, long buccal, or lingual) may lead to direct intracranial extension. For this reason, whenever the mandible is resected for control of carcinoma, the inferior dental bundle should be taken as high as possible. Similarly, whenever a rim resection is being considered, the excised portion of the mandible must include the inferior dental canal.

Invasion of vessels

Intravascular tumor cells are usually seen as small clumps lying either freely in the vessel lumen or within thrombi. Close et al[47] demonstrated a significant correlation between vascular invasion and the incidence of nodal metastases, and extended this work to show a correlation between microvascular invasion and survival from oral and oropharyngeal cancer.[48] The assessment of microvascular invasion in stage determination may therefore be important, and has been discussed earlier. Paradoxically, no consistent association has been established between penetration of the internal jugular vein and the presence of systemic blood-borne metastases.

Invasion of arteries is rare. Infiltrating carcinomas tend to grow around arteries, leaving a distinct periadventitial clear zone. Even in patients with carotid rupture, infiltration of the arterial wall is rare. The main predisposing factors are previous irradiation of the neck, necrosis of skin flaps, infection, and salivary fistulas.

Thrombi containing tumor cells are not seen in lymphatics and neither is direct permeation along the lumen. It is not understood how tumors metastasize from one level of lymph node to the next.

Invasion of bone

The principal mode of access to the facial bones is by direct extension. Invasion is facilitated by anatomical openings such as the inferior dental canal and incisive and palatine foramina. Access of tumor by periosteal lymphatics is probably not important. Despite the dense cortical plates, mandibular invasion is more common than maxillary invasion. This may perhaps be due to persistence of nutrient vessels running vertically and perforating the crest of the alveolar ridge, even in the edentulous mandible. Reference has already been made to the mylohyoid muscle acting as a barrier to deep invasion. This observation that invasion spreads downwards from the alveolar crest indicates that rim resection of the mandible is a sound procedure in selected cases, provided that the resection includes the inferior dental canal and its contents throughout its length.

The mechanism of bone invasion is mainly by induction of host osteoclasts. Direct erosion of bone by tumor cells is only a very late feature. The osteoclasts are stimulated by a combination of osteolytic factors, such as prostaglandins E_2 and F_2 and others such as interleukin-2. These mediators are formed both by the tumor cells and also by host tissues. There is no correlation between the extent of bone destruction or the presence of distant skeletal metastases with hypercalcemia. There is presumptive evidence that such tumors produce humoral calcium-mobilizing factors.

Preoperative assessment of early bone involvement is difficult. Gilbert et al[49] have compared the value of clinical assessment, radiography, and bone scans, and correlated the frequency of mandibular involvement with spread to lymph nodes. A possible reason for the difficulties in assessing the extent of bone involvement is that it is produced in different ways. Lukinmaa et al[50] have shown that oral cancers invade bone either by nonuniform infiltration or on a broad front, and that the extent of infiltration of bone can considerably exceed their superficial dimensions. By contrast, some large tumors with clinical fixation to the mandible may not have invaded bone. There was also no clear correlation between the degree of differentiation and bone invasion.

As to visualizing the extent of bone invasion, Millesi et al[51] correlated the findings of conventional radiography, sonography, computed tomography (CT), magnetic resonance imaging (MRI), and technetium scintigraphy, and concluded that ultrasonography provided the most reliable diagnosis in most areas of the mandible. Bahadur[52] also compared radiography, CT, and isotope scans, but found none of them to be completely reliable and recommended resection of the superior margin of the mandible for all carcinomas close to, even when not visibly involving, the bone. By contrast, Ator et al[53] claim that using T_1 and T_2 sequences on a small group of patients, MRI was the most reliable method of determining the full extent of mandibular marrow invasion and was superior to CT scanning and conventional imaging methods.

Metastases to regional lymph nodes

Clinical assessment of cervical lymph nodes is unreliable. As long ago as 1906, Crile[54] observed that 'palpable glands may be inflammatory and impalpable glands may be carcinomatous.' However, the distribution of nodal metastases from cancers of the mouth and jaws is reasonably predictable. Cancers of the tongue, floor of the mouth, and alveolar ridges metastasize principally to the ipsilateral submandibular, jugulodigastric, and middle deep cervical nodes. Cancers of the retromolar trigone spread to the submandibular, jugulodigastric, and upper and middle deep cervical nodes. The parapharyngeal nodes may also be invaded, but are not accessible to conventional radical neck dissection. Cancers of the lip and tip of the tongue spread to submental and submandibular nodes. Lesions of the tongue, lip, and floor of mouth close to the midline metastasize to nodes on both sides of the neck.

The number of nodes involved is usually small, but extensive involvement of nodes along the entire length of the jugular chain is more frequent with aggressive tongue cancers, which also spread to nodes in the posterior triangle.

Important prognostic factors are multiple involved nodes, metastases in the low cervical nodes and extension of carcinoma beyond the node capsule. The degree of histological differentiation in nodal metastases and in the primary tumor is usually similar, and both are equally sensitive, or resistant, to radiotherapy. Extranodal spread results in infiltration of local muscles, the carotid sheath and its contents, bone, salivary glands, skin, and prevertebral fascia.

BEHAVIOR AND MANAGEMENT

The main options are total excision, radiotherapy, or both. Frequently, oral cancer is treated by surgery combined with radiotherapy ('multimodality therapy'). Surgery is typically preferred

for: small carcinomas, which can be easily excised; carcinomas involving bone, because of the risk of later radionecrosis after radiotherapy; and tumors that have failed to respond or have recurred after radiotherapy. The aim is to excise the carcinoma with as wide a margin as possible, ideally 1 cm or more. Modern surgical methods allow excision, reconstruction, grafting, or by-passing of almost any structure in the oral regions. However, a margin of more than a few millimeters is rarely achieved in practice, because the carcinoma may be too extensive and its margin may be difficult to identify at operation. Also, wider excision may make reconstruction difficult. Such a small margin is insufficient to guarantee removal of the carcinoma, which may recur at the original site.

Dental disease must be dealt with before starting treatment, particularly if irradiation is to be given. Dental infection or extractions may lead to extensive osteomyelitis in irradiated bone because of its poor vascularity, and it is very resistant to treatment.

Irradiation provides more acceptable cosmetic and functional results than major surgery, but causes considerable discomfort during a long course of treatment and has unwanted effects in the long term. These include distressing xerostomia, mucosal and skin atrophy, fibrosis of tissues, and the risk of osteomyelitis (osteoradionecrosis).

Radiotherapy is carried out by implantation of radioactive material into and around the neoplasm (brachytherapy), or by beams of X-rays or γ-rays from X-ray generators or radioactive isotopes such as cobalt-60 (teletherapy).

Reconstructive surgery is normally performed at the same operation as excision, in order to obtain a better cosmetic and functional result.

Recurrence after treatment may be at the primary site or in lymph nodes. Primary-site recurrence usually signifies a poor prognosis because either a full course of radiotherapy or as large an excision as practical will already have been performed. Recurrence in lymph nodes usually appears within 2 years after treatment. The metastases probably arise from microscopic deposits of carcinoma already in the lymph nodes at the time of initial therapy (occult metastases). They may be treated surgically by block dissection or by radiotherapy, and do not necessarily indicate failure of treatment. Block dissection of clinically normal cervical lymph nodes is sometimes performed to remove occult metastases, but this is a controversial procedure.

A recent approach to treatment is photodynamic therapy. In principle, a light sensitizing drug is administered and localizes to the tumor site. Exposure of the tumor to light of an appropriate wavelength triggers a photochemical reaction, which should kill the cancer cells. One problem is to find a drug that allows a sufficiently selective effect, and the method overall requires long-term assessment of its value.

Palliative treatment is given to patients who have advanced tumors or for treatment failures. Radiotherapy is the most practical method for palliative care, but surgery is occasionally used when a large tumor compromises the airway or becomes grossly necrotic. Chemotherapy is little used in the UK, being

Table 33.2 Some factors that adversely affect survival from oral cancer

Delay in treatment
Advanced age
Male gender
Tumor size
Posterior location
Lack of histological differentiation
Lymph node spread

reserved for widespread metastases or salvage therapy. It causes serious complications and may not improve survival.

SURVIVAL FROM ORAL CANCER

Duration of survival after treatment depends on many factors (Table 33.2). In comparison with malignant neoplasms at other body sites, oral carcinoma has a poor prognosis. The quality of life in the terminal stages is also poor.

The poorer survival of older people is probably because they are less able to withstand radiotherapy or surgery. The reason for the poorer survival rates for males is uncertain, although later presentation seems likely. Tumor stage at the start of treatment depends both on its growth rate and on the delay in diagnosis. Some small (early) carcinomas are fast-growing and aggressive, but large tumours, even if slow-growing, are more difficult to manage. In either case, delay in treatment allows further tumor spread and leads to a poorer chance of long survival.

The highest mortality from oral cancer is in the first 2 years. The disease then continues to claim victims, but at a slower rate, and those few that survive for 10 years have a reasonable chance of having been cured. As a guide to survival rates, nearly 90% of males with early-stage disease, survive the first year, about 65% survive for up to 5 years, while just under 55% survive for 10 years. Of males with late-stage disease, well under 45% survive the first year, about 16% survive for 5 years, and 12% survive for 10 years.

As to the site of the growth (see Table 33.1), the extremes are seen in cancer of the lip, where the 5-year survival rate for males is over 77%. For cancer of the tongue the survival rate is 26%, and in the mesopharynx it is only 17.6%. Tumors of the tongue, particularly of the posterior third, are not readily detectable and are more difficult to excise. In general, therefore, the more posterior the tumor is, the poorer the survival. For some sites, particularly when bone is involved, surgery is usually required, whereas for the tongue in particular, where retention of good function is critical, radiotherapy may be preferred. Surgery may, however, be contraindicated because of unsuitability of the patient for anesthesia or because of its mutilating effects. However, if surgery is considered to be the most appropriate form of treatment for a particular patient, it is important that there is a reasonable prospect of cure, the entire tumor can be removed, and the final result will be cosmetically acceptable to the patient. The considerable advances

in reconstructive techniques are important in making the results of extensive surgery tolerable by the patient.

Chemotherapy has its advocates, but many regard it as a treatment of last resort. Despite anecdotal reports of cures, there is not as yet any evidence that chemotherapy, either alone or in combination with surgery and/or radiotherapy, confers any benefit. The toxic effects of chemotherapy itself also confer a significant mortality, and Stell[55] has shown that it actually shortens survival when compared with conventional treatment.

REFERENCES

1. Binnie WH, Cawson RA, Hill GB, Soaper AE 1972 Oral cancer in England and Wales. A national study of morbidity, mortality, curability and related factors. Office of Population Censuses and Surveys. Studies on Medical and Population Subjects No. 23. HMSO, London
2. Waterhouse J, Muir C, Correa P et al (eds) 1976 Cancer incidence in five continents. International Agency for Research on Cancer, Lyon, vol IV
3. Boyle P, Macfarlane GJ, Scully C 1993 Oral cancer: necessity for prevention strategies. Lancet 342: 1129
4. Hindle I, Downer MC, Speight PM 1994 Necessity for prevention strategies for oral cancer. Lancet 343: 178–179
5. Chen J, Eisenberg E, Krutchkoff DJ, Katz RV A 1991 Changing trends in oral cancer in the United States, 1935 1985; a Connecticut study. J Oral Maxillofac Surg 49: 1152–1158
6. Goldberg HI, Lockwood SA, Wyatt SW, Crossett LS 1994 Trends and differentials from cancers of the oral cavity and pharynx in the United States, 1973–1987. Cancer 74: 565–572
7. National Cancer Institute 1990 Cancer Statistics Review, 1973–1987 (NIH publication No. (PHS) 90–2789). US Department of Health and Human Services, Public Health Service, Bethesda, MD
8. Hindle I, Downer MC, Speight PM 1996 The epidemiology of oral cancer. Br J Oral Maxillofac Surg 34: 471–476
9. Moore C, Catlin D 1976 Anatomic origins and locations of cancer. Am J Surg 114: 150–153
10. Ogus HD, Bennett MH 1978–1979 Carcinoma of the dorsum of the tongue: a rarity or misdiagnosis. Br J Oral Surg 16: 115–124
11. Bouquot JE, Weiland LH, Kurland LT 1988 Leukoplakia and carcinoma in situ synchronously associated with invasive oral/pharyngeal carcinoma in Rochester, Minn., 1935–1984. Oral Surg Oral Med Oral Pathol 65: 199–207
12. Hogewind WFC, van der Waal I, van der Kwast, Snow GB 1989 The association of white lesions with oral squamous cell carcinoma. A retrospective study of 212 patients. Int J Oral Maxillofac Surg 18: 163–164
13. Anderson DL 1971 Cause and prevention of lip cancer. J Can Dent Assoc 37: 138–143
14. Belamarie J 1969 Malignant tumours in Chinese. Intl J Cancer 4: 560–564
15. Dorn HF, Cutler SJ 1969 Morbidity from cancer in the United States. (Public Health Monograph No. 56). US Department of Health, Education, and Welfare, Washington, DC, p 1–11
16. Lindqvist C, Teppo L 1978 Epidemiological evaluation of sunlight as a risk factor of lip cancer. Br J Cancer 37: 983–987
17. Caniff JP, Harvey W, Harris M 1986 Oral submucous fibrosis: its pathogenesis and management. Br Dent J 160: 429–434
18. Murti PR, Bhonsle RB, Pindborg JJ, Daftary DK, Gupta PC, Mehta FS 1985 Malignant transformation rate in oral submucous fibrosis over a 17-year period. Community Dent Oral Epidemiol 13: 340–341
19. Mehta FS, Pindborg JJ, Daftary DK et al 1969 Oral leukoplakia among Indian villagers. The association with smoking habits. Br Dent J 127: 73–77
20. Wynder EL, Bross IJ, Feldman RM 1957 A study of the aetiological factors in cancer of the mouth. Cancer 10: 1300–1318
21. Keller AZ 1967 Cirrhosis of the liver, alcoholism and heavy smoking associated with cancer of the mouth and pharynx. Cancer 20: 1015
22. Martinez I 1969 Factors associated with cancer of the oesophagus, mouth and pharynx in Puerto Rico. J Natl Cancer Inst 42: 1069–1073
23. Graham S, Dayal H, Rohrer T 1977 Dentition, diet, tobacco and alcohol in the epidemiology of oral cancer. J Natl Cancer Inst 59: 1611–1621
24. Pindborg JJ, Roed-Petersen B, Renstrup G 1972 Role of smoking in floor of the mouth leukoplakias. J Oral Pathol 1: 22–27
25. Hoffman D, Sanghvi LD, Wynder EL 1974 Comparative chemical analysis of Indian bidi and American cigarette smoke. Intl J Cancer 14: 49–54
26. Pindborg JJ, Kiaer J, Gupta PC et al 1967 Studies in oral leukoplakia, prevalence of leukoplakia among 10 000 persons in Lucknow, India, with special reference to use of tobacco and betel nut. Bull WHO 37: 109–124
27. Link JO, Kaugars GE, Burns JC 1992 Comparison of oral carcinomas in smokeless tobacco users and nonusers. J Oral Maxillofac Surg 50: 452–455

28. Larsson A, Axéll T, Andersson G 1991 Reversibility of snuff dippers' lesion in Swedish moist snuff users: a clinical and histologic study. J Oral Pathol Med 20: 258–264

29. Winn DM, Blot WJ 1985 Second cancer following cancers of the buccal cavity and pharynx in Connecticut, 1935–1982. Natl Cancer Inst Monogr 68: 25–48

30. Hirayama T 1996 An epidemiological study of oral and pharyngeal cancer in central and south-east Asia. Bull WHO 34: 41–47

31. Jaftarey J, Zaidi SHM 1976 Carcinoma of the oral cavity and oropharynx in Karachi (Pakistan). An appraisal. Trop Doct 6: 63–67

32. Wynder EL, Bross IJ, Feldman RM 1957 A study of the etiological factors in cancer of the mouth. Cancer 10: 1300–1323

33. Lemon FR, Walden RT, Woods RW 1964 Cancer of the lung and mouth in Seventh Day Adventists. Preliminary report on a population study. Cancer 17: 486–492

34. Binnie WH, Cawson RA, Hill GB, Soaper A 1972 Oral cancer in England and Wales. A national study of morbidity, mortality, curability and related factors. Office of Population Censuses and Surveys, HMSO, London

35. Binnie WH 1976 Epidemiology and aetiology of oral cancer in Britain. Proc R Soc Med 69: 737–740

36. Protzel M, Giardina AC, Albano EH 1964 The effect of liver imbalance on the development of oral tumours in mice following the application of benzypyrene in tobacco tar. Oral Surg 18: 622–626

37. Cawson RA, Rajasingham KC 1972 Ultrastructural features of the invasive phase of *Candida albicans*. Br J Dermatol 87: 535–543

38. Cawson RA 1973 Induction of epithelial hyperplasia by *Candida albicans*. Br J Dermatol 89: 497–503

39. Cawson RA 1966 Chronic oral candidiasis and leukoplakia. Oral Surg Oral Med Oral Pathol 22: 582–591

40. Cawson RA, Binnie WH 1980 *Candida* leukoplakia and carcinoma: a possible relationship. In Mackenzie I C, Dabelsteen E, Squier C A (eds) Oral premalignancy. Proceedings of the first Dow Symposium). University of Iowa, Iowa, p 59–66

41. Kennedy AW, Hart WR 1982 Multiple squamous cell carcinomas in Fanconi's anaemia. Cancer 50: 811–814

42. Alter BP 1996 Fanconi's anemia and malignancies. Am J Hematol 53: 99–110

43. Ogden GR, Kiddie RA, Lunny DP, Lane DP 1992 Assessment of p53 protein expression in normal, benign and malignant oral mucosa. J Pathol 166: 389–394

44. Piffko J, Bankfalvi A, Ofner D et al 1995 Expression of p53 protein in oral squamous cell carcinomas and adjacent non-tumourous mucosa of the floor of the mouth: an archival immunohistochemical study using wet autoclave pretreatment for antigen retrieval. J Oral Pathol Med 24: 337–342

45. Renstrup G, Smulow JB, Glickman I 1962 Effect of chronic mechanical irritation of chemically-induced carcinogenesis in the hamster cheekpouch. J Am Dent Assoc 64: 770–775

46. Graham S, Dayal H, Rohrer T 1977 Dentition diet, tobacco and alcohol in the epidemiology of oral cancer. J Nat Cancer Inst 59: 1611–1621

47. Close LG, Burns DK, Reisch J, Schaefer SD 1987 Microvascular invasion in cancer of the oral cavity and oropharynx. Arch Laryngol Head Neck Surg 113: 1191–1195

48. Close LG, Brown PM, Vuitch MF, Reisch J, Schaefer SD 1989 Microvascular invasion and survival in cancer of the oral cavity and oropharynx. Arch Laryngol Head Neck Surg 115: 1304–1309

49. Gilbert S, Tzadik A, Leonard G 1986 Mandibular involvement by oral squamous cell carcinoma. Laryngoscope 96: 96–101

50. Lukinmaa P-L, Hietanen J, Söderholm A-L, Lindquist C 1992 The histologic pattern of bone invasion by squamous cell carcinoma of the mandibular region. Br J Oral Maxillofac Surg 30: 1990 2–7

51. Millesi W, Prayer L, Helmer M, Gritzman N 1990 Diagnostic imaging of tumor invasion of the mandible. Intl J Oral Maxillofac Surg 19: 294–298

52. Bahadur S 1990 Mandibular involvement in oral cancer. J Laryngol Otol 104: 968–971

53. Ator GA, Abemayer E, Lufkin RB, Hanafee WN, Ward PH 1990 Evaluation of mandibular tumor invasion with magnetic resonance imaging. Arch Otolaryngol Head Neck Surg 116: 454–459

54. Crile G 1906 Excision of cancer of the head and neck with special reference to the plan of dissection based on 132 operations. J Amer Med Assoc 47: 1780–1784

55. Stell PM 1990 Adjuvant chemotherapy in head and neck cancer. Clin Otolaryngol 15: 193–195 [editorial]

Uncommon types of carcinoma

34

Verrucous carcinoma

This uncommon variant of squamous cell carcinoma characteristically appears as a raised or cauliflower-like white warty lesion, and is less aggressive than the more common squamous cell carcinoma. Elderly males are most commonly affected. In the USA in particular, verrucous carcinoma is typically seen as a consequence of prolonged tobacco chewing or snuff dipping.

MICROSCOPY

Verrucous carcinoma typically has a heavily keratinized, or parakeratinized, irregular clefted surface with parakeratin extending deeply into the clefts. The prickle cell layers show bulbous hyperplasia but, for a considerable time at least, the tumor has a well-defined lower border and basal lamina. Atypia is minimal, and there is usually a subepithelial inflammatory infiltrate (Figs 34.1 and 34.2).

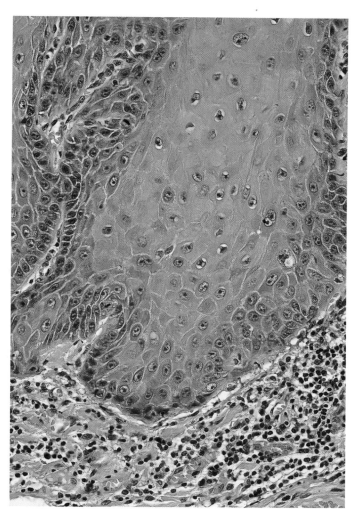

Fig. 34.2 Verrucous carcinoma. Higher power view shows the typical bland cytology.

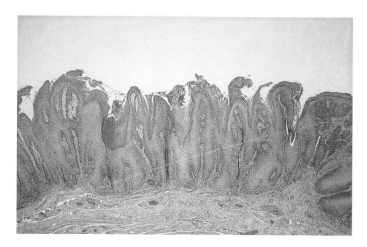

Fig. 34.1 Verrucous carcinoma. There is typical hyperkeratosis, clefting of the epithelium, a well-defined, 'pushing' deep margin, and inflammatory infiltrate.

VERRUCOUS HYPERPLASIA

A distinction has been made between verrucous hyperplasia and verrucous carcinoma.[1] Verrucous hyperplasia is said not to extend more deeply than, or is superficial to, the surrounding normal

241

epithelium. Verrucous carcinoma, by contrast, extends more deeply and pulls down the adjacent normal epithelium at its margins. However, verrucous hyperplasia is said to show dysplasia in the majority of cases, and can develop into verrucous carcinoma or squamous cell carcinoma, and it is widely agreed that the two – if they are indeed separate entities – cannot be reliably distinguished, or may coexist. The distinction does not seem to be of any great significance, even if it can be made, and in practical terms the management is the same.

BEHAVIOR AND TREATMENT

Verrucous carcinoma grows slowly, becomes invasive only later, and metastasizes later still. The regional lymph nodes may be enlarged, but usually as a result of inflammation. Ultimately, if neglected or mismanaged, deeper tissues are invaded and metastases appear.

Wide surgical excision should be curative. Despite earlier claims, it has not been confirmed that radiotherapy induces dedifferentiation and invasive behavior of verrucous carcinomas. However, any individual palpable lymph nodes should be removed, but block dissection is not justified except on the rare occasions when involvement is confirmed histologically.

Keratoacanthoma ('self-healing carcinoma')

Keratoacanthoma is a relatively common lesion of the skin and sometimes of the lips, but rarely affects the oral cavity. Habel et al[2] in a review of intraoral keratoacanthomas, found patients' ages to range from 12 to 80 years, and of 10 reported cases six patients were less than 40 years old. There also appeared to be a strong predilection for males.

CLINICAL FEATURES

Clinically, the lesion appears as a painless cratered nodule. Even more rare is the eruptive variant which lacks the keratin-filled crater and more closely resembles a neoplastic ulcer clinically. Spontaneous regression over a period of 4–6 months leaving a small scar is characteristic, but unusual confidence is required to leave such a lesion untreated.

MICROSCOPY

At low power, keratoacanthoma has a characteristic goblet shape with normal mucosa forming the lips of the cup, and showing an abrupt change to the carcinoma-like epithelium. There is typically, significant epithelial atypia and, despite the absence of deep invasion, there is poor demarcation of the peripheral epithelium from the stroma (Figs 34.3 and 34.4).

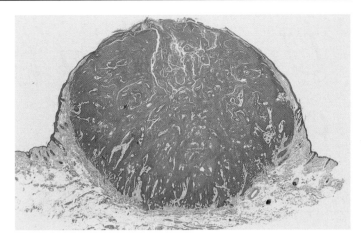

Fig. 34.3 Keratoacanthoma. Low-power view shows the typical goblet shape, the partial epithelial covering and punctum, and well-defined deep margins.

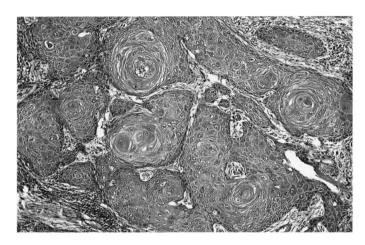

Fig. 34.4 Keratoacanthoma. Higher power view shows the strong resemblance to a squamous cell carcinoma but, in this case, lack of epithelial atypia.

Habel et al,[2] in reporting what may be the first case of an intraoral eruptive keratoacanthoma, confirmed the difficulty of reliably distinguishing the central part of these lesions from a squamous cell carcinoma microscopically. They considered the most distinctive microscopic features to be the elevation of the normal mucosa at the margin of the lesion and the abrupt change to hyperplasia.

In view of possible difficulties in differentiating keratoacanthoma from squamous cell carcinoma histologically, account should also be taken of the clinical features of the former, in particular its more rapid growth, which usually extends over 6–12 weeks, and its more frequent appearance in children or young adults.

Basaloid squamous cell carcinoma

Basaloid squamous cell carcinoma is uncommon. Hellquist et al[3] reported the first case involving the palate and found that approximately 100 cases had been reported since the tumor was first described in the upper aerodigestive tract by Wain et al in 1986.[4] It has a strong predilection for the base of the tongue, hypopharynx, and supraglottic larynx. The floor of the mouth may also be affected.

CLINICAL FEATURES

Clinically, basaloid squamous carcinomas form exophytic tumors without any distinguishing features. However, nodal or distant metastases at the time of presentation have been a frequent finding.

MICROSCOPY

The tumor is bimorphic with co-existence of basaloid cell proliferation and a smaller squamous component. The basaloid cells are moderately pleomorphic and form nests, cords, or cribriform configurations, frequently with palisading. Mitoses and comedo-type necrosis may be frequent. Squamous differentiation, occasionally with keratin pearl formation, is seen within basaloid cell areas. Sometimes there are separate small nodules of frank carcinoma adjacent to the main areas of basaloid cell proliferation (Figs 34.5–34.7).

Continuity with or origin from the overlying mucosa, which is likely to be dysplastic, may be seen. Perineural invasion is a frequent finding. Banks et al[5] described the differential diagnosis from adenoid cystic carcinoma, and the value of negative staining for muscle-specific actin typical of basaloid squamous carcinoma.

BEHAVIOR AND MANAGEMENT

Basaloid squamous carcinoma behaves aggressively. Of the 40 patients described by Banks et al,[5] only 13 were alive without

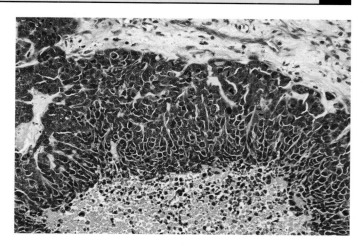

Fig. 34.6 Basaloid squamous cell carcinoma. Higher power view shows darkly staining cells with scanty cytoplasm and mitotic activity with central comedo-like necrosis within the tumor island.

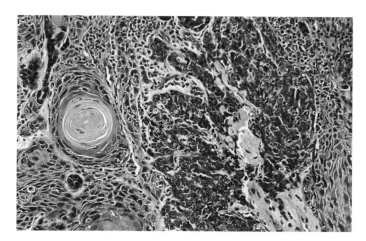

Fig. 34.7 Basaloid squamous cell carcinoma. Higher power view shows basaloid tumor merging with better differentiated squamous cell carcinoma.

evidence of tumor after 1 year. They considered that the relatively advanced stage at presentation was the main factor determining the poor prognosis and that, stage for stage, the behavior and treatment of basaloid squamous carcinoma and squamous cell carcinoma were similar.

Spindle cell carcinoma

Spindle cell carcinomas predominantly affect the upper aerodigestive tract and are rare in the oral cavity. The main diagnostic problem has been its differentiation from mesenchymal tumors. Ellis & Corio[6] were able to present 59 cases and concluded that males were predominantly affected at a mean age of 57 years. The lower lip (42%), tongue (20%), and the alveolar ridge of the gingiva (19%) were the most frequently affected sites.

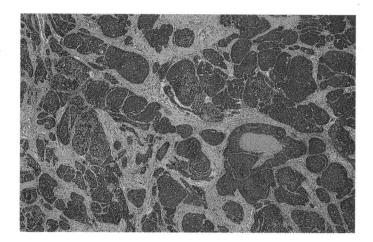

Fig. 34.5 Basaloid squamous cell carcinoma. Low-power view shows islands of small darkly staining epithelial cells.

CLINICAL FEATURES

Clinically, spindle cell carcinoma is unlikely to present anything to differentiate it from squamous cell carcinoma, although tumors in the nasopharynx are mainly polypoid.

MICROSCOPY

The tumor is pleomorphic and sometimes dimorphic, with areas showing transition from recognizable squamous cell carcinoma. In the absence of the latter, differentiation may depend on immunohistochemistry.

Typically, spindle cells dominate the microscopic picture, but sometimes there is transition to more anaplastic cells and occasionally admixture with giant cells. In densely cellular areas, spindle cells may form fascicles. In less densely cellular areas, slender spindle and stellate cells may produce a myxoid appearance. Keratin staining of the spindle cells is positive and Tse et al[7] have shown desmosomal structures by electron microscopy (Figs 34.8–34.10).

BEHAVIOR AND MANAGEMENT

There is no definitive protocol of treatment, due to the paucity of cases. Variations in the histological picture do not appear to be of any value in prognosis. Radical surgery has been found to be the most effective measure, and radiotherapy has been found to be ineffective. Overall, however, growth is typically rapid, and metastases may spread to regional lymph nodes. Ellis & Corio[6] found that of 45 patients on whom follow-up data were available, 55% died from their disease in a mean time of less than 2 years.

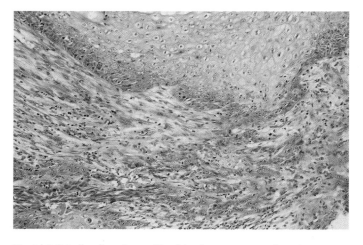

Fig. 34.8 Spindle cell carcinoma. Transition from squamous cell carcinoma to spindle cells.

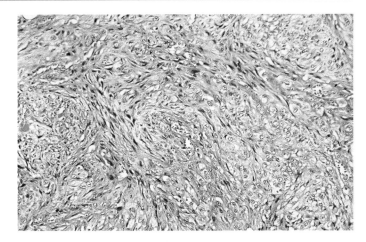

Fig. 34.9 Spindle cell carcinoma. Higher power view shows an almost entirely spindle cell configuration.

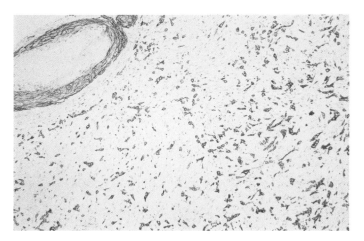

Fig. 34.10 Spindle cell carcinoma. Immunohistochemistry with pancytokeratin monoclonal antibody (MNF 116) confirms the epithelial nature of the spindle cells.

Merkel cell and other neuroendocrine carcinomas

Merkel cells are neuroendocrine cells that have synaptic associations with intraepidermal and dermal nerve endings, but their function is unknown. Merkel cell carcinomas are rare but aggressive tumors, which mainly affect sun-damaged skin in elderly patients (mean age 75 years). Approximately 40% of these tumors arise in the skin of the head and neck region, and most of the remainder in the skin of the limbs. A few cases have been reported in the oral cavity. Vigneswaram et al[8] found reports of 12 oral examples, of which 11 were in males. Consistent with the predilection of the tumors for areas vulnerable to actinic damage, 10 were in the lips. Only one was in the buccal mucosa and one other was in the mucobuccal fold. Another example, reported by Hayter et al,[9] arose just beneath the buccal mucosa in a 73-year-old man.

CLINICAL FEATURES

Clinically, oral Merkel cell carcinomas form small, painless nodules, which grow rapidly, may ulcerate, and may become painful.

MICROSCOPY

Merkel cell carcinomas usually consist of uniform cells with little cytoplasm, but large round basophilic nuclei with one or two small nucleoli and prominent nuclear membranes. When in sheets, these cells have a lymphoma-like appearance. Otherwise they may form trabeculae, whorls, or strands of cells spreading between collagen fibers, and do not initially involve the surface epithelium (Figs 34.11 and 34.12). Intermediate and small cell Merkel cell carcinomas with worse prognoses have also been described. Differentiation from other small cell tumors, particularly metastases, may be difficult. Immunohistochemistry shows a characteristic staining with CAM 5.2 and other low-molecular-

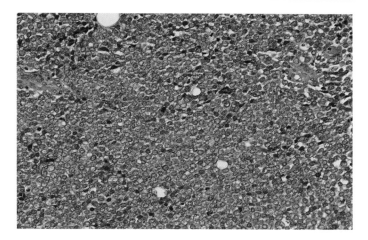

Fig. 34.12 Merkel cell carcinoma. Higher power view shows the densely packed tumor cells with scanty cytoplasm and typical 'watery' nuclei.

weight, but not high-molecular-weight, cytokeratin antibodies. Vigneswaram et al[8] suggest that this type of cytokeratin staining, together with globular paranuclear staining with antibody to neurofilament proteins, is unique to Merkel cells. Approximately 50% of these tumors are also positive for neuron-specific enolase or chromogranin, but in cases of doubt electron microscopy may be required. Ultrastructurally, Merkel cells contain dense membrane-bound neurosecretory granules and paranuclear whorls of intermediate filaments.

Undifferentiated oat cell carcinomas with neuroendocrine features are also rare, and usually are hormonally silent. They have sometimes not been distinguished from Merkel cell carcinomas, and are also highly invasive and aggressive. Yoshida et al[10] have reported an example where the blood sugar fell after treatment.

BEHAVIOR AND MANAGEMENT

Eight of the 12 oral Merkel cell tumors reviewed by Vigneswaram et al[8] metastasized to lymph nodes or distant sites, and three patients died from their tumors within 1–11 months. The periods of follow-up of most of the remaining reported cases were short.

The treatment of choice appears to be wide surgical excision followed by radiotherapy, to which these tumors are sensitive. Prophylactic irradiation of the regional nodes is also advised. Vigneswaram et al[8] quote a recommended dose of 50 Gy in 25 fractions. With this regimen, their patient was disease-free after a year. Complete clinical remission has also been reported with chemotherapy by Wynne et al.[11] Nevertheless, the aggressiveness of these tumors is shown by the report by Hayter et al[9] of a patient who, after surgery and radiotherapy (50 Gy), developed a metastasis and pathological fracture in the upper arm. Despite radiotherapy to the humerus and a course of chemotherapy, multiple metastases were found in many sites after the patient had died from other causes, only 8 months after the initial diagnosis.

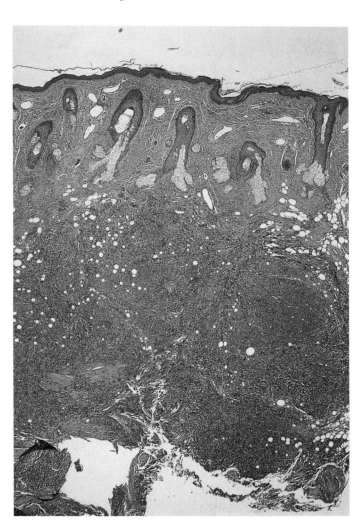

Fig. 34.11 Merkel cell carcinoma of skin. Low-power view shows lobules of small basophilic cells in the typical dermal location.

Adenoid squamous carcinoma

This variant of oral carcinoma is also uncommon. Jones et al[12] reported three examples, and in reviewing the literature found reports of 23 involving the oral cavity. The term 'adenoid squamous carcinoma' is given to squamous cell carcinoma in which gland-like spaces are created by acantholysis in islands of tumor cells. It is a different entity from *adenosquamous carcinoma*, which is composed of both squamous and glandular structures, as discussed below.

CLINICAL FEATURES

Clinically, these carcinomas are as varied in appearance as squamous cell carcinomas, and can be verrucous, ulcerated, nodular, or hyperkeratotic. The lips were most frequently affected (81% of cases), and in particular the lower lip (65% of cases). This finding is consistent with the role of solar keratosis, as with adenoid squamous carcinoma of the skin. Patients' ages ranged from 40 to 75 years, and males heavily predominated.

MICROSCOPY

The infiltrating neoplasm shows transition from squamous to adenoid or ductal structures deeply. Duct-like structures are lined by a single or double layer of atypical cuboidal epithelial cells, which show nuclear pleomorphism, hyperchromatism, and mitotic activity. Acantholytic and dyskeratotic cells may be present in the lumens. With lip tumors, adjacent squamous epithelium may show solar keratosis with acantholysis. Jones et al[12] found two of their three cases to be AE1/AE3 and EMA positive and FVIIIAG negative (Fig. 34.13).

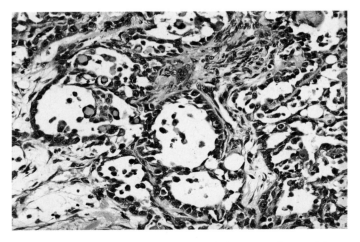

Fig. 34.13 Adenoid squamous carcinoma. Acantholysis gives it the typical duct-like appearance.

BEHAVIOR AND MANAGEMENT

Confirmation of the diagnosis is by biopsy. Lip tumors tend to be recognized early and have a good prognosis if excised entire. Intraoral examples tend to be recognized later and to be aggressive. Of earlier reported intraoral tumors, several patients died from their disease despite radiotherapy, surgery, or chemotherapy. However, too little is known of the behavior of these tumors to make any useful practical comments, except to advise wide excision in the first instance.

Adenosquamous carcinoma

Adenosquamous carcinoma is an exceptionally uncommon oral tumor which has been defined by the World Health Organization as a malignant tumor with histological features of both adeno-carcinoma and squamous cell carcinoma. The glandular and squamous components are in close proximity to one another, but are generally distinct.

Napier et al[13] have reported an adenosquamous carcinoma arising on the maxillary alveolar ridge, and found reports of 58 cases arising in the mouth or tonsillar region.

CLINICAL FEATURES

The patient (a 61-year-old woman) reported by Napier et al[13] presented with a rapidly growing mass, which extended from the maxillary alveolar ridge into the buccal sulcus. It was dark red, fleshy and bled easily.

MICROSCOPY

Adenosquamous carcinoma shows variable proportions of the squamous and glandular components. In the case reported by Napier et al[13] the mucin-producing adenocarcinomatous component formed less than 5% of the bulk of the excision specimen. Immunoperoxidase staining showed the squamous component to be positive for high-molecular-weight keratins (LP34), and negative for both low-molecular-weight keratins (CAM 5.2) and carcinoembryonic antigen, while the reverse was true for the glandular component.

Napier et al[13] point out that there are no criteria for the diagnosis of adenosquamous carcinoma in terms of the quantities of the different components and that some cases may have been misdiagnosed because a small area of glandular tumor had been missed. Buckley et al[14] in their study of carcinoma of the uterine cervix found that what they initially termed 'squamous carcinoma with mucus secretion' had a similar prognosis to adenosquamous carcinomas, in which the glandular component made up at least a third of the tumor. They therefore considered that such a distinction was invalid, and that any squamous carcinoma that showed any trace of mucus secretion should be regarded as an adenosquamous carcinoma (Fig. 34.14).

BEHAVIOR AND MANAGMENT

Unlike its counterparts in the hypopharynx, larynx, and nasal cavities, oral adenosquamous carcinoma is an aggressive tumor with a poor prognosis. Napier et al[13] found that there was adequate follow-up data for only six reported cases. All these tumors metastasized widely, and five patients died from their tumor. In their own case, despite a hemimaxillectomy, a submandibular lymph node metastasis was noted within 4 weeks and the patient died with tumor in the neck 26 weeks after diagnosis and radiotherapy.

Therefore, exceptionally aggressive treatment of oral adenosquamous carcinoma appears to be necessary. The main requirements are probably to carry out as wide a resection as possible, followed by radiotherapy.

Epidermoid carcinoma of salivary glands

Epidermoid carcinoma can very occasionally arise from minor oral salivary glands, forming about 1% of tumors there. Unless its origin can be seen to be from salivary tissue rather than from surface epithelium, such tumors are not likely to be distinguishable from the usual type of squamous cell carcinoma, and indeed the distinction is not likely to be of clinical significance.

Basal cell carcinoma

Basal cell carcinoma is a skin tumor and does not arise in the oral

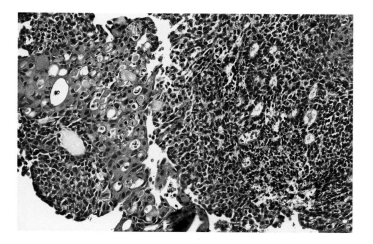

Fig. 34.14 Adenosquamous carcinoma. In contrast with the previous specimen there is ductal differentiation contiguous with typical squamous cells.

mucosa. However, other tumors such as adenoid cystic carcinomas of salivary glands and an occasional variant of ameloblastoma may have a basaloid appearance (see Chs 52 and 3).

Metastases to the oral mucosa

Metastases to the oral mucosa from distant neoplasms are uncommon, but are usually readily distinguished from primary mucosal tumors (see Ch. 55).

Carcinoma of the maxillary antrum

Carcinoma of the antrum is so uncommon that it does not have an individual entry in national cancer statistics; rather, it is included with nose, nasal cavities, middle ear, and other sinuses. All these together account for only about one-third as many cases as cancer of the mouth. Only a few (about 15%) of these rare carcinomas spread through the floor of the antrum to appear as oral tumors.

Microscopically, carcinoma of the antrum is, with rare exceptions, squamous cell carcinoma, often well differentiated and therefore not distinguishable from carcinomas arising from the oral mucosa.

BEHAVIOR AND MANAGEMENT

Confirmation of the diagnosis depends on finding the antral mass and destruction of the antral floor. Wide excision and radiotherapy are the usual lines of treatment.

Juxtaoral organ of Chievitz

The organ of Chievitz is probably a vestigial structure, occasionally found in the tissues on the medial surface of the mandibular ramus close to the site of injection for inferior alveolar nerve blocks. Its importance is the possibility of it being mistaken for a carcinoma.

Danforth & Baughman[15] found 25 examples from 24 stillbirths and adult autopsy material. The appearances varied from nests of squamous cells with intercellular bridges and bordered by basal-type cells, to duct-like with the appearance of secretions. Numerous small myelinated nerve fibers were interspersed among the epithelial nests. The possibility therefore exists of this structure being mistaken for a carcinoma showing perineural invasion. It is not known to be of any importance otherwise (Fig. 34.15).

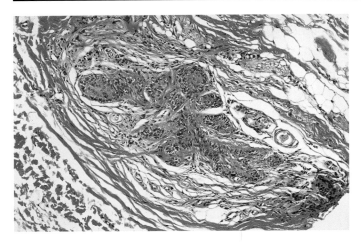

Fig. 34.15 Juxta-oral organ of Chievitz. The lobes of epithelium in a fibrous stroma could readily be mistaken for an epithelial neoplasm.

REFERENCES

1. Shear M, Pindborg JJ 1980 Verrucous hyperplasia of the oral mucosa. Cancer 46: 1855–1862
2. Habel G, O'Regan B, Eissing A, Khoury F, Donath K 1991 Intra-oral keratoacanthoma: and eruptive variant and review of the literature. Br Dent J 170: 336–339
3. Hellquist HB, Dahl F, Karlsson MG, Nilsson C 1994 Basaloid squamous cell carcinoma of the palate. Histopathology 25: 178–180
4. Wain SL, Kier R, Vollmer RT, Bossen EH 1986 Basaloid squamous carcinoma of the tongue, hypopharynx and larynx. Report of 10 cases. Hum Pathol 17: 1158–1166
5. Banks ER, Frierson HF, Mills SE, George E, Zarbo RJ, Swanson PE 1992 Basaloid squamous cell carcinoma of the head and neck. A clinicopathologic and immunohistochemical study of 40 cases. Am J Surg Pathol 16: 939–946
6. Ellis gl, Corio RL 1980 Spindle cell carcinoma of the oral cavity: a clinicopathologic assessment of fifty-nine cases. Oral Surg Oral Med Oral Pathol 50: 523–534
7. Tse JJ, Aughton W, Zirkin RM, Herman GE 1987 Spindle cell carcinoma of oral mucosa: case report with immunoperoxidase and electron microscopic studies. J Oral Maxillofac Surg 45: 267–270
8. Vigneswaram N, Müller S, Lense E, Stacey B, Hewan-Lowe K, Weathers DW 1992 Merkel cell carcinoma of the labial mucosa. An immunohistochemical and ultrastructural study with a review of the literature on Merkel cell carcinomas. Oral Surg Oral Med Oral Pathol 74: 193–200
9. Hayter JP, Jacques K, James KA 1991 Merkel cell tumour of the cheek. J Oral Maxillofac Surg 29: 114–116
10. Yoshida H, Onizawa K, Hirohata H 1995 Neuroendocrine carcinoma of the tongue: report of a case. J Oral Maxillofac Surg 53: 823–827
11. Wynne C, Kearsley J 1988 Merkel cell tumor: a chemosensitive skin cancer. Cancer 62: 28–31
12. Jones AC, Freedman PD, Kerpel SM 1993 Oral adenoid squamous carcinoma: a report of three cases and review of the literature. J Oral Maxillofac Surg 51: 676–681
13. Napier SS, Gormley JS, Newlands C, Ramsay-Baggs P 1995 Adenosquamous carcinoma. A rare neoplasm with an aggressive course. Oral Surg Oral Med Oral Pathol 79: 607–611
14. Buckley CH, Beards CS, Fox H 1988 Pathological prognostic indicators in cervical cancer with particular reference under the age of 40 years. Br J Obstet Gynaecol 95: 47–56
15. Danforth RA, Baughman RA 1979 Chievitz's organ: a potential pitfall in oral cancer diagnosis. Oral Surg Oral Med Oral Pathol 48: 231–236

Mesenchymal tumors

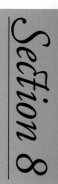

Benign fibrous tumors

35

The vast majority of mesenchymal soft tissue tumors and tumor-like lesions of the oral and perioral region are benign.

Fibromas and fibrous nodules

The current view is that true fibromas of the mouth are exceedingly rare and in any case cannot necessarily be distinguished with certainty from non-neoplastic fibrous hyperplastic lesions. Rarely, fibromas may be confused with neurofibromas or, more important, with well-differentiated fibrosarcomas. From the practical viewpoint, however, the vast majority of fibrous swellings in the mouth are benign. Daley et al[1] retained the term *epulis* for four types of gingival overgrowth. From their analysis of 1298 major epulides they found that fibrous hyperplasias comprised 61%, peripheral ossifying fibromas 22%, pyogenic granulomas 12%, and peripheral giant cell granuloma 5%.

FIBROUS NODULES (EPULIDES, DENTURE-INDUCED HYPERPLASIA, AND OTHERS)

Hyperplastic fibrous nodules are the most common tumor-like swellings in the mouth. They mostly appear to result from low-grade trauma.

CLINICAL FEATURES

Clinically, these lesions all form pinkish nodules, unless the surface has been injured and has ulcerated. Fibrous epulides form on the gingival margin in relation to anterior teeth, denture-induced hyperplasias form under the flanges of dentures ('epulis fissuratum'), or sometimes in the vault of the palate, while fibrous ('fibroepithelial') polyps form on the buccal mucosa, edges of the tongue or other sites.

MICROSCOPY

Fibrous nodules consist of irregularly interlacing bundles of collagenous fibrous tissue in continuity with the corium, and lack any capsule or pseudocapsule. The epithelium is usually mildly acanthotic. The area of an epulis in contact with gingival plaque is usually inflamed. However, nodules related to dentures may show no inflammation unless ulcerated or superficially infected by *Candida albicans*. Bilateral, symmetrical fibrous overgrowths of the maxillary tuberosities, which appear to be a developmental anomaly, are structurally similar.

Dystrophic or metaplastic calcification, osteoid, or bone formation is common, particularly in fibrous epulides, and was seen in 46.5% of 204 fibrous nodules by Zain & Wei.[2] Fibrous epulides containing calcifications of various types are also described by some as *peripheral ossifying fibromas*. Buchner & Hansen,[3] for example, analyzed the histomorphologic spectrum of 207 cases and, in particular, the various patterns of calcification and ossification. Although some of these lesions were sometimes highly cellular and resembled an ossifying fibroma microscopically, they emphasized that these nodules were *not* a counterpart of the endosteal ossifying fibroma, and were reactive in nature (Figs 35.1 and 35.2).

BEHAVIOR AND MANAGEMENT

The growth potential of these lesions is not known for certain, as few are left untreated. However, patients' histories often suggest that some of these lumps can remain stationary for several years. Excision is necessary to confirm the diagnosis and is usually curative, but recurrence can follow, particularly if any irritant such as a badly fitting denture, rough restoration, or calculus has not been removed.

Small denture-induced lesions may sometimes regress if the denture is trimmed adequately, but excision is required to confirm the diagnosis.

NEOPLASTIC EPULIDES

'Epulis' is a useful clinical term defining the site of a lesion, but it has no specific histological connotations. It is important therefore to appreciate that, although most epulides are benign, malignant

251

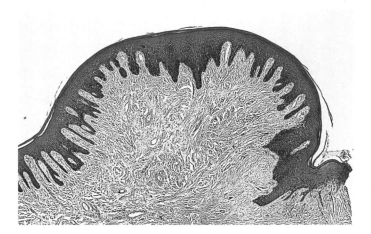

Fig. 35.1 Fibrous polyp. Irregular bundles of fibrous tissue merge with the lamina propria, and the epithelium is mildly hyperplastic.

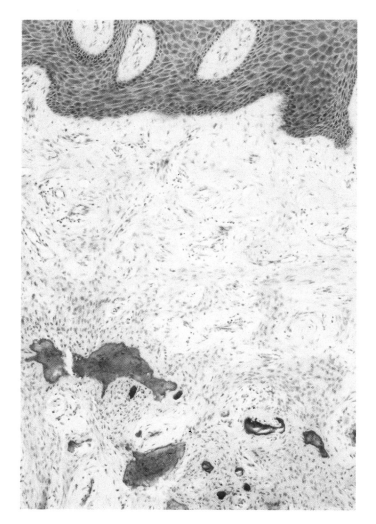

Fig. 35.2 Ossification in a fibrous epulis ('peripheral ossifying fibroma').

(particularly metastatic) tumors can produce lesions clinically mimicking a simple (non-neoplastic) epulis.

Hirshberg et al[4] were able to find 157 reports of metastases to oral soft tissues. The most frequent oral site was the gingiva (54.8%) (see Ch. 55).

CLINICAL FEATURES

Clinically, a gingival deposit resembles a benign hyperplastic lesion, such as a pyogenic granuloma or giant cell epulis, and ulcerates infrequently. In 20%, the oral lesion was the first sign of neoplastic disease.

MICROSCOPY

Metastases resemble the primary tumors histologically, and the majority are therefore adenocarcinomas of various types, usually covered by intact epithelium.

BEHAVIOR AND MANAGEMENT

In most cases, the presence of a distant primary neoplasm is known and it will be clear that the oral lesion is a metastasis. In a minority, where the primary has not been recognized, microscopy may indicate the site of origin. Although this should lead to the discovery of the primary tumor, the fact that it has metastasized usually indicates a poor prognosis. Excision of the oral deposit canot be expected to have any effect on the progress of the disease. A possible exception is that of renal cell carcinoma, where metastases frequently precede symptoms from the primary neoplasm and, rarely, treatment of both the primary and the metastasis have been effective.

Uncommon though these metastases may be, they make it mandatory to biopsy all apparently hyperplastic oral nodules.

Giant cell fibroma

The giant cell fibroma is a common minor histological variant with distinctive microscopic and clinical features. It was first described by Weathers & Callihan,[5] who found them to account for 108 of 2000 oral fibrous nodules.

CLINICAL FEATURES

Huston's review[6] of 464 cases showed that nearly 60% of giant cell fibromas develop in the first three decades, and nearly 60% are in women with an average age of 26 years. The single most common site (50%) is on the lower gingiva; other sites together account almost equally for most of the remainder.

Unlike the more common fibrous lesions, the giant cell fibroma is typically pedunculated. About 60% have a warty or nodular surface and may be mistaken clinically for a papilloma.

MICROSCOPY

The giant cell fibroma has a distinctive pattern of arcuate or sinuous bundles of collagenous connective tissue, which surround but are clearly separated from stellate, rather than multinucleate, giant cells. The nuclei of the giant cells are large and vesicular, while the cytoplasm may have prominent dendritic processes and contain melanin granules. Blood vessels, particularly capillaries, are prominent (Figs 35.3 and 35.4). These features are therefore quite different from the typical giant cell epulis described below.

Ultrastructural studies by Weathers & Campbell[7] suggested that the mononuclear giant cells were atypical fibroblasts, and

that the multinucleate cells formed by fusion of the latter. The giant cells contained numerous intracellular microfibrils, and so the authors postulated a viral origin for these lesions, which had many histological features in common with the virus-induced fibroblastoma of deer.

Odell et al[8] examined the giant cells in 16 giant cell fibromas by immunohistochemistry using a large panel of reagents. All giant cells reacted positively for vimentin and prolyl-4-hydroxylase, indicating a functional fibroblast phenotype.

BEHAVIOR AND MANAGEMENT

The giant cell fibroma is benign and complete excision is curative.

Pyogenic granuloma and pregnancy epulis

Oral pyogenic granulomas usually develop on the gingival margins, and less frequently at other sites. In an analysis of 175 hyperplastic gingival lesions, Anneroth & Sigurdson[9] found that pyogenic granulomas and pregnancy epulides together accounted for 59 cases, and were as frequent as fibrous nodules. They also found that pyogenic granulomas were considerably more frequent in women than men in all age groups, but that pyogenic granulomas in nonpregnant women were slightly more frequent than pregnancy epulides. By contrast, Daley et al[1] found that pregnancy epulides accounted for only 42 of 757 epulides of all types.

CLINICAL FEATURES

Clinically, they form pink or red, soft nodules.

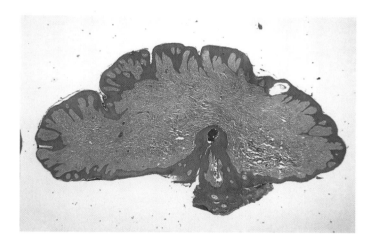

Fig. 35.3 Giant cell fibroma. Low-power view shows the nodular surface.

MICROSCOPY

Pyogenic granulomas consist of a loose edematous and mucinous stroma containing large thin-walled blood vessels, and are typically infiltrated throughout by leucocytes. However, inflammatory infiltration is not invariable, and the vascular nature of the lesion becomes obvious. The blood vessels are so numerous that the alternative term for cutaneous pyogenic granulomas is *granuloma telangiectaticum*, and Enzinger & Weiss[10] categorize them as polypoid capillary hemangiomas. Regezi et al[11] found that mitotic activity and nuclear atypia in pyogenic granulomas was as frequent as in extensive Kaposi's sarcomas in those infected with the human immunodeficiency virus (HIV). The thin epithelial covering is frequently ulcerated, and there is then a more intense inflammatory infiltrate and fibrinous exudate on the surface (Figs 35.5–35.7).

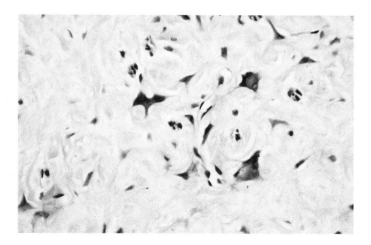

Fig. 35.4 Giant cell fibroma. Higher power view shows the angular giant cells with only a few vesiculated nuclei in a stroma of short, tangled collagenous fibers.

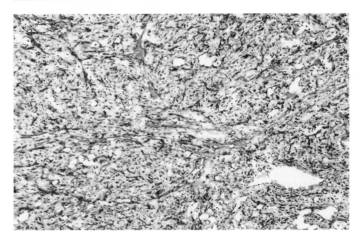

Fig. 35.5 Pyogenic granuloma/pregnancy epulis. In the absence of superimposed inflammation the lesion can be seen to consist largely of thin-walled blood vessels of varying size and strands of endothelial cells.

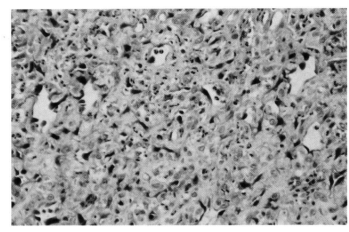

Fig. 35.7 Pyogenic granuloma/pregnancy epulis. Higher power view shows an unusual degree of pleomorphism and hyperchromatism of the endothelial cells, but this does not indicate malignancy.

There is no evidence to suggest that pyogenic granulomas are a stage in the development of fibrous nodules or are merely inflamed fibrous nodules; rather, they are vascular proliferations.

BEHAVIOR AND MANAGEMENT

Excision is typically curative.

Pregnancy epulis

The so-called 'pregnancy epulis' is indistinguishable clinically and histologically from a pyogenic granuloma. However, there is an enhanced tendency to develop a proliferative gingivitis and gingival pyogenic granulomas during pregnancy. Like pyogenic granulomas in nonpregnant women, inflammation may be minimal or absent, but vascular proliferation is occasionally so active as to suggest a neoplasm. Nevertheless, the behavior is benign.

BEHAVIOR AND MANAGEMENT

Gingival hyperplasia of pregnancy should be treated by meticulous oral hygiene. A pregnancy epulis persisting after parturition should be excised. As these lesions are often a cause of anxiety to the pregnant patient, it may be necessary to excise them during pregnancy if reassurance fails.

Peripheral odontogenic fibroma

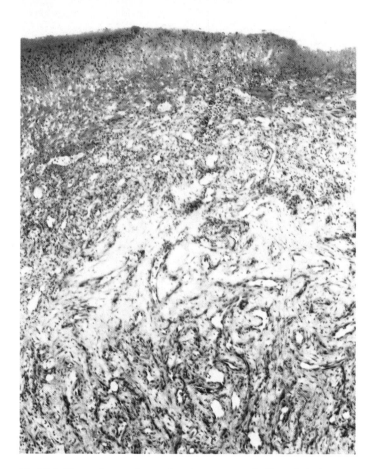

Fig. 35.6 Ulcerated pyogenic granuloma/pregnancy epulis. Beneath the lost area of epithelium there is a concentrated but localized inflammatory infiltrate. Deeply, the lesion shows its essential vascular character.

Although clinically indistinguishable from the common fibrous oral nodules, the peripheral odontogenic fibroma is a distinct entity, with the same histological features as the central type (see Ch. 10).

Ossifying fibromyxoid tumor

Ossifying fibromyxoid tumor was first described by Enzinger et al in 1989.[12] It usually forms a painless, slowly growing sub-cutaneous mass in the limbs or limb girdles in adults. In the cases reviewed by Enzinger et al,[12] patients were predominantly males. Williams et al[13] have described nine cases in the head and neck region in patients aged between 29 and 75 years. Two of these nine tumors were beneath the gingival and palatal mucosae. Williams et al[14] reported a further case in the parotid region.

MICROSCOPY

Goodlad & Fletcher[15] suggest that the microscopic appearances of ossifying fibromyxoid tumor give an initial impression of a myoepithelial or salivary gland tumor. There is a dense hyaline pseudocapsule through which tumor may occasionally extend. The capsule usually contains lamellar bone, either scanty in amount or so extensive as to form a complete shell. Within the capsule, the tumor typically consists of lobules, but sometimes strands or whorls of uniform, rounded or spindle-shaped cells with indistinct or pale eosinophilic cytoplasm and vesiculated nuclei. The stroma is myxoid or sometimes hyaline, and contains thin-walled branching vessels or sometimes fibrous septa. These extend inwards from the capsule and may also show ossification.

Goodlad & Fletcher[15] found that the tumor cells were usually S-100 protein positive, desmin positive in 70%, and focally actin positive in 50%. GFAP was occasionally positive, but cytokeratins hardly ever so. Goodland & Fletcher[15] noted that rare cases showed cytological features of malignancy, but were uncertain whether these were in fact malignant ossifying fibromyxoid tumors, unusual malignant schwannomas, or extraosseous osteosarcomas.

BEHAVIOR AND MANAGEMENT

Ossifying fibromyxoid tumor usually appears to be benign, but undoubtedly has a propensity for recurrence. One of the tumors reported by Williams et al[13] that had been categorized as a malignant ossifying fibromyxoid tumor underwent multiple local recurrences, while the later tumor reported by Williams et al[14] recurred three times over a period of 24 years. Goodlad & Fletcher[15] noted that a single example of ossifying fibromyxoid tumor had metastasized. The ability of the tumor to extend through the capsule is probably the main factor leading to recurrence after excision, which therefore should be wide.

Focal mucinosis

This rare myxoid lesion is considered to be the oral counterpart of cutaneous focal mucinosis. It was first described in the mouth by Tomich,[16] and Saito et al[17] presented two further cases.

Oral focal mucinosis is non-neoplastic, of unknown etiology, and may be the result of overproduction of hyaluronic acid by fibroblasts at the expense of collagen production.

CLINICAL FEATURES

Clinically, these asymptomatic nodular swellings are commonly mistaken for fibromas or mucoceles. Although this lesion has been found in various oral sites, there is a predilection for the mucosa overlying bone. The cases reported by Saito et al[17] formed epulis-like gingival swellings.

MICROSCOPY

Focal mucinosis consists of a well-circumscribed collection of myxomatous connective tissue which is sharply delimited by fibrous connective tissue on its lateral and deep margins. The myxomatous zone may extend directly to the covering epithelium, or may be separated from it by a thin band of fibrous tissue (Fig 35.8).

In contrast to myxomas, reticulin fibers (apart from those associated with the few blood vessels) are absent throughout, and the myxoid tissue does not infiltrate the surrounding tissues.

BEHAVIOR AND MANAGEMENT

Local surgical excision is adequate and recurrence is unlikely.

Nasopharyngeal (juvenile) angiofibroma

Enzinger & Weiss[10] consider it debatable whether this tumor should be classified as fibrous or vascular. Although they include it among the fibrous tumors because of the predominance of the fibrous component, in practice it has to be treated as a vascular tumor because of the risk of severe hemorrhage. It is therefore discussed with other vascular tumors (see Ch. 42).

Spindle cell and pseudomesenchymal tumors of salivary glands

Occasionally pleomorphic adenomas consist predominantly of spindle (myoepithelial) cells (see Ch. 51). Rarely, malignant

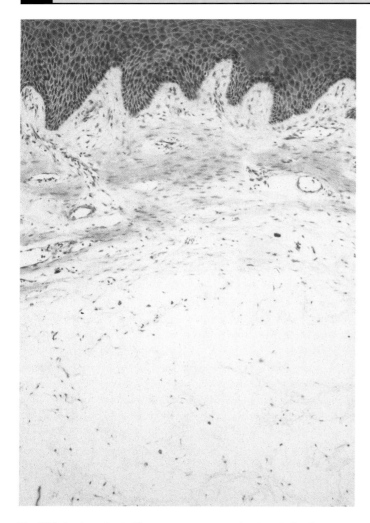

Fig. 35.8 Focal mucinosis. The myxomatous connective tissue is sharply circumscribed and separated from the covering epithelium by a thin band of fibrous tissue.

myoepithelial tumors (malignant myoepitheloma, myoepithelial carcinoma) can have a sarcomatous appearance (see Ch. 52). Differential diagnosis from true mesenchymal tumors of salivary glands may depend on finding recognizable epithelial elements but, if this fails, the myoepithelial cells should be identifiable by immunostaining for S-100 protein, keratin, actin, and vimentin.

Chondromyxoid fibroma

This tumor is discussed with the cartilaginous tumors (see Ch. 28) because of the problem of differential diagnosis from chondrosarcoma.

REFERENCES

1. Daley TD, Wysocki GP, Wysocki PD, Wysocki DM 1990 The major epulides: clinicopathological correlations. J Canad Dent Assoc 56: 627–630
2. Zain RB, Fei YJ 1990 Fibrous lesions of the gingiva: a histopathologic analysis of 204 cases. Oral Surg Oral Med Oral Pathol 70: 466–470
3. Buchner A, Hansen LS 1987 The histomorphologic spectrum of peripheral ossifying fibroma. Oral Surg Oral Med Oral Pathol 63: 452–461
4. Hirshberg A, Leibovich P, Buchner A 1993 Metastases to the oral mucosa: analysis of 157 cases. J Oral Pathol Med 22: 385–390
5. Weathers DR, Callihan MD 1974 Giant cell fibroma. Oral Surg Oral Med Oral Pathol 37: 374–384
6. Houston GD 1982 The giant cell fibroma. A review of 464 cases. Oral Surg 53: 582–587
7. Weathers DR, Campbell WG 1974 Ultrastructure of the giant cell fibroma of the oral mucosa. Oral Surg Oral Med Oral Pathol 38: 550–556
8. Odell E, Lock C, Lombardi T 1994 Phenotypic characterisation of stellate and giant cells in giant cell fibroma by immunocytochemistry. Oral Pathol Med 23: 284–287
9. Anneroth G, Sigurdson A 1983 Hyperplastic lesions of the gingiva and alveolar mucosa. A study of 175 cases. Acta Odontol Scand 41: 75–86
10. Enzinger FM, Weiss SW 1995 Soft tissue tumors, 3rd edn. C V Mosby, St Louis
11. Regezi JA, MacPhail LA, Daniels TE et al 1993 Oral Kaposi's sarcoma: a 10-year retrospective histopathologic study. J Oral Pathol Med 11: 292–297
12. Enzinger FM, Weiss SW, Liang CY 1989 Ossifying fibromyxoid tumour of soft parts. A clinicopathologic analysis of 59 cases. Am J Surg Pathol 13: 817–827
13. Williams SB, Ellis Gl, Meis JM, Heffner DK 1993 Ossifying fibromyxoid tumour (of soft parts) of the head and neck region: a clinicopathological and immunohistochemical study of nine cases. J Laryngol Otol 107: 75–80
14. Williams RW, Case CP, Irvine GH 1994 Ossifying fibromyxoid tumour of soft parts – a new tumour of the parotid/zygomatic arch region. Br J Oral Maxillofac Surg 32: 174–177
15. Goodlad JR, Fletcher CDM 1995 Recent developments in soft tissue tumours. Histopathology 27: 103–120
16. Tomich CE 1974 Oral focal mucinosis. Oral Surg 38: 714–718
17. Saito I, Ide F, Enomoto T, Kudo I 1985 Oral focal mucinosis. J Oral Maxillofac Surg 43: 372–374

Fibromatoses and fasciites 36

Fibromatoses

Fibromatoses are proliferative lesions of connective tissue that infiltrate surrounding tissues, have a strong tendency to recur, but are non-neoplastic and do not metastasize. Nothing certain is known of their etiology, and they do not appear to be reactive.

INCIDENCE

The more common superficial fibromatoses, such as Dupuytren's contracture or Peyronie's disease, have specific site distributions, while the deep fibromatoses (desmoids) affect the abdomen, particularly after childbirth. The extra-abdominal fibromatoses far more frequently involve the limbs or chest wall, and an analysis by Enzinger & Weiss[1] of 376 extra-abdominal fibromatoses (seen over a period of 20 years) found only seven (2%) involving the head region.

Overall, fibromatoses mainly affect adults, but oral and perioral fibromatoses, although uncommon, most frequently appear between the ages of 0 and 9 years.

Valli & Altini[2] found reports of 28 cases in the oral or perioral tissues. They added three new examples and nine new cases of the intraosseous counterpart, desmoplastic fibroma of the jaws, and retrieved 51 earlier reports.

Of 27 oral or perioral fibromatoses, Valli & Altini[2] confirmed that the majority (16) developed within the first 9 years of life, eight appeared between the ages of 10 and 19 years, and only three between the ages of 20 and 29 years. The mean age at diagnosis was 8 years.

CLINICAL FEATURES

Fibromatoses typically form relatively slow-growing, usually painless, poorly circumscribed, tumor-like masses. They may be entirely within soft tissue, such as muscle, or be periosteal and cause bone erosion. Later, if the growth has involved nerve fibers, it can cause pain. Rarely, fibromatoses can be multifocal.

The most common site was in the paramandibular region. In addition to those few arising within the mouth, fibromatoses originating in the neck can spread to the jaw or floor of the mouth.

MICROSCOPY

Fibromatoses consist of proliferating fibrous tissue, which ranges in appearance from mature fibrous tissue with abundant collagen to highly cellular tissue consisting of tumor-like fibroblasts alone. The collagen fibers in the more fibrous specimens tend to form short bundles, which lack the streaming patterns of and are less well defined than those of fibrosarcomas. These appearances can vary between one specimen and another and also within a single specimen (Fig. 36.1).

The fibroblast nuclei may contain two or three nucleoli, but tend to be small and uniform in size. A few mitoses may be seen in the more cellular areas, but are never atypical. Within the fibrous tissue, the blood vessels often form slit- or cleft-like spaces. Inflammation is typically slight or absent, but when present is due to superimposed infection and can alter the microscopic appearances.

Particularly characteristic of these lesions is their tumor-like infiltration of surrounding tissues, including, occasionally, bone

Fig. 36.1 Fibromatosis. In this moderately cellular example the fibroblasts have uniform-sized nuclei and form ill-defined interweaving strands.

and envelopment of nerve and muscle fibers. Despite this property and the cellular appearances, fibromatoses do not metastasize. The current belief is that previously reported metastases were of fibrosarcomas rather than fibromatoses. Evidence for the value of microscopy for predicting behavior is conflicting.

In children, fibroblastic proliferation may be more active; fibromatoses may therefore appear even more alarming microscopically than in adults, and be interpreted as sarcomas (Fig. 36.2).

In an attempt to distinguish fibromatosis and fasciitis from fibrosarcoma, Oshiro et al[3] used proliferating cell nuclear antigen (PCNA), DNA flow cytometry, and p53 positivity. They found that fibrosarcoma was more likely to show aneuploidy, abnormal p53 expression and a high proliferative index. Nodular fasciitis and fibromatosis showed neither aneuploidy nor abnormal p53 expression, and had a lower proliferative index than the majority of fibrosarcomas. Nevertheless, 26% of fibrosarcomas were not aneuploid, a similar number showed no abnormal p53 expression, and 14 of 19 were both p53 negative and had a low proliferative index. The results were not therefore clear-cut, but p53 positivity was probably indicative of a poor prognosis.

BEHAVIOR AND MANAGEMENT

Surgical control of fibromatoses in the oral or perioral area is difficult because of their close proximity to vital structures, their infiltrative nature and the limited room for maneuver.

The current consensus is that the treatment should be by as wide an excision as possible, but as fibromatoses are not truly malignant, mutilating operations should be avoided. Recurrence rates may range from 25% to 65%, depending on the aggressiveness of the lesion and the completeness of excision, but the recurrence rate for oral and perioral fibromatoses appears to be lower than for those in other sites. Although there was superficial erosion of the underlying bone of the jaw in 16 of the 29 cases reported by Valli & Altini,[2] all showed similar histological features. These workers considered that there was no valid distinction

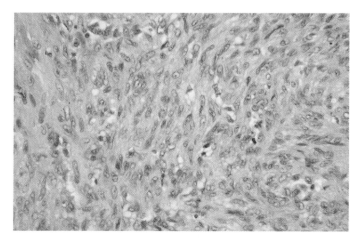

Fig. 36.2 Infantile fibromatosis. High-power view shows actively proliferating fibroblasts with vesiculated nuclei in a fine fibrous stroma.

between the so-called adult and infantile aggressive types of fibromatoses. Overall, they found a recurrence rate of 22%, and Fowler et al[4] from a study of 31 oral and paroral cases confirmed these findings and a recurrence rate of 23.8%. Nevertheless, in many sites infantile fibromatoses have, overall, less tendency to recur, despite more aggressive histologic appearances, and may rarely regress spontaneously. Thus, Hoffman et al[5] reported, in a 2-year-old boy, aggressive infantile fibromatosis which underwent spontaneous regression over a 3-year period, and noted reports of earlier cases where lesions had remained static or regressed after incomplete resection. None of the reported oral lesions metastasized or (unlike fibromatoses in other sites) had a fatal outcome, despite their proximity to vital structures.

In view of the limited opportunities for total excision of oral or perioral fibromatoses, the likelihood of recurrence must be accepted. A possible alternative to such treatment, suggested by Hoffman et al,[5] is to take advantage of possible spontaneous regression. They advocated noninterventional treatment in cases where

- pain and functional disturbance were absent, but resection would have to be extensive and would require reconstruction
- local infiltration posed no danger to the patient
- absence of malignancy was unequivocally confirmed histologically
- there was no doubt about the availability of the patient for regular long-term follow-up.

If this choice is made, follow-up must be close and the patient seen monthly during the active phase of the disease. Radiographs or, preferably, computed tomography scans or magnetic resonance imaging should be done every 3 months until regression becomes apparent. Once the lesion becomes static, examination can be at 6-month intervals, but the possibility of recurrence after 5 years or more must be taken into account.

The value of megavoltage irradiation has not been widely confirmed and, as always with such treatment, there is the risk of inducing malignant change.

In all cases, prolonged follow-up is necessary. Rarely, recurrences have appeared as long as 10 years after initial treatment. Therefore, it may be unwise to interpret treatment as being curative unless there has been a long disease-free period.

DESMOPLASTIC FIBROMA

Desmoplastic fibroma of the jaw is another form of fibromatosis.

INCIDENCE

Approximately 75% of patients are below the age of 30 years, and 50% are between the ages of 10 and 20 years. The mandible, usually at the junction between the ramus and body, is the most common site in the head and neck region. Donohue et al[6] reported a case involving the maxilla and noted 73 earlier cases involving the jaws. Of these, 13 were in the maxilla. Of 49 reported lesions in the jaws reviewed by Hashimoto et al,[7] only six were in the maxilla.

CLINICAL FEATURES

The main manifestation is gradual expansion of the jaw, but occasionally there is aching pain. Unusually, the palatal lesion reported by Donohue et al[6] fungated through the mucosa after the first biopsy.

RADIOGRAPHY

Desmoplastic fibroma gives rise to an area of radiolucency that is usually well circumscribed and may be multilocular with a honeycomb or trabeculated appearance, or, less frequently, unilocular. Roots of related teeth may be resorbed and, rarely, the margins suggest infiltration of the surrounding bone. The margins are therefore less well circumscribed than suggested by the radiographic appearances, and merge with the surrounding bone histologically.

MICROSCOPY

The main microscopic features of fibromatosis have been described in the previous section. As mentioned, strong p53 reactivity may indicate a poor prognosis.

BEHAVIOR AND MANAGEMENT

Desmoplastic fibroma is aggressive and progressive but, as mentioned earlier, does not metastasize. It must be distinguished histologically from myofibromatosis, which is less aggressive and more amenable to treatment. Myofibromatosis can be distinguished by the slightly different microscopic appearances (see below) and the staining of the cells for smooth muscle actin. Fibromatosis must also be distinguished from fibrosarcoma, which is both more destructive locally and can metastasize. However, differentiation of highly cellular fibromatosis from low-grade fibrosarcoma may be more difficult, and some believe there to be a continuous spectrum of appearances between the two.

Because of its infiltrative character, curettage or local excision of desmoplastic fibroma may be followed by recurrence in up to 30% of cases. Neither microscopic findings nor site are predictive of recurrence. Of 12 cases in the maxilla reviewed by Donohue et al,[6] three recurred after excision. By contrast, two cases in infants, reported by Carr et al,[8] were initially aggressive but underwent spontaneous regression after incomplete excision.

Excision with an adequate margin of normal bone is generally regarded as the treatment of choice. Wider excision is necessary for lesions that have extended into the soft tissues. Mutilating

surgery is not justified, as any recurrences are purely local and can be controlled when they appear. As for soft tissue fibromatoses, the possibility of spontaneous regression should not be dismissed, and an expectant policy may be justified under certain circumstances.

Malignant change has been reported after radiotherapy, which is therefore contraindicated.

MYOFIBROMATOSIS

This uncommon lesion was termed *infantile myofibromatosis* by Chung & Enzinger,[9] but can also affect adults. Speight et al[10] have described three oral cases (one in an adult), together with the immunohistochemical and ultrastructural findings, and reviewed reports of oral and perioral cases. Jones et al[11] reported 13 cases, of which three were in the jaws, and also reviewed the literature.

CLINICAL FEATURES

Myofibromatosis is usually solitary. It can occasionally be multifocal and may be fatal by involving vital structures. Solitary lesions in the oral cavity typically consist of firm, painless lumps of a few weeks or months duration. Infants and children are predominantly, but not exclusively, affected.

MICROSCOPY

Myofibromatosis is biphasic and consists of spindle and round cells. The configurations include spindle cells with eosinophilic cytoplasm and long, blunt-ended nuclei, arranged either in diffuse sheets or in streaming, fascicular patterns, sometimes interlacing or in whorls. Small cells are rounded or polygonal and have large nuclei relative to the amount of cytoplasm, which is weakly eosinophilic. The small cells form foci in areas of spindle cells, but elsewhere can be close packed and surround slit-like or dilated blood vessels to give an hemangiopericytoma-like appearance. There are occasional normal mitoses (Figs 36.3–36.5).

Speight et al[10] noted myofibromatous cells within the lumen of veins and degenerating or reactive muscle fibers within the lesion, as a result of infiltration of adjacent tissue. Nevertheless, infiltration is typically limited and localized. They also noted that many of the cells were PTAH positive, and some showed conspicuous longitudinal striation. Immunohistochemistry showed the cells to be positive for vimentin and smooth muscle actin, but S-100 and desmin negative. The ultrastructural features were also typical of myofibroblasts.

The varied appearances have in the past led to misdiagnoses of myofibromatosis as neural tumors, leiomyomas, leiomyosarcomas, or hemangiopericytomas. Myofibromatosis can also be mistaken for fibromatosis. However, as summarized by Speight et al,[10] fibromatosis is more frequently intramuscular and more aggressively infiltrative. In addition, it does not produce the

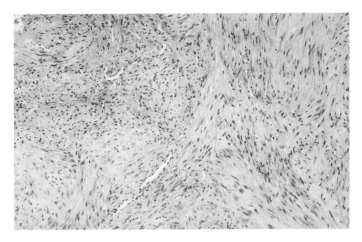

Fig. 36.3 Myofibromatosis. Low-power view shows ill-defined fascicles of spindle cells interspersed with small cells.

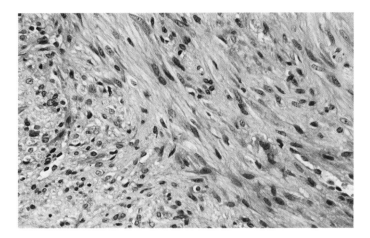

Fig. 36.4 Myofibromatosis. Higher power shows the eosinophilic staining of the cytoplasm of the spindle cells with eosinophilic cytoplasm and their long, blunt-ended nuclei in streaming, fascicular patterns. The small cells are concentrated to one side in this area.

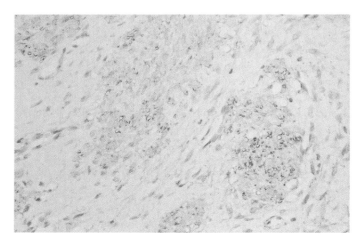

Fig. 36.5 Myofibromatosis. Positive staining for smooth muscle actin.

hemangiopericytoma-like configurations or hyalinized areas seen in myofibromatosis.

BEHAVIOR AND MANAGEMENT

Myofibromatosis is benign and may sometimes regress spontaneously. Conservative excision is currently the treatment of choice, but may occasionally have to be repeated. Enzinger & Weiss[1] consider that myofibromatoses are probably hamartomas of myofibroblasts; if this is so, mutilating surgery should be avoided.

MYOFIBROMATOSIS OF THE JAWS

Myofibromatosis of the mandible has been reported by Matthews et al,[12] Vigneswaran et al,[13] and Jones et al,[14] who in reviewing earlier reports noted that no cases involving the maxilla had been described in children and no examples in either jaw had been described in adults.

CLINICAL FEATURES

Myofibromatosis affects infants or children, causing a painless expansion of the mandible.

RADIOGRAPHY

Myofibromatosis causes a well-demarcated uni- or multilocular area of radiolucency, which may be associated with tilting of related teeth.

MICROSCOPY

The microscopic appearances are the same as those of soft tissue myofibromatosis.

BEHAVIOR AND MANAGEMENT

Diagnosis depends on exposing the lesion and incisional or excisional biopsy. Some examples can be readily enucleated, and others can be curetted out. Myofibromatosis is less aggressive than desmoplastic fibroma and there appear to be no reports of recurrences. Spontaneous regression has also been seen.

GINGIVAL FIBROMATOSIS

Enzinger & Weiss[1] include gingival fibromatosis among the fibrous tumors of infancy and childhood. However, gingival fibromatosis is not a fibromatosis of the type described earlier. It can be congenital (familial) or acquired. The latter is typically a result of treatment with phenytoin or, less often, cyclosporin, nifedipine, or other calcium-channel blockers.

Familial gingival fibromatosis (typically, an autosomal dominant trait) is generalized, may completely bury the teeth (pseudo-anodontia), and can affect the deciduous dentition. Unlike drug-induced gingival hyperplasia, the fibrous overgrowth extends uniformly along the alveolar ridge. Thickening of the facial features until they may resemble acromegaly, hypertrichosis, and sometimes epilepsy, or, rarely, mental defect may be associated. Despite the deep false pocketing, there may be little gingival inflammation.

Drug-induced gingival fibromatosis tends to be exacerbated by poor oral hygiene, and particularly affects the interdental papillae, which become bulbous and separated from each other by pseudoclefts. Typically, the gingival stippling is enhanced, giving the tissue an orange-peel texture.

MICROSCOPY

Fibrous gingival hyperplasia shows dense collagenous fibrous tissue, often with elongation of the rete ridges of the overlying epithelium. The appearances of the drug-induced and familial types are similar (Fig. 36.6).

BEHAVIOR AND MANAGEMENT

Meticulous oral hygiene may control this hyperplasia to some extent, but is unlikely to cause it to resolve. Gingivectomy may be justifiable, particularly for cosmetic reasons, but in the familial type should preferably be delayed until after puberty, when regrowth of the fibrous tissue is likely to be slower. Gingivectomy may then be necessary, and may have to be repeated at intervals.

Fasciites

Fasciites are benign proliferative lesions of fibroblasts. Their etiology is unknown, but they are thought to be reactive rather than neoplastic, even though a stimulus is unlikely to be identifiable. Despite their name, fasciites are not inflammatory and do not necessarily arise from fascial tissue.

In the body as a whole, fasciites are said by Enzinger & Weiss[1] to be the most common tumor-like lesion of fibrous tissue. However, such statements probably take no account of the innumerable hyperplastic fibrous nodules in the mouth.

Fasciites tend to affect the limbs and are rare in the region of the mouth. Barnes[15] found that, among 225 reported cases of nodular fasciitis, 11 were in the mouth and a further four had been described as being in the 'jaw and cheek.'

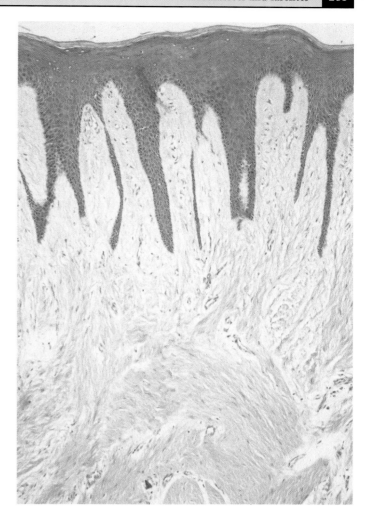

Fig. 36.6 Gingival fibromatosis. This example is cyclosporin induced. It shows the typical appearance of all types, namely the elongated 'drawn down' rete ridges and dense fibrous connective tissue of the body of the lesion.

Fasciitis presents the paradox of rapid tumor-like growth and, often also, microscopic appearances that have frequently been mistaken for poorly differentiated sarcomas ('pseudosarcomatous fasciitis'), but are considerably less aggressive than the fibromatoses and have little or no tendency to recur after limited excision.

The two main types of fasciitis most relevant to the mouth are nodular and proliferative fasciitis.

BEHAVIOR AND MANAGEMENT

The essential consideration is that fasciites are benign. They have limited growth potential, less tendency to recur and extend than fibromatoses, and may also resolve spontaneously.

The treatment of choice is limited excision. This should also provide the pathologist with the junction between the lesion and surrounding tissue. Since the rapid growth of fasciitis is likely to lead to early treatment (especially in the mouth where even minute lumps cause symptoms) fasciites will usually be small, and readily excised.

It is particularly important that the surgeon should not be misled by the rapid growth of these lesions into overhasty mutilating operations.

NODULAR FASCIITIS

In-keeping with the tumor-like microscopic features, nodular fasciitis produces a rapidly growing localized mass, typically reaching a few centimeters in diameter in 1–3 weeks.

INCIDENCE

Adults aged 20–35 are predominantly affected, and in this group the upper extremity is the most frequent site. Although nodular fasciitis is uncommon in children, the head and neck region may be relatively more frequently affected.

MICROSCOPY

Fasciites are poorly circumscribed and consist essentially of short irregular interlacing bundles of fibrous tissue characteristically forming feathery patterns as a result of abundant mucopolysaccharide ground substance, but also contain small amounts of mature collagen. The fibroblast nuclei are plump, vesiculated and with large nucleoli. Mitoses are common, but are usually normal. Lymphocytes and erythrocytes are often scattered in the fibrous tissue (Figs 36.7 and 36.8).

PAROSTEAL FASCIITIS

This rare variant originates from periosteum and may result in destruction of cortical bone and reactive subperiosteal new bone formation. Microscopically, the appearances are those of nodular fasciitis, and it is therefore distinguishable from sclerosing periostitis.

PROLIFERATIVE FASCIITIS

Proliferative fasciitis differs from nodular fasciitis in that a slightly older age group (40–70 years) tends to be affected and about 60% of cases are in the arm or leg. Head or neck lesions are certainly no more common and may even be more rare than those of nodular fasciitis.

CLINICAL FEATURES

The usual history is of a firm subcutaneous or submucosal lesion

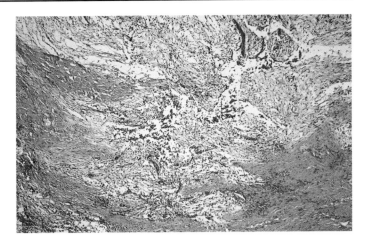

Fig. 36.7 Nodular fasciitis. The proliferating fibroblasts in an abundant mucopolysaccharide ground substance produce a characteristically feathery appearance and lack a well-defined margin.

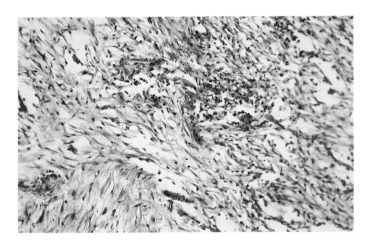

Fig. 36.8 Nodular fasciitis. Higher power view shows the plump nuclei of the fibroblasts, which are spread apart by the ground substance, and inflammatory cells.

that has developed within a few weeks and is painless. In the mouth, it may ulcerate.

MICROSCOPY

The mass is poorly circumscribed, and may extend into underlying muscle. The connective tissue forming the mass has no discernible pattern, and consists of immature fibroblasts, including bizarre hyperchromatic giant forms, and can be mistaken for a sarcoma. There are fine reticulin fibers, but little or no mature collagen is apparent, and the stroma is predominantly mucoid (Figs 36.9–36.11).

As the lesion matures, it becomes less abundantly cellular, giant nuclei are fewer or absent, and there is more collagen. Maturation can be rapid and may develop between the time of an initial biopsy and definitive excision.

Fibrosarcoma

37

Fibrosarcoma of soft tissues

Malignant soft tissue tumors in the oral and perioral regions, apart from being uncommon, do not differ histologically from those in other sites, but may be more difficult to manage because of the proximity of vital structures. Their infrequency means that reliable data on their behavior are difficult to obtain, but some tumors may possibly behave differently from those in other sites. Sarcomas of salivary glands, for example, appear to have a worse prognosis than those that form elsewhere, despite the possibility of their earlier recognition. However, this too may be a reflection of the difficulties of adequate excision from such a site.

Microscopically, some sarcomas present special problems. First, there is the long-standing difficulty of determining the diagnoses of tumors the light microscopic appearances of which frequently differ little from one another. However, this difficulty has been ameliorated by the use of immunohistochemistry, electron microscopy, and identification of cytogenetic abnormalities.[1] Such methods also help to identify many benign soft tissue tumors and tumor-like lesions that have been, and may still sometimes be, mistaken for sarcomas.

Identification of chromosomal abnormalities is assuming growing importance in soft tissue tumor diagnosis, as reviewed by Sreekantaiah et al.[2] However, with many tumors specific cytogenetic abnormalities have yet to be defined.

Staging of soft tissue sarcomas, as a guide to treatment and prognosis, is also difficult because of the lack of any universally accepted staging system.[3] The rarity of soft tissue sarcomas in the head and neck region, and particularly in the oral regions, has also made it even more difficult to establish treatment protocols or factors determining prognosis. Furthermore, of course, the proximity of vital structures frequently makes wide excision of these tumors difficult or impossible. Unfortunately, mutilating surgery does not necessarily prolong life greatly.

Fibrosarcoma is particularly rare in the mouth, but can occasionally be a consequence of irradiation of the region. Eversole et al[4] were able to find 20 cases of fibrosarcomas of the oral soft tissues reported between 1921 and 1951. Four tumors involved the mandible; one of these also involved the mastoid, tongue, and hard palate. By contrast, among 29 fibrosarcomas of the head and neck region seen over a period of 32 years, Mark et al[5] noted only one each in the tongue and cheek, respectively.

INCIDENCE

The peak age incidence of oral fibrosarcomas is probably between 35 and 55 years.

CLINICAL FEATURES

Oral fibrosarcomas form initially smooth, sometimes lobulated, firm swellings, but later the surface may ulcerate.

MICROSCOPY

The malignant fibroblasts can be well differentiated, and form close-packed, spindle-shaped cells with large but uniform nuclei, in long interlacing bundles streaming through the mass and producing small amounts of collagen (Figs 37.1 and 37.2).

At the other extreme, the fibroblast nuclei can be pleomorphic,

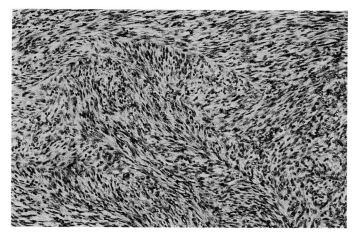

Fig. 37.1 Fibrosarcoma. Low-power view shows the typical herringbone pattern of the interlacing fascicles of fibroblasts.

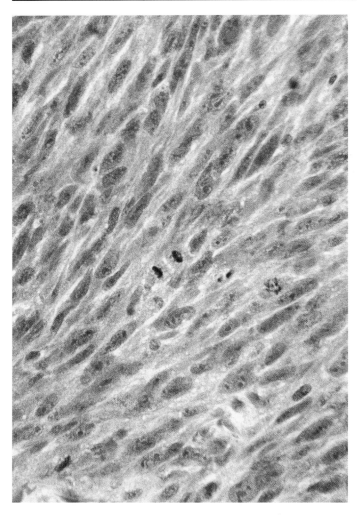

Fig. 37.2 Fibrosarcoma. The neoplastic fibroblasts have large but relatively uniform nuclei, with some mitotic activity but relatively little cytoplasm.

vary in size, and show frequent mitoses, and little intercellular matrix is produced.

BEHAVIOR AND MANAGEMENT

Only a minority, even of poorly differentiated fibrosarcomas, metastasize, but radical excision at the earliest possible stage is essential. This may be very difficult in the head and neck region, and may explain the poorer prognosis for tumors in this site. Well-differentiated (grade I) tumors appear to have a far better prognosis than grade IV tumors, but no clinical feature such as age of onset or duration of symptoms appears to affect the issue. Mark et al[5] suggest that radiotherapy should be used for patients with positive surgical margins and may be helpful in controlling high-grade tumors. There is, as yet, no firm evidence for the value of chemotherapy as ancillary treatment, although it has frequently been used.

Because of the rarity of these tumors, reported 5-year survival rates vary widely, from 83% for well-differentiated tumors to

0–36% for poorly differentiated fibrosarcomas from all parts of the body. Of the 20 cases reviewed by Eversole et al,[4] 12 patients were known to be alive and well for periods between 8 months and 18 years.

Death is mainly from local recurrence and spread. Greager et al[6] reported the results of treatment of 14 fibrosarcomas of the head and neck region (precise sites not stated), and found the 5- and 10-year survival rates to be 57% and 50%, respectively. Wide excision was used as primary treatment, and re-excision was considered for local recurrences. The prognosis did not appear to be related to tumor stage, but the median survival was significantly better for those with low-grade tumors.

General considerations affecting management of soft tissue sarcomas

Soft tissue sarcomas of the oral and perioral regions are heterogeneous and vary in their potential for metastasis. Kraus et al[7] have attempted to determine prognostic factors, but point out the difficulties in generalizing about this group of uncommon tumors and the paucity of data on individual histological types. From a database of 1400 adult soft tissue sarcomas, only 60 involved the head and neck and of these only eight were in the oral cavity. Rhabdomyosarcomas were excluded because of their different treatment requirements.

Krauss et al[7] concluded that wide excision was the first essential, with the use of computed tomography scanning or magnetic resonance imaging to aid in defining tumor extent. Gadolinium enhancement further improved the accuracy of staging. After surgery, imaging was of little value in identifying residual tumor because of edema or scarring. However, microscopic evidence for failure to clear the margins was regarded as an indication for radiotherapy. Kraus et al[7] also reviewed previous, larger studies of prognostic factors and survival. The latter also represented longer periods of study (15–26 years) than that of Kraus et al.[7] All agreed that tumor grade and clear excision margins were significant factors relating to survival. All the earlier studies, but not the one by Kraus et al,[7] agreed also that tumor size was the third determinant of survival.

Fibrosarcoma of bone

Fibrosarcomas of bone account for less than 5% of primary malignant bone tumors. The most frequent sites are the metaphyseal region of the medulla of a bone of the leg. In approximately 20% of cases fibrosarcoma is secondary to some other bone lesion such as Paget's disease or a giant cell tumor, or a complication of previous radiotherapy of a soft tissue lesion.

INCIDENCE

Approximately 15% of fibrosarcomas of bone are in the head and neck region, with a predilection for the skull or jaws. The mandible, particularly the body, is affected more frequently than the maxilla in a ratio of 3 : 1 to 4 : 1. Males are slightly more frequently affected than females; most patients are aged between 30 and 40 years, but there is a wide age range.

CLINICAL FEATURES

Fibrosarcoma of the jaws causes pain, swelling, and loosening of teeth. Radiographically it causes an ill-defined radiolucent area with no distinctive features or, rarely, a relatively well-circumscribed area of radiolucency.

MICROSCOPY

Fibrosarcoma of bone appears similar to its soft tissue counterpart with long interlacing fascicles of spindle-shaped fibroblasts and some collagen formation. The chief difficulty in differential diagnosis is with desmoblastic fibroma (described earlier).

BEHAVIOR AND MANAGEMENT

The treatment is radical surgical excision, possibly supplemented by radiotherapy. The tumor may metastasize to the lungs or other bones, but although data on fibrosarcomas of the jaws are limited, these tumors are thought to have a better prognosis than osteosarcomas or chondrosarcomas. About 30% of fibrosarcomas arise from the periosteum and appear to have a better prognosis than intramedullary fibrosarcomas. Five-year survival rates for fibrosarcomas of the bones of the head and neck range from 27% to 40%. The prognosis is affected by the extent of the tumor at operation and the degree of dedifferentiation. Fibrosarcomas of bone secondary to other diseases generally also have a worse prognosis.

REFERENCES

1. Angervall L, Kindblom L-G 1993 Principles of pathologic–anatomic diagnosis and classification of soft tissue sarcomas. Clin Orthopaed Rel Res 289: 9–18
2. Sreekantaiah C, Ladanyi M, Rodriquez E, Chaganti RSK 1994 Chromosomal abnormalities in soft tissue tumors. Relevance to diagnosis, classification and molecular mechanisms. Am J Pathol 144: 1121–1134
3. Peabody TD, Simon MA 1993 Principles of staging of soft-tissue sarcomas. Clin Orthopaed Rel Res 289: 19–31
4. Eversole LR, Schwartz D, Sabes WR 1973 Central and peripheral fibrogenic and neurogenic sarcoma of the oral regions. Oral Surg 36: 49–62
5. Mark RJ, Sercarz JA, Tran L, Selch M, Calcaterra TC 1991 Fibrosarcoma of the head and neck. Arch Otolaryngol Head Neck Surg 117: 396–401
6. Greager JA, Reichard K, Campana JP, Das Gupta TK 1994 Fibrosarcoma of the head and neck. Am J Surg 167: 437–439
7. Kraus DH, Dubner S, Harrison LB et al 1994 Prognostic factors for recurrence and survival in head and neck soft tissue sarcomas. Cancer 74: 697–702

Fibrohistiocytic tumors and malignant fibrous histiocytoma

38

Fibrohistiocytic tumors

The term 'fibrohistiocytic tumor' is used by Enzinger & Weiss[1] for a diverse group of tumors and tumor-like lesions, which can be benign, malignant, or intermediate in behavior. Within this broad category are the xanthomas and xanthogranulomas, which can be difficult to distinguish from sarcomas but are benign or even self-limiting. Fibrohistiocytic tumors predominantly affect the skin or skeletal muscles and are rare in the mouth, where fewer than a dozen cases have probably been reported. The single most characteristic microscopic feature of these tumors is a storiform (knotted or tangled) pattern to the spindle cells, but the appearances are very variable, with xanthomatous or myxoid areas, or many giant cells. Ultrastructural and tissue culture studies have largely supported the belief that these tumors arise from a tissue histiocyte that has fibroblastic properties and gives rise to both histiocyte-like and fibroblastic cells histologically.

Malignant fibrous histiocytoma

Lesions earlier reported as fibrosarcomas or other sarcomas have been found on reassessment to be malignant fibrous histiocytomas. These tumors are predominantly soft tissue tumors, but a minority are intraosseous. From the few reports of fibrous histiocytomas arising in oral or perioral tissues no useful generalizations about the clinical features can be made.

INCIDENCE

Adults are affected, and in the case of the most common type (in the lower extremity) the peak age is in the seventh decade. The tumor can develop in the soft tissues or bone, as described later. Nuamah & Browne[2] have reported a submasseteric malignant fibrous histiocytoma, which presented as an abscess.

CLINICAL FEATURES

Grossly, the tumor typically forms a multilobulated fleshy mass.

MICROSCOPY

Typical features are short bundles of spindle cells forming storiform, matted or cartwheel patterns. However, fibrosarcoma-like patterns may also be seen, as well as giant cells and pleomorphic areas with plumper histiocyte-like cells and variable numbers of mitoses (Figs 38.1–38.3).

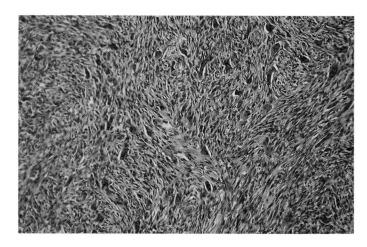

Fig. 38.1 Malignant fibrous histiocytoma. The densely packed spindle cells have formed a typical matted pattern.

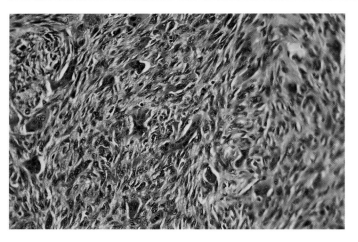

Fig. 38.2 Malignant fibrous histiocytoma. Close-packed malignant spindle cells showing prominent nuclei and some mitotic activity, but scanty collagen, form tangled bundles surrounding some giant cells.

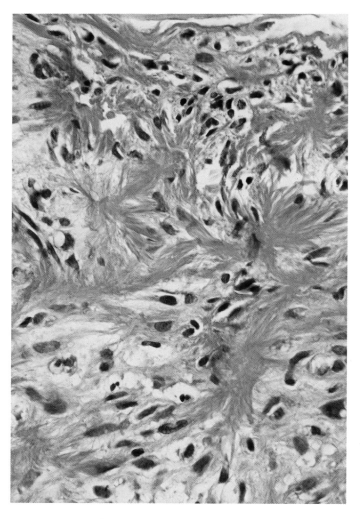

Fig. 38.3 Malignant fibrous histiocytoma. Higher power view shows the characteristic knotted (storiform) pattern of fibers.

GIANT CELL VARIANT OF MALIGNANT FIBROUS HISTIOCYTOMA

This tumor, which has also been termed *malignant giant cell tumor of soft tissues*, consists of histiocytes, fibroblasts and osteoclast-like cells As a consequence it may closely resemble a giant cell tumor of bone, apart from the lack of osteoid or osseous tissue. As this variant is considerably less common than the storiform type of malignant fibrous histiocytoma, little is known about its behavior, but there is nothing to suggest that it is any more benign.

BEHAVIOR AND MANAGEMENT

Malignant fibrous histiocytoma is actively invasive and spreads particularly along tissue planes. Unlike other sarcomas, it has a tendency to involve lymph nodes.

Treatment of fibrous histiocytoma is by radical excision. Regional lymph nodes should also be cleared, as the tumor metastasizes in over 40% of cases, sometimes when microscopic features indicative of malignancy are minimal. There is some evidence that postoperative radiotherapy improves the prognosis. In the case presented by Nuamah & Browne,[2] treatment consisted of wide local excision and neck dissection, which revealed involvement of a single node. Postoperative radiotherapy was given, but within 8 months the tumor had metastasized to the small intestine and the patient died 4 months later of disseminated abdominal and pelvic disease, despite resection of the small intestine and chemotherapy.

MALIGNANT FIBROUS HISTIOCYTOMA OF THE JAWS

Block et al[3] were able to find reports of 16 cases affecting the maxilla and added another, while Anavi et al[4] identified from the literature 13 cases involving the mandible. Fibrous histiocytomas of the jaws after irradiation of the region have been described by Ireland et al,[5] who reported two cases, and by Lin et al,[6] who identified five examples.

CLINICAL FEATURES

Malignant fibrous histiocytomas of the jaws do not show any distinctive features to distinguish them from other malignant tumors. Pain, swelling, an area of radiolucency, and loosening of teeth are typical.

BEHAVIOR AND MANAGEMENT

Diagnosis depends on microscopy. The microscopic features are as described above. Fibrous histiocytomas, even if histologically benign, should be widely excised. One patient reported by Besly et al[7] required exenteration of the orbit. The possibility of lymph node involvement should also be considered and neck dissection carried out if necessary. The prognosis appears to be remarkably poor, and none (apart from one lost to follow-up) of the 16 patients reviewed by Block et al[3] survived. The longest known period of disease-free survival was only 27 months, and eight patients soon died from their tumors or had metastases. Adjuvant radiotherapy, chemotherapy, or both have frequently been given, but their value is uncertain.

REFERENCES

1. Enzinger FM, Weiss SW 1995 Soft tissue tumors, 3rd edn. C V Mosby, St Louis
2. Nuamah IK, Browne RM 1995 Malignant fibrous histiocytoma presenting as perioral abscess. Int J Oral Maxillofac Surg 24: 158–159.
3. Block MS, Cade JE, Rodriguez FH 1986 Malignant fibrous histiocytoma of the maxilla. J Oral Maxillofac Surg 44: 404–412
4. Anavi Y, Herman GE, Craybill S, MacIntosh RB 1989 Malignant fibrous histiocytoma of the mandible (review). Oral Surg Oral Med Oral Pathol 68: 436–443
5. Ireland AJ, Eveson JW, Leopard PJ 1988 Malignant fibrous histiocytoma: a report of two cases arising in sites of previous irradiation. Br J Oral Maxillofac Surg 165: 445–460
6. Lin SK, How SW, Wang JT, Liu BY, Chiang CP 1994 Oral postradiation malignant fibrous histiocytoma: a clinicopathological study. J Oral Pathol Med 23: 324–329
7. Besly W, Wiesenfeld D, Kleid S, Poker I 1993 Malignant fibrous histiocytoma of the maxilla – a report of two cases. Br J Oral Maxillofac Surg 31: 45–48

Benign tumors of neural tissue

39

Traumatic neuroma

Traumatic neuromas are uncommon in the mouth. They usually result from accidental operative damage. Although seven examples reported by Rasmussen[1] had followed extractions or more minor dental operations, this number is negligible in relation to the number of extractions that are carried out.

Clinically, traumatic neuromas may give rise to neuralgic pain, particularly if irritated, for example by a denture, and of 45 cases reported by Peszkowski & Larsson,[2] 15 were painful. Eight of the latter had followed extractions or other trauma, and trauma was suspected in six others. Women accounted for 75% of patients with painful neuromas, which were more frequently encountered in patients older than 50 years. Twenty-five per cent of 31 traumatic neuromas reported by Sist & Green[3] were painful, and all of these were in women. The majority of traumatic neuromas are therefore painless, and are found only as small nodules in the tissues.

Peszkowski & Larsson[2] found that traumatic neuromas were rare before the age of 20 years and the peak frequency was between the ages of 40 and 49 years, with a gradually declining frequency thereafter. The single most common site was within the jaws (11 cases), but the tongue, mental foramen, lower lip, and gingival sulcus together accounted for many more cases.

MICROSCOPY

Traumatic neuromas consist of tangled bundles of nerve fascicles in a dense fibrous stroma (Fig. 39.1).

Both Sist & Greene[3] and Peszkowski & Larsson[2] found that an inflammatory infiltrate was significantly more frequently present in painful traumatic neuromas.

BEHAVIOR AND MANAGEMENT

Surgical excision is curative. However, Rasmussen[1] found that severe pain persisted in two of seven cases (in one case for 16 years) after excision. Peszkowski & Larsson[2] also found that pain was

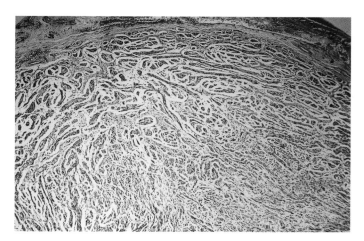

Fig. 39.1 Traumatic neuroma. Tangled bundles of nerve fascicles in a dense fibrous stroma.

completely relieved after excision in only four of 15 cases. In one case pain was still present 10 years later.

Neurilemmoma (Schwannoma)

Schwann cells are neuroectodermal cells that ensheath the axons. Individual peripheral nerves, which consist of a group of axons, are surrounded by a sheath of concentric layers of perineural (Schwann) cells and also collagen fibers. The epineurium ensheathes a group of nerve fascicles in a larger peripheral nerve and consists only of fibrous connective tissue.

Typical neurilemmomas are readily recognizable histologically but, as Hadju[4] has pointed out, there are several more or less pathologically distinct types of benign nerve sheath tumor, and not all malignant nerve sheath tumors are recognizable by microscopy alone.

According to Enziger & Weiss,[5] neurilemmomas have a predilection for the head and neck region where, Williams et al[6] state, 25–48% of them are found. Neurilemmomas may form either in the oral soft tissues or within the jaws (Fig. 39.3).

The ages of 12 patients reported by Williams et al[6] ranged from 16 to 60 years (mean 39.5 years). All the neurilemmomas were in the oral soft tissues, and nine of them had arisen from terminal branches of the trigeminal nerve. All but two of these 12 cases were in males.

In the mouth, neurilemmomas usually form small, painless, nondescript nodules. Only one of the tumors reported by Williams et al[6] was painful. Most were less than 10 mm in maximum dimension, including two examples that had been present for 10 years. However, if neglected, neurilemmomas can grow to a large size, and a painless one 10 cm in maximum dimension in the submandibular space has been reported.[7] Another large neurilemmoma mimicked a submandibular salivary gland tumor.[8]

MICROSCOPY

Neurilemmomas are encapsulated and consist of two types of tissue. Antoni A tissue usually predominates and forms a closely interwoven pattern of elongated spindle-shaped cells, the nuclei of which are often palisaded or regimented. They produce a

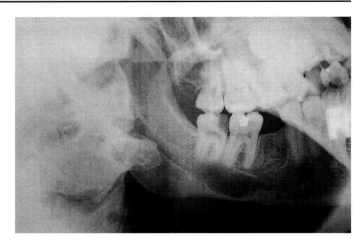

Fig. 39.3 Neurilemmoma of the inferior dental nerve. The tumor has caused fusiform expansion of the inferior dental canal.

distinctive picture, especially when they surround acellular eosinophilic structures (Verocay bodies) (Fig. 39.2).

Ultrastructurally, Verocay bodies consist of interdigitated cytoplasmic processes and reduplicated basement membrane. Reticulin fibers are also abundant. Type B tissue is loose with relatively scanty, scattered spindle cells with pleomorphic nuclei. Some of these may be so large and hyperchromatic as to suggest malignancy. Degenerative changes in Antoni B tissue are associated with the presence of large dilatated blood vessels. Exceptionally uncommonly, neurilemmomas can be multinodular.

Strong positive reactivity for S-100 protein is seen in the Antoni A tissue and is considerably stronger in neurilemmomas than in neurofibromas (Figs 39.4–39.6).

Nahass & Penneys[9] have reported that Merkel cells, identified by immunohistochemical staining for cytokeratin 8 with CAM 5.2, were more frequently found in the epithelium overlying cutaneous neurilemmomas than over neurofibromas. Merkel cells were found in greater numbers in a linear array along the basal cell layer overlying neurilemmomas, but only as isolated cells over neurofibromas.

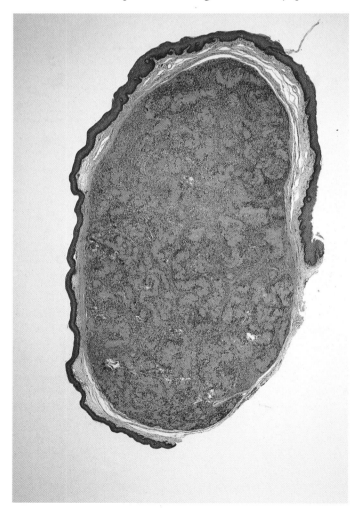

Fig. 39.2 Neurilemmoma. Low-power view shows the circumscribed nature of the tumor and, even at this power, many Verocay bodies.

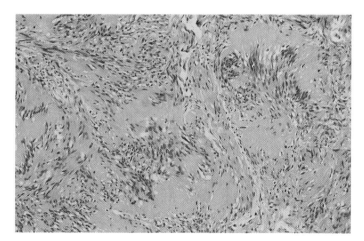

Fig. 39.4 Neurilemmoma. Palisading of nuclei and Verocay bodies are prominent (Antoni A tissue).

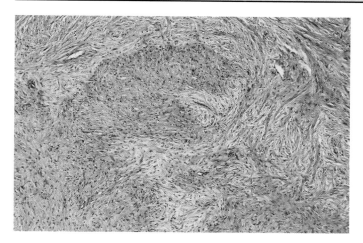

Fig. 39.5 Neurilemmoma. Antoni B tissue showing the spindle cells surrounding a focus of Antoni A tissue.

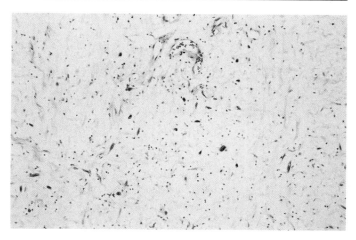

Fig. 39.7 Degenerated schwannoma. Low-power view shows a sparsely cellular tumor with some pleomorphic and hyperchromatic nuclei.

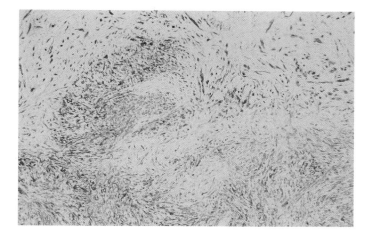

Fig. 39.6 Neurilemmoma. Positive S-100 staining of Antoni B tissue.

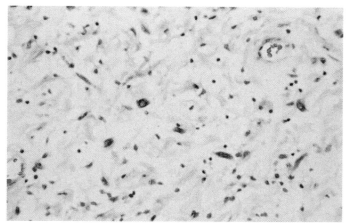

Fig. 39.8 Degenerated schwannoma. Higher power view shows some bizarre nuclear forms having a misleading appearance of atypia.

BEHAVIOR AND MANAGEMENT

If completely excised, neurilemmomas do not recur. Unlike neurofibromas, malignant change is virtually unknown, although a single example has been reported by Carstens & Schrodt.[10]

Degenerated (ancient) Schwannoma

Ancient schwannomas are usually long-standing, neglected tumors. Reports of intraoral ancient neurilemmomas are scanty. Eversole & Howell[11] are credited with first reporting a case, while McCoy et al[12] in reporting another have also illustrated the ultrastructural findings.

MICROSCOPY

The tumor is sparsely cellular, and only small groups of cells with a suggestion of nuclear palisading are sometimes seen. Individual cells have eosinophilic cytoplasm but indistinct cell margins. Calcifications, cyst formation, and hyalinization may be seen. Usually, there is infiltration by many histiocytes and siderophages. More important, the Schwann cells show a misleading degree of atypia, with large, hyperchromatic, often multilobed nuclei (Figs 39.7 and 39.8).

McCoy et al[12] have confirmed that the cells of an ancient schwannoma are essentially similar to typical schwannoma cells. They showed that the bulk of the tumor was composed of many reduplications of basal lamina, which accompanied thin cytoplasmic processes, rather than of type III collagen as had previously been thought. Perivascular hyaline was also found to be largely composed of basal lamina material. Submicroscopic calcified spherules were scattered among the basal lamina material.

BEHAVIOR AND MANAGEMENT

Despite the histologic suggestion of atypia, ancient neurilemmomas behave like their conventional counterparts, and resection is curative.

Neurofibroma

Solitary intraoral neurofibromas are more uncommon than neurilemmomas, and when an oral neurofibroma is found the patient should be investigated for neurofibromatosis. Among 37 neurogenic tumors of the maxillofacial region, Krause et al[13] found only five solitary neurofibromas but 23 typical or ancient schwannomas. By contrast, Chen & Miller[14] found that neurofibromas accounted for 49 of 55 intraoral neurogenic tumors.

CLINICAL FEATURES

Neurofibromas form painless smooth nodules. Occasionally, one develops in the inferior dental nerve, and is seen radiographically as a fusiform expansion of the inferior dental canal. Loutfy et al[15] have reported a neurofibroma of the main trunk of the trigeminal nerve that caused localized destruction in the region of the foramen ovale.

MICROSCOPY

Neurofibromas consist of cells with elongated, bent, or sinuous nuclei separated by abundant, fine, and equally sinuous collagen fibers. Reticulin fibers, by contrast, are scanty. Sharma et al[16] have confirmed by electron microscopy that neurofibromas are composed of Schwann cells, fibroblast-like cells, and intermediate cells in almost equal proportions (Fig. 39.9).

Isaacson[17] showed and Johnson et al[18] confirmed that mast cells are frequently found among the fibers and typically are more numerous than in neurilemmomas. Mast-cell products may contribute to the growth of neurofibromas, neurofibromatosis, and traumatic neuromas.[19]

Johnson et al[18] also showed, by UCHL-1, LN-1 or LN-2 immunoreactivity, that lymphocytic infiltration was heavier than conventional staining suggested.

Sharma et al[16] have confirmed that reactivity for S-100 protein is patchy and variable in neurofibromas, and that nerve sheath tumors in general do not show reactivity for myelin basic protein (MBP).

BEHAVIOR AND MANAGEMENT

When a neurofibroma is identified, neurofibromatosis should be excluded. Neurofibromas also have a potential for malignant change, particularly when a feature of neurofibromatosis. Otherwise, solitary neurofibromas are benign and complete excision should be curative.

Neurothekeoma (nerve sheath myxoma)

This rare tumor appears to arise from perineural cells. It more frequently forms in the skin in the head and neck area but, rarely, appears in the mouth. Rodriguez-Peralto & El-Naggar[20] reported a neurothekeoma in the buccal mucosa, but could find reports of only seven earlier examples involving the oral cavity. Three of these involved the tongue, two the buccal mucosa, and one each the palate or retromolar area. The mean age at presentation was 33 years, and women were more frequently affected.

MICROSCOPY

Neurothekeoma consists of well-defined lobules of myxoid tissue separated by fibrous septa. The degree of cellularity varies and the cells appear stellate or rounded. Multinucleate cells may also be present. Staining for S-100 protein is variable, but when positive may help to distinguish neurothekeomas from other myxoid tumors (Figs 39.10 and 39.11).

BEHAVIOR AND MANAGEMENT

All reported oral neurothekeomas have been 1 cm or less in diameter. They are benign and respond to excision. No recurrences have been reported.

Palisaded encapsulated neuroma

Palisaded encapsulated neuromas (PENs) are probably more common than is generally appreciated. Reed et al,[21] who first

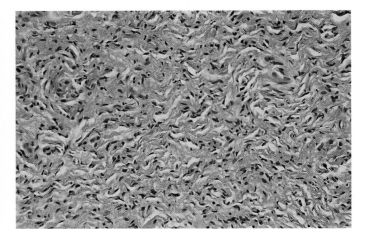

Fig. 39.9 Neurofibroma. Both the nuclei and spindle cells have a typical serpentine appearance.

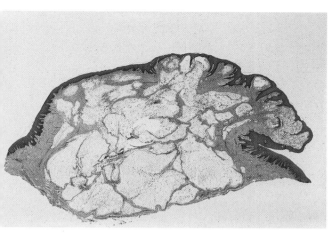

;. 39.10 Neurothekeoma. Well-defined lobules of myxoid tissue are separated
fibrous septa.

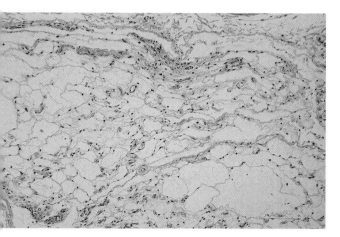

;. 39.11 Neurothekeoma. Higher power view shows a predominance of
xoid tissue, which contains some inconspicuous nerve bundles.

scribed and named this tumor, were able to analyze the find-
gs in 44 examples. Twenty years later, Dakin et al[22] commented
at palisaded encapsulated neuroma remained **underdiagnosed**
d even unrecognized on many occasions. Chauvin et al[23] in
eir review of previous reports, considered that Tomich & Moll[24]
ere the first to report an oral palisaded encapsulated neuroma,
nich in this case was on the lower lip. The distinction from
her nerve sheath tumors is important because of the lack of any
sociation between palisaded encapsulated neuroma and
urofibromatosis.

LINICAL FEATURES

lisaded encapsulated neuromas most frequently affect the facial
perioral skin, usually between the fourth and sixth decades.
owever, the 13 intraoral examples presented by Chauvin et al[23]
rmed approximately 22% of intraoral neural tumors, with the

palate as site of predilection. These tumors form smooth firm,
sessile nodules 2–3 mm in diameter. Ten of the 13 patients were
men, and the mean age was 51 years.

MICROSCOPY

Palisaded encapsulated neuromas are circumscribed and sometimes
have capsules that are continuous with the perineurium of a
peripheral nerve on their deep aspect. Despite their name, Dakin
et al[22] point out that encapsulation of these tumors is frequently
incomplete. The bulk of the tumor consists of fascicles of spindle-
shaped cells with sinuous outlines and prominent nuclei. Relatively scanty connective tissue is interspersed between the tumor
cells. The nuclei have a tendency to palisade, sometimes sufficiently to cause the tumor to resemble a schwannoma, but
Verocay bodies are typically absent. However, in the 81 facial
palisaded encapsulated neuromas surveyed by Dover et al,[25]
palisading was not prominent (Figs 39.12 and 39.13).

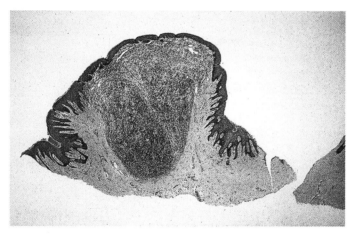

Fig. 39.12 Palisaded encapsulated neuroma. Low-power view shows a sharply
circumscribed aggregate of neural tissue in the submucosa.

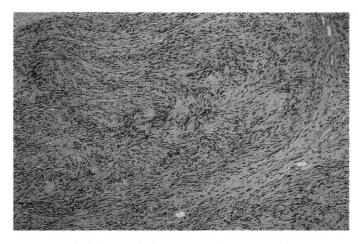

Fig. 39.13 Palisaded encapsulated neuroma. Higher power view shows
conspicuous palisading, but an absence of Verocay bodies.

Chauvin et al[23] reported that most of the lesional cells were strongly S-100 positive, antibodies to neurofilaments show peripheral nerve axons within the mass, and the perineural cells of the capsule are EMA positive.

The presence of nerve axons in palisaded encapsulated neuromas distinguishes them from a schwannoma. The dominance of Schwann cells and the EMA-positive capsule distinguish palisaded encapsulated neuroma from diffuse neurofibroma.

BEHAVIOR AND MANAGEMENT

Palisaded encapsulated neuroma is benign. Moreover, from their ultrastructural finding of changes resembling axonal regeneration, Dover et al[25] suggested that it could be traumatic in origin. The appearance of palisaded encapsulated neuroma on oral sites (palate and lips) that have been subjected to trauma also caused Chauvin et al[23] to suggest that the lesion might be reactive rather than neoplastic. Excision is curative.

Plexiform neurofibromas

Plexiform neuromas are exceedingly rare in the mouth. They consist of poorly organized mixtures of nerve fibrils, which are usually unmyelinated and tangled, but normal or hypertrophied nerve fibers are sometimes present. There is diffuse proliferation of spindle cells of neural origin, myxoid areas and, often, fat. Mast cells, as in many other fibroproliferative disorders, are conspicuous and appear to contribute to the overgrowth of neural fibrous tissue. Compact bundles of cells apparently originating from the peri- or epineurium proliferate into the surrounding tissues (Figs 39.14 and 39.15).

BEHAVIOR AND MANAGEMENT

Plexiform neurofibromas are typically a sign of von Recklinghausen's disease or multiple endocrine neoplasia syndrome, which need to be investigated. That aside, excision should be curative.

Neurofibromatosis

Neurofibromatosis is one of the phakomatoses ('neurodermatoses'), which are genetically determined hamartomatous or neoplastic diseases of the skin and nervous system.

Peripheral and central neurofibromatoses are genetically and phenotypically distinct. The peripheral type (NF I; von Recklinghausen's disease) is associated with changes in the long arm of chromosome 17 and accounts for over 90% of cases. The

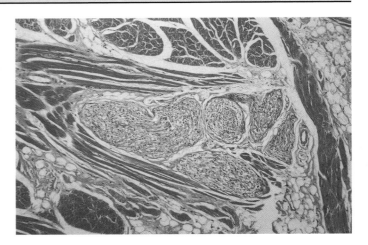

Fig. 39.14 Plexiform neurofibroma. Within the body of the tongue are well-defined bundles of neural tissue.

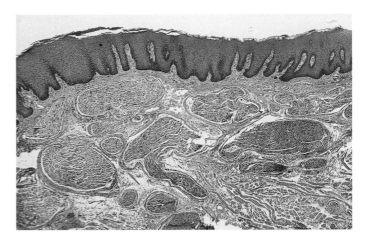

Fig. 39.15 Mucosal neuroma in endocrine adenoma syndrome (MEN III). A typical submucosal plexiform neuroma.

central type (NF II) is associated with a defect near the center of the long arm of chromosome 22, is characterized by bilateral acoustic neuromas, and accounts for the remainder. Neurofibromatosis type I is one of the most common autosomal dominant disorders, and the prevalence of the disease may approach 1 in 3000 of the population. Seven other types of neurofibromatosis are currently recognized.

CLINICAL FEATURES

The following account refers to type I neurofibromatosis, except where stated otherwise.

The characteristic features of peripheral neurofibromatosis are multiple coffee-colored (café-au-lait) macules, subcutaneous and sometimes skeletal neurofibromas, and Lisch nodules (brownish, dome-shaped hamartomas of the iris). The severity of the disease ranges from inconspicuous to grossly disfiguring tumorous deformities. The skin tumors start to develop at or near puberty, and frequently cause itching while actively growing, which may possibly result from degranulation of the many mast cells. In severe cases cutaneous tumors can form in hundreds or even thousands.

The café-au-lait spots typically start to appear within the first year of life. They resemble freckles but appear in sites shielded from sunlight, such as the axillae. In the absence of neurofibromas the diagnosis of the disease depends on finding multiple café-au-lait spots and Lisch nodules.

Neurofibromas affect the head and neck region in over 25% of cases. Intraoral tumors were thought to be uncommon, but Shapiro et al[26] detected oral soft tissue neurofibromas in six of 22 patients, while D'Ambrosio et al[27] found intraoral lesions in 92% of 38 patients with neurofibromatosis. The most common abnormality, present in 53% of these patients, was enlargement of the filiform papillae. Intraoral neurofibromas were found in 26% and macroglossia was also sometimes seen. Geist et al[28] have reviewed the findings in both types of neurofibromatosis, but the single patient with suspected type II disease showed only a single nodule on the dorsum of the tongue. The nodule was thought, but not histologically confirmed, to be a neurofibroma or neurilemmoma.

Bones can be involved as a result of tumors growing from nerve fibers and forming subperiosteal or more central, cyst-like areas of radiolucency. D'Ambrosio et al[27] noted enlargement of the mandibular foramen in 34%, enlargement of the mandibular canal in 29%, and branching of the mandibular canal in 24% of 38 patients. Other abnormalities of the jaws have been reviewed by Vincent & Willams.[29] Facial asymmetry can result from involvement of the facial bones, as described by, for example, Neville et al.[30] Bone destruction may also result from formation of fibroma-like masses containing giant cells. White et al,[31] in their survey of the head and neck manifestations of 257 cases of neurofibromatosis (type not specified, but mainly type I disease), found that bony abnormalities were the most common and were present in 50% of patients. Macrocephaly was present in 30%.

However, the grotesque abnormalities, particularly the enormous, distorted skull of the famous Elephant Man described by Frederick Treves, are now known not to have resulted from severe neurofibromatosis, but were recognized by Tibbles & Cohen[32] to have been due to the more recently recognized proteus syndrome. Major features of the latter, as reviewed by Samlaska et al,[33] include hemihypertrophy, macrodactyly, exostoses, epidermal naevi, scoliosis, and subcutaneous masses due to a variety of lipomatous or hamartomatous tumors, usually with an angiomatous component.

MICROSCOPY

Plexiform neurofibromas are strongly suggestive, if not diagnostic, of von Recklinghausen's disease or of multiple endocrine neoplasia syndrome, which may be associated.

Neurofibromas are even more common than plexiform lesions, but are not distinguishable from those not associated with von Recklinghausen's disease. Neurilemmomas may sometimes also be found.

The café-au-lait spots show melanin hyperpigmentation of both keratinocytes and melanocytes, usually with scattered abnormally large melanin granules (giant melanosomes).

BEHAVIOR AND MANAGEMENT

Isolated tumors can be excised for functional or cosmetic reasons and recurrence is unusual. A major concern is the risk of sarcomatous change which, as suggested by Neville et al,[30] may develop in 5% of cases of type I neurofibromatosis but is relatively uncommon in the head and neck region. Ducatman et al[34] found 18% of 62 sarcomas developing in neurofibromatosis in the head and neck region, while Guccion & Enzinger[35] found only 9% of them to involve this region. As a consequence, Neville et al[30] were able to find only sporadic reports of this complication in the oral cavity. They reported two other patients, both of whom died from their disease within a year, while in five reported cases four died within 1–2.8 years and the fifth had a massive recurrence when last seen.

Other serious complications of type I neurofibromatosis include disfigurement, mental handicap, or other neurological disease (such as epilepsy or paraplegia) due to spinal neurofibromas. Skeletal abnormalities and central nervous system tumors, particularly gliomas of the optic nerves or chiasma, may also develop. As mentioned earlier acoustic neuromas are the main manifestation of neurofibromatosis type II but, contrary to earlier descriptions, are rarely associated with peripheral neurofibromatosis (type I). However, type III neurofibromatosis is a mixed form of the disease, with features of both type I and type II.

Mucosal neuromas in endocrine adenoma syndromes

Oral mucosal neuromas, particularly along the lateral borders of the tongue, are a feature of multiple endocrine adenoma syndrome type III (Williams and Pollock syndrome), in which they are associated with medullary carcinoma of the thyroid and phaeochromocytoma.

Neuromas in this syndrome resemble the plexiform or traumatic types, but may be more fibrotic if traumatized.

The recognition of one of these unusual tumors in the mouth is an indication for investigation for endocrine adenoma syndrome, which they may antecede.

REFERENCES

1. Rasmussen OC 1980 Painful traumatic neuromas of the oral cavity. Oral Surg Oral Med Oral Pathol 46: 191–195
2. Peszkowski MJ, Larsson A 1990 Extraosseous and intraosseous oral traumatic neuromas and their association with tooth extraction. J Oral Maxillofac Surg 48: 963–967

3. Sist TC, Green GW 1981 Traumatic neuromas of the oral cavity. Oral Surg Oral Med Oral Pathol 51: 394–398
4. Hajdu SI 1993 Peripheral nerve sheath tumours. Histogenesis, classification and prognosis. Cancer 72: 3549–3552
5. Enzinger FM, Weiss SW 1988 Soft tissue tumors, 2nd edn. C V Mosby, St Louis
6. Williams HK, Cannell H, Silvester K, Williams DM 1993 Neurilemmoma of the head and neck. Br J Oral Maxillofac Surg 31: 32–35
7. Bochlogyros PN, Kanakis P, Tsikou-Papafrangou N, Chase D 1992 A large, painless mass in the submandibular space. J Oral Maxillofac Surg 50: 1213–1216
8. Mair S, Lermain G 1989 Benign neurilemmoma (Schwannoma) masquerading as a pleomorphic adenoma of the submandibular salivary gland. Acta Cytolog 33: 907–911
9. Nahass GT, Penneys MS 1994 Merkel cells in neurofibromas and neurilemmomas. Br J Dermatol 131: 664–666
10. Carstens H, Schrodt G 1969 Malignant transformation of a benign encapsulated neurilemmoma. Am J Surg Pathol 51: 144–148
11. Eversole LR, Howell RM 1971 Ancient neurilemmoma of the oral cavity. Oral Surg Oral Med Oral Pathol 32: 340–343
12. McCoy M, Mincer HH, Turner JT 1983 Intraoral ancient neurilemmoma (ancient schwannoma). Oral Surg Oral Med Oral Pathol 56: 174–184
13. Krause H-R, Hemmer J, Kraft K 1993 The behaviour of neurogenic tumours of the maxillofacial region. J Cranio-Maxillo Fac Surg 21: 258–261
14. Chen S-Y, Miller AS 1979 Neurofibroma and schwannoma of the oral cavity. A clinical and ultrastructural study. Oral Surg Oral Med Oral Pathol 47: 522–538
15. Loutfy WG, Ryan DE, Toohill RJ, Meyer GA 1990 Trigeminal nerve neurofibroma: case report. J Oral Maxillofac Surg 48: 650–654
16. Sharma SS, Sarkar C, Mathur M, Dinda AK, Roy S 1990 Benign nerve sheath tumors: a light microscopic, electron microscopic and immunohistochemical study of 102 cases. Pathology 22: 191–195
17. Isaacson P 1976 Mast cells in benign nerve sheath tumours. J Pathol 119: 193–196
18. Johnson MD, Kamso-Pratt J, Federspiel CF, Whetsell WO 1989 Mast cell and lymphoreticular infiltrates in neurofibromas. Comparison with nerve sheath tumours. Arch Pathol Lab Med 113: 1263–1270
19. Giorno R, Claman HN 1989 Mast cells and neurofibromatosis. Neurofibromatosis 2: 35–41
20. Rodriguez-Peralto JL, El-Naggar AK 1992 Neurothekoma of the oral cavity: case report and review of the literature. J Oral Maxillofac Surg 50: 1224–1226
21. Reed RJ, Fine RM, Meltzer HD 1972 Palisaded encapsulated neuromas of the skin. Arch Dermatol 106: 865–870
22. Dakin MC, Leppard B, Theaker JM 1992 The palisaded encapsulated neuroma (solitary circumscribed neuroma). Histopathology 20: 405–410
23. Chauvin PJ, Wysocki GP, Daley TD, Pringle GA 1992 Palisaded encapsulated neuroma of oral mucosa. Oral Surg Oral Med Oral Pathol 73: 71–73
24. Tomich CE, Moll MC 1976 Palisaded encapsulated neuroma of the lip. J Oral Surg 34: 265–268
25. Dover JS, From L, Lewis A 1989 Palisaded encapsulated neuromas. A clinicopathologic study. Arch Dermatol 125: 386–389
26. Shapiro SD, Abramovitch K, van Dis ML 1984 Neurofibromatosis: oral and radiographic manifestations. Oral Surg Oral Med Oral Pathol 58: 493–498
27. D'Ambrosio JA, Langlais RP, Ord RA 1988 Jaw and skull changes in neurofibromatosis. Oral Surg Oral Med Oral Pathol 66: 391–396
28. Geist JR, Gander DL, Stefanac SJ 1992 Oral manifestations of neurofibromatosis types I and II. Oral Surg Oral Med Oral Pathol 73: 376–382
29. Vincent SD, Williams TP 1983 Mandibular abnormalities in neurofibromatosis. Case report and literature review. Oral Surg Oral Med Oral Pathol 55: 253–257
30. Neville BW, Hann J, Narang R, Garen P 1991 Oral neurofibrosarcoma associated with neurofibromatosis. Oral Surg Oral Med Oral Pathol 72: 456–461
31. White AK, Smith RJH, Bigler CR, Brooke WF, Schauer PR 1986 Head and neck manifestations of neurofibromatosis. Laryngoscope 96: 732–737
32. Tibbles JAR, Cohen Jr MM 1986 Proteus syndrome: the Elephant Man diagnosed. Br Med J 293: 683–685
33. Samlaska CP, Levin SW, James WD, Benson PM, Walker JC, Perlik PC 1989 Proteus syndrome. Arch Dermatol 125: 1109–1114
34. Ducatman BS, Scheithauer BW, Piepgras DG, Reiman HM, Ilstrup DM 1986 Malignant peripheral nerve sheath tumors: a clinicopathologic study of 120 cases. Cancer 57: 2006–2021
35. Guccion JG, Enzinger FM 1979 Malignant sshwannoma associated with von Recklinghausen's disese. Virchows Arch [A] 383: 43–57

Malignant nerve sheath tumors 4

Malignant tumors of nerve sheath origin may be malignant schwannomas or neurofibrosarcomas. However, there is no universally agreed terminology, so that Piatelli et al[1] found no fewer than 19 synonyms for these tumors. There also is no clear evidence that such distinctions affect the prognosis.

Malignant nerve sheath tumors are undoubtedly uncommon, particularly in the mouth or jaws. In a survey of 4550 soft tissue sarcomas in adults, Lawrence et al[2] found that only 8.9% were in the head or neck region, and that malignant nerve sheath tumors formed between 3% and 4% of all sarcomas. Greager et al,[3] in a survey of 53 soft tissue sarcomas of the head and neck in adults, found only eight to be neurogenic, although they were the second most frequent type after fibrosarcomas. However, in an analysis of 164 sarcomas of the head and neck, Tran et al[4] found malignant schwannomas and neurofibrosarcomas together to account for nearly 10%.

As for the mouth and jaws, in a survey of 352 soft tissue sarcomas of the head and neck Freeman et al[5] found only three neurogenic sarcomas in the oropharyngeal region. Eversole et al[6] reviewed 19 cases of neurogenic sarcoma and presented another. DiCerbo et al[7] were able to retrieve information on 36 intraoral or perioral neurogenic sarcomas reported since 1930, and presented another.

The diagnostic difficulties in recognizing some malignant nerve sheath tumors before the era of monoclonal antibodies or recognition of chromosomal abnormalities, suggests the possibility that these tumors were underrepresented in the earlier studies. Punjabi et al,[8] who reported an example in the parotid gland, have discussed the diagnosis and differential diagnosis.

CLINICAL FEATURES

From the limited data available, Eversole et al[6] suggest that those tumors in the oral soft tissues more frequently affect the cheek or lip, where they form nondescript soft masses. Therefore, the diagnosis is not usually made until after excision. Intraosseous malignant nerve sheath tumors more frequently affect the mandible and can cause paresthesia, anesthesia, or pain.

MICROSCOPY

Appearances are variable. Plump spindle-shaped cells may be arranged in bundles, which may be whorled or interlacing. A matrix of looser fibroblastic cells or of a more mucinous nature may be seen. In well-differentiated tumors Antoni type A tissue may be recognizable, but in all types excessive cellularity, nuclear hyperchromatism, and mitoses are typical. A characteristic finding is an area of necrosis surrounded by elongated cells with a palisaded arrangement. Staining for S-100 protein is positive in up to 50% of these tumors.

Other tumors tend to resemble fibrosarcomas so closely that their neural origin may not be recognizable unless they can be seen to be in continuity with neural tissue or a typical area of neurofibroma. The tumors are usually composed of interlacing bundles of spindle-shaped cells, but looser and shorter than those of fibrosarcomas and with bent nuclei. The cells are either densely aggregated in streaming or swirling patterns, or more loosely arranged in a mucinous or myxoid matrix. Nuclei are typically plump or ovoid and vesiculated. Mitoses are often numerous. The malignant nature of the tumor may be obvious from the cellularity and nuclear changes, but in other cases mitoses may be scanty and the cells lack any significant nuclear abnormalities. However, at the periphery in particular, invasion or tissue destruction may be seen.

DiCerbo et al[7] have summarized previous findings that aid diagnosis (Figs 40.1–40.3), namely:

- association with von Recklinghausen's disease
- origin of the neoplasm within the anatomical compartment of a nerve
- close association of the origin of the tumor in another with the pattern of a neurofibroma
- origin of the neoplasm in the site of a previously excised neurofibroma
- microscopic characteristics as already described, but in particular extreme pleomorphism, numerous mitoses, hypercellularity, and areas of necrosis.

Malignant nerve sheath tumors are associated with the chromosomal abnormalities 17p13 in the region of the p53 tumor

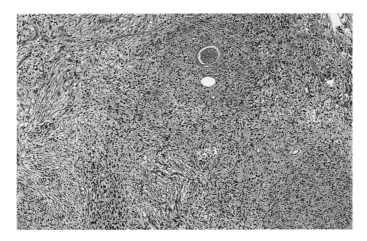

Fig. 40.1 Malignant nerve sheath tumor. Low-power view shows the highly cellular nature of this tumor and conspicuous nuclear pleomorphism and hyperchromatism. A nerve fibril, from which the tumor may have originated, is enclosed.

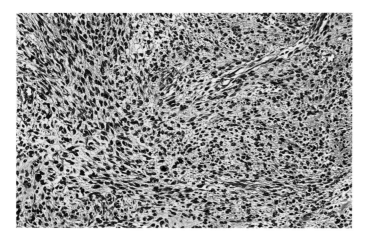

Fig. 40.2 Malignant nerve sheath tumor. Higher power view shows a highly cellular tumor with pleomorphic and hyperchromatic nuclei and abnormal mitoses.

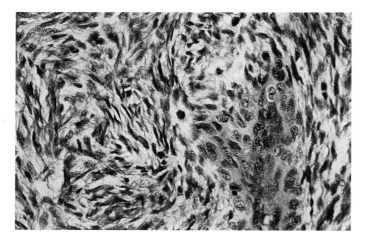

Fig. 40.3 Malignant nerve sheath tumor. The cells retain a sinuous appearance, but mitotic activity is prominent.

suppressor gene and 17q11 near the neurofibromatosis I gene.[9] This may assist diagnosis in difficult cases. Otherwise, resort to electron microscopy may be necessary to identify Schwann cells by recognition of their characteristic basal membrane.

Melanotic malignant schwannoma can cause difficulties of microscopic diagnosis. Two cases involving the oral cavity were reported by Grätz et al,[10] who reviewed the literature. They found reports of 126 malignant schwannomas of the oral cavity, but of only two other melanotic tumors.

The patients reported by Grätz et al[10] were males aged 62 and 79 years. The tumors consisted of elongated spindle cells forming interlacing bundles in a neural pattern. Most of the nuclei showed only mild polymorphism, but there were some atypical cells with bizarre nuclei and showing mitotic activity. There was local palisading and myxoid stromal change. Both tumors contained thickened irregular nerves with enlarged hyperchromatic nuclei. Many cells contained unevenly distributed melanin granules. Reactivity to S-100 protein was only focal, but was intense in both pigmented and nonpigmented cells. No other immunohistochemical stains then available were positive, apart from a diffuse but weak desmin positivity. Use of MMA (melanoma-associated antigen) and HMB-45 may help to distinguish these tumors from melanomas.

BEHAVIOR AND MANAGEMENT

Most malignant nerve sheath tumors are aggressive and pursue a rapid course. However, there are few follow-up data on oral and perioral tumors. In the survey by Eversole et al,[6] most of the patients had been followed up for a matter of months. One patient with a maxillary tumor died within 4 months and another after 1 year. Three patients died after 5 years. The longest survival without recurrence was 4 years. All three patients reported by Neville et al[11] died from their disease, but the patient reported by DiCerbo et al[7] was disease-free after 7 years.

Too little information exists to determine whether the grade of the tumor significantly affects the prognosis, but in the oral and perioral region the tumor stage is likely to be the determining factor.

Radical excision is the treatment of choice. However, the recurrence rate is high, as the tumor may infiltrate along the nerve sheath or spread via the bloodstream. The value of radiotherapy is controversial. Spread to lymph nodes is uncommon.

MALIGNANT TRITON TUMOR

'Malignant Triton* tumor' is the term given to malignant nerve sheath tumors with rhabdomyoblastic differentiation. Approxi-

---

* Triton, the son of the sea god Poseidon, had the advantages of a man's head and trunk but a fish's tail. Triton is also the name given to marine gastropods with large spiral shells and to the nucleus of the tritium atom. How appropriate this term is to the tumor in question is less clear.

mately 60% of malignant Triton tumors are associated with neurofibromatosis type I, and from a review of 27 reported and nine new cases Brooks et al[12] found that 59% were in the head and neck region. However, these tumors have rarely been reported in the oral region and have no distinctive clinical features. One example in the palate was reported by Shotton et al.[13]

MICROSCOPY

Malignant Triton tumors show variable numbers of rhabdomyoblasts scattered in a stroma that is otherwise typical of a malignant nerve sheath tumor. The rhabdomyoblasts typically stand out from the pale neural cells because of their abundant eosinophilic cytoplasm. They may be tadpole-shaped and show cross-striations. They are desmin positive and myoglobin may be demonstrable in the more mature cells.

BEHAVIOR AND MANAGEMENT

Brooks et al,[12] from their analysis of 36 cases, found that there was a high risk of local recurrence and that the 5-year survival rate was 12%.

The rarity of malignant Triton tumors is such that there is little that can be said about the optimal treatment, but it is based on the same principles as that for malignant nerve sheath tumors.

REFERENCES

1. Piatelli A, Angelone A, Pizzicannella G et al 1984 Malignant schwannoma of the tongue: report of a case and review of the literature. Acta Stomatol Belg 81: 213–217
2. Lawrence W, Donegan WL, Natarajan N, Mettlin C, Beart R, Winchester S 1987 Adult soft tissue sarcomas. Ann Surg 205: 349–359
3. Greager JA, Patel MK, Briele HA, Walker MJ, Gupta TKD 1985 Soft tissue sarcomas of the adult head and neck. Cancer 56: 820–824
4. Tran LM, Mark R, Meier R, Calcaterra TC, Parker RG 1992 Sarcomas of the head and neck. Cancer 70: 160–177
5. Freeman AM, Reiman HM, Woods JE 1989 Soft tissue sarcomas of the head and neck. Am J Surg 158: 367–372
6. Eversole LR, Schwartz WD, Sabes WR 1973 Central and peripheral fibrogenic and neurogenic sarcomas of the oral regions. Oral Surg Oral Med Oral Pathol 36: 49–62
7. DiCerbo M, Sciubba JJ, Sordill WC, DeLuke DM 1992 Malignant schwannoma of the palate: a case report and review of the literature. J Oral Maxillofac Surg 50: 1217–1221
8. Punjabi AP, Haug RH, Chung-Park MJA, Likavek M 1996 Malignant peripheral nerve sheath tumor of the parotid gland: report of a case. J Oral Maxillofac Surg 54: 765–769
9. Fletcher JA, Weidner N, Corson JM 1990 Laboratory investigation and genetics in sarcomas. Curr Sci 2: 467–473
10. Grätz KW, Makek M, Sailer HF 1991 Malignant melanotic schwannoma of the oral cavity. J Oral Maxillofac Surg 20: 236–238
11. Neville BW, Hann J, Narang R, Garen P 1991 Oral neurofibrosarcoma associated with neurofibromatosis type I. Oral Surg Oral Med Oral Pathol 72:456–461
12. Brooks JS, Freeman M, Enterline HL 1985 Malignant 'Triton' tumors: natural history and immunohistochemistry of nine new cases and literature review. Cancer 55: 2543–2549
13. Shotton JC, Stafford ND, Breach NM 1988 Malignant Triton tumour of the palate – a case report. Br J Oral Maxillofac Surg 26: 120–123

Neuroectodermal and related small cell tumors

4

Olfactory neuroblastoma (Aesthesioneuroblastoma)

This rare malignant neoplasm originates from the olfactory membrane of the upper nasal cavity or, very occasionally, from ectopic olfactory tissue in the lower nasal cavity, maxillary antrum, or nasopharynx. It is invasive and can metastasize. Though frequently described in textbooks of oral pathology, it rarely involves the oral cavity.

CLINICAL FEATURES

Olfactory neuroblastoma can appear at almost any age, but may have a bimodal peak incidence in the second and fifth decades. It usually causes nasal symptoms such as stuffiness, congestion, rhinorrhea, headache, and epistaxis. Radiographically there is an expanding mass which can be mistaken for a nasal mucocoele or polyp.

Involvement of the oral cavity is rare and only occasional examples have been reported.[1-3] Feifel et al[4] have reported extension of the tumor into the maxillary alveolar ridge with oral instead of nasal symptoms. Olfactory neuroblastoma can also loosen teeth or cause toothache-like pain, paresthesia, or anesthesia, as reviewed by Myers et al.[5] They reported a case in a 79-year-old woman who had expansion of the upper molar alveolar ridge and a granulomatous-looking soft tissue mass associated with a perforation into the maxillary antrum. This tumor was also producing ectopic arginine vasopressin and gave rise to inappropriate antidiuretic hormone production.

MICROSCOPY

Olfactory neuroblastomas display a neural pattern and a lobular architecture of close-packed small round cells with little cytoplasm, in a neurofibrillary matrix. Rosette or pseudorosette formation is common. However, little differentiation may be apparent. Immunohistochemistry may then be helpful. Nonspecific enolase is the most consistently positive marker. S-100 staining is sometimes also positive, as may be synaptophysin and chromogranin to a variable degree. Staining for vimentin, neurofilaments, and keratins is also variable (Figs 41.1–41.3).

BEHAVIOR AND MANAGEMENT

Classification of olfactory neuroblastomas into grades I to IV according to the degree of cellular dysplasia has some bearing on prognosis. The tumor is slow-growing but, in addition to local invasion, the tumor can metastasize to regional lymph nodes, lungs, or bone in 20–40% of cases and also to the orbit or brain. If the brain is involved, the resulting cerebral symptoms can dominate the picture.

Treatment is usually with a combination of surgical excision and radiotherapy, if required. In the series of 15 olfactory neuroblastomas reported by O'Connor et al,[6] only two patients (13%) presented with nodal involvement. They stressed that local control of the primary site by successful surgical resection followed by radiotherapy is the treatment of choice and is unlikely to be followed by distant spread.

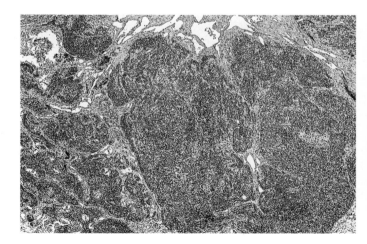

Fig. 41.1 Olfactory neuroblastoma. The lobular pattern of close-packed small round cells with little cytoplasm is typical.

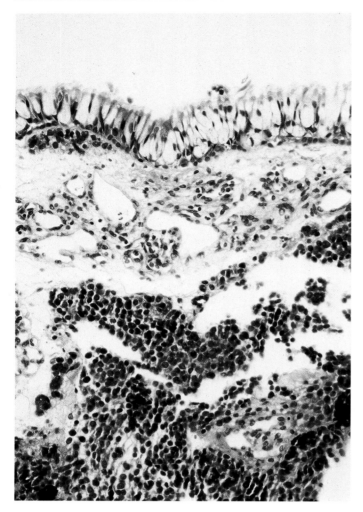

Fig. 41.2 Olfactory neuroblastoma. The round tumor cells are in their typical location beneath a nasal cavity lining.

Cervical paragangliomas (chemodectomas, 'glomus' tumors)

Paragangliomas arise from neuroendocrine cells associated with autonomic ganglia. Paragangliomas in the head and neck include (in order of frequency) carotid body (chemodectoma), jugulotympanic (glomus jugulare and glomus tympanicum), intravagal (glomus vagale), laryngeal, nasal, and orbital tumors. True glomus tumors (glomangiomas) are described in Chapter 42.

Ten per cent are multiple and in 8% other neural crest tumors are associated. Usually these tumors are benign, but up to 6% may be frankly malignant and capable of metastasizing.

Overall, paragangliomas comprise only 0.01% of head and neck tumors. However, they can be important in the differential diagnosis of masses in this area. Glomus jugulare tumors may masquerade as deep or, rarely, as superficial lobe parotid tumors.[7,8] One of the four cervical paragangliomas reported by Wood et al[9] caused distortion of a submandibular gland sialogram. Carotid body tumors may mimic deep lobe parotid tumors, branchial cysts, or cervical lymphadenopathy. Lustman & Ulmansky[10] have reported a paraganglioma causing a rubbery exophytic lump on the tongue, but could find only two other reports of paragangliomas in the mouth.

MICROSCOPY

In paragangliomas, the cells are grouped in clusters or nests, which are often sharply demarcated. The tumor cells typically have rounded nuclei and prominent cytoplasm that ranges from conspicuously granular to clear, and sometimes have well-defined cell membranes. Argyrophil neurosecretory granules can usually be identified by Grimelius staining, but if this fails electron microscopy may be required (Figs 41.4–41.8).

The correlation between the histologic appearances and malignancy is poor. Central necrosis of the cell nests, mitotic activity,

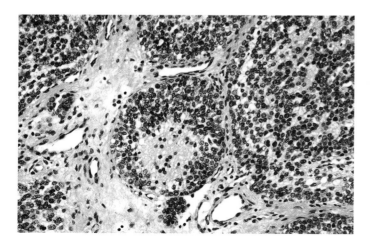

Fig. 41.3 Olfactory neuroblastoma. Higher power view shows the lobules of round cells in a fine fibrillary matrix.

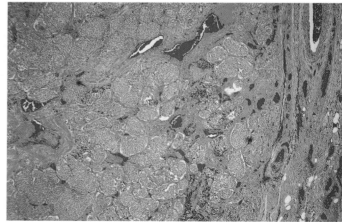

Fig. 41.4 Paraganglioma. A carotid body tumor showing the typical thecal configuration and the prominent vasculature.

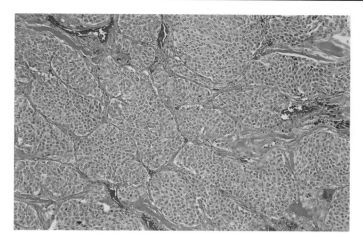

Fig. 41.5 Paraganglioma. Higher power view shows the round nuclei of the tumor cells in the lobular configuration.

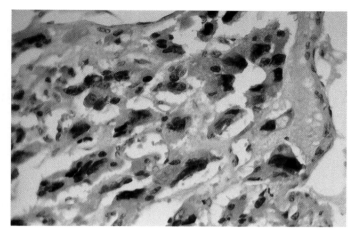

Fig. 41.8 Paraganglioma. The gross nuclear pleomorphism in this tumor does not denote malignancy.

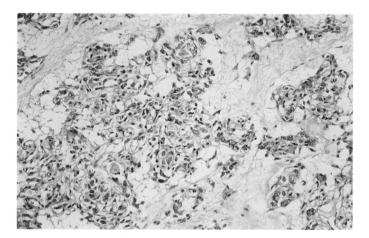

Fig. 41.6 Paraganglioma. In this variant there is prominent vacuolization of the tumor cells, giving some of them a lipoblast-like appearance.

and invasion of vascular spaces suggest malignancy, but can sometimes also be seen in benign paragangliomas.

BEHAVIOR AND MANAGEMENT

Paragangliomas are slow-growing – a 78-year-old woman reported by Wood et al[9] had been aware of the swelling in her neck for 7 years. If a paraganglioma is suspected, computed tomography (CT) scans and angiography are valuable. These tumors are so vascular that, unless very small, angiograms will show their location, vascular supply, and extent. As pressure from these tumors causes turbulence in the carotid blood flow, Doppler ultrasound imaging can aid diagnosis and has the advantage of being noninvasive. Carotid body tumors lying between the internal and external carotid arteries spread them apart, whereas glomus jugulare tumors usually displace them forwards. However, a paraganglioma in an unusual site such as the tongue is unlikely to be suspected, and such investigations would not be considered. Unfortunately also, their vascularity is such that incisional biopsy can cause considerable bleeding.

Despite the microscopic atypia, only about 5% of carotid paragangliomas are malignant, and malignancy in jugulotympanic paragangliomas is virtually unknown. Treatment is by surgical excision. Some tumors are so vascular as to cause troublesome bleeding at operation. The example reported by Brandrick et al[8] was originally thought to be a deep lobe parotid tumor, but unusually severe bleeding at operation led this astute surgeon to suspect a paraganglioma. Incomplete excision is followed by recurrence. Radiotherapy is probably not of value, as the majority of these tumors appear to be relatively radioresistant.

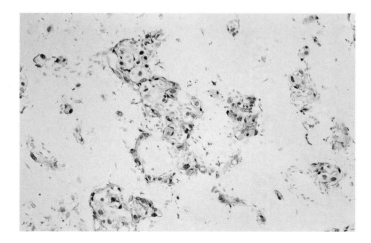

Fig. 41.7 Paraganglioma. S-100 staining of the lipoblast-like cells confirms their neural nature.

Heterotopic brain tissue tumors

These are discussed in Chapter 54.

Ewing's sarcoma

Ewing's sarcoma comprises 10–15% of all primary sarcomas of bone, but fewer than 3% are in the jaws. It predominantly affects the legs or pelvis, but of those that affect the head and neck region the mandible is affected twice as frequently as the maxilla.

The histogenesis of Ewing's sarcoma has long been controversial, but immunocytochemistry has shown that the cells stain for neural markers, particularly neuron-specific enolase or Leu-7 or both. Moreover, the tumor cells may form rosette-like patterns as seen in neuroblastoma and retinoblastoma. Although Ewing's sarcoma cells may stain for vimentin and have been thought to be pluripotential, it is generally accepted that this tumor is neuroectodermal and shares cytogenetic abnormalities with primitive neuroectodermal tumor.[11]

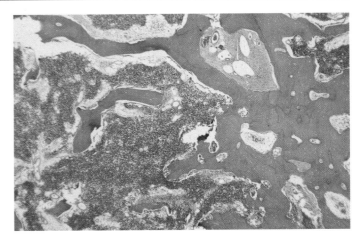

Fig. 41.9 Ewing's sarcoma. Low-power view showing invasion of bone.

CLINICAL FEATURES

The majority of patients are white males, usually aged 5–20 years, and rarely are over 30 years.

Typical symptoms are bone swelling and often pain, progressing over a period of months. Teeth may become loosened and the overlying mucosa ulcerated.

RADIOGRAPHY

Radiographically, Ewing's sarcoma appears as an irregular osteolytic lesion with or without cortical expansion. The onion-skin appearance due to the periosteal reaction that is sometimes seen in long bones is rare in the jaws. The clinical and radiographic findings in 105 reported cases have been reviewed by Wood et al.[12]

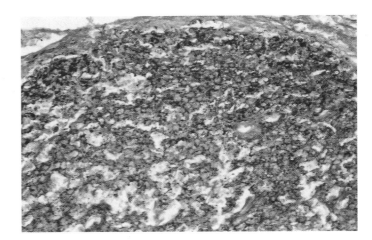

Fig. 41.10 Ewing's sarcoma. Higher power view shows the lymphoma-like cell with vacuolation.

MICROSCOPY

Ewing's sarcoma cells resemble, but are about twice the size of, mature lymphocytes having a darkly staining nucleus surrounded by a rim of cytoplasm, which is typically vacuolated. The tumor cells are in diffuse sheets or in loose lobules, separated by septa. Grouping of tumor cells around blood vessels and areas of hemorrhage and necrosis may be seen (Figs 41.9–41.12).

Important diagnostic features are the presence of intracellular glycogen in approximately 75% of cases, but absence of reticulin from the stroma.

Ewing's sarcoma may be difficult to differentiate from metastatic neuroblastoma or a lymphoma unless intracellular glycogen is detectable. Alcohol fixation is useful for improving the reliability of staining for glycogen. Small cell osteosarcoma may also appear similar, except for small foci of osteoid.

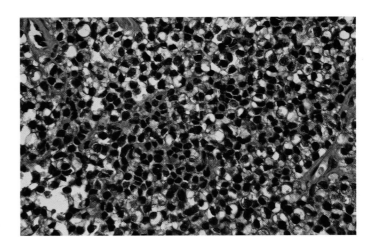

Fig. 41.11 Ewing's sarcoma. PAS stain showing glycogen-rich cells.

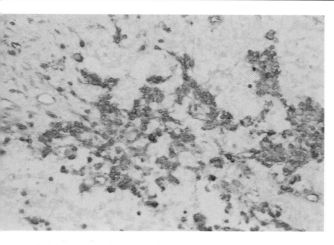

41.12 Ewing's sarcoma showing positive staining for HBA-71.

The cytogenetic abnormality t(11;22)(q24;q12) is found in [?]% of cases. It is of diagnostic value, but fresh tissue is required. [?]etschmer[13] recommends as an alternative the monoclonal anti[bo]dy HBA-71, which reacts with the Ewing-specific antigen [M]C2 and has a sensitivity of up to 98%.

[BE]HAVIOR AND MANAGEMENT

[Th]e most common sites for metastases are the lungs and other [bo]nes. Since Ewing's sarcoma is so rare as a primary tumor in the [jaw]s, the possibility that such a tumor is a metastasis from another [bo]ne may need to be investigated by a skeletal survey. Lymph [no]des are involved in 10–20% of cases. Fever, leucocytosis, raised [ES]R, and anemia indicate a poor prognosis.

[C]urrently, the initial treatment of choice is probably as wide [an] excision as possible, together with megavoltage irradiation and [mu]lti-agent chemotherapy. This combination treatment appears [to] have improved the 5-year survival rate from about 10% to 60% [or] more. However, there is a significant increase in second (par[ticu]larly lymphoreticular) tumors as a consequence of the chemo[the]rapy, and there is insufficient information as to the effec[tiv]eness of multimodal treatment of Ewing's sarcoma of the jaws.

Melanotic neuroectodermal tumor of infancy

[Th]is uncommon tumor was thought in the past to be odonto[gen]ic and was termed *melanotic adamantinoma* because of its [de]velopment in close proximity to the teeth. However, it appears [to] originate from the neural crest.

[C]LINICAL FEATURES

[Me]lanotic neuroectodermal tumors develop in the first year of [lif]e. Mosby et al[14] identified reports of 195 cases, of which 64%

were in the maxilla, 11% in the mandible, 5% in the brain, and isolated examples in almost any other site. In the maxilla it forms an expansile mass, stretching but not ulcerating through the overlying mucosa, which appears bluish because of the underlying pigmentation. Radiographs show an area of bone destruction, with irregular margins and sometimes displacement of teeth.

MICROSCOPY

The tumor consists of slit-like or larger spaces lined by cuboidal, melanin-containing cells in a fibrous stroma. Small round cells, which are nonpigmented, form clusters in the stroma or lie in the alveolar spaces. These round cells resemble those of a neuroblastoma, and may be associated with neurofibrillary material resembling glia (Figs 41.13–41.15).

Ultrastructurally the pigmented cells show both epithelial and melanocytic features. The rounded, nonpigmented cells have

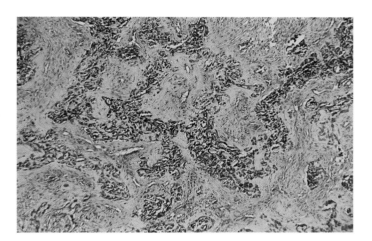

Fig. 41.13 Neuroectodermal tumor of infancy. Slit-like and larger spaces are lined by cuboidal melanin-containing cells in a fibrous stroma.

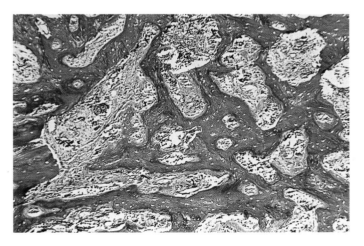

Fig. 41.14 Neuroectodermal tumor of infancy. There is diffuse infiltration of the maxillary bone.

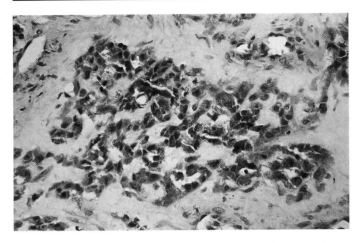

Fig. 41.15 Neuroectodermal tumor of infancy. Melanin granules are prominent in the tumor cells as well as nonpigmented cells lining an alveolar space.

slender cell processes and cytoplasmic neurofilamentous material that suggest a neuroblastic origin. Slootweg[15] has reviewed the immunocytochemistry and confirmed that, unlike melanomas, none of the cells are S-100 positive.

BEHAVIOR AND MANAGEMENT

Radiographs, CT scans, and magnetic resonance imaging are not diagnostic in themselves, but the appearance of a destructive maxillary tumor in the maxilla in an infant together with submucosal pigmentation and high levels of urinary vanillomandelic acid is distinctive. Melanotic neuroectodermal tumor is widely thought to be benign, but up to 15% of cases may recur, and a few have metastasized. Radical excision may be indicated, but where this was not feasible radiotherapy and/or chemotherapy has been used.

REFERENCES

1. Chaudry AP, Haar JG, Koul A, Nickerson PA 1979 Olfactory neuroblastoma (esthesioneuroblastoma): a light and ultrastructural study of two cases. Cancer 44: 564–579
2. Meyrowitz MR, Mauro JV, Mintz S, Schiro W 1984 Olfactory neuroblastoma: report of a case. J Am Dent Assoc 108: 199–201
3. Mills SE, Frierson HF 1985 Olfactory neuroblastoma: a clinicopathologic study of 21 cases. Am J Surg Pathol 9: 317–327
4. Feifel H, Riediger D, Gärtner H-V 1992 Esthesioneuroblastoma. A case report. Int J Oral Maxillofac Surg 21: 292–294
5. Myers SL, Hardy DA, Wiebe CB, Schiffman J 1994 Olfactory neuroblastoma invading the oral cavity in a patient with inappropriate antidiuretic hormone secretion. Oral Surg Oral Med Oral Pathol 77: 645–650
6. O'Connor TA, McLean P, Juillard GJF, Parker RG 1989 Olfactory neuroblastoma. Cancer 63: 2426–2428
7. Rood JP, Landon JD, Rapidis AD, Caruana PE 1982 Carotid sheath tumor – a diagnostic challenge. Oral Surg Oral Med Oral Pathol 53: 554–556
8. Brandrick JT, Das Gupta AR, Singh R 1988 Jugulotympanic paraganglionoma (glomus jugulare tumour) presenting as a parotid neoplasm. J Laryngol Otol 102: 741–744
9. Wood GA, Pogrel MA, Hardman FG 1986 Cervical paragangliomas: a report of four cases. Br J Oral Maxillofac Surg 24: 169–177
10. Lustman J, Ulmansky M 1990 Paraganglioma of the tongue. J Oral Maxillofac Surg 48: 1317–1319
11. Dehner LP 1993 Primitive neuroectodermal tumour and Ewing's sarcoma. Am J Surg Pathol 17: 1–13
12. Wood RE, Nortje CJ, Hesseling P, Grotepass F 1990 Ewing's tumor of the jaw. Oral Surg Oral Med Oral Pathol 69: 120–127
13. Kretschmer CS 1994 Ewing's sarcoma and the 'peanut' tumors. New Engl J Med 331: 325–326
14. Mosby EL, Lowe MW, Cobb CM, Ennis RL 1992 Melanotic neuroectodermal tumor of infancy: review of the literature and report of a case. J Oral Maxillofac Surg 50: 886–894
15. Slootweg PJ 1992 Heterologous elements in melanotic neuroectodermal tumor of infancy. J Oral Pathol Med 21: 90–92

Tumors of blood and lymphatic vessels

42

Hemangiomas

Most hemangiomas are malformations or hamartomas of blood vessels. They are usually either congenital, capillary-type vascular nevi, cavernous, or, frequently, mixed. Unlike most of these, the senile or cherry angioma forms on the lips or other sites late in life. Some hemangiomas, particularly those of bone, can extend during pregnancy, as do pyogenic granulomas.

Hemangiomas form flat or prominent, soft purplish lesions, which characteristically blanch under pressure and can bleed if traumatized. Cavernous hemangiomas may grow in size with age. Extensive congenital cutaneous hemangiomas (port wine stains) of the face can also involve the underlying oral tissues, as discussed below. Large hemangiomas are an occasional cause of macroglossia or macrocheilia. Hemangiomas (usually cavernous or mixed type) can, rarely, form intraosseous tumors, as also discussed below.

MICROSCOPY

Capillary hemangiomas consist of a dense mass of capillaries or imperforate rosettes of endothelium, particularly in infants. Cavernous hemangiomas consist of dilated, blood-filled vascular spaces with endothelial linings, and are frequently poorly circumscibed (Figs 42.1–42.3).

Thromboses may be followed by organization and fibrosis. This can lead to gradual replacement of the vascular component by fibrous tissue containing lipid- and hemosiderin-containing histiocytes. Such a lesion has been termed a *sclerosing hemangioma*, but the term should be avoided as it has also been misapplied to the benign cutaneous fibrous histiocytoma.

BEHAVIOR AND MANAGEMENT

Mucosal hemangiomas should be recognizable clinically and treatment can usually be avoided. Removal of prominent cavernous

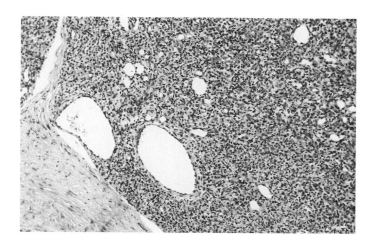

Fig. 42.1 Hemangioma. This capillary type shows the multiplicity of minute vessels.

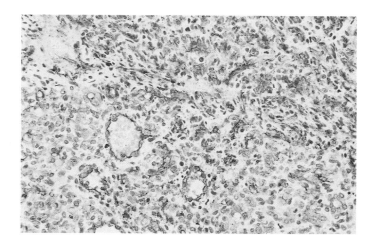

Fig. 42.2 Hemangioma. Capillary hemangioma stained for factor VIII-related antigen shows well-formed as well as small rosettes of endothelial cells without lumens.

hemangiomas should be considered only if there has been significant or recurrent hemorrhage. In such cases, selective embolization may be needed to control bleeding at operation. Angiography may be required to determine the extent of exceptionally large hemangiomas and to identify feeder vessels.

293

Small predominantly capillary lesions, respond well to cryo-therapy, laser ablation, or injection of sclerosing agents. These methods may give better cosmetic results than surgical excision in such sites as the lips.

INTRAMUSCULAR HEMANGIOMA

The intramuscular hemangioma is uncommon. Rossiter et al[1] in their literature review noted that 14–22% of hemangiomas were in the head and neck region and that the masseter muscle was the site of predilection for 36% in this area. They are probably congenital, but are not usually recognized until the second or third decades. They form slow-growing, firm or compressible swellings and may be painful. The diagnosis is unlikely to be made clinically but, if superficial, the overlying skin can become purplish red and warm to the touch or, rarely, undergo pressure necrosis. Of 10 intramuscular hemangiomas of the head and neck region reported by Rossiter et al,[1] five were in the masseter muscle, but only one showed any skin discoloration.

The vascular nature of these tumors may be suggested by calcifications or phleboliths seen on plain radiographs in areas devoid of venous plexuses.

BEHAVIOR AND MANAGEMENT

Intramuscular hemangiomas, unlike some other types, do not appear to regress spontaneously. They can be shown by computed tomography (CT) scanning, but are more clearly delineated by magnetic resonance imaging (MRI) particularly T_2-weighted images. The diagnosis can be substantiated by angiography if necessary, but the latter is probably only indicated when large vascular connections are suspected. Surgical excision is the treatment of choice and effectively also confirms whether or not a malignant tumor is present. It is particularly indicated for cosmetic reasons or uncontrollable pain. Preoperative hemorrhage is a hazard and preoperative embolization may be required. Normal muscle beyond the gross margins of the tumor usually must also be excised, and great care is needed to avoid damage to the facial nerve. Rossiter et al[1] quote recurrence rates of 20%, 9% and 28% for capillary, cavernous, and mixed types, respectively, recurrence being mainly as a consequence of incomplete excision.

MUCOCUTANEOUS ANGIOMATOSIS AND OTHER ANGIOMATOUS SYNDROMES

Vascular nevi of the skin may be part of a syndrome such as the *Sturge Weber syndrome*. The latter comprises angiomatosis within the distribution of the trigeminal nerve and of the ipsilateral leptomeninges. Meningeal involvement leads to epilepsy or hemiparesis and, usually, mental defect. A more limited form consists only of a diffuse vascular nevus of the face and of the underlying oral tissues, including the gingivae. This type may have sharply defined lower and midline boundaries.

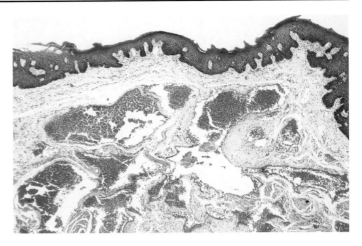

Fig. 42.3 Cavernous hemangioma. Poorly circumscribed, large, dilated blood vessels are within the oral mucosa.

When the gingivae are involved, the swollen tissue can cause false pocketing and inflammation. Rarely, local trauma can induce the formation of a rapidly growing, sarcoma-like mass.

These nevi are developmental anomalies and usually consist of grossly dilated vessels. There may be a genetic component in their etiology, as suggested by several syndromes of which they are a feature. Similar lesions can also be induced by the drug thalidomide given during pregnancy, or be a feature of the fetal alcohol syndrome.

Isolated nevi are rarely of clinical significance unless they are disfiguring. Ugly angiomas of the face can be treated by skin grafting, liquid nitrogen cryotherapy, or laser-induced fibrosis. Management of false pocketing due to hemangioma-induced gingival hyperplasia is by conventional periodontal therapy.

Hereditary hemorrhagic telangiectasia (Osler–Rendu–Weber syndrome) is transmitted as an autosomal dominant trait. It is characterized by multiple telangiectases of skin and mucous membranes. Despite the hereditary nature of the disease, cutaneous telangiectases do not usually become apparent until the age of about 30 years. The cutaneous lesions appear as red macules, small nodules, or spidery capillary networks. Oral lesions appear as red or purplish-red spots, particularly on the lips and tongue.

Microscopically, telangiectases appear as minute knots or loops of dilated vessels with an attenuated lining of endothelium, projecting up immediately beneath the epithelium.

Epistaxis from telangiectases in the nasal mucosa is common and can precede the appearance of cutaneous telangiectases, but significant bleeding from oral telangiectases is rare.

Maffucci's syndrome is a congenital, but not hereditary, disease which comprises multiple enchondromas and hemangiomas, particularly of the skin and sometimes of the oral mucosa. In the patient reported by Kennedy,[2] who reviewed earlier reports, a capillary hemangioma of the tongue was associated with intracranial chondromatosis. The chief hazard of Maffucci's syndrome is the development of malignant tumors, particularly chondrosarcomas in those with extensive skeletal enchondromatosis.

Ataxia telangiectasia is a neurocutaneous disorder in which telangiectasia is associated with progressive cerebellar ataxia, abnormalities of many organs, immunodeficiency, and a greatly raised incidence of lymphomas or, less frequently, carcinomas. Moghadam et al[3] reported a case with oral involvement. They reviewed the condition in detail and earlier reports of oral vascular lesions.

HEMANGIOMAS OF BONE

Hemangiomas form fewer than 1% of tumors of bone, but a high proportion are in the head and neck region. Of these, about 30% are in the jaws with the mandible involved twice as frequently as the maxilla. Women are twice as frequently affected as men, but the tumor can be seen at virtually any age. Hemangiomas of bone present problems of clinical diagnosis and considerable difficulties of management but not of histological diagnosis once the tissue becomes available.

CLINICAL FEATURES

Hemangiomas of the jaw give rise to progressive painless swellings. When the overlying bone becomes sufficiently thinned, the swelling may become pulsatile, teeth may be loosened, and there may be spontaneous bleeding, particularly from gingival margins involved by the tumor. Some of these tumors behave aggressively and rapidly erode surrounding bone. Rarely, a rapidly expanding hemangioma can be associated with the Kasabach–Merritt syndrome[4] of thrombocytopenia, hemorrhagic tendencies, microangiopathic hemolytic anemia, and consumption coagulopathy.

Radiographically, a hemangioma appears as a generally rounded or pseudoloculated area of radiolucency with ill-defined margins and often a soap-bubble appearance.

In view of their overall rarity and in the absence of bleeding or superficial signs of a vascular tumor, the possibility of an intraosseous hemangioma is unlikely to be suspected from the clinical or radiographic appearances. Under such circumstances, there is a significant hazard of hemorrhage at operation. One of the few warning signs is the appearance of a bluish swelling when the periosteum is elevated. Theoretically, hemangioma should be considered in the differential diagnosis of radiolucent lesions of the jaws, particularly those having the radiographic features described earlier. Though it is not feasible to carry out angiography on every doubtful case, the hazards of intraosseous hemangiomas are probably the strongest argument for aspiration of cyst-like lesions of uncertain nature.

MICROSCOPY

Hemangiomas of bone are essentially similar to their soft tissue counterparts. They are usually cavernous, rarely capillary or may be mixed (Fig. 42.4). However, those which are most likely to bleed severely are usually arteriovenous vascular malformations

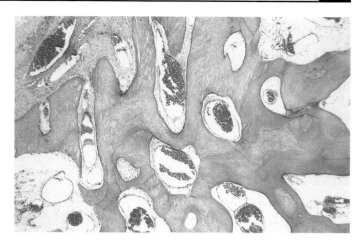

Fig. 42.4 Haemangioma of bone. The more common cavernous type.

rather than true neoplasms. Histologically, the appearances of the latter vary, but there may be large thick- and thin-walled blood vessels in close apposition to each other, sometimes with other areas resembling a capillary hemangioma.

BEHAVIOR AND MANAGEMENT

Opening a hemangioma or extracting a related tooth can give rise to torrential bleeding, which has sometimes proved fatal. Lamberg et al[5] reviewed 11 such cases, where death occurred despite carotid artery ligation in six of them. Larson & Peterson[6] have also reviewed this problem and its management.

Arteriovenous (high-flow) hemangiomas have one or more large feeder arteries, tend to be the most rapidly expanding, and are most likely to bleed profusely when opened. When there are identifiable feeder vessels, selective arterial embolization makes any subsequent resection very much easier and safer. Surgery should follow embolization as soon as possible, and certainly within 3 days, as collateral vessels quickly open up. Wide block resection with margins of normal bone is the only practical method of dealing with high-flow hemangiomas, as recommended by Bunel & Sindet-Pedersen,[7] who also reviewed the variable clinical manifestations and treatment options. Larsen & Peterson[6] have described the hemodynamics of high-flow lesions and means of controlling the development of collateral vessels before surgery.

Hemangioendothelioma

In infants there may be proliferation of the endothelial lining of capillary hemangiomas so that the endothelial cells appear rounded and the lesion consists of thin capillary channels and solid cords of cells. Such lesions are sometimes called *benign hemangioendotheliomas* (Fig. 42.5).

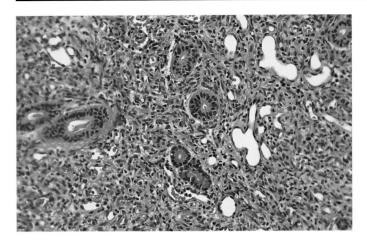

Fig. 42.5   Juvenile haemangioendothelioma. Proliferation of plump endothelial cells has produced some thick-walled vessels among thin-walled capillary channels in this parotid gland tumor.

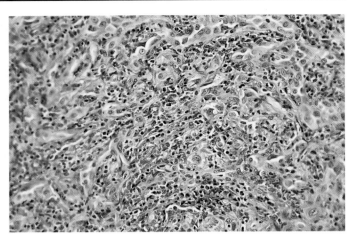

Fig. 42.6   Epithelioid haemangioma. Low-power view shows the epithelioid endothelial cells surrounding small vascular spaces containing blood cells.

However, Enzinger & Weiss[8] otherwise regard hemangioendotheliomas as an ill-defined group of borderline or intermediate malignancy, of which the main type is the epithelioid hemangioendothelioma.

EPITHELIOID HEMANGIOENDOTHELIOMA

Epithelioid hemangioendothelioma was first described by Weiss & Enzinger in 1982.[9] Ellis & Kratochvil[10] reported 12 examples in the head and neck region. Marrogi et al[11] reported two oral epithelioid hemangioendotheliomas and reviewed a total of five others.

Clinically, oral epithelioid hemangioendotheliomas have appeared as pinkish swellings, which sometimes ulcerate. Those reviewed by Marrogi et al[11] were 2–15 mm in size, and three of the five affected the gingivae.

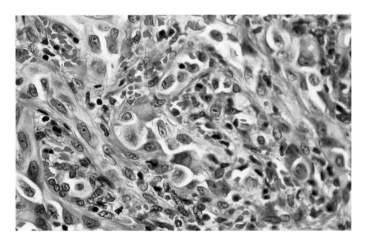

Fig. 42.7   Epithelioid haemangioma. Higher power view shows the conspicuously epithelioid appearance of the endothelial cells and small vascular spaces.

MICROSCOPY

Epithelioid hemangioendotheliomas consist of round to more elongated cells forming short strands or solid nests. Some primitive, poorly formed, vascular channels may be seen, but larger, distinct blood vessels are uncommon. Many cells are vacuolated and contain intracytoplasmic lumina, which may inflate them. There is little mitotic activity and the tumor cells usually show no atypia. They may be closely packed or surrounded by more abundant stroma, which is sometimes hyaline, myxoid, or chondroid in appearance with a high content of sulfated acid mucins similar to those found in normal vessel walls (Figs 42.6 and 42.7).

Reticulin stains outline individual or small clusters of endothelial cells. Reactivity to factor VIII and *Ulex europaeus* are positive but, unlike pyogenic granulomas, staining for smooth muscle actin is negative. There is little or no inflammatory component, but there may be a peripheral lymphoplasmacytic infiltrate.

The epithelioid appearance of the tumor cells can cause them to be confused with a carcinoma and, in particular, intracytoplasmic lumina can mimic those in adenocarcinomas, especially as epithelioid hemangioendothelioma may not be obviously vascular.

BEHAVIOR AND MANAGEMENT

Enzinger & Weiss[8] categorize epithelioid hemangioendothelioma as being of intermediate malignancy, but quote a 13% mortality overall and 65% for those in the lung. By contrast, where information was available, four of the five epithelioid hemangioendotheliomas reviewed by Marrogi et al[11] responded to wide excision without recurrence within periods of 1–4 years.

EPITHELIOID HEMANGIOMA, ANGIOLYMPHOID HYPERPLASIA WITH EOSINOPHILS, AND KIMURA'S DISEASE

Epithelioid hemangioma was first described in 1969 by Wells & Whimster[12] as *angiolymphoid hyperplasia* with *eosinophilia*. Although peripheral eosinophilia is only occasionally found in patients in the West, it is characteristic of Kimura's disease, which shares some features, and causes confusion between these disorders, as discussed below.

Epithelioid hemangiomas typically appear between the ages of 20 and 40 years and affect females more frequently than males. The skin of the head and neck region is most frequently affected and the cutaneous lesions first appear as dull red pruritic plaques. Later, scratching causes excoriation, bleeding, and crusting. Oral lesions are only occasionally encountered, and may resemble pyogenic granulomas or may ulcerate.[13,14]

MICROSCOPY

Proliferation of blood vessels leads to formation of thick-walled capillaries. These vessels are lined by large endothelial cells, which have been likened (somewhat fancifully) to tombstones, and which protrude into the lumen. Often there are noticeable gaps between these cells. There may also be conspicuous smooth-muscle proliferation, producing irregular sheaves of muscle cells between the vessels. Lymphoid proliferation with formation of germinal follicles is most conspicuous at the periphery of the mass. There is a dense stromal inflammatory response, in which eosinophils are typically numerous and may form dense foci with central necrosis. This picture is subject to considerable variation in terms of blood-vessel proliferation and stromal inflammatory reaction (Figs 42.8–42.9).

KIMURA'S DISEASE

This is rare in the West but common in China, Japan, and

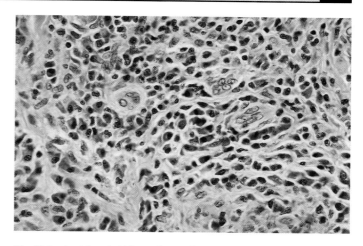

Fig. 42.9 Angiolymphoid hyperplasia with eosinophils. Higher power view to show the characteristic blood-vessel changes and the stromal eosinophil infiltrate.

Singapore. The lesions form deeper masses rather than mucosal or cutaneous nodules and can be mistaken for lymphomas. Involvement of the parotid and submandibular glands and of cervical lymph nodes are typical manifestations.

Microscopically, the lesions are somewhat similar to epithelioid hemangioma, but in the original description by Kimura et al[15] emphasis was laid on the lymphoproliferation rather than the vascular abnormalities. Kuo et al[16] have detailed the differences between Kimura's disease and angiolymphoid hyperplasia with eosinophilia in Taiwanese patients. Both disorders have a predilection for the head and neck region, a tendency to recur, and some histological features in common, as already described. Angiolymphoid hyperplasia with eosinophilia was more frequent in older patients, tended to form cutaneous or mucosal nodules and, despite its name, eosinophilia was frequently absent. Histologically, Kimura's disease lacked epithelioid endothelial cells and frequently showed eosinophilic folliculolysis in the lymphoid tissue, formation of eosinophilic microabscesses, and perinodal eosinophilic infiltrates. Peripheral blood eosinophilia is typically present, serum immunoglobulin (IgE) levels are frequently raised, and IgE deposits may be detected in germinal centers.

BEHAVIOR AND MANAGEMENT

Excision of epithelioid hemangiomas is curative but may have to be repeated.

Intravascular papillary endothelial hyperplasia (Masson's pseudoangiosarcoma)

Intravascular papillary endothelial hyperplasia, despite some similarities in appearance to angiosarcoma, is more probably an

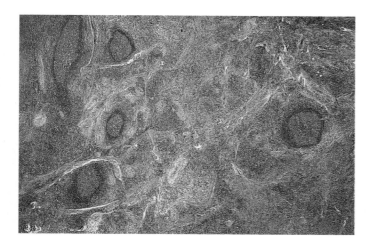

Fig. 42.8 Angiolymphoid hyperplasia with eosinophils. Immensely thick-walled vessels are interspersed by lymphoid follicles.

unusual development of an organizing thrombus. Attention was drawn to the lesion by Rosai & Ackerman in 1974.[17] Since then, Luce et al[18] have described the clinical features and histology in detail, and in reviewing 96 cases found that 21% were in the head and neck region and 13% in the mouth. Females were more commonly affected (52%) than males, and the average age was 40 years. Intravascular papillary endothelial hyperplasia is usually subcutaneous, but Buchner et al[19] were able to report 16 oral examples and also review the condition in detail.

CLINICAL FEATURES

The age of the 16 patients reported by Buchner et al[19] ranged from 30 to 63 years, with a mean of 53 years. Fifty-six per cent of these tumors were in women. The lower lip was most frequently involved (six cases); other sites were the tongue, buccal mucosa, mandibular vestibule, and upper lip. The lesions varied from soft to firm in consistency, were usually bluish, and ranged in size from 0.5 to 1.8 cm in diameter. They resembled mucoceles, varices, or hemangiomas. Their duration varied from 1 month to 6 years.

Wendell et al[20] reported intravascular papillary endothelial hyperplasia that formed a painful submandibular mass that waxed and waned over a 2-year period.

MICROSCOPY

Two types of intravascular papillary endothelial hyperplasia may be seen. A pure type forms within a dilated vascular space, while a mixed type forms as a focal change in a pre-existing vascular lesion such as a hemangioma. However, the microscopic appearances of the two types are the same.

The characteristic histological appearance is that of multiple papillary structures apparently floating freely in vascular spaces. The papillae arise from one or more stalks attached to the vessel wall and are covered by plump endothelial cells, which are uniform in size but are sometimes hyperchromatic. The papillary cores consist of fibrous connective tissue, which is sometimes hyalinized or may contain deposits of hemosiderin. Thrombi in varying degrees of organization can usually be seen and appear to merge with the papillary structures (Figs 42.10–42.12).

Sometimes, variations of these typical appearances have caused intravascular papillary endothelial hyperplasia to be mistaken for an angiosarcoma. Thrombus is occasionally absent, and in some areas the papillae appear to fuse to form slender, anastomosing vascular channels. In other cases proliferation of endothelial cells can lack the typical papillary configuration. Unlike angiosarcomas, intravascular papillary endothelial hyperplasia is typically confined within a vascular space and associated with thrombus formation. The papillae are covered by only by one or two layers of endothelium that lacks nuclear atypia or frequent mitoses. Necrosis is also absent.

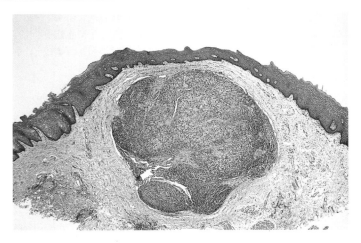

Fig. 42.10　Intravascular papillary endothelial hyperplasia. Low-power view.

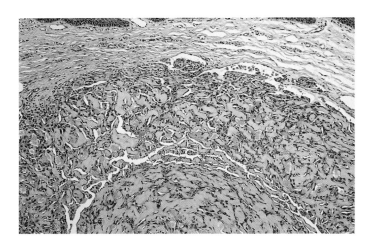

Fig. 42.11　Intravascular papillary endothelial hyperplasia. The remnants of the parent blood vessel, its endothelial lining, and a few erythrocytes are just visible (above right).

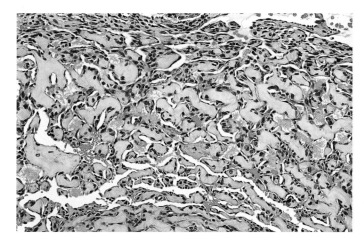

Fig. 42.12　Intravascular papillary endothelial hyperplasia. The multiple hyaline papillary structures have an endothelial covering with plump active-looking nuclei.

BEHAVIOR AND MANAGEMENT

Intravascular papillary endothelial hyperplasia is a benign reactive process and responds to local excision.

Nasiogaryngeal (juvenile) angiofibroma

As noted in Chapter 35, Enzinger & Weiss[8] consider it debatable whether this tumor should be classified as fibrous or vascular, but in practical terms it is a vascular tumor in which surgery can lead to potentially fatal bleeding.

Nasopharyngeal angiofibroma is uncommon, but occasionally involves the oral cavity. With rare exceptions it affects males, usually during adolescence, and is exceptionally uncommon before the age of 10 years. This age and gender distribution suggests a hormonal influence, as reviewed by Weprin & Siemers.[21] Iannetti et al[22] consider that the age of clinical onset may represent asymptomatic growth from the vascular structures of the basosphenoid region, starting at an early period and with symptoms presenting at a late stage of development of the tumor in early adolescence.

CLINICAL FEATURES

Nasopharyngeal angiofibroma typically forms a soft polypoid mass in the nasal cavity or sinuses. It grows both expansively and by peripheral infiltration. Typical early signs are nasal obstruction, infection and bleeding (epistaxes), which can occasionally be life-threatening, or painful. Erosion of the palate can produce an intraoral swelling or bulging of the face, with loss of the nasolabial fold, which may bring the patient to seek attention.

RADIOGRAPHY

Typical features are a soft tissue mass in the nasopharynx, causing forward bulging of the posterior wall of the antrum. The bony margins are usually clearly defined, but may be eroded.

MICROSCOPY

The histology and immunohistochemistry of 32 angiofibromas has been reported by Beham et al.[23] These tumors typically consist of cleft-like or wider vascular spaces in a connective tissue stroma. The walls of the vascular spaces are of variable thickness and have a variable muscle content. They are lined by a single layer of endothelial cells and most lack an elastic lamina. In some places the endothelium is separated from the stroma by only a single attenuated layer of contractile cells; in others there are pad-like

thickenings of the muscle coat. The stroma consists of plump spindle, angular, or stellate cells, with varying amounts of collagen (Figs 42.13 and 42.14).

Beham et al[23] reported that all vessel walls stained for vimentin and smooth-muscle actin. Only a few desmin-positive cells were present and these were mainly seen in vessels with thicker muscle coats. Stromal cells were positive for vimentin only, but in some more fibrotic hyaline areas there was reactivity for smooth muscle actin. These findings highlighted the irregular thickness of the vessel walls, lack of elastic laminae, and lack of stromal elastic fibers, which together seemed likely to be responsible for the strong tendency of these tumors to bleed profusely.

BEHAVIOR AND MANAGEMENT

The microscopic appearances often do not give sufficient indication of the potential for torrential bleeding. Even when an

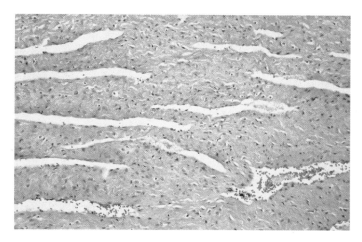

Fig. 42.13 Juvenile angiofibroma. Vascular spaces range from mere clefts to gaping sinusoid-like spaces in a densely fibrous stroma.

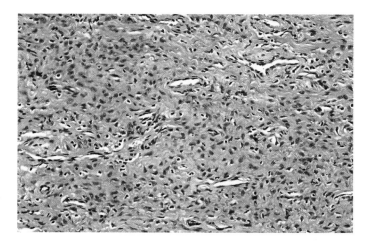

Fig. 42.14 Juvenile angiofibroma. The endothelial lining of vascular spaces is so attenuated as to appear incomplete and separated from the stroma by little in the way of an elastic lamina.

angiofibroma is suspected, the clinical or radiographic picture may be difficult to distinguish from a malignant tumor. However, the risk of dangerous hemorrhage is such that even biopsy is so hazardous that it should be avoided. Reliance is usually therefore placed on the clinical picture and CT scanning, MRI, and angiography. However, if biopsy is considered, it should only be carried out after admission to hospital and in anticipation of heavy bleeding.

Because of the risk of otherwise uncontrollable hemorrhage, bilateral control of the external carotid arteries before excision is essential. Preoperative embolization has been recommended by Siniluoto et al,[24] who found that it limited blood loss to a third of that in previous cases. There were also fewer recurrences, presumably because fuller control of bleeding allowed more complete excision.

Angiofibromas usually behave aggressively and invade surrounding tissues. Iannetti et al[22] recommend a variety of osteotomies for access to angiofibromas, according to their position. Complete excision may require facial reconstruction.

Cryosurgery, radiotherapy, or both are other options, but unless destruction of the tumor is complete the risk of recurrence is high. The hazards of irradiation in the young and the risk of inducing sarcomatous change must also be considered. Moreover, it is not certain that irradiation will cause the fibrous component to regress, but in the short term at least it is likely to control symptoms and cause the tumor to shrink after a single course of 30–35 Gy.

With current imaging techniques, surgery is therefore the treatment of choice, but should only be undertaken with a clear appreciation of the hazards.

In contrast to the dangers of treatment, Weprin & Siemers[21] have reported spontaneous regression of a juvenile angiofibroma over a 12-year period, in a boy whose parents refused consent to surgery. Weprin & Siemers[21] also reviewed earlier reports of spontaneous regression of these tumors after incomplete excision. Whenever possible, therefore, an expectant approach to the management of these tumors should be considered.

Perivascular tumors

HEMANGIOPERICYTOMA

Hemangiopericytoma is a rare tumor. It most frequently arises in the subcutaneous tissues and only occasionally in the mouth. Brockbank[25] found reports of 34 intraoral hemangiopericytomas, of which eight were in the tongue. Kwon et al[26] considered that only one more case involving the tongue had been reported since then. Lesions usually form solitary, firm nodules. Any age may be affected, but infantile hemangiopericytoma as reported by Baker et al[27] may be a different entity, as discussed below.

MICROSCOPY

Hemangiopericytomas vary in appearance, but typically consist of small closely packed cells with ill-defined cytoplasm and darkly staining nuclei. Interspersed among them are many vascular spaces, which may be slit-like or sinusoidal. Occasionally, the pericytes may have a palisaded configuration or may show interstitial mucoid degeneration. Positive silver staining of the capillary basement membrane shows the tumor cells to lie outside it and helps to differentiate pericytomas from tumors of endothelial origin (Figs 42.15–42.17).

Immunohistochemistry shows hemangiopericytoma cells to be variably positive for vimentin, and sometimes focally positive for smooth-muscle actin. However, Baker et al[27] failed to demonstrate myofibrils or dense bodies by electron microscopy. Staining for epithelial and neural markers was also negative.

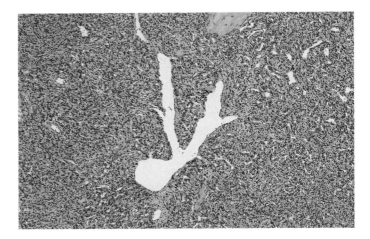

Fig. 42.15 Haemangiopericytoma. Low-power view shows the highly cellular appearance with many small vascular spaces and a typical irregular (staghorn-shaped) space.

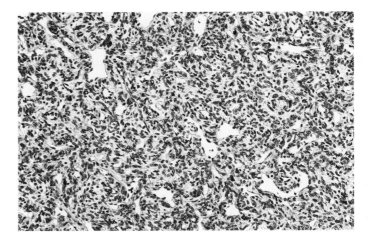

Fig. 42.16 Haemangiopericytoma. The closely packed cells with ill-defined cytoplasm are interspersed with vascular spaces. Some of the pericytes may have a suggestion of a palisaded configuration.

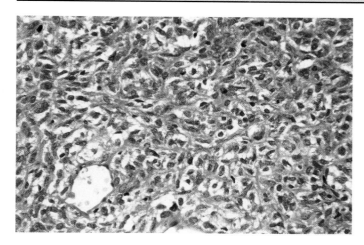

Fig. 42.17 Haemangiopericytoma. Higher power view shows the small closely packed pericytes with ill-defined cytoplasm and darkly staining nuclei, but only a single obvious vascular space.

Other tumors, such as mesenchymal chondrosarcomas or synovial sarcomas, may have extensive hemangiopericytoma-like areas and may be mistaken for the latter.

Rare, more obviously malignant hemangiopericytomas are more cellular, show cellular pleomorphism and mitotic activity, and sometimes areas of hemorrhage or necrosis.

Infantile hemangiopericytomas differ from those in adults in being multilobular and, despite a high mitotic rate, necrosis and hemorrhage, having a benign prognosis. Baker et al,[27] who reported an intraoral infantile hemangiopericytoma, found reports of only four others.

BEHAVIOR AND MANAGEMENT

The behavior of hemangiopericytomas is unpredictable; most are benign but some are infiltrative and can metastasize. Some follow-up information was available for 27 of the 34 cases reviewed by Brockbank,[25] but six recurred after excision and three metastasized.

Some hemangiopericytomas present obviously malignant histological features, but benign histological appearances are not a guarantee of benign behavior.

Adequate excision is the treatment of choice, as these tumors are not radiosensitive. The value of chemotherapy for the more malignant variants has not been widely confirmed.

GLOMUS TUMOR

True glomus tumors arise from specialized arteriovenous shunts involved in body-temperature regulation. Glomus tumors may, to some degree, resemble paragangliomas ('glomus jugulare' etc.) microscopically, but they are distinct entities. Oral glomus tumors are rare, but isolated examples have been reported, for example, by Saku et al[28] who described their immunohistochemical findings, Ficarra et al,[29] and Moddy et al,[30] who also reported immuno-histochemical findings in a glomus tumor of the lip and in 19

other examples. Geraghty et al[31] reported a case and reviewed 14 previous examples.

MICROSCOPY

Glomus tumors are typically circumscribed with a dense fibrous pseudocapsule. They consist of small dark cells with conspicuous punched-out nuclei and pale cytoplasm, surrounding dilated vascular channels lined by endothelium which, unlike the glomus cells, is factor VIII positive. The most common pattern is of solid sheets of cells interspersed with vascular spaces of various sizes, or vascular spaces that break up the tumor cells into a network of strands. Small groups of cells surrounded by dense reticulin fibers can assume a thecal configuration, and individual cells can be shown to be surrounded by basal lamina material forming a chicken-wire appearance. Blood vessels with hypertrophic walls may be scattered randomly within the tumor (Figs 42.18 and 42.19).

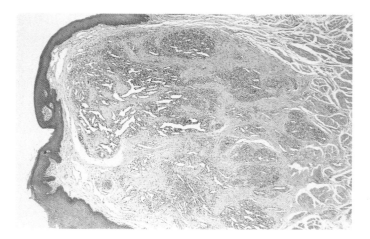

Fig. 42.18 Glomus tumor. Small dark cells surround vascular channels. They are circumscribed by dense fibrous tissue, covered in turn by oral mucosa.

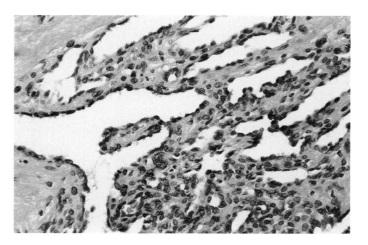

Fig. 42.19 Glomus tumor. Higher power view shows the punched-out nuclei with pale cytoplasm surrounding endothelium-lined vascular channels.

The cell of origin appears to be a modified smooth-muscle cell. It stains for vimentin, myosin, and smooth-muscle actin.

Enzinger & Weiss[8] also distinguish glomus tumors proper, as described above, from glomangiomas and glomangiomyomas, which are less common. Glomangiomas are less well circumscribed, contain dilated vascular spaces and relatively few glomus cells, and resemble hemangiomas clinically. Glomangiomyomas show gradual transition of glomus cells to mature smooth-muscle cells.

BEHAVIOR AND MANAGEMENT

Simple excision is usually effective and recurrence is rare.

LYMPHANGIOMAS

Lymphangiomas are more uncommon than hemangiomas but, like them, may be superficial or deep and capillary or cavernous.

Superficial lymphangiomas are pale or pink, translucent, and may have a finely nodular surface. They may blacken when traumatized as a consequence of bleeding into the lymphatic spaces. Deep lymphangiomas particularly affect the tongue and are another rare cause of macroglossia, or can affect the lip, causing macrocheilia.

A rare variant is the lymphangioma of the alveolar ridge of neonates.

MICROSCOPY

Lymphangiomas differ little histologically from their hemangiomatous counterparts and consist of capillary or cavernous lymphatic channels, but these appear empty or filled with eosinophilic colloidal material (Figs 42.20 and 42.21).

Capillary lymphangiomas frequently cannot be distinguished from hemangiomas if there has been pre- or perioperative bleeding into the capillary spaces. 'Cystic hygroma' is a term given to cavernous lymphangiomas with unusually large, cyst-like lymphatic spaces; it is most common in the neck.

BEHAVIOR AND MANAGEMENT

Lymphangiomas need only to be treated if frequently traumatized, with resulting inflammation and swelling. However, lymphangiomatous macroglossia may interfere with swallowing, cause drooling and, when traumatized, enlarge and become infected. Excision is then necessary. Small lesions can be resected completely. Limited resection, sufficient to restore normal function, can be carried out on large lesions, and there is a good chance that the lesion will remain static after growth is complete. Large lymphangiomas in the neck require very extensive dissection which, if possible, is best delayed until growth is completed.

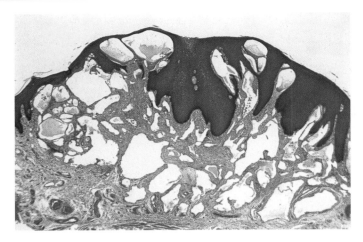

Fig. 42.20   Lymphangioma. Cavernous lymphatic spaces extend superficially into the oral mucosa.

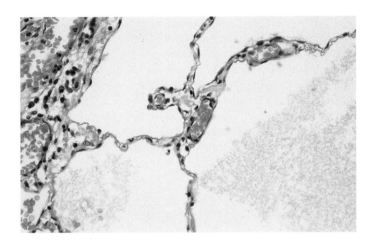

Fig. 42.21   Lymphangioma. The lymphatic spaces are surrounded by septa containing blood vessels. The delicacy of these septa is such that slight trauma causes bleeding into the lymphatic spaces.

LYMPHANGIOMAS OF THE ALVEOLAR RIDGES OF NEONATES

Levin et al[32] have described previously unrecognized lymphangiomas of the alveolar ridges of neonates. They were found in 3.7% of 1470 black neonates, but not in any of 582 whites. These lymphangiomas formed blue-domed, fluid-filled swellings on the posterior crest of the maxillary alveolar ridge and posterior lingual surface of the mandibular ridge. They could be unilateral or bilateral, in either or both jaws.

Microscopy

All specimens consisted of numerous slit-like spaces lined by what appeared to be endothelium with scanty intervening connective tissue stroma without any inflammatory infiltrate. Better defined vascular channels with endothelial lining were sometimes evident. The spaces sometimes contained red blood cells, which probably extravasated during excision.

REFERENCES

1. Rossiter JL, Hendrix RA, Tom LWC, Potsic WP 1993 Intramuscular hemangioma of the head and neck. Otolaryngol Head Neck Surg 108: 18–26
2. Kennedy JG 1973 Dyschondroplasia and haemangiomata (Mafucci's syndrome). Report of a case with oral and intracranial lesions. Br Dent J 135: 18–21
3. Moghadam BKH, Yadeh JY, Gier RE 1993 Ataxia-telangiectasia. Review of the literature and a case report. Oral Surg Oral Med Oral Pathol 75: 791–797
4. Kasabach HH, Merritt KK 1940 Haemangioma with exensive purpura. Am J Dis Child 59: 1063–1067
5. Lamberg MA, Tasanen A, Jääskeläinen J 1979 Fatality from central hemangioma of the mandible. J Oral Surg 37: 578–584
6. Larson PE, Peterson LJ 1993 A systematic approach to management of high-flow vascular malformations of the mandible. J Oral Maxillofac Surg 51: 62–69
7. Bunel K, Sindet-Pedersen S 1993 Central hemangioma of the mandible. Oral Surg Oral Med Oral Pathol 75: 565–570
8. Enzinger FM, Weiss SW 1995 Soft tissue tumors, 3rd edn. St Louis: C V Mosby
9. Weiss SW, Enzinger FM 1982 Epithelioid haemangioendothelioma: a vascular tumor often mistaken for a carcinoma. Cancer 50: 970–981
10. Ellis GL, Kratochvil FJ 1986 Epithelioid haemangioendothelioma of the head and neck: a clinicopathologic report of twelve cases. Oral Surg Oral Med Oral Pathol 61: 61–68
11. Maroggi AJ, Boyd D, El-Mofty SK, Waldron C 1991 Epithelioid haemangioendothelioma of the oral cavity: report of two cases and review of literature. J Oral Maxillofac Surg 49: 633–636
12. Wells GC, Whimster I 1969 Subcutaneous angiolymphoid hyperplasia with eosinophilia. Br J Dermatol 81: 1–5
13. Razquin S, Mayoyo E, Citores MA, Alvira R 1991 Angiolymphoid hyperplasia with eosinophilia of the tongue: report of a case and review of the literature. Hum Pathol 22: 837–839
14. Toeg A, Kermish M, Grishkin A, Temkin D 1993 Histiocytoid hemangioma of the oral cavity. J Oral Maxillofac Surg 51: 812–814
15. Kimura T, Yoshimora S, Tshikawa E 1948 On the unusual granulation combined with hyperplastic changes of lymphoid tissue. Trans Soc Pathol (Jpn) 37: 179–183
16. Kuo T-T, Shih L-Y, Chan H-L 1988 Kimura's disease. Involvement of regional lymph nodes and distinction from angiolymphoid hyperplasia with eosinophilia. Am J Surg Pathol 12: 843–854
17. Rosai J, Ackerman LR 1974 Intravascular atypical vascular proliferation. Arch Dermatol 109: 714–717
18. Luce EB, Montgomery MT, Redding SW, Aufdemorte TB 1988 Intravascular angiomatosis (Masson's lesion). J Oral Maxillofac Surg 46: 736–741
19. Buchner A, Merrell PW, Carpenter WM, Leider AS 1990 Oral intravascular papillary endothelial hyperplasia. J Oral Pathol Med 19: 419–422
20. Wendell AE, High CL, Fowler CB, Finn RA 1994 Well-circumscribed recurring facial mass. J Oral Maxillofac Surg 52: 177–182
21. Weprin LS, Siemers PT 1991 Spontaneous regression of juvenile nasopharyngeal angiofibroma. Arch Otolaryngol Head Neck Surg 117: 796–797
22. Iannetti G, Belli E, De Ponte F, Cicconetti A, Delfini R 1994 The surgical approaches to nasopharyngeal angiofibroma. J Cranio Max Fac Surg 23: 311–316
23. Beham A, Fletcher CDM, Kainz J, Schmid C, Humer U 1993 Nasopharyngeal angiofibroma: an immunohistochemical study of 32 cases. Virchows Arch A Pathol Anat 423: 281–285
24. Siniluoto TMJ, Luotonen JP, Tikkakoski TA, Leinonen ASS, Jokinen KE 1993 Value of pre-operative embolization in surgery for nasopharyngeal angiofibroma. J Laryngol Otol 107: 514–521
25. Brockbank J 1979 Hemangiopericytoma of the oral cavity: report of case and review of the literature. J Oral Surg 37: 659–664
26. Kwon H-J, Browne GA, Posalaky IP, Waite DE 1984 Hemangiopericytoma of the tongue: report of a case. J Am Dent Assoc 109: 583–585
27. Baker DL, Oda D, Myall RWT 1992 Intraoral infantile hemangiopericytoma. Oral Surg Oral Med Oral Pathol 73: 596–602
28. Saku T, Okabe H, Matsutani K, Sasaki M 1985 Glomus tumor of the cheek: and immunohistochemical demonstration of actin and myosin. Oral Surg Oral Med Oral Pathol 60: 65–71
29. Ficarra G, Merrell PW, Johnston WH, Hansen LS 1986 Intraoral solitary glomus tumor (glomangioma): case report and literature review. Oral Surg Oral Med Oral Pathol 62: 306–311
30. Moody GH, Myskow M, Musgrove C 1986 Glomus tumor of the lip. A case report and immunohistochemical study. Oral Surg Oral Med Oral Pathol 62: 312–318
31. Geraghty JM, Thomas RWN, Robertson JM, Blundell JW 1992 Glomus tumour of the palate: case report and review of the literature. Br J Oral Maxillofac Surg 30: 398–400.
32. Levin LS, Jorgenson RJ, Jarvey BA 1976 Lymphangiomas of the alveolar ridges in neonates. Pediatrics 58: 881–884

Kaposi's sarcoma, bacillary angiomatosis, and angiosarcoma

43

Kaposi's sarcoma

Classical (sporadic) Kaposi's sarcoma was described by Moritz Kaposi in 1872[1] in Central Europe among elderly persons of Mediterranean or Jewish origin, as a multiple pigmented sarcoma of the skin. It is predominantly cutaneous, mainly affects the lower extremities, and visceral lesions are rarely clinically apparent. Head and neck involvement is exceedingly rare. Kaposi's sarcoma with broadly similar characteristics is also common in Africa, particularly in Zaire, where it formed about 12% of all malignant tumors in the pre-AIDs era.

From being a rarity in the Western world, Kaposi's sarcoma has become epidemic with the spread of HIV infection, and is sometimes also seen in organ-transplant patients as a consequence of deep immunosuppression. However, the tumor is predominantly seen in homosexual or bisexual males or in those who have had sexual relations with them.[2] It is associated with a CD4 lymphocyte count of less than 200 cells/μl. Rarely, Kaposi's sarcoma has been seen in homosexual or bisexual males who are HIV-negative.[3,4] There are thus strong reasons for regarding Kaposi's sarcoma as a sexually transmitted disease.

In such patients the tumor has changed in its sites of predilection, and in some areas of the USA, for example, has become the most common malignant tumor of the oral cavity. It is this type of Kaposi's sarcoma that is mainly discussed here. Its clinical features, microscopy, and pathogenesis have been reviewed in detail by Wang et al.[5]

CLINICAL FEATURES

AIDS-related Kaposi's sarcoma frequently involves the head and neck. Lamster et al[6] found oral Kaposi's sarcoma in nearly 5% of 63 HIV-positive, male homosexuals and no cases among 57 HIV-positive intravenous drug users. Overall, probably 12–25% HIV-positive homosexual males present with Kaposi's sarcoma. It can sometimes be the initial manifestation of HIV infection, as noted by, for example, Epstein & Silverman,[7] or appear later in the course of AIDS. However, oral Kaposi's sarcoma is frequently associated with other manifestations of HIV infection, such as candidosis, hairy leukoplakia, or HIV-associated gingivitis. It may be the cause of early symptoms, but the tumor is usually multifocal, with lesions affecting skin, lymph nodes, and viscera. At autopsy most organs are frequently found to be involved.

Otherwise, the site may be oropharyngeal, cutaneous, or in the cervical lymph nodes. Within the mouth the palate is most frequently affected, and the tumor typically produces a flat or nodular purplish lesion. It can have a similar site of predilection in immunosuppressed patients, but is a relatively rare complication of such treatment in the West. The clinical differential diagnosis is from oral purpura, bacillary angiomatosis and pyogenic granulomas, from which it can be distinguished by microscopy. Primary intraosseous Kaposi's sarcoma is rare, but two cases have been reported by Langford et al.[8]

Kaposi's sarcoma is associated with a high rate of second neoplasms, particularly lymphomas, and clinical suspicion of the diagnosis of Kaposi's sarcoma is also strengthened by coexisting or a history of opportunistic infections.

A viral cause has long been suspected and the current candidate is human herpes virus 8 (HHV-8). HHV-8 DNA can be found in Kaposi's sarcoma cells, and patients with both HIV and HHV-8 infection appear to have a high risk of developing Kaposi's sarcoma.[9]

MICROSCOPY

Kaposi's sarcoma originates in endothelial cells, as shown by immunoreactivity for factor VIII and CD34.

The tumor produces florid angiomatoid proliferation, with some resemblance to granulation tissue. Recognition of the tumor may therefore be difficult, particularly in the early stages.

In the earliest ('presarcomatous') stage there is angiomatous proliferation, with formation of irregular slit-like vascular spaces and perivascular cuffing by lymphocytes and plasma cells. In the intermediate stage the angiomatoid changes are more widespread with irregular vascular spaces, together with perivascular proliferation of spindle-shaped and angular cells. Finally, the picture becomes increasingly dominated by proliferation of the interstitial spindle-shaped and angular cells, and mitoses may be prominent. There is typically also extravasation of erythrocytes and deposition of hemosiderin, and there may be central necrosis (Figs 43.1–43.3).

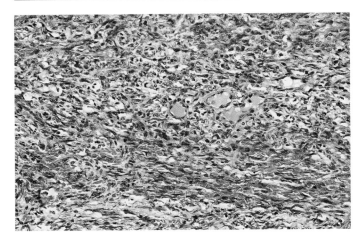

Fig. 43.1 Kaposi's sarcoma. The florid angiomatoid proliferation bears some resemblance to granulation tissue.

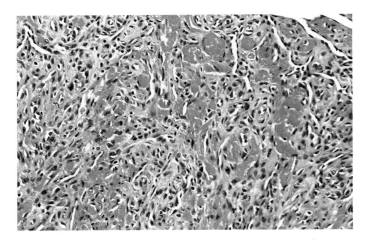

Fig. 43.2 Kaposi's sarcoma. In this area, there are few vascular spaces. Spindle cells predominate and show some mitotic activity.

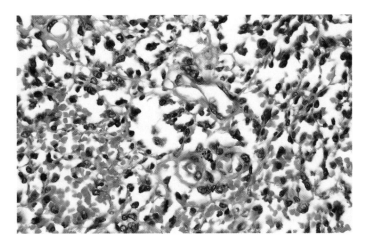

Fig. 43.3 Kaposi's sarcoma. Higher power view of the spindle and angular cells some of which surround vascular spaces.

These appearances vary with the stage of development of the tumor. In a 10-year retrospective study of 120 oral Kaposi's sarcomas, Regezi et al[10] found that the tumors fell into two categories: small, well-delineated lesions, and larger infiltrative lesions. Small lesions had an intact surface and, microscopically, the flat surface reflected the macular appearance clinically. The tumors were confined to the superficial submucosa, separated from the epithelium by a connective tissue band, but had mild, scattered lymphocytic infiltration.

Small lesions typically consisted of inconspicuous proliferation of spindle- to oval-shaped cells, which often formed ill-defined vascular spaces. The latter were usually lined by spindle cells, but oval or polygonal cells were also seen. Occasionally, capillaries were seen towards the periphery. The spindle and oval cells were usually seen in patches, but occasionally formed isolated nodules. Extravasated red cells were seen among the spindle cells in 94% of tumors, but deposits of hemosiderin were seen in only 42%. Hyaline globules (phagocytosed erythrocytes) were seen in 45%. Nuclear atypia (hyperchromatism and pleomorphism) was infrequently noted and mitoses were seen in 26%.

Nearly half the patients with small circumscribed lesions had multifocal disease, which frequently progressed to nodular lesions.

Larger, infiltrative lesions consisted of spindle-shaped cells, which formed slit-like vascular spaces. The vessels frequently formed sharp angles or multiple branches, or dilated spaces particularly in the zone immediately beneath the surface. Extravasated red cells were invariably present, while hemosiderin deposits and hyaline globules were as frequently seen as in small lesions. Mitotic figures were noted in 62% of large lesions and varied in number from 1 to 14 per high power field.

Immunoreactivity for CD34 antigen was positive in most spindle cells in all cases of Kaposi's sarcoma, irrespective of size. CD34 immunoreactivity was seen in cells lining vascular spaces or inconspicuous vascular slits in small lesions, and in endothelium of surrounding vessels. CD34 reactivity appears to be the most reliable marker of endothelial progenitor cells and is valuable in the diagnosis of Kaposi's sarcoma. This has been confirmed, in fixed paraffin sections, by Russell Jones et al,[11] who found it more satisfactory than CD31 but that the relative reactivity varied with the stage of the tumor. Both CD34 and CD31 were more reliable than other markers such as *Ulex europaeus* (UEA-1) and factor-VIII-related antigen.

The differential diagnosis of Kaposi's sarcoma from the considerably more uncommon bacillary angiomatosis is discussed in the following section.

BEHAVIOR AND MANAGEMENT

In 'classical' (sporadic) Kaposi's sarcoma, radiotherapy is the accepted treatment for localized disease, while combined, cytotoxic chemotherapy is used for disseminated disease.

In the case of epidemic (AIDS-associated) Kaposi's sarcoma, a great variety of treatment regimens such single-agent, combined chemotherapy, or zidovudine with interferon-α and radiotherapy have been tried.[12] The short-term prognosis of the tumor itself as a result of such treatment is often good, and death is usually from associated opportunistic infections. Circumscribed lesions localized within the mouth and associated with a CD4 T-lymphocyte count of more than 500 cells/μl may be treated by excision, cryotherapy, or even sclerotherapy, or with two or three fractions of radiotherapy, to which they rapidly respond. At a CD4 level of fewer than 200 cells/μl systemic chemotherapy and antiretroviral treatment is advisable, while for intermediate CD4 counts interferon with zidovudine may be appropriate.

The prognosis of Kaposi's sarcoma deteriorates greatly with spread to the lungs or other viscera and CD4 counts of fewer than 100/cells/μl.

Bacillary (epithelioid) angiomatosis

Bacillary angiomatosis is an uncommon angioproliferative lesion that particularly affects patients with HIV infection. It causes purplish papulonodular lesions, which can be mistaken clinically for Kaposi's sarcoma.[13] However, the causative bacteria can be identified. It is essential to make the distinction, as bacillary angiomatosis is potentially curable with antimicrobial treatment.

Bacillary angiomatosis is caused by a small plemorphic Gram-negative bacillus that can only be visualized in lesions by use of a silver stain such as Warthin–Starry[14] and is difficult to culture. It has been identified as *Bartonella henselae*.[15] 16S ribosomal sequencing for the bacterial protein can be used as an alternative method of diagnosis.

B. henselae also causes cat-scratch disease, a common cause of lymphadenopathy in immunocompetent persons in the USA, and about 70% of patients with bacillary angiomatosis give a history of contact with a cat. However, the mode of transmission is uncertain, as many cats have asymptomatic *Bartonella* bacteremia, and the bacterium can also be found in their fleas. *B. henselae* is closely related to *Bartonella quintana*, which causes trench (quintan) fever, and either species seems to be able to cause bacillary angiomatosis.

CLINICAL FEATURES

Bacillary angiomatosis usually causes multiple, tender, red skin lesions resembling pyogenic granulomas in appearance. They usually blanch on pressure, and often grow very rapidly. Perioral lesions may be seen, and liver or spleen involvement is also possible. Although intraoral lesions are uncommon, oral bacillary angiomatosis in the absence of cutaneous lesions has been reported as the first sign of HIV infection by Speight et al.[16] A febrile illness is typically associated. Liver involvement can lead to *peliosis hepatis* (blood-filled liver cysts).

MICROSCOPY

Lesions of bacillary angiomatosis consist of (Fig. 43.4):

- Lobular proliferation of small blood vessels: these are lined by large endothelial cells, sometimes termed 'epithelioid' or 'tombstone' cells, which protrude into the lumens.
- Epithelial collarettes.
- An edematous stroma containing scattered neutrophils and leucoclastic debris.
- Clumps of amorphous, eosinophilic, granular material that can be shown to consist of masses of the causative bacteria by Warthin–Starry staining or electron microscopy.

In the differential diagnosis from Kaposi's sarcoma, attention is drawn to the circumscribed and multilobular configuration of bacillary angiomatosis, with its prominent epithelioid endothelial cells protruding into the lumens of small blood vessels, but with an absence of spindle-cell proliferation with vascular slits and the causative bacteria appearing as clumps of amorphous eosinophilic material. The diagnosis can be confirmed by demonstration of *Bartonella* by appropriate staining, 16S ribosomal sequencing, electron microscopy, or serology.

BEHAVIOR AND MANAGEMENT

Since bacillary angiomatosis is not neoplastic, it is clearly essential to exclude Kaposi's sarcoma, as described above. Bacillary angiomatosis should be treated by antimicrobial chemotherapy. Currently, erythromycin appears to be the most effective drug, and bacillary angiomatosis appears to respond better than cat-scratch disease to it. Alternatives are trimethoprim–sulfamethoxazole, rifampicin, or doxycycline. In the event of relapse, a 3-month course of one of the alternative antibiotics is required. Deaths from bacillary angiomatosis have mainly been secondary.

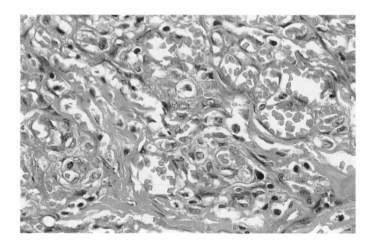

Fig. 43.4 Bacillary angiomatosis. Small blood vessels are lined by large endothelial cells.

Angiosarcoma

ANGIOSARCOMA OF SOFT TISSUES

Attempts to divide angiosarcomas into subcategories have been unsatisfactory so that Enzinger & Weiss[17] use the term *angiosarcoma* for malignant tumors of endothelial cells, whether these are of capillaries or lymphatics.

Angiosarcomas are distinctly uncommon, particularly in the oral cavity. Hodgkinson et al,[18] in reporting 13 patients with cutaneous angiosarcomas, noted one example in the lower lip. In an analysis of 366 angiosarcomas seen over a 10-year period, Enzinger & Weiss[17] found that only 4% were in the oral cavity, pharynx or nasal sinuses. By contrast, the skin of the head and neck region is the single most frequent site of these tumors.

Oliver et al[19] have reported a rare example of an intraoral angiosarcoma in a 69-year-old Vietnamese woman. It caused extreme tenderness of the floor of the mouth, dysphagia, and hemorrhage on minor trauma. Within the mouth the tumor appeared as an obvious hemorrhagic lesion involving the anterior floor of the mouth, lateral border of the tongue, and extending back to the right tonsillar fossa.

MICROSCOPY

Angiosarcomas range from those with capillary-like spaces lined by plump endothelial cells showing few mitoses (grade I) to those where vascular formation can only be recognized by reticulin staining to show malignant endothelial cells within its sheath (grade III). These cells are mitotically active, have prominent nucleoli, and there are foci of necrosis. Lymphocytes and eosinophils can sometimes be so numerous in the stroma as to lead to misdiagnosis if the biopsy is inadequate (Fig. 43.5).

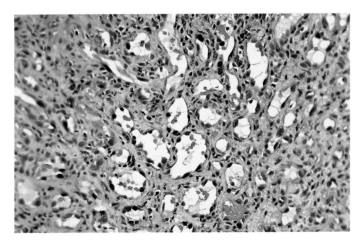

Fig. 43.5   Angiosarcoma. A moderately well-differentiated tumor with plump endothelial cells with large vesiculated nuclei, and prominent nucleoli lining small vascular spaces.

Poorly differentiated endothelial cells may fail to react for factor-VIII-related antigen, but may be identified by more sensitive markers such as *Ulex europaeus 1* lectin and for CD34.

BEHAVIOR AND MANAGEMENT

The prognosis appears to depend greatly on the degree of differentiation; well-differentiated examples (grade I; sometimes termed *hemangioendotheliomas*) are less likely to metastasize. The treatment of choice appears to be wide surgical excision with radiotherapy for any inaccessible areas of tumor. The patient reported by Hodgkinson et al[18] died from her disease within 5 years, despite surgical removal of the lesion and radiotherapy.

ANGIOSARCOMA OF BONE

Angiosarcoma is a particularly rare bone tumor. In reviewing 133 reported cases, Barnes et al[20] could identify only seven examples reported in the mandible.

Dull pain and swelling are typical symptoms and, like other malignant tumors, angiosarcoma can loosen teeth. If neglected, the tumor can erode through the bone and spread into the soft tissues. Radiographically, there is a poorly circumscribed area of radiolucency without any distinguishing features.

MICROSCOPY

The microscopic appearances are essentially the same as those of the soft tissue counterpart.

BEHAVIOR AND MANAGEMENT

Data on the prognosis of angiosarcomas of the jaws are extremely limited, but it is likely to be poor.

REFERENCES

1. Kaposi M 1872 Idiopathisches multiple pigmentsarkom der Haut. Arch Dermatol Syphilis 4: 265–273 (Chem Abs 1982; 32: 342–347)
2. Beral V, Peterman TA, Berkelman RL, Jaffe HW 1990 Kaposi's sarcoma among persons with AIDS: a sexually transmitted infection. Lancet 335: 123–128
3. Marquart KH, Engst R, Oehlschaegel G 1991 An 8-year history of Kaposi's sarcoma in an HIV-negative bisexual male. AIDS 5: 346–347
4. Vandercam B, Tennstedt D, Gala JL, Bodeus M, Louwagie J, Burtonboy G 1991 Kaposi's sarcoma in a human immunodeficiency virus-negative homosexual man. J Infect Dis 164: 214–218
5. Wang C-Y E, Schroeter, AL, Su W P D 1995 Acquired immunodeficiency syndrome-related Kaposi's sarcoma. Mayo Clin Proc 70: 869–879
6. Lamster IB, Begg MD, Mitchell-Lewis D et al 1994 Oral manifestations of HIV infection in homosexual men and intravenous drug users. Study design and relationship of epidemiologic, clinical and immunologic parameters to oral lesions. Oral Surg Oral Med Oral Pathol 78: 163–174
7. Epstein JB, Silverman S 1992 Head and neck malignancies associated with HIV infection. Oral Surg Oral Med Oral Pathol 73: 193–200
8. Langford A. Pohle H-D, Reichart PA 1991 Primary intraosseous AIDS-associated Kaposi's sarcoma. Report of two cases with initial jaw involvement. Int J Oral Maxillofac Surg 20: 366–368

9. Rickinson AR 1996 Changing seroepidemiology of HHV-8. Lancet 348: 1110–1111

10. Regezi JA, MacPhail LA, Daniels TE et al 1993 Oral Kaposi's sarcoma: a 10-year retrospective histopathologic study. J Oral Pathol Med 11: 292–297

11. Russell Jones R, Orchard G, Zelger B, Wilson Jones E 1995 Immunostaining for CD31 and CD34 in Kaposi sarcoma. J Clin Pathol 48: 1011–1016

12. Northfelt DW 1994 Treatment of Kaposi's sarcoma. Current guidelines and future perspectives. Drugs 48: 569–582

13. Glick M, Cleveland DB 1993 Oral mucosal bacillary epithelioid angiomatosis in a patient with AIDS associated with rapid alveolar bone loss: case report. J Oral Pathol Med 22: 235–239

14. Cotell SL, Noskin GA 1944 Bacillary angiomatosis. Clinical and histologic features, diagnosis and treatment. Arch Intern Med 154: 524–554

15. Tompkins LS 1994 *Rochalimaea* infections. Are they zoonoses? JAMA 271: 553–554

16. Speight PM, Zakrzewska J, Fletcher CDM 1990 Epithelioid angiomatosis affecting the oral cavity as the first sign of HIV infection. Br Dent J 171: 367–370

17. Enzinger FM, Weiss SW 1995 Soft tissue tumors, 3rd edn. C V Mosby, St Louis.

18. Hodgkinson DJ, Soule EH, Woods JE 1979 Cutaneous angiosarcoma of the head and neck. Cancer 44: 1106–1113

19. Oliver AJ, Gibbons SD, Radden BG, Busmains I, Cook RM 1991 Primary angiosarcoma of the oral cavity. Br J Oral Maxillofac Surg 29: 38–41.

20. Barnes L 1985 Diseases of the bones and joints. In: Barnes L (ed). Surgical pathology of the head and neck. Marcel Dekker, New York, pp. 883–1044.

Tumors and tumor-like diseases of striated muscle

44

MUSCLE DEGENERATION AND REGENERATION

Muscle degeneration and regeneration are most likely to be seen as a result of trauma or involvement of muscle in infections or malignant tumors.

Muscle degeneration is characterized by hyaline change with loss of cross-striations, vacuolation and, ultimately, necrosis. Infiltration by inflammatory cells and phagocytosis are early consequences.

Regeneration frequently follows muscle damage and is characterized by: basophilia of the fibers; indistinct striations; increased number and size of nuclei, sometimes with prominent nucleoli (sarcolemmal giant cells); and formation of variably sized but often small fibers. Sarcolemmal giant cells may give the misleading impression of a neoplasm, are seen in some of the tumor-like diseases of muscle, but are a normal feature of muscle regeneration.

Myositis

PROLIFERATIVE MYOSITIS

This uncommon pseudosarcomatous disorder, which may be related to proliferative fasciitis, occasionally affects muscles of the head and neck region to produce a firm, rapidly growing tumor-like swelling. Dent et al[1] have reported the light and electron microscopic findings in a case affecting the tongue in a 70-year-old male, and reviewed the literature. They concluded that, of 50 reported cases, 10 involved the head and neck. Adults aged over 45 years are chiefly affected.

MICROSCOPY

Proliferative myositis consists of loosely arranged, highly pleomorphic cells in an infiltrative growth pattern. Giant cells with basophilic or amphophilic cytoplasm, and binucleate or multinucleate cells, sometimes with conspicuous nucleoli, may be prominent and resemble ganglion cells or rhabdomyoblasts. They

are separated by loose, edematous, proliferating spindle cells; inflammatory cells are scanty or absent. Remnants of degenerating muscle fibers may be seen particularly near the periphery (Figs 44.1–44.3).

Fujiwara et al,[2] on the basis of their finding in an oral specimen, state that the ganglion-like cells did not stain for desmin or myo-

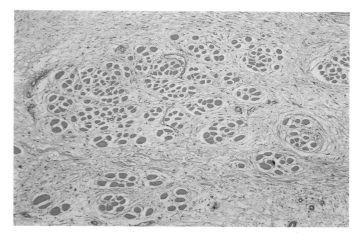

Fig. 44.1 Proliferative myositis. Low-power view showing degenerating muscle fibers.

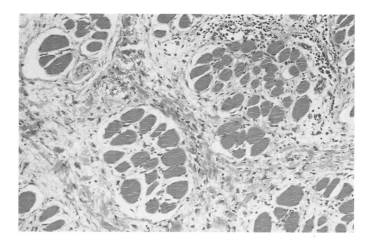

Fig. 44.2 Proliferative myositis showing sarcolemmal giant cells and nuclear abnormalities.

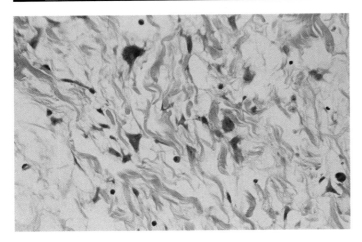

Fig. 44.3 Proliferative myositis showing sarcolemmal giant cells in cross-section and nuclear abnormalities, at higher power.

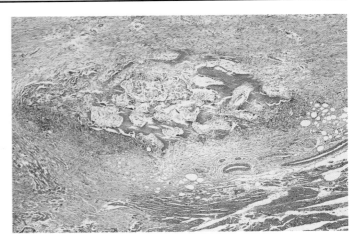

Fig. 44.4 Myositis ossificans. Low-power view showing fibrous and osseous replacement of muscle.

globin, and suggested that they were of myofibroblastic or macrophage origin. Dent et al[1] concluded that ultrastructural findings suggested that they were myofibroblasts.

Surrounding tissues are infiltrated and, hardly surprisingly, a diagnosis of malignancy and particularly of rhabdomyosarcoma was initially made in 14 of the 33 cases reviewed by Enzinger & Dulcey.[3] Nevertheless, proliferative myositis is completely benign, as shown by its tendency to regress spontaneously.

Biopsy is essential to establish the diagnosis, but surgical intervention may be necessary, mainly for cosmetic reasons. At most, limited local reduction of the mass is required; none of the 10 cases quoted by Dent et al[1] recurred, even after incomplete resection.

MYOSITIS OSSIFICANS

This rare, benign proliferative process can be confused histologically with osteosarcoma. Solitary myositis ossificans (traumatic or ossifying myositis) may follow chronic trauma or an isolated blow to a muscle, but in at least 50% of cases there is no history of injury. Experimentally, trauma to muscle does not reproduce the pathologic features of this condition.

CLINICAL FEATURES

The masseter or temporalis muscle, usually in a teenager or young adult, can be affected, and a localized, painful nodule develops within it. A faint, delicate pattern of ossification typically starts to appear after about 3 weeks and may, rarely, cause ankylosis (see Ch. 7). Woolgar et al[4] have reported myositis ossificans of the sternomastoid muscle that mimicked a cervical lymph node metastasis, in a man with carcinoma of the larynx.

MICROSCOPY

There is, typically, initial reactive fibroblastic proliferation and

organization of any hematoma present. In the developed lesion, there is usually characteristic zoning, with a border of irregular trabeculae of cellular osteoid and woven bone surrounding a highly vascular central mass of proliferating, immature fibroblasts, which are typically pleomorphic with prominent mitoses (Fig. 44.4).

The picture is readily mistaken for sarcomatous change, but the process is benign and self-limiting. Sarcomatous change that has occasionally been reported in ossifying myositis does not seem to have been authenticated fully. However, it is important to emphasize the fact that, although pseudosarcomatous diseases have been described above, true osteosarcomas or chondrosarcomas can also develop in soft tissues. Therefore, care must be taken not to dismiss osteosarcoma-like or chondrosarcoma-like changes as benign merely because they are within soft tissues.

Treatment is by wide surgical excision. Recurrences are very common, but systemic bisphosphonates may help to prevent them.

Rhabdomyoma

Cardiac rhabdomyomas are relatively common. They are usually associated with one of the phakomatoses, particularly tuberous sclerosis. By contrast, the extracardiac rhabdomyoma is one of the most uncommon of all tumors. From a review of the world literature, Ferlito & Frugoni[5] estimated that there had been only about 50 reports. Corio & Lewis[6] were able to identify 13 additional intraoral examples from the Armed Forces Institute of Pathology files, but could find reports of only 16 other cases. However, in reporting a case of sublingual rhabdomyoma large enough to cause gross upward displacement of the tongue, Napier et al[7] concluded that approximately 110 extracardiac cases had been reported and that 77% of these had affected the head and neck region.

Occasionally, rhabdomyomas can be multifocal. Gardner & Corio[8] reviewed reports of nine histologically verified cases, including one of their own. Seven of these were in males aged between 58 and 82 years. Most of the lesions were extraoral. Two cases of multifocal fetal rhabdomyomas were also reported. Schlosnagle et al[9] reported another case in a 65-year-old female. This mass, in the position of the sublingual gland, had been present for 20 years and consisted of approximately 20 distinct nodules of rhabdomyoma with typical light and electron microscopic appearances.

INCIDENCE

Oral rhabdomyomas affect men at least twice as frequently as women, with a peak incidence between ages 50 and 60 years. Napier et al[7] stated that 33% of head and neck rhabdomyomas were in the tongue or sublingual region, 8% in the soft palate, and the remainder in extraoral sites (such as the larynx, pharynx, anterior neck, or postauricular area), and were occasionally multifocal.

CLINICAL FEATURES

The tumor typically forms a slow-growing, painless firm swelling.

MICROSCOPY

Rhabdomyomas are well circumscribed or encapsulated and consist of large cells with eosinophilic cytoplasm. They often contain such large vacuoles as to appear fatty, and sometimes cause the granular eosinophilic cytoplasm to have a spidery appearance. The cell membranes are sharply defined. In hematoxylin and eosin stained sections, cross-striations can, with careful examination, be found, but these are more readily demonstrable using PTAH (Figs 44.5 and 44.6).

Periodic acid/Schiff (PAS) staining shows glycogen in the cytoplasm and in the peripheral vacuoles. Cleveland et al[10] investigated the immunohistochemistry of five adult rhabdomyomas, but did not detect reactivity to pancytokeratin, S-100 protein, or vimentin. Positive reactions were seen to antibodies against muscle-specific actin (in 5–25%), desmin (in 50–90%), and myoglobin (90–95%). Argyrophil nuclear organizer regions (AgNORs), quantified in three of the five tumors showed low counts consistent with a benign process.

Cleveland et al[10] confirmed previous ultrastructural findings, namely mitochondria, patchy aggregation of glycogen particles, and nemaline bodies, as prominent cytoplasmic components. Myofilaments, mainly actin-like filaments, were interconnected with dense nemaline bodies, which are the abortive form of the Z bands of striated muscle fibers. Some nemaline bodies showed fine periodicity. Frequently they were aligned in irregular rows corresponding to the irregular cross-striations seen by light microscopy.

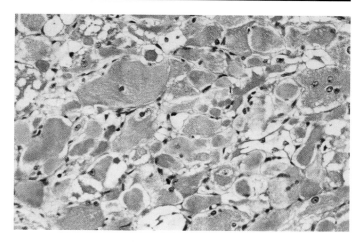

Fig. 44.5 Rhabdomyoma. Vacuolated cells give the tumor a fatty appearance and have a large area of eosinophilic cytoplasm.

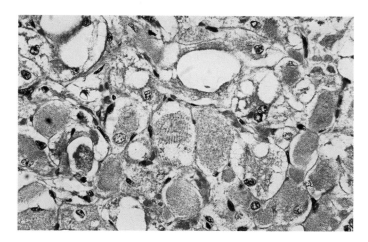

Fig. 44.6 Rhabdomyoma. Higher power view shows prominent cross-striations.

Diagnosis depends on showing cross-striations and the absence of any features of malignancy.

BEHAVIOR AND MANAGEMENT

At operation, a rhabdomyoma may shell out readily. Recurrence is uncommon unless the tumor is so large that complete excision cannot be achieved. There appears to be no potential for malignant change.

FETAL RHABDOMYOMA

Fetal rhabdomyomas are particularly uncommon; Gardner & Corio[11] concluded that only five oral cases had previously been reported. The importance of these tumors is the possibility of mistaking them for sarcomas.

INCIDENCE

Fetal rhabdomyomas affect infants and, despite their name, adults also, over a wide age range. The two peaks of incidence for those in the head and neck region (unlike those of the vulvovaginal region) are 0–3 years and 50–60 years. Males are predominantly affected, but the numbers have been so small that this finding may not be significant.

CLINICAL FEATURES

These tumors form painless soft swellings, which may be pedunculated.

MICROSCOPY

The two variants of fetal rhabdmyoma are the myxoid and cellular. Myxoid fetal rhabodymomas are well circumscribed or encapsulated and consist of haphazardly scattered skeletal muscle cells interspersed with round, lymphocyte-like undifferentiated cells and separated by a myxoid stroma. However, the latter may be

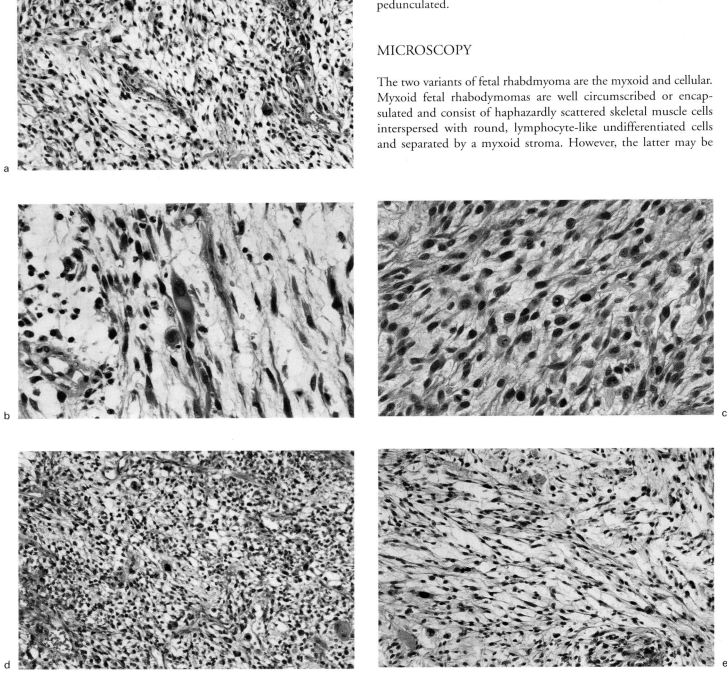

Fig. 44.7 Rhabdomyosarcoma, embryonal type. **a** Elongated cells with eosinophilic cytoplasm and bizarre nuclei in a myxoid stroma. **b** Higher power view shows, in particular, a strap-shaped binucleate rhabdomyoblast. **c** Tadpole cells and mitotic activity. **d** Prominent mitoses. **e** Loose myxoid stroma.

scanty or almost absent so that the tumor is highly cellular. The muscle cells are frequently strap-shaped and show distinct cross-striations, particularly when stained with PTAH.

Cellular fetal rhabdomyomas are, as the name implies, highly cellular and consist mainly of interwoven bundles of spindle cells with scanty stroma. There is mild nuclear pleomorphism and there may be a herring-bone pattern and nuclear palisading. These spindle cells are frequently not immediately recognizable as immature muscle cells. Cross-striations can sometimes be seen, but a careful search may be necessary. There are also scattered, round eosinophilic cells, which may be recognizable as myoblasts. The main features helping to distinguish these benign tumors from sarcomas are their circumscription and the paucity of mitotic activity.

BEHAVIOR AND MANAGEMENT

The main consideration, as already implied, is not to mistake these tumors for sarcomas, by appreciation that fetal rhabdomyomas can be seen in the oral cavity and by recognition of their histological features. Excision is effective.

Rhabdomyosarcoma

Although rare overall, rhabdomyosarcomas are among the most common sarcomas found in the mouth and second only to AIDS-related Kaposi's sarcoma.

These tumors form rapidly growing, soft swellings, which (apart from the botryoid form which is unlikely to be seen in the mouth) are nondescript in character. In Dito & Batsakis' series[12] of 49 oropharyngeal and nasopharyngeal rhabdomyosarcomas, there were 30 in the palate or tongue and 31 in the nasopharynx. Of these patients, 79% were under 12 years of age.

MICROSCOPY

Rhabdomyosarcomas are categorized as embryonal, alveolar, and pleomorphic types, depending upon the predominant pattern. The embryonal type is the most common and accounts for about 75% of all cases. It is particularly common in the head and neck area, and most examples are seen in children under the age of 12 years. Alveolar rhabdomyosarcoma tends to affect a somewhat older age group and is more frequently found in the soft tissues of the extremities. Pleomorphic rhabdomyosarcoma is rare and most often forms in the large muscles of the extremities in adults aged over 45 years, but many authorities believe that many tumors formerly thought to be adult pleomorphic rhabdomyosarcomas should be recategorized as malignant fibrous histiocytomas.

Embryonal rhabdomyosarcoma consists of sheets of ovoid or spindle cells, which may be tightly packed or interspersed in a loose myxoid stroma. Some of the round and spindle cells have eosinophilic cytoplasm, which may stream out to form racquet- or strap-shaped cells. Cross-striations may be seen, but their presence is not essential for diagnosis. Glycogen is also present in the better differentiated cells, but is usually dissolved out in processing to leave multivacuolate, spider-web cells. Some embryonal rhabdomyosarcomas are highly pleomorphic and contain foci of varying size of larger bizarre cells (Fig. 44.7).

The botryoid variant of embryonal rhabdomyosarcoma most frequently arises in the mucosa of hollow organs such as the nasal cavity, bile duct, or urinary bladder, or in the vagina. It is rare in the oral cavity, but an example resembling a bunch of grapes, on the palate of 16-year-old boy, was reported by Chen et al.[13]

Histologically, botryoid rhabdomyosarcoma has a polypoid configuration and typically shows an abundance of mucoid stroma with scattered spindle-shaped or round rhabdomyoblasts. There is sometimes a cell-rich superficial zone, and the overlying epithelium may occasionally undergo pseudoepitheliomatous hyperplasia (Fig. 44.8).

Alveolar rhabdomyosarcoma tends to affect a somewhat older age group; it is considerably less common than the embryonal type and only occasionally seen in the mouth. It consists of ill-defined nests of ovoid or round cells around central alveolar spaces. The individual alveoli are separated by fibrous septae. Multinucleated tumor giant cells are often also present (Figs 44.9 and 44.10).

Pleomorphic rhabdomyosarcoma, which most often affects adults over the age of 45 years, consists of pleomorphic large round, or polygonal cells of variable size and with varying amounts of cytoplasm, which may be eosinophilic. No pattern is recognizable. Some may be racquet- or tadpole-shaped, but rarely show cross-striations. Many tumors previously thought to be adult pleomorphic rhabdomyosarcomas are probably malignant fibrous histiocytomas (Figs 44.11–44.13).

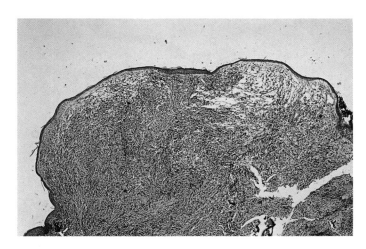

Fig. 44.8 Rhabdomyosarcoma. Low-power view of a mucosal botryoid tumor, which appeared as a soft polypoid mass with haphazard masses of spindle and strap-shaped rhabdomyoblasts microscopically.

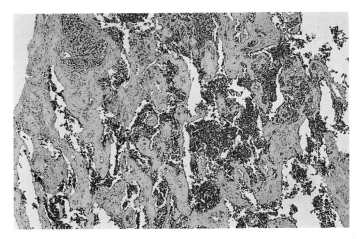

Fig. 44.9 Rhabdomyosarcoma. Alveolar type showing ill-defined nests of darkly staining rhabdomyoblasts in and hanging from the walls of alveolar spaces.

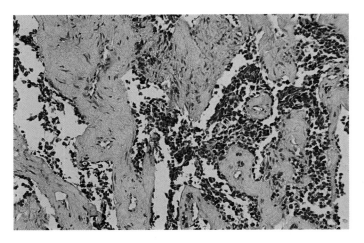

Fig. 44.10 Rhabdomyosarcoma. Higher power view of the same section as in Figure 44.9.

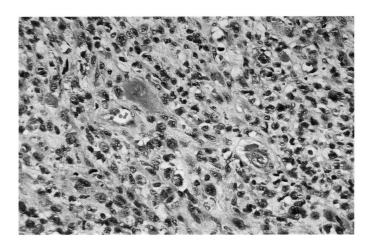

Fig. 44.11 Rhabdomyosarcoma. Pleomorphic type. The tumor is highly cellular and shows, in particular, a large cell with granular eosinophilic cytoplasm and another with vesiculation of the cytoplasm giving a spider-web appearance.

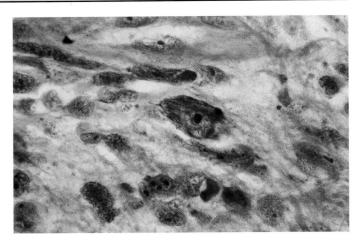

Fig. 44.12 Rhabdomyosarcoma. Pleomorphic type. PTAH-stained section shows a single striated cell.

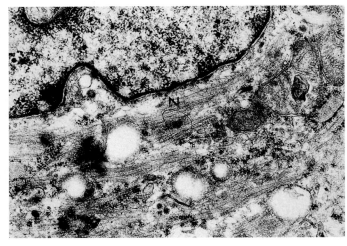

Fig. 44.13 Rhabdomyosarcoma. Pleomorphic type. The electron micrograph shows the characteristic Z-line density.

Diagnosis of rhabdomyosarcoma can be difficult and depends primarily on the identification of neoplastic rhabdomyoblasts. However, cells with cross-striation are present in only 20–60% of cases and are mainly seen in the embryonal type. Myoglobin is the most specific marker, but is usually negative in poorly differentiated tumors. Immunostaining for desmin, myosin, and sarcomeric actin are widely used, and when positive serve to differentiate poorly differentiated rhabdomyosarcomas from other, small round-cell tumors such as Ewing's sarcoma. Nevertheless, Rangdaeng & Truong[14] found that up to 17% of nonmyogenic tumors stained with muscle-specific actin or desmin or both. El Naggar et al[15] reported that of 13 rhabdomyosarcomas of the head and neck all stained positively with antibodies to HHF-35 muscle-specific actin, 12 to D33 desmin, and 11 with DER-11 anti-desmin. Alveolar rhabdomysarcomas show a characteristic cytogenetic abnormality, namely t(2;13)(q35–37;q13),[16] which is of diagnostic value.

El Naggar et al[15] have also reported that flow cytometry of 17 rhabdomyosarcomas of the head and neck showed that 92.7% of the 13 primary tumors were aneuploid, as were all of four recurrent tumors. All these patients except two died from their disease after periods of 2–72 months.

The histogenesis of rhabdomyosarcoma is problematical, as shown by an example reported by Tanaguchi et al,[17] which had apparently arisen from the stroma of a long-standing amelo-blastoma in a 65-year-old male. Many rhabdomyosarcomas do not arise in striated muscle, and Enzinger & Weiss[18] suggest that rhabdomyosarcomas form from primitive and undifferentiated mesenchyme or from embryonal muscle tissue displaced during the early stages of development.

BEHAVIOR AND MANAGEMENT

As already described, the prognosis is poor, with local recurrence or distant metastases in many cases. Lymph nodes, often at a distance, may be involved in up to 50% of cases, but favored sites of metastases are the bones or lungs.

The first line of treatment is radical excision, and this is usually supplemented by radiotherapy. It is believed that adjuvant combination chemotherapy may greatly improve the prognosis. However, of the six adults with rhabdomyosarcomas of the head and neck treated by surgery, radiotherapy, and chemotherapy, reported by El Naggar et al,[15] all but one died from their disease within periods of 15–78 months. Of four patients with embryonal rhabdomyosarcomas reported by Chen et al,[13] three died with metastases to lungs or bone within 17 months, while the fourth patient had been observed for less than a year. By contrast, Meehan et al[19] have reported a 21-year-old woman with an embryonal rhabdomyosarcoma of the floor of the mouth which grew to 8 cm × 8 cm × 8 cm, filling and extruding from her mouth after her refusal to complete an earlier course of chemotherapy.

Treatment of the recurrence with adriamycin, local irradiation, and debulking surgery was carried out and, when last seen 6 years later, only scar tissue remained in the tumor area.

REFERENCES

1. Dent CD, DeBoom GW, Hamlin ML 1994 Proliferative myositis of the head and neck. Report of a case and review of the literature. Oral Surg Oral Med Oral Pathol 78: 354–358
2. Fujiwara K, Watanabe T, Katsuki T, Ohyama S, Goto M 1987 Proliferative myositis of the buccinator muscle: a case with immunohistochemical and electron microscopic analysis. Oral Surg Oral Med Oral Pathol 63: 597–601
3. Enzinger FM, Dulcey F 1967 Proliferative myositis. Report of thirty three cases. Cancer 20: 2213–2223
4. Woolgar JA, Beirne JC, Trianafyllou A 1995 Myositis ossificans of the sternocleidomastoid muscle presenting as cervical lymph-node metastasis. Int J Oral Maxillofac Surg 42: 170–173
5. Ferlito A, Frugona P 1975 Rhabdomyoma purum of the larynx. J Laryngol 89: 1131–1141
6. Corio RL, Lewis DM 1970 Intraoral rhabdomyomas. Oral Surg 48: 525–531
7. Napier SS, Pagni CG, McGimpsey JG 1991 Sublingual adult rhabdomyoma. Report of a case. Int J Oral Maxillofac Surg 20: 201–203
8. Gardner DG, Corio RL 1984 Multifocal adult rhabdomyoma. Oral Surg Oral Med Oral Pathol 56: 76–78
9. Schlosnagle DC, Kratochvil AFJ, Weathers DR, McConnel FMS 1983 Intraoral multifocal adult rhabdomyoma. Arch Pathol Lab Med 107: 638–642
10. Cleveland DB, Chen S-Y, Allen CM, Ahing SI, Svirsky JA 1994 Adult rhabdomyoma. A light microscopic, ultrastructural, virologic and immunologic analysis. Oral Surg Oral Med Oral Pathol 77: 147–153
11. Gardner DG, Corio RL 1983 Fetal rhabdomyoma of the tongue, with a discussion of the two histologic variants of this tumor. Oral Surg 56: 293–300
12. Dito WR, Batsakis, JG 1962 Rhabdomyosarcoma of the head and neck. An appraisal of the biologic behavior in 170 cases. Arch Surg 84: 112–118
13. Chen S-Y, Thakur A, Miller AS, Harwick RD 1995 Rhabdomyosarcoma of the oral cavity. Report of four cases. Oral Surg Oral Med Oral Pathol Oral Radiol Endod 80 (192): 192–201
14. Rangdaeng S, Truong LD 1991 Comparative immunocytochemical staining for desmin and muscle-specific actin. A study of 576 cases. Am J Clin Pathol 96: 32–45
15. El Naggar AK, Batsakis JG, Ordonez NG, Luna MA, Goepfert H 1993 Rhabdomyosarcoma of the adult head and neck: a clinicopathological and DNA ploidy study. J Laryngol Otol 107: 716–720
16. Turc-Carel C, Lizard-Nacol S, Justrao E, Favrot M, Philip T, Tabone E 1986 Consistent chromosomal translocation in alveolar rhabdomyosarcoma. Cancer Genet Cytogenet 19: 361–362
17. Tanaguchi K, Okamura K, Matsuura H et al 1995 Rhabdomyosarcoma arising in the course of long-standing ameloblastoma. Oral Surg Oral Med Oral Pathol Oral Radiol Endod 80: 202–206
18. Enzinger FM, Weiss SW 1995 Soft tissue tumors, 3rd edn. CV Mosby, St Louis
19. Meehan S, Davis V, Brahim JS 1994 Embryonal rhabdomyosarcoma of the floor of the mouth. A case report. Oral Surg Oral Med Oral Pathol 78: 603–606

Tumors of smooth muscle 45

Leiomyoma and angiomyoma

Leiomyomas are rare in the mouth and, because of the paucity of smooth muscle in the oral tissues, mainly arise from muscle cells in the walls of blood vessels. Damm & Neville[1] considered that these tumors were less uncommon than generally believed, and traced reports of 55 intraoral examples. Svane et al[2] believed that a total of 113 oral leiomyomas had been reported and of these 84 were angiomyomas. In 111 cases where the gender had been recorded, males and females were equally represented. However, intraosseous leiomyomas are undoubtedly rare.

These tumors are termed *angiomyomas* (or *angioleiomyomas*) if their vascular origin is apparent or *leiomyomas* if they are solid. The lips, particularly the lower, were affected in 16, the tongue in 13, and the cheek in 11 of the 62 cases analyzed by Giles & Gosney.[3] The lesions form slow-growing nondescript swellings, which are usually painless. Angiomyomas may have a bluish color due to the prominent vascular component.

MICROSCOPY

Leiomyomas consist of interlacing bundles or whorls of spindle-shaped cells of smooth-muscle origin interspersed with collagen fibers, which may sometimes predominate. Small vascular channels are scattered within the mass. The nuclei of the muscle cells are typically elongated and blunt-ended. Differentiation from other spindle-cell tumors, such as neurofibromas, may be difficult. Myofibrils can be demonstrated by PTAH staining, but diagnosis may depend on electron microscopy to demonstrate myofibrils. Immunohistochemistry may be helpful, but neurogenous tumors may also stain positively for desmin, actin, and vimentin.

Angiomyomas consist of blood vessels with their walls thickened by smooth muscle proliferation. They are interspersed with bundles of smooth muscle (Figs 45.1 and 45.2).

BEHAVIOR AND MANAGEMENT

Leiomyomas and angiomyomas are benign and respond to conservative excision.

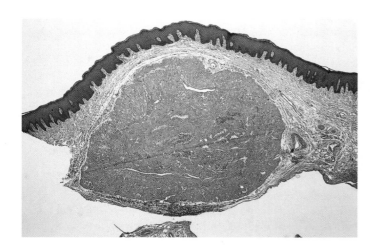

Fig. 45.1 Leiomyoma. Low-power view of a mucosal tumor, showing a solid appearance and curcumscription.

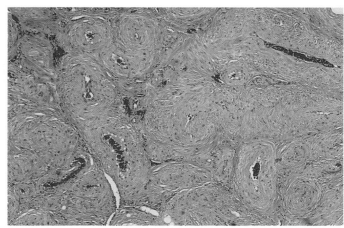

Fig. 45.2 Angiomyoma. Proliferation of smooth muscle has produced gross thickening of the vessel walls.

LEIOMYOMATOUS HAMARTOMA

Semba et al[4] reported what they considered to be the first example of a gingival leiomyomatous hamartoma in the English literature. They categorized this lesion as a hamartoma because of its presence at birth, midline site, and intermingling of smooth muscle and nerve fibers. They noted reports of four other cases in the Japanese literature.

INTRAOSSEOUS LEIOMYOMAS

MacLeod et al[5] considered that of 116 reported oral leiomyomas only three were intraosseous. However, White et al[6] found five reports of central leiomyomas, and Burke[7] reported another. The ages of those affected have ranged from 3.5 to 71 years. The body of the mandible is the most frequent site.

RADIOGRAPHY

Central leiomyomas appear as circumscribed, sometimes multilocular areas of radiolucency, and are usually asymptomatic.

MICROSCOPY

Intraosseous leiomyomas may be solid or angiomyomatous and do not differ from their soft-tissue counterparts. Of four cases reviewed by White et al,[6] and for which follow-up data were available, there had been no recurrence after enucleation or currettage for periods ranging from 2 to 6 years.

Leiomyosarcomas

Leiomyosarcomas are also distinctly uncommon in the mouth. Poon et al[8] could find only 24 documented cases in the preceding 75 years. Schenberg et al[9] reviewed the findings in 34 reported cases and added four more.

Clinically, Schenberg et al[9] noted that 59% of these leiomyosarcomas had formed in the jaws, of these, 32% were in the maxilla. The cheek was involved in 13% and the tongue in 11%. The tumor formed a mass, which was painful in 61%. Those in the jaws formed nondescript smooth swellings, while some of the soft-tissue examples formed more irregular masses that sometimes ulcerated.

The age at presentation ranged from 10 months to 88 years and males accounted for 63%.

MICROSCOPY

Leiomyosarcomas typically form interlacing bundles of spindle cells. The latter are elongated and weakly eosinophilic with

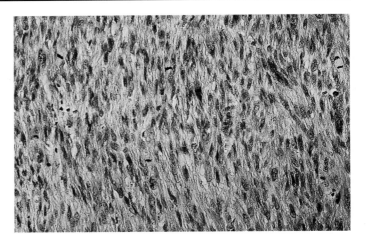

Fig. 45.3 Leiomyosarcoma. The spindle-shaped eosinophilic cells have blunt-ended nuclei, some of which show pleomorphism and mitotic activity.

blunt-ended nuclei like leiomyomas, but show hyperchromatism, cellular pleomorphism, and mitotic activity. Well-differentiated examples show well-defined intersecting fascicles of spindle cells, while poorly differentiated tumors show a more disordered pattern. The margins are aggressively infiltrative (Fig. 41.3).

Differentiation from other spindle-cell sarcomas is frequently difficult with routine stains. Positive staining for smooth-muscle-specific actin and desmin is helpful, but some leiomyosarcomas fail to react. Enzinger & Weiss[10] claim that most leiomyosarcomas stain for muscle-specific actin (HHF35). Alternatively, myofilaments and deeply clefted nuclei may be demonstrable by electron microscopy.

BEHAVIOR AND MANAGEMENT

Treatment is by wide surgical excision at the earliest possible moment. This is more easily achieved with soft tissue than with intraosseous tumors. Surgery may be supplemented by radiotherapy, but Schenberg et al[9] found that there was no consensus as to its value. Chemotherapy is generally reserved for palliation of inoperable tumors or metastatic disease. Metastasis of intraoral leiomyosarcomas has been reported in 39% of cases, most frequently to the lungs, but to regional lymph nodes in 15%, usually in association with distant spread. Schenberg et al[9] found that only 23% of patients were disease-free after 5 years and 69% had died from their disease by this time.

LEIOMYOSARCOMA OF BONE

Leiomyosarcoma is another rare tumor but, as noted earlier, Schenberg et al[9] found that 59% of 38 reported cases had arisen in the maxilla or mandible.

CLINICAL FEATURES

Intraosseous leiomyosarcomas form bony swellings and are locally destructive and often painful. They are not clinically or radiographically distinguishable from many other malignant tumors.

MICROSCOPY

The microscopic features are essentially the same as those of the soft-tissue counterpart described earlier.

BEHAVIOR AND MANAGEMENT

Treatment is by radical surgical excision. Maxillectomy or wide mandibular resection is required, but the prognosis is poor.

EPITHELIOID LEIOMYOSARCOMA

Freedman et al[11] have reported what they believed to be the first two cases of this variant in the oral cavity. Both examples were in black females. One had a gingival mass, and the other had nasal obstruction and orbital swelling from a tumor, which appeared to have originated between the upper second and third molars.

MICROSCOPY

Epithelioid leiomyoblasts with round cells with ovoid nuclei and eosinophilic or clear cytoplasm, are the characteristic feature, and may predominate. Interlacing fascicles of spindle-shaped smooth muscle cells intermingle with the epithelioid cells. They formed

only a minor component of the tumors reported by Freedman et al,[11] but suggested the diagnosis.

BEHAVIOR AND MANAGEMENT

Too little information is available to determine whether the response to treatment of intraoral epithelioid leiomyosarcomas is any different from the more common types. The first patient reported by Freedman et al[11] died from disseminated disease 21 months after initial examination. The second failed to respond to chemotherapy and, despite maxillectomy and exenteration of the orbit, was left with residual disease.

REFERENCES

1. Damm DD, Neville BW 1979 Oral leiomyomas. Oral Surg Oral Med Oral Pathol 47: 343–348
2. Svane TJ, Simith BR, Consentino BJ, Cundiff EJ, Ceravolo JJ 1986 Oral leiomyomas. Review of the literature and report of a case of palatal angiopleiomyoma. J Periodontol 57: 433–435
3. Giles AD, Gosney MBE 1982 Oral angiomyoma: a case report. Br J Surg 20: 142–146
4. Semba I, Kitano M, Mimura T 1993 Gingival leiomyomatous hamartoma: immunohistochemical and ultrastructural observations. J Oral Pathol Med 22: 468–470
5. MacLeod SPR, Mitchell DA, Miller ID 1993 Intraosseous leiomyoma of the mandible: report of a case. Br J Oral Maxillofac Surg 31: 187–188
6. White DK, Selinger LR, Miller AS, Behr MM, Damm DD 1985 Primary angioleiomyoma of the mandible. J Oral Maxillofac Surg 43: 640–643
7. Burke JJ 1995 Vascular leiomyoma of the mandible: report of a case. J Oral Maxillofac Surg 53: 65–66
8. Poon C-K, Kwan N-T, Yin N-Y, Chao S-Y 1987 Leiomyosarcoma of gingiva: report of a case and review of the literature. J Oral Maxillofac Surg 45: 888–892
9. Schenberg ME, Slootweg PJ, Koole R 1993 Leiomyosarcomas of the oral cavity. Report of four cases and review of the literature. J Cranio-Maxillo-Fac Surg 21:342–347
10. Enzinger FM, Weiss SW 1995 Soft tissue tumors, 3rd edn. C V Mosby, St Louis
11. Freedman PD, Jones AC, Kerpel SM 1993 Epithelioid leiomyosarcoma of the oral cavity: report of two cases and review of the literature. J Oral Maxillofac Surg 51: 928–932

Tumors of adipose tissue 46

Lipomas occasionally form within the mouth, particularly from the buccal fat pad or lip, or, rarely, within the parotids or other major salivary glands.

Vindenes[1] reported six examples of oral lipomas, which formed soft fluctuant swellings with a distinctive creamy color when submucosal. Deeply situated tumors are more difficult to recognize clinically, but Cottrell et al[2] have shown that computed tomography or magnetic resonance imaging may enable the diagnosis to be made. In approximately 5% of cases lipomas are multiple. The tendency to develop multiple lesions is sometimes inherited as a simple autosomal dominant trait, and may also be seen in neurofibromatosis, Gardner's syndrome, and Dercum's disease (painful subcutaneous lipomas and obesity).

MICROSCOPY

Lipomas consist of mature fat cells enclosed within fine areolar tissue and surrounded by a fibrous capsule (Fig. 46.1). Those which contain fibroblasts intermingled with the fat cells are known as *fibrolipomas*; these are rare in the oral cavity.

BEHAVIOR AND MANAGEMENT

Excision of lipomas is curative. Enzinger & Weiss[3] state that they have never encountered malignant change in a lipoma, but point out that morphologic variations in the microscopic appearances of lipomas could sometimes lead lipomas to be mistaken for incipient liposarcomas.

SPINDLE CELL AND OTHER LIPOMA VARIANTS

McDaniel et al[4] reported the first case of spindle-cell lipoma of the oral cavity and described the ultrastructural findings. Since then further examples have been reported.[5-7]

MICROSCOPY

Spindle-cell lipomas consist of variable numbers of adipocytes

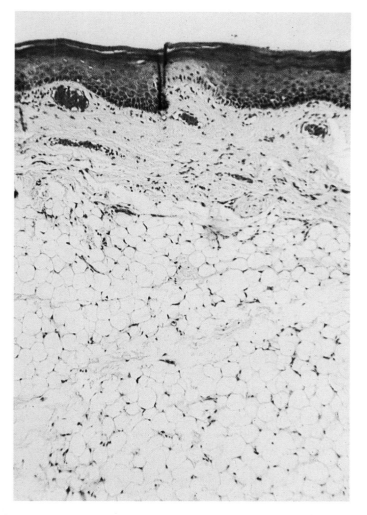

Fig. 46.1 Lipoma. Fat cells are confined by delicate areolar tissue.

surrounded by fibroblast-like cells, which may be relatively few or so many as to dominate the picture. Lombardi & Odell,[7] when reviewing four earlier reports, confirmed that the spindle cells failed to stain with antibody against S-100, α smooth muscle actin, or desmin (Fig. 46.2).

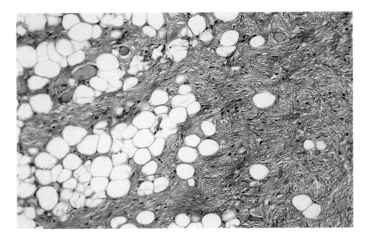

Fig. 46.2 Spindle-cell lipoma. Fat globules and adipocytes are interspersed with a dense stroma of spindle cells.

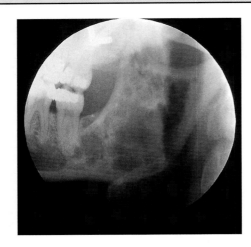

Fig. 46.3 Liposarcoma of the mandible. The radiograph shows multiple areas of bone destruction in the region of the ramus.

Other lipoma variants that are rare in the mouth include the *angiolipoma* and *myolipoma*. Unlike conventional lipomas, angiolipomas are sometimes painful or tender. Microscopically, angiolipomas consist of mature fat cells separated by blood vessels with minute or inconspicuous lumens. Occasionally the vascular component is so extensive that the tumor can be mistaken for Kaposi's sarcoma.

BEHAVIOR AND MANAGEMENT

Excision is normally curative. However, some angiolipomas, although benign, are infiltrative. These require wide excision, and bleeding at operation may be brisk. Flaggart et al[8] quote a 50% recurrence rate.

Liposarcoma

Enzinger & Weiss[3] state categorically that liposarcoma is one of the most common soft-tissue tumors of adult life. They noted that 5.6% of 1076 liposarcomas seen at the Armed Forces Institute of Pathology were in the head and neck region. Liposarcomas have also been estimated to form 4% of sarcomas of the head and neck region,[9] but McCulloch et al,[10] who reported a case, could identify only 76 cases in that area, reported between 1911 and 1990. Undoubtedly also, liposarcomas are rare tumors in the mouth. Baden & Newman[11] reported an example and another in the pharynx. In a review of 35 of these tumors in the head and neck region seen between 1911 and 1977, they found nine involving the floor of the mouth, cheek, lip, or soft palate. Most were well-differentiated myxoid liposarcomas, but one was poorly differentiated and another was of mixed cell type. Liposarcomas have also been reported in the cheek (presumably arising in the buccal fat pad)[12,13] and in the tongue.[14] Zheng & Wang[15] report-

ed 10 cases in the oral and maxillofacial region. Of these, two were in the oral soft tissues and one was in the mandible (Fig. 46.3). Eight of these 10 tumors were in women (mean age 33 years). Friedman et al[16] described, in an 18-year-old woman, a pleomorphic liposarcoma of the pterygomandibular space, which they believed was only the second example of this tumor involving the maxilla. Minec[17] concluded that 28 liposarcomas affecting the oral tissues had been reported, and added four more: two had formed in the submandibular space, one was in the tongue and the other in the hard palate. Golledge et al,[18] reviewing the findings in 76 patients with head and neck liposarcomas, noted that 8% were in the mouth.

CLINICAL FEATURES

Liposarcomas have a variable presentation and clinical course. Almost any age can be affected, but the mean is 43 years. Typically, liposarcomas form nondescript swellings, but are frequently slow-growing, painless at first, and interpreted as benign. The buccal fat pad is the most frequent oral site. Later, growth accelerates, the mass becomes painful and may bleed or ulcerate.

MICROSCOPY

Liposarcomas show a wide variety of appearances. Enzinger & Weiss[3] classify well-differentiated types as lipoma-like, inflammatory, or sclerosing. They point out that, like developing fat, lipoblasts of liposarcomas range from primitive mesenchymal cells containing only minute cytoplasmic droplets of lipid, to signet ring cells the cytoplasm of which is filled with a single large, sharply defined droplet of fat, which distorts the nucleus as it expands.

Well-differentiated liposarcomas can thus be recognized microscopically by obvious fat formation, foamy fat-containing lipoblasts, and signet ring cells. Characteristic, irregularly shaped giant cells with foamy cytoplasm may also be present. Myxoid, round cell, dedifferentiated, and pleomorphic liposarcomas are also recognized.

Liposarcomas are sometimes so cellular as to obscure their lipoblastic origin. When fat is present, it usually resembles embryonal adipose tissue and consists of fat cells in myxoid tissue. In unblocked material it may stain with a fat stain such as Sudan red. Liposarcomas that consist entirely of embryonal adipose tissue resemble myxomas (Figs 46.4–46.6; see also Fig. 36.13).

Critical to diagnosis is recognition of adipocytes and lipoblasts. They stain for vimentin and S-100 protein, but may not express these antigens if poorly differentiated. Some of the tumor cells may also stain for smooth-muscle actin.

BEHAVIOR AND MANAGEMENT

Radical excision is the treatment of choice, but margins are

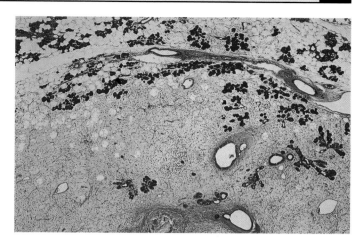

Fig. 46.6 Liposarcoma, myxoid type. This example has infiltrated the parotid gland.

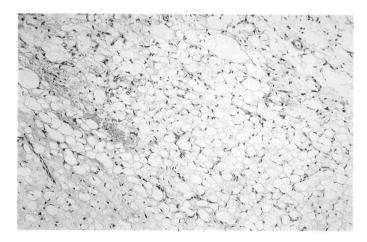

Fig. 46.4 Liposarcoma. At low power this well-differentiated example looks little different from a lipoma apart from its greater cellularity.

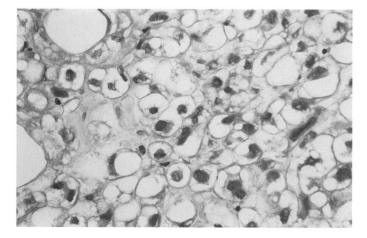

Fig. 46.5 Liposarcoma. The adipose nature of the tumor is still evident, but the cells show pleomorphic, hyperchromatic nuclei and some are binucleate.

frequently difficult to define. Neck dissection is required if regional lymph nodes are involved. Radiotherapy may be useful postoperatively or for palliation if surgery fails. The value of chemotherapy is uncertain, but Friedman et al[16] reported a patient who refused surgery, but whose tumor remained localized, under treatment with adriamycin, for the 18 months available for follow-up, but continued to grow.

Recurrence is common and largely related to the degree of differentiation. Well-differentiated and myxoid liposarcomas have the best prognosis. The myxoid type rarely metastasizes but can recur locally. The round-cell type is more aggressive, and pleomorphic liposarcomas have a strong tendency to metastasize and are potentially lethal. However, the size of the tumor at presentation is an important factor affecting survival.

Survival data on oral liposarcomas are extremely limited, but Minic[17] concluded that a predominance of myxoid and well-differentiated tumors in the oral tissues resulted in a generally favorable prognosis. One patient had five recurrences over a period of 10 years, but only five patients died from their tumors. By contrast, in their review of 76 liposarcomas of the head and neck region, Golledge et al[18] found that, although myxoid liposarcomas overall had a 5-year survival rate of 73%, those in the mouth had the worst prognosis (5-year survival rate 50%), but data were available on only four cases.

REFERENCES

1. Vindenes H 1978 Lipomas of the oral cavity. Int J Oral Surg 7: 162–166
2. Cottrell DA, Norris LH, Doku C 1993 Orofacial lipomas diagnosed by CT and MRI. J Am Dent Assoc 124: 110–115
3. Enzinger FM, Weiss SW 1995 Soft tissue tumors, 3rd edn. C V Mosby St Louis
4. McDaniel RK, Newland JR, Chiles DG 1984 Intraoral spindle cell lipoma: case report with correlated light and electron microscopy. Oral Surg Oral Med Oral Pathol 57: 52–57
5. Christopoulos B. Nicolatou O, Patrikiou A 1989 Spindle cell lipoma. Report of a case. Int J Oral Maxillofac Surg 18: 208–209
6. Levy FE, Goding GS 1989 Spindle cell lipoma: an unusual presentation. Otolaryngol Head Neck Surg 101: 601–603
7. Lombardi T, Odell EW 1994 spindle cell lipoma of the oral cavity: report of a case. J Oral Pathol Med 23: 237–239

8. Flaggart JJ, Heldt LV, Keaton WM 1986 Angiolipoma of the palate. Report of a case. Oral Surg Oral Med Oral Pathol 60: 333–336

9. Farhood AI, Hajdu SI, Shiu MH, Strong EW 1990 Soft tissue sarcomas of the head and neck in adults. Am J Surg 160: 365–369

10. McCulloch TM, Makielski KH, McNutt MA et al 1992 Head and neck liposarcoma: histologic reevaluation of reported cases. Arch Otolaryngol Head Neck Surg 118: 1045–1049

11. Baden E, Newman R 1977 Liposarcoma of the oropharyngeal region. Review of the literature and report of two cases. Oral Surg Oral Med Oral Pathol 40: 889–902

12. Eidinger G, Katsikeris N, Gullane P 1991 Liposarcoma; report of a case and review of the literature. J Oral Maxillofac Surg 48: 984–988

13. Charnock DR, Jett T, Heise G, Taylor R 1991 Liposarcoma arising in the cheek: report of a case and review of the literature. J Oral Maxillofac Surg 49: 258–300

14. Guest PG 1992 Liposarcoma of the tongue: a case report and review of the literature. Br J Oral Maxillofac Surg 30: 268–269

15. Zheng J-W, Wang Y 1994 Liposarcoma in the oral and maxillofacial region: an analysis of 10 consecutive patients. J Oral Maxillofac Surg 52: 595–598

16. Friedman JL, Bistriz JI, Robinson MJ 1995 Pleomorphic liposarcoma of the pterygomandibular space involving the maxilla. Oral Surg Oral Med Oral Pathol Oral Radiol Endod 79: 488–491

17. Minec AJ 1995 Liposarcomas of the oral tissues: a clinicopathologic study of four tumors. J Oral Pathol Med 24: 180–184

18. Golledge J, Fisher C, Rhys-Evans P 1995 Head and neck liposarcoma. Cancer 76: 1051–1058

Benign pigmented lesions and melanomas 47

Factors affecting human melanocyte growth, differentiation, and pigment production have been reviewed by Yaar & Gilchrest.[1] Melanocytes arise from the neural crest and migrate to the basal cell layer of epithelia. There they form melanin, which is transferred via dendritic processes to adjacent keratinocytes. More rapid synthesis and formation of coarser granules of melanin (as in colored races), or proliferation of melanocytes, or both, results in deeper pigmentation.

Junctional activity is the term given to proliferation of melanocytes at the epitheliomesenchymal junction and protrusion of foci of melanocytes into the corium. In adults, junctional activity suggests the possibility of malignant change.

Compound nevi show both junctional activity and clusters of nevus cells in the corium. In such cases, melanocytes appear to be dropping down from the basal layer. Compound nevi of the skin are sometimes benign, but intraoral malignant melanomas are invariably compound (Figs 47.1–47.3).

Pigmented nevi far more frequently affect the skin than the mouth, but Buchner & Hansen[2] have reported the findings in 36 oral pigmented nevi of all types and reviewed 155 more from the literature. They found intramucosal nevi to account for 55% and common blue nevi to account for 32% of 191 benign pigmented lesions. Compound nevi accounted for 6%, junctional nevi for 5%, and combined nevi for 2%.

Eisen & Voorhees[3] have reviewed the spectrum of melanomas and other pigmented lesions seen in the oral cavity.

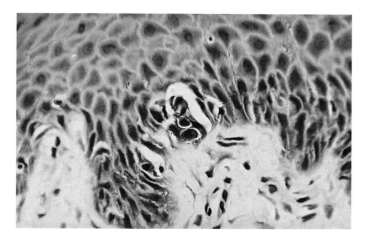

Fig. 47.2 Junctional activity. The nevus cells are confined to the basal layer; there is no evidence of cell or nuclear atypia.

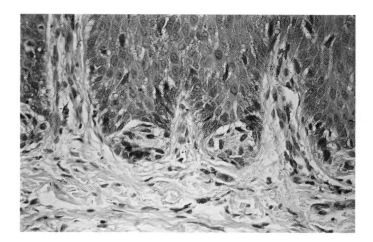

Fig. 47.1 Junctional nevus. Nests of nevus cells fill the tips of the rete ridges.

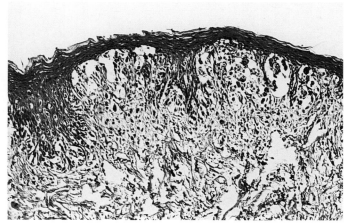

Fig. 47.3 Compound nevus. Low-power view showing conspicuous junctional activity with nevus cells, which are also seen in the superficial lamina propria.

327

Intramucosal melanotic nevi

Oral melanocytic nevi can be congenital or develop later. However, it is often impossible to know whether a melanocytic nevus, being asymptomatic, has recently arisen or has merely been noticed for the first time.

INCIDENCE

The buccal mucosa and the palate were the most common sites, and women accounted for 60% of the patients.[2]

CLINICAL FEATURES

Melanocytic nevi are well circumscribed and usually slightly raised or sometimes macular, but only very rarely polypoid. They can be brown, bluish, gray, or almost black, but 13% may be unpigmented and reddish.[2]

MICROSCOPY

Most melanotic nevi are intramucosal and show nevus cells that are usually pigmented, in circumscribed groups (theques) in the depths of the epithelium or immediately subjacent to the basal cell layer.

Gazit & Daniels[4] state that the round cells of melanotic nevi express S-100 more intensely than HMB-45.

Compound mucosal nevi are rare and may be difficult to distinguish from malignant melanoma if trauma has induced proliferative cellular activity. Junctional nevi of the oral mucosa are even more uncommon, as described earlier (Figs 47.4–47.6).

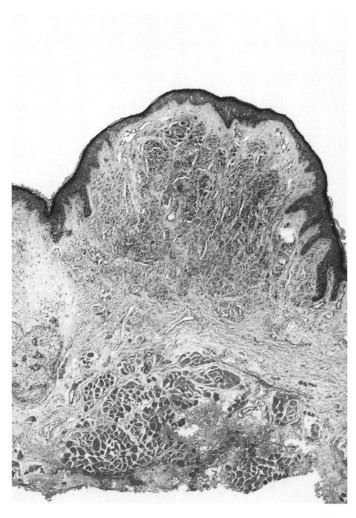

Fig. 47.4 Intramucosal nevus. Low-power view showing a symmetrical, nodular appearance. Pigmentation is not prominent in this lesion.

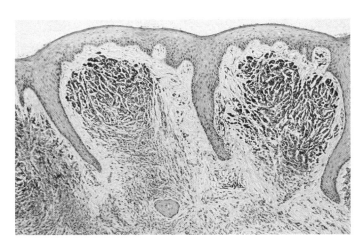

Fig. 47.5 Intramucosal nevus. Low-power view of a pigmented lesion showing downward maturation.

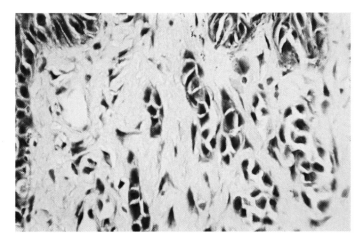

Fig. 47.6 Intramucosal nevus. High-power view of nests of plump nevus cells showing no evidence of atypia.

Blue nevi

Blue nevi form about a third of all oral nevi and resemble other pigmented lesions clinically apart from the bluish tinge.

MICROSCOPY

Blue nevi are covered by normal epithelium, but spindle-shaped pigmented melanocytes and melanin-containing macrophages (melanophages) are loosely grouped together in the corium and are typically well separated from the epithelial basal layer by connective tissue. Gazit & Daniels[4] have reported that the spindle cells of blue nevi express both S-100 and HMB-45 strongly (Figs 47.7 and 47.8).

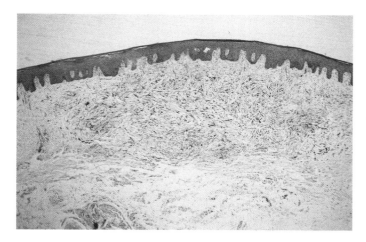

Fig. 47.7 Common blue nevus. A low-power view reveals a demarcated aggregate of pigmented cells within the lamina propria of palatal mucosa. The overlying epithelium is normal.

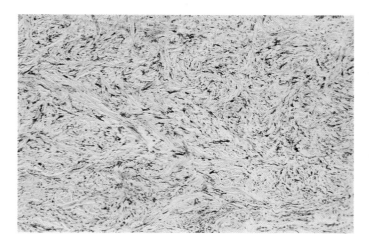

Fig. 47.8 Common blue nevus. At high power, the spindle and dendritic morphology of the lesional cells is apparent.

Oral melanocytic nevus combined with blue nevus (combined nevus) is rare, as noted earlier. Combined nevi have been reported by Ficarra et al.[5]

Oral melanotic macule

These freckle-like, brown to black pigmented macules are most commonly seen on the lip or buccal mucosa. Kaugars et al[6] analyzed the findings in 353 cases. These represented 0.4% of their 86 202 accessions over 22 years. The mean age of patients was 43.1 years (range 1–80 years), 63.5% were female, and 83.5% were white. The lower lip was involved in 33%, the palate and gingiva in approximately 20% each, and the buccal mucosa in 18%; 16.5% of cases were multiple macules. No mention was made of infection with human immunodeficiency virus (HIV) in any of these patients but oral and labial melanotic macules may be seen in 2–6% of patients with HIV infection, as discussed below. Barrett et al[7] have reported the development of oral melanotic macules after a course of external radiation to the cervical lymph nodes. No other cause for the pigmentation other than the radiotherapy was apparent, but they were unable to find any other reports of this phenomenon apart from radiation-associated esophageal melanosis.

MICROSCOPY

Overproduction of melanin is confined to the basal cell layer or immediately adjacent keratinocytes, but the epithelium and corium are otherwise normal. Prominent melanocytic activity is absent (Fig. 47.9).

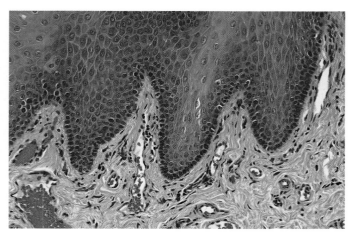

Fig. 47.9 Oral melanotic macule. There is focal hypermelanosis only in the basal and immediately suprabasal keratinocytes.

BEHAVIOR AND MANAGEMENT

Excision biopsy of melanotic macules is necessary for diagnosis but those in HIV-negative persons are more likely to enlarge and recur after excision. Increasing numbers of oral melanotic macules, particularly those that enlarge or recur after excision, may therefore be a sign of HIV infection.

ORAL MELANOTIC MACULES ASSOCIATED WITH HIV INFECTION

Langford et al[8] noted oral melanotic macules in 2.4% of 250 HIV-positive persons. Ficarra et al[9] found that oral melanotic macules developed in 6.4% of 217 HIV-positive persons over a 2-year period and were present in 3.6% of seronegative persons. The difference was not statistically significant, but the frequency of melanotic macules appears to rise with the severity of HIV infection. Cohen & Callen[10] have reported increasing numbers of oral melanotic macules in a patient 4 years before HIV infection was detected.

Histologically, these lesions show vacuolation of the spinous cells, either in large clusters or throughout the thickness of the epithelium. Excess melanin deposition is present in the basal cell layer and upper portion of the lamina propria.

The vacuolated cells resemble the koilocyte-like cells of hairy leukoplakia, but EBV DNA was found in only two specimens. The cause of the melanotic macules was unclear but in two patients they followed administration of zidovudine (AZT).

Lentigo simplex

Lentigo simplex of the oral mucosa resembles a melanotic macule clinically. Trodahl & Sprague[11] found 11 examples among 135 pigmented lesions of the oral mucosa, while Buchner et al[12] reported three examples in females aged 15–56 years.

MICROSCOPY

Microscopically, lentigo simplex shows long, slender rete ridges with an excess of melanocytes in the basal layer. Junctional activity is occasionally seen.

BEHAVIOR AND MANAGEMENT

Lentigo simplex is benign, but malignant lentigo can develop, particularly in sunburnt skin.

Melanoacanthoma

Melanoacanthoma is an exceptionally uncommon pigmented lesion. The cutaneous type was described by Mishima & Pinkus[13] and the oral variant was reviewed by Buchner et al,[12] who considered that approximately 20 acceptable examples had been reported at that time. Melanoacanthomas have mostly been seen in blacks, and women have been affected three times as frequently as men.

CLINICAL FEATURES

Melanoacanthomas have appeared as unilateral, sharply demarcated, deeply pigmented macules or may be more proliferative and appear warty. They form in areas subject to trauma, and may regress after removal of the trauma or incomplete excision. Melanoacanthoma may, therefore, be reactive rather than neoplastic.

MICROSCOPY

The epithelium is acanthotic and contains clear cells and large melanin-producing melanocytes with dendritic processes, which are made more obvious by silver staining. There is no nuclear pleomorphism or atypia (Figs 47.10 and 47.11).

MANAGEMENT

All oral pigmented lesions need to be treated by excision biopsy to exclude malignant melanoma. As most benign lesions are small, excision is curative. As a general guide, nevi are more common in younger people (up to 40 years), are usually small, and appear to be static.

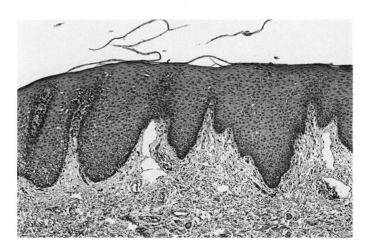

Fig. 47.10 Melanoacanthoma. Low-power view shows rete and melanocytic hyperplasia.

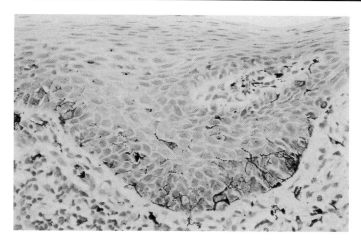

Fig. 47.11 Melanoacanthoma. High-power view. Pleomorphic, hyperchromatic melanocytes with dendritic processes, staining positively for S-100 and melanin. S-100 immunoperoxidase/Masson Fontana stain.

Malignant melanoma

Intraoral melanomas are uncommon but have a poor prognosis, as emphasized by van der Waal et al,[14] due to the long asymptomatic period. The peak age incidence is between 40 and 60 years; nearly 50% of these melanomas are on the hard palate, and about 25% are on the upper gingivae. Men are slightly more frequently affected. About 30% of melanomas are preceded by an area of hyperpigmentation, often by many years. Pigmentation varies from black to brown. Rare nonpigmented melanomas (15% of oral melanomas) are red. Oral melanomas may be flat, but are usually raised or nodular, and asymptomatic initially, but may later become ulcerated, painful or may bleed. Tanaka et al[15] on the basis of 20 new cases and a review of 140 others, have defined five types:

- pigmented nodular
- nonpigmented nodular
- pigmented macular
- pigmented mixed type
- nonpigmented mixed type.

Because of their rapid growth, most oral melanomas are at least 1 cm across, and approximately 50% of patients have metastases at presentation. Metastases spread to regional lymph nodes, lungs, liver, brain, and bones. Clinical aspects, microscopy, and management have been reviewed by Strauss & Strauss,[16] who point out that mucosal melanomas are more common in India, Africa, and Japan, but cutaneous melanomas are less frequent in those countries. Tanaka et al[15] suggest that oral melanomas account for up to 12% of all melanomas in Japan, as compared with 0.2–8% in Europe and the USA.

MICROSCOPY

Malignant melanocytes invade both epithelium and connective tissue. Melanoma cells may be round, spindle-shaped, or both, and there may be associated pseudoepitheliomatous hyperplasia.

Superficially spreading melanomas, which are considerably more uncommon in the mouth than on the skin, have a pre-invasive phase when atypical melanocytes with clear areas of cytoplasm (pagetoid cells) are clustered along the epitheliomesenchymal junction. Growth is radial rather than invasive, and there may be a few scattered melanocytes in the superficial corium associated with a sparse inflammatory cellular infiltrate. Active invasion follows after a variable period.

Anaplastic, nonpigmented malignant melanomas can readily be confused with other mesenchymal tumors, and can be sarcoma-like. Diagnosis is greatly helped by immunohistochemistry. Melanomas are typically S-100, melanoma-associated antigen (MMA), and HMB-45 positive, as reported by Gazit & Daniels.[4] HMB-45 and NKI/C3 are currently regarded as being more specific for malignant melanoma than is reactivity for S-100 protein. However, in a clinicopathologic and immuno-histochemical analysis of nine oral malignant melanomas, which showed the same general features as in previous series, Barrett et al[17] found that each of them individually showed features of each type of cutaneous melanoma. None of them stained for cytokeratins. All expressed S-100, but two that were strongly positive for S-100 did not stain with either HMB45 or NKI/C3. Therefore, Barrett et al[17] suggested that oral malignant melanoma, on the basis of its clinicopathologic and immuno-histochemical features, should be regarded as a separate entity from cutaneous melanoma (Figs 47.12–47.20).

BEHAVIOR AND MANAGEMENT

Oral melanomas are highly malignant and have a high mortality. Chiu & Weinstock,[18] from a study of 109 oral and 60 nasal melanomas, found that the median survival was 2 years and the 5-year survival rate was 25%. Biopsy is essential to confirm the diagnosis. Clinically, size and rapid growth, particularly if associated with destruction of underlying bone or presence of metastases, are indicators of a poor outcome.

Microscopically, tumor thickness, measured in millimeters from the granular cell layer to the deepest identifiable melanocyte (the Breslow thickness), is the main guide to prognosis. With cutaneous melanomas the 5-year survival rate is inversely proportional to the Breslow thickness. The poor prognosis of oral melanomas is probably due to their later detection than for more conspicuous skin tumors, but some consider them to be more aggressive and possibly deserving of a separate category in classification.

Other indicators of a poor prognosis are malignant melanocytes in blood vessels, and multiple, or atypical, mitoses, and metastasis to regional nodes or other sites. The morphology of the melanocytes or the amount of melanin does not appear to affect the outcome.

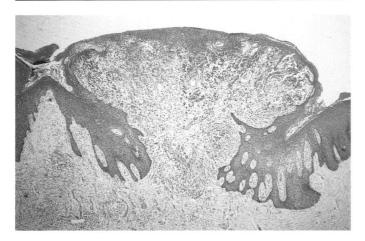

Fig. 47.12 Malignant melanoma. Vertical growth phase showing a nodular, ulcerated, exophytic neoplasm with a cuff of mucosa covered by hyperplastic epithelium.

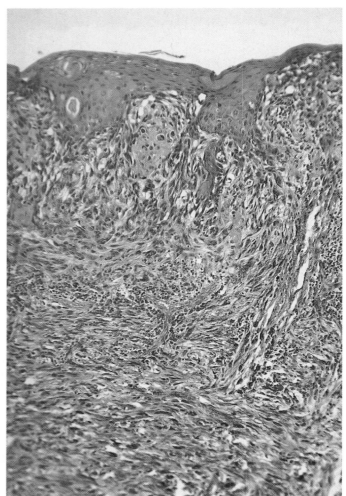

Fig. 47.14 Malignant melanoma. Pleomorphic, hyperchromatic melanocytes at the tips of the rete ridges with sheets of pigmented spindle cells and melanophages in the superficial lamina propria.

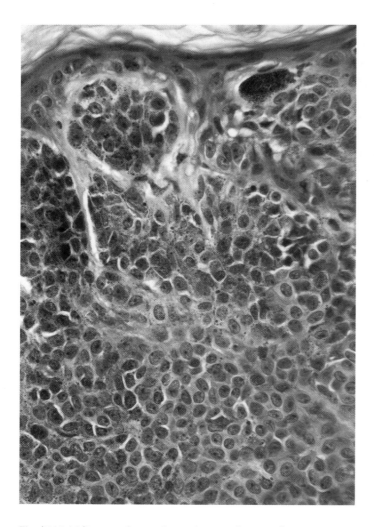

Fig. 47.13 Malignant melanoma. Pagetoid groups of tumor cells are present in the suprabasal epithelium.

Once the diagnosis has been confirmed, the only hope of cure is provided by wide excision with a 2–5 cm margin, followed by radical radiotherapy. Tanaka et al[15] quote reports to the effect that malignant melanoma is radioresistant and that radiotherapy is only palliative, but found it to be effective in their own cases. Block dissection of any clinically involved lymph nodes may also be necessary. There is no wide confirmation as yet that chemotherapy is of significant value except for palliation, although there are many chemotherapeutic regimens under trial. However, Umeda & Shimada[19] claim success for treatment of 11 patients with surgical excision, neck dissection of clinically involved nodes, and chemotherapy. Survival for up to 2 years without evidence of disease was achieved for nine of their 11 patients.

Immunotherapy with, for example, interferon, and gene therapy are also under trial. Strauss & Strauss[16] quote reported 5-year survival rates ranging from 4.5% to 29%, with a median

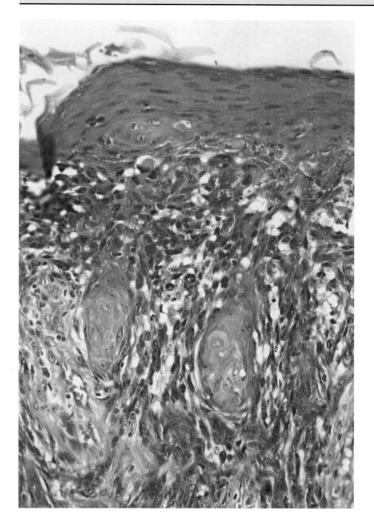

Fig. 47.15 Malignant melanoma. High-power view showing pleomorphic malignant melanocytes and the epithelium has extended deeply to give a pseudoepitheliomatous appearance.

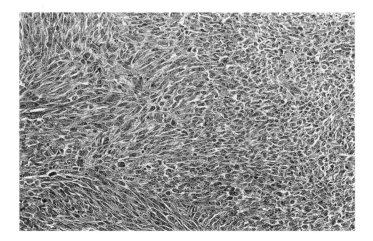

Fig. 47.16 Malignant melanoma. Sheets of epithelioid melanocytes are intermingled with spindle-shaped melanocytes.

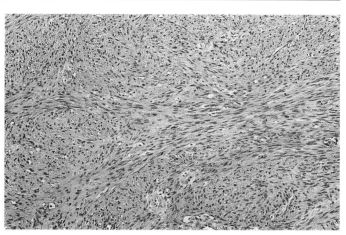

Fig. 47.17 Malignant melanoma showing sarcomatous, 'swarming' pattern.

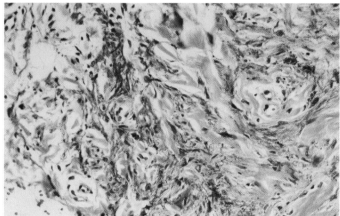

Fig. 47.18 Malignant melanoma. High-power view of pigmented, sarcoma-like spindle cells.

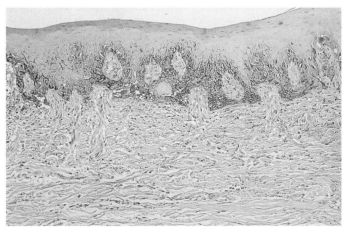

Fig. 47.19 Malignant melanoma. Radial growth phase showing abundant positive basal and suprabasal, superficially migrating cells. Peroxide bleach followed by S100 immunoperoxidase.

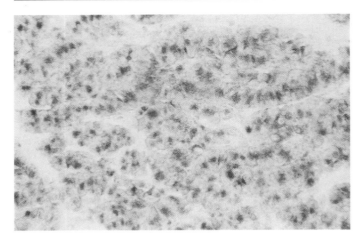

Fig. 47.20 Malignant melanoma. Immunohistochemistry showed the tumor cells to be HMB45-positive.

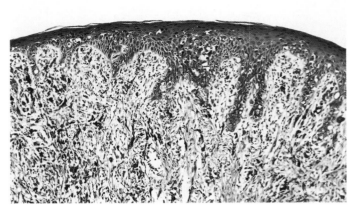

Fig. 47.21 Lentigo maligna. The epithelium has the typical honeycomb appearance with neoplastic melanocytes within the epithelium and spread along the basal layer.

survival of 18.5 months after initial diagnosis. The value of interferon remains uncertain, as discussed by Yoshida et al.[20]

LENTIGO MALIGNA MELANOMA

This variant is relatively common on the facial skin, where it may have a radial growth phase for many years. It is exceptionally uncommon in the oral cavity and cannot be distinguished clinically from the more common types of intraoral melanoma.

MICROSCOPY

Lentigo maligna is distinguishable by proliferation of atypical dendritic melanocytes along the basal layer of the epithelium, with little tendency to invade the upper layers. Fixation artifact causes melanocytes to appear with clear halos. Pigmentation is sometimes abundant and may spread through the full thickness of the epithelium. Progression to invasive melanoma is characterized by proliferation of malignant melanocytes, which are typically spindle-shaped and parallel with the surface both in junctional nests and more deeply in the corium (Fig. 47.21).

Acral lentigo maligna, which can also occasionally be seen in the mouth, shows even more inconspicuous changes, initially with angular, atypical melanocytes scattered along the basal layer of a hyperplastic epithelium. Cutaneous lentigo maligna melanoma has an exceptionally slow peripheral growth. However, no better prognosis for this variant when in the mouth has been confirmed. Strauss & Strauss[16] have pointed out that oral melanomas that resemble lentigo maligna melanoma histologically have an initial radial growth phase, but the vertical growth phase is aggressive with a strong potential for widespread metastasis.

DESMOPLASTIC MALIGNANT MELANOMA

Anstey et al[21] have analyzed the clinicopathologic features of 25 cases of cutaneous desmoplastic malignant melanoma, and noted that the diagnosis was made without significant delay in only eight of these cases. Unlike other melanomas, males are predominantly affected, and desmoplastic malignant melanoma more frequently arises in the elderly. It is exceptionally uncommon in the oral cavity, but Kurihara et al,[22] who could find reports of only two earlier cases, described an example involving the gingiva. This tumor, in a 58-year-old male, formed an epulis-like swelling with a smooth surface, and two adjacent smaller, brown verrucous swellings associated with macular pigmentation. Kilpatrick et al[23] have added three new cases and emphasized the diagnostic difficulties. The site of predilection appears to be the maxillary alveolar ridge, and the tumor is typically nonpigmented.

MICROSCOPY

Desmoplastic malignant melanoma consists of a fibrotic mass containing melanocytes. In most of the cutaneous cases reported by Anstey et al[21] and the oral case reported by Kurihara et al,[22] there was melanocytic junctional proliferation superficially. The melanoma cells were spindle shaped, nonpigmented, and showed moderate atypia and occasional mitoses. Morphologically, melanoma cells were difficult to distinguish among the fibrous tissue with conventional staining. Being amelanotic they were also negative with Masson–Fontana stain. The adjacent verrucous lesions showed non-neoplastic papillary proliferation and intraepithelial nests of melanocytes. The latter showed moderate atypia and occasional mitoses, but no vertical invasion. The desmoplastic melanoma and the verrucous melanoma cells were strongly positive for S-100 protein, but only mildly or moderately positive for nonspecific enolase. The three tumors reported by

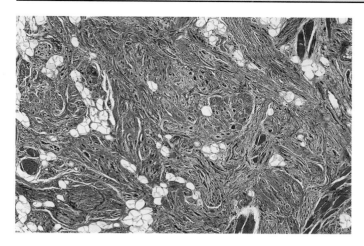

Fig. 47.22 Desmoplastic melanoma. Isolated nests and strands of tumor cells are seen buried in a dense tangled fibrous stroma.

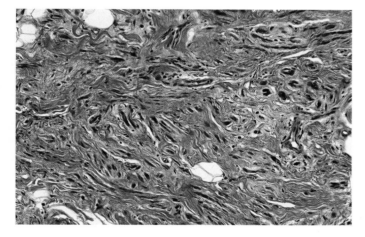

Fig. 47.23 Desmoplastic melanoma. Even at higher power, melanoma cells are difficult to discern with hematoxylin and eosin staining.

Kilpatrick et al[23] showed fibrosarcoma- or neurosarcoma-like areas, absence of melanin pigment, and only one showed positive reactivity for HMB-45. However, all were S-100 positive (Figs 47.22 and 47.23).

Anstey et al[21] had also noted that melanin was not identifiable in typical areas of desmoplastic melanoma in any of their specimens.

BEHAVIOR AND MANAGEMENT

Some of the cutaneous desmoplastic malignant melanomas reported by Anstey et al[21] grew rapidly. After surgical excision, only 13 of 25 patients were alive and without evidence of tumor 9 months to 10 years later. The oral example reported by Kurihara et al[22] grew slowly over a year. It recurred 18 months after partial maxillectomy. The recurrence showed a much higher

mitotic rate and cellularity, but some of the tumor cells were S-100 negative. In reviewing the outcome in seven cases of oral desmoplastic malignant melanoma where information was available, Kilpatrick et al[23] found that four patients had died from their disease within periods of 4 months to 2.5 years

Therefore, aggressive treatment of desmoplastic malignant melanoma seems to be necessary.

METASTATIC MELANOMAS

Metastatic melanomas have very occasionally been reported in the oral cavity and in the parotid gland. Patton et al[24] analyzed records of 809 cases of metastases of malignant melanoma documented at the National Institutes of Health and found that 15 had been in the oral soft tissues or jaws. The mean age at the time of diagnosis of the primary melanoma was approximately 40 years (range 16–60 years). Diagnosis of oral metastases followed 5 months to 12 years later. The tongue was the single most frequently affected oral site, and in many cases there were multiple other sites of metastases. Nine patients died 8 months to 10 years after diagnosis of the primary tumor, but six survived for 0.9–10 years. Billings et al[25] suggested that 0.6–9.3% of cutaneous melanomas metastasized to the mucosa of upper aerodigestive tract and appeared 2–7 years after the cutaneous lesion. Junctional activity in overlying or adjacent mucosa was useful for distinguishing primary malignant melanoma from metastases in which the mucosa was typically intact.

If nonpigmented and anaplastic, metastatic melanomas may be difficult to recognize if the possibility is not suspected and immunostaining is not carried out.

A note of caution about the accuracy of diagnosis of pigmented lesions has also been sounded by Farmer et al,[26] who described the low level of agreement shown by a panel of expert pathologists who were presented with 37 cases judged to be 'classical.' There was unanimous agreement as to whether or not the melanocytic neoplasms were malignant in only 30% of cases.

REFERENCES

1. Yaar M, Gilchrest BA 1991 Human melanocyte growth and differentiation: a decade of new data. J Invest Dermatol 97: 611–617
2. Buchner A, Hansen LS 1987 Pigmented nevi of the oral mucosa: a clinicopathologic study of 36 cases and review of 155 cases from the literature. Oral Surg Oral Med Oral Pathol 63: 566–572
3. Eisen D, Voorhees JJ 1991 Oral melanoma and other pigmented lesions of the oral cavity. J Am Acad Dermatol 24: 527–537
4. Gazit D, Daniels TE 1994 Oral melanocytic lesions: differences in expression of HMB-45 and S-100 antigens in round and spindle cells of malignant and benign lesions. J Oral Pathol Med 23: 60–64
5. Ficarra G, Hansen LS, Engbretson S, Levin LS 1987 Combined nevus of the oral mucosa. Oral Surg Oral Med Oral Pathol 63: 196–201
6. Kaugars GE, Heise AP, Riley WT, Abbey LM, Svirsky JA 1993 Oral melanotic macules. A review of 353 cases. Oral Surg Oral Med Oral Pathol 76: 59–61
7. Barrett AW, Porter SR, Scully C, Eveson JW, Griffiths MJ 1994 Oral melanotic macules that develop after radiation therapy. Oral Surg Oral Med Oral Pathol 77: 431–434
8. Langford A, Pohle HD, Gelderblom H et al 1989 Oral hyperpigmentation in HIV-infected patients. Oral Surg Oral Med Oral Pathol 67: 301–307
9. Ficarra G, Shillitoe EJ, Adler-Storthz K et al 1990 Oral melanotic macules associated with HIV. Oral Surg Oral Med Oral Pathol 70: 301–307

10. Cohen LM, Callen JP 1992 Oral and labial melanotic macules in a patient infected with human immunodeficiency virus. J Am Acad Dermatol 26: 653–654

11. Trodahl JN, Sprague WG 1970 Benign and malignant melanocytic lesions of the oral mucosa: an analysis of 135 cases. Cancer 25: 12–23

12. Buchner A, Merrell PW, Hansen LS, Leider AS 1991 Melanocytic hyperplasia of the oral mucosa. Oral Surg Oral Med Oral Pathol 71: 58–62

13. Mishima Y, Pinkus H 1960 Benign mixed tumor of melanocytes and malpighian cells. Arch Dermatol 81: 539–550

14. van der Waal RI, Snow GB, Karim AB, van der Waal I 1994 Primary malignant melanoma of the oral cavity: a review of eight cases. Br Dent J 176; 185–188

15. Tanaka N, Amagasa T, Iwaki H et al 1994 Oral malignant melanoma in Japan. Oral Surg Oral Med Oral Pathol 78: 81–90

16. Strauss JE, Strauss SI 1994 Oral malignant melanoma: a case report and review of literature. J Oral Maxillofac Surg 52: 972–976

17. Barrett AW, Bennett JH, Speight PM 1995 A clinicopathological and immunohistochemical analysis of primary oral malignant melanoma. Eur J Cancer B: Oral Oncol 31: 100–115

18. Chiu NT, Weinstock MA 1996 Melanoma of oronasal mucosa. Population-based analysis of occurrence and mortality. Arch Otolaryngol Head Neck Surg 122: 985–988

19. Umeda M, Shimada K 1994 Primary malignant melanoma of the oral cavity – its histological classification and treatment. Br J Oral Maxillofac Surg 32: 39–47

20. Yoshida H, Mizukami M, Hirohata H, Hagiwara T 1994 Response of primary oral malignant melanoma: report of two cases. J Oral Maxillofac Surg 53: 506–510

21. Anstey A, Mc Kee P, Wilson Jones E 1993 Desmoplastic malignant melanoma: a clinicopathological study of 25 cases. Br J Dermatol 129: 359–371

22. Kurihara K, Sanada E, Yasuda S, Yamasaki H 1992 Desmoplastic malignant melanoma. Oral Surg Oral Med Oral Pathol 74: 201–205

23. Kilpatrick SE, White WL, Brown JD 1996 Desmoplastic malignant melanoma of the oral cavity. An underrecognised diagnostic pitfall. Cancer 78: 383–389

24. Patton LL, Brahim JS, Baker AR 1994 Metastatic malignant melanoma of the oral cavity. A retrospective study. Oral Surg Oral Med Oral Pathol 78: 51–56

25. Billings KR, Wang MB, Secarz JA, Fu YS 1995 Clinical and pathological distinction between primary and metastatic melanoma of the head and neck. Otolaryngol Head Neck Surg 112: 700–706

26. Farmer ER, Gonin R, Hanna MP 1996 Discordance in the histopathologic diagnosis of melanoma and melanocytic nevi between expert pathologists. Hum Pathol 27: 528–531

Soft tissue tumors of uncertain nature

48

Geranular cell tumor ('myoblastoma')

This tumor, was considered to be a disease of muscle by Abrikossoff.[1] However, from their ultrastructural and histochemical findings, Fisher & Wechsler[2] proposed that it originated from Schwann cells or their precursors. Reports of positive staining with neuron-specific enolase by Rode et al[3] and S-100 ('brain-specific') protein by Armin et al[4] appeared to confirm this view, and Thompson[5] found that granular cell tumors of the tongue failed to stain for myoglobin. However, other ultrastructural reports have suggested an origin from undifferentiated mesenchymal cells and, in any case, S-100 protein is not specific for neural cells.

Stewart et al[6] found that skeletal muscle stained weakly and that 50% of rhabdomyomas also stained positively for S-100 protein. They also found that 70% of granular cell tumors were invested by muscle and only 5% by nerve. In one of their cases examined by electron microscopy, the granular cells showed a direct evolution from muscle fibers. Baden et al[7] reviewed the histochemical findings up to 1990, and noted that, unlike granular cell tumors, Schwann cells did not stain positively with neural crest markers such as NSE or NK1/C3. Whereas Schwann cells stained positively for GFAP, granular cell tumors did not. Mentzel et al[8] reported the immunohistochemical findings on smooth-muscle tumors that showed granular cytoplasmic change. They concluded that granular cytoplasmic change was no more than a cytological phenotype, which apparently represented a particular metabolic change that was not exclusively associated with Schwann cell tumors, and that the granular cell tumor was not a specific entity.

INCIDENCE

Baden et al,[7] in their review of the literature, considered that over 1200 granular cell tumors had been reported, with about 50% of them in the head and neck region. Of these, approximately 60% were in the tongue, which is the most common single site. There was a female preponderance of 2 : 1 and a predilection for blacks. The age range of those affected is wide, but there is a peak in the fourth to sixth decades. Multiple tumors comprised 7–16% of cases and formed synchronously or metachronously over the course of several years.

CLINICAL FEATURES

Granular cell tumors often form small circumscribed lumps or firm areas just under the surface, particularly in the tongue. Occasionally, the lesion is large and prominent, or resembles a carcinoma clinically. Rarely they may develop in the midline of the tongue and then be mistaken for median rhomboid glossitis or even a carcinoma.

MICROSCOPY

The appearances are difficult to reconcile with a neural origin as the large granular cells frequently appear to merge with muscle fibers. The granules, which are eosinophilic and periodic acid Schiff (PAS) positive, may be so coarse as to make the cells conspicuous, or so fine as to be difficult to see. The cell membranes are typically well defined. Frequently, the overlying epithelium undergoes pseudoepitheliomatous hyperplasia, which may be mistaken for a carcinoma and be treated as such[9] (Figs 48.1–48.3 and 48.6).

A rare desmoplastic variant in which small nests of granular cells are embedded in a dense collagenous stroma is recognized, but only a single example has so far been reported(Figs 48.4 and 48.5).[10]

Granular cell tumors respond to local excision but can recur if excision is inadequate.

BEHAVIOR AND MANAGEMENT

Excision is the treatment of choice and, if complete, is curative.

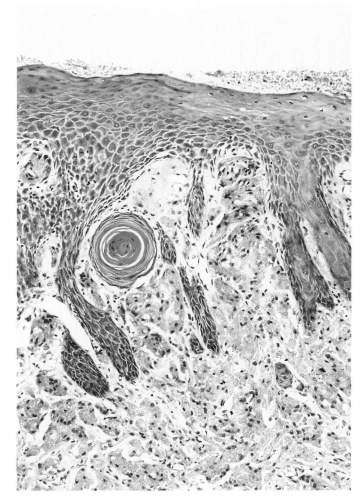

Fig. 48.1 Granular cell tumor. Pseudoepitheliomatous hyperplasia with prominent cell nests. A typical appearance of oral examples of this tumor.

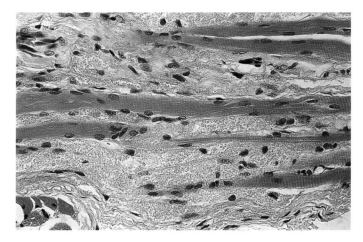

Fig. 48.2 Granular cell tumor. The merging of muscle fibers of the tongue with granular cells gives credence either to a muscle fiber origin to the tumor or that it is a nonspecific degenerative change.

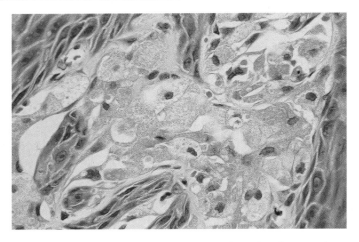

Fig. 48.3 Granular cell tumor. Higher power view of granular cells among the proliferating epithelium.

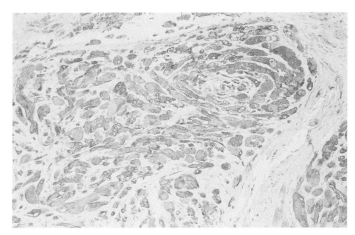

Fig. 48.4 Granular cell tumor. The granular cells are strongly positive for S-100 protein.

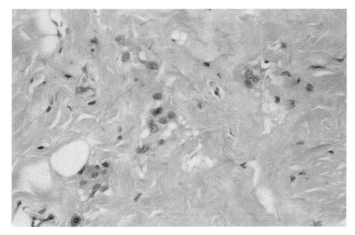

Fig. 48.5 Granular cell tumor. Desmoplastic variant with granular cells embedded in a dense collagenous stroma.

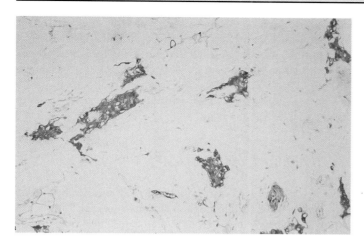

Fig. 48.6 Desmoplastic granular cell tumor. S-100 positive cells are seen in the collagenous stroma

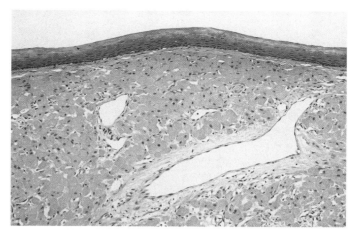

Fig. 48.7 Congenital granular cell epulis. In contrast to the granular cell tumor, the granular cells are covered by flattened stratified squamous epithelium and there are prominent dilated vessels within the mass.

Congenital granular cell epulis (gingival granular cell tumor)

This uncommon entity is found on the alveolar ridge of the newborn. Zuker & Buenchea,[11] in reviewing the literature since 1972, found reports of 195 examples. The maxilla is affected in 65%, and 85% of affected infants are female.

A congenital epulis forms a soft rounded swelling a few millimeters across, or may be so large as to protrude from the mouth. Such cases can cause neonatal respiratory obstruction but can be visualized in utero by ultrasonography.[12] Immediate postnatal treatment is thus possible.

MICROSCOPY

The mass consists of closely packed granular cells with prominent cell membranes and among which is a delicate network of capillaries. Rarely, small odontogenic rests may be present. Unlike granular cell tumor, the overlying epithelium is thin and flat and the granular cells are invested by muscle fibers (Figs 48.7 and 48.8).

Unlike the granular cell tumor, congenital epulis cells are S-100 negative, but may stain positively for myogenous markers such as myosin and actin. The ultrastructural findings of Rohrer & Young[13] indicated an origin from pericytes, and those of Zarbo et al[14] indicated an origin from a primitive gingival mesenchymal cell with the potential for smooth-muscle cytodifferentiation. Damm et al[15] used a large panel of immunohistochemical stains on five congenital epulides. Unlike several earlier workers they found that none of these epulides stained positively for epithelial markers, α1 antitrypsin, carcinoembryonic antigen, desmin, factor VIII, KP-1, leucocyte common antigen, muscle-specific actin, OKT6, or S-100 protein. The only positive results (four of five specimens) were with neuron-specific enolase and vimentin.

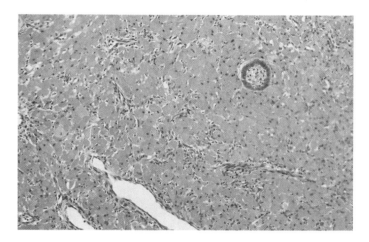

Fig. 48.8 Congenital granular cell epulis. The granular cells are well defined and contain an eccentric nucleus. The mass also contains an island of odontogenic epithelium.

In contrast to the histochemical findings, Zarbo et al[16] and Damm et al[15] found contractile elements and evidence of smooth muscle differentiation by electron microscopy. There was also active production of extracellular collagen. The granular appearance seen by light microscopy was due to widespread autophagocytosis. Damm et al[15] suggested, therefore, that the tumor cells had pericytic and myofibroblastic features.

BEHAVIOR AND MANAGEMENT

Treatment is by excision, but the congenital epulis does not apparently recur even if excision is incomplete, and may sometimes regress spontaneously. This suggests that the lesion is a hamartoma. In the case reported by MacMahon & Mintz[12] a KTP (potassium, titanyl phosphate) laser (532 nm wavelength) was used and led to rapid healing.

Alveolar soft part sarcoma

This uncommon tumor was formerly considered to be a malignant form of the granular cell tumor, but immunohistochemical findings have been inconsistent. It is of debatable histogenesis, but the most favored possibilities are that it is of neural crest or myogenic origin.

Alveolar soft part sarcomas account for fewer than 1% of all soft tissue sarcomas. A review by Enzinger & Weiss[17] of 143 cases at the Armed Forces Institute of Pathology showed that 27% of these tumors were in the head and neck area, particularly in the orbital region (16 cases) or the tongue (10 cases). In the head and neck region these tumors most often affect children, whereas those in the lower extremities (the single most frequent site) are usually found in adults. The peak frequency is at a mean age of 25 years and in younger patients; females are more frequently affected. However, Carson et al[18] reported an alveolar soft part sarcoma of the tongue in a 64-year-old man, which is in sharp contrast to the ages of the 41 patients that they reviewed. Marker et al[19] reported another case in the mouth and reviewed the findings in 11 other oral examples. Nine of these were in the tongue.

Even more uncommon is metastasis of alveolar soft part sarcoma to the oral tissues, as reported by Porter et al[20] who described an example in the tongue secondary to a primary tumor in the brachialis muscle.

CLINICAL FEATURES

Alveolar soft part sarcomas form nondescript, painless swellings without distinctive features, although they are sometimes so richly vascular as to cause a bruit or even to be pulsatile.

MICROSCOPY

Alveolar soft part sarcoma shows an organoid pattern consisting of tumor cells in rounded nests outlined by delicate or dense fibrovascular septa. The pattern is similar to that of a paraganglioma. The tumor cells are large, rounded, or polygonal with finely granular cytoplasm. The nuclei are large with prominent nucleoli. Loss of intercellular adhesion can lead to the formation of a pseudoalveolar pattern.

A characteristic diagnostic feature is the presence of PAS-positive, diastase-resistant, rod-shaped granules in the cytoplasm of the tumor cells. Electron microscopy shows membrane-bound granules and crystalloids, some of which are of remarkably regular rhomboid shape with a linear paracrystalline substructure.

Carson et al[18] found that their specimen stained positively only for neuron-specific enolase, as did only two other reported cases that they reviewed. This review included the findings of eight previous reports and made apparent the variability of the immunohistochemical staining patterns of this tumor. Sciot et al[21] reported strongly positive staining for desmin and weakly positive staining for vimentin, but negative staining for neural markers. They also identified a chromosomal abnormality with involvement of 17q25, and considered that their findings supported a myogenic origin.

BEHAVIOR AND MANAGEMENT

Alveolar soft part sarcomas grow slowly but tend to metastasize early, particularly to the lungs, brain, and skeleton, sometimes before the primary tumor has been detected. Marker et al[19] quote estimated survival rates of 62% after 5 years, 43% after 10 years, and 8% after 20 years. The main route of spread is hematogenous, and tumor cells may be found in blood vessels sometimes, even at an early stage. Metastases may therefore be present when the patient is first seen. Thus, the patient reported by Carson et al[18] had a large tongue mass and involvement of regional lymph nodes. Despite an unresectable mass and poor response to radiotherapy and chemotherapy, this patient survived for nearly 3 years before succumbing to widespread metastatic disease. Radical surgical excision is indicated, but the long-term prognosis is poor and most patients die as a result of their disease. However, the patient reported by Marker et al[19] was still free from disease 19 years after radical surgery.

Benign mesenchymoma

Mesenchymomas consist of a mixture of two or more mesenchymal elements such as fat, smooth muscle, blood vessels, and cartilage or bone, but contain no epithelial elements. Choristomas, by contrast, contain only a single ectopic tissue, such as cartilage, in the soft tissues. Mesenchymomas are found in the extremities, urogenital tract, or breast; they are particularly uncommon in the oral cavity. Daly & Gutenberg[22] were able to trace reports of 20 mesenchymomas of the oral cavity, while Micheau et al[23] found only one case of mesenchymoma among 2109 tumors of the tongue. Takenoshita et al[24] reported a mesenchymoma of the tongue in an 88-year-old woman and, in reviewing the literature, considered it to be only the eighth case of mesenchymoma of the tongue to have been reported.

CLINICAL FEATURES

Mesenchymomas have usually been found in children or young adults up to the age of 25 years. The example in an 88-year-old woman reported by Takenoshita et al[24] is therefore exceptional, and they produced additional evidence suggesting that mesenchymomas are neoplasms rather than hamartomas.

Oral mesenchymomas typically form dome-shaped, smooth-surfaced, painless swellings. They are usually less than 2 cm in diameter when first noticed, soft or firm in texture, and pink, yellowish, or grey in color, depending on the predominant mesenchymal elements.

MICROSCOPY

Mesenchymomas are not encapsulated. The mesenchymal components are distributed haphazardly and may extend slightly into or entrap adjacent normal structures such as a few muscle fibers. Typical components are mature cartilage, bone, adipose tissue, striated or smooth muscle, blood vessels, and peripheral nerve tissue. There is considerable variation in the appearance and the number of mesenchymal components present. Thus, a mesenchymoma consisting mainly of cartilage may mimic a chondroma or cartilaginous choristoma.

It may be noted that Enzinger & Weiss[17] only recognize malignant mesenchymoma as an entity, and suggest that the term *benign mesenchymoma* has been used as an alternative term for such tumors as lipomas with cartilaginous or osseous metaplasia, or intramuscular haemangiomas with overgrowth of fatty tissue.

BEHAVIOR AND MANAGEMENT

The reported rate of growth of benign mesenchymomas appears to vary widely. For example, the mesenchymoma of the lower lip reported by Couwenhoven et al[25] had been noticed only 4 weeks earlier, while the example on the tongue reported by Takenoshita et al[24] had been growing gradually for at least 12 years.

Stout[26] reported a single case of a mesenchymoma that underwent sudden malignant change, but no such cases have as yet been reported in the oral cavity.

Excision is the treatment of choice. Takenoshita et al[24] quote a recurrence rate of 20%. This probably reflects the ability of mesenchymomas to extend into the surrounding tissues. Excision should therefore include an adequate margin of normal tissue, and prolonged follow-up should be maintained.

Synovial sarcoma

Paradoxically, synovial sarcoma affects tissues adjacent to or unrelated to joints rather than joints themselves. The extremities, particularly the lower, are most commonly involved. Enzinger & Weiss[17] in their analysis of 345 cases noted that 9% were in the head and neck region, although only the neck, pharynx, or larynx were involved. Shmookler et al[27] reported 11 cases in the orofacial regions; of these only two were in the tongue. Nevertheless, oral and perioral regions such as the soft palate,[28] tongue,[29,30] and other sites[31] can be affected, as can the temporo-

mandibular joint[32] on rare occasions. Overall, the tongue appears to be the single most frequently affected site in the mouth. Carrillo et al[33] reported one case and reviewed six others. The base of the tongue was involved in five of them. A rare possibility is metastasis of synovial sarcoma to the jaws, of which two examples have been reported.[34]

CLINICAL FEATURES

Synovial sarcoma frequently forms an insidiously growing, deep soft tissue mass, which may eventually become painful and, if related to a joint, limit movement.

MICROSCOPY

Classical synovial sarcoma is biphasic, with both spindle cell and epithelial elements. The spindle cells are fibroblast-like, while the epithelial cells, which stain positively with epithelial cell markers, are typically cuboidal or tall and columnar.

The spindle cells usually form the bulk of the tumor and are usually uniform, with plump nuclei and indistinct cytoplasm. They may form well-oriented streams of cells resembling a well-differentiated fibrosarcoma. Mast cells are typically present and are particularly numerous in the spindle-cell areas. Less cellular areas can show collagen formation, myxoid change, or calcification. Varying degrees of calcification or even ossification develops in about 40% of these tumors, and is an important radiological feature.

The epithelial cells can form a variety of arrangements, such as whorls or solid cords, or they may confer a gland-like appearance to an area. Sometimes they may line clefts or cyst-like spaces and thus may resemble normal synovium. An uncommon variation is squamous differentiation with the formation of occasional cell nests.

In the monophasic type of synovial sarcoma, epithelial elements are scanty and difficult to find. The bulk of the tumor therefore consists of spindle-shaped cells in the same configurations as seen in biphasic tumors (Figs 48.9 and 48.10).

Variable numbers of these spindle cells may stain for epithelial markers. The characteristic cytogenetic abnormality, that is, t(x;18)(p11.2;q11.2), is of diagnostic value.

Although the main types of synovial sarcoma have been described, many variations on these configurations may be seen.

BEHAVIOR AND MANAGEMENT

Metastases, most frequently to the lungs, form in about 50% of cases, and can sometimes appear 10 years or more after initial treatment. Metastases to lymph nodes are seen in only 10–20% of cases.

The prognosis of synovial sarcoma is related to its extent at diagnosis and to the degree of differentiation, rather than to the

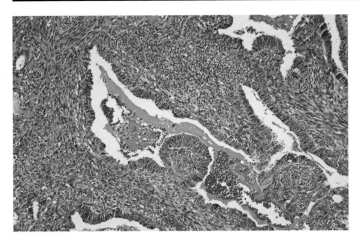

Fig. 48.9 Synovial sarcoma. Unlike epithelioid sarcoma, the appearance is clearly biphasic, with streaming fascicles of spindle cells covered by cuboidal and columnar epithelial cells, surrounding clefts and giving an appearance resembling synovium.

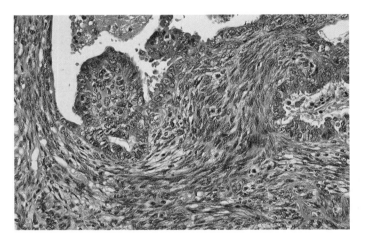

Fig. 48.10 Synovial sarcoma. Higher power view shows a densely cellular tumor and the contrast between the spindle and epithelial cells.

relative amounts of the cellular components. Despite its slow growth, the tumor has a poor prognosis. Reported 5-year survival rates vary between 25% and 50%, but late metastases cause the survival rate to fall significantly thereafter. Of the seven cases reviewed by Carillo et al,[33] four were alive and well 1–3 years later, and one was alive and well 8 years later.

Wide excision is necessary, and adjunctive radiotherapy should probably also be given. However, it is difficult to assess cure rates, as recurrences may be so greatly delayed.

Epithelioid sarcoma

Epithelioid sarcoma predominantly affects the superficial or deep soft tissues of the distal extremities of young adults and can

ulcerate through the skin. Chase & Enzinger[35] analyzed in detail the findings in 241 cases, and reviewed the diagnosis and prognostic indicators. Of 202 cases where the site was known, only three were in the head and neck region. However, Enzinger & Weiss,[17] found 4% of 215 epithelioid sarcomas to be in the head and neck region. The only case of oral epithelioid sarcoma appears to be that reported by Jameson et al.[36] In this case the tumor presented as a 1 cm chronic painless ulcer with heaped up edges in the anterior palate of a 20-year-old black male.

MICROSCOPY

A conspicuous feature is the formation of solid nodules, frequently with central necrosis. Confluence of the nodules gives rise to a mass with scalloped margins.

The cells are typically plump and polygonal, with moderately abundant eosinophilic cytoplasm and ill-defined cell membranes. The nuclei are rounded and vesicular with conspicuous nucleoli. These epithelioid cells merge with spindle-shaped cells with elongated nuclei, rather than showing a distinct biphasic pattern that is more typical of synovial sarcoma. The varied appearances range from those mimicking squamous cell carcinoma to that of an angiosarcoma (Figs 48.11–48.15). In the case reported by Jameson et al,[36] cellular atypia was inconspicuous, although there were some areas of nuclear pleomorphism. No vascular or lymphatic permeation was seen. There was positive immuno-reactivity with CAM 5.2 and vimentin, but not to factor VIII or S-100 protein. The immunohistochemical findings of seven extraoral epithelioid sarcomas reported by Fisher[37] were that all were vimentin-positive. All but one reacted strongly for keratins, and most were strongly EMA and CAM 5.2 positive. Ultra-structurally, these tumor cells showed a spectrum of differentiation up to fully developed epithelial features, while fibroblasts and myofibroblasts were seen at the periphery of the tumor nodules.

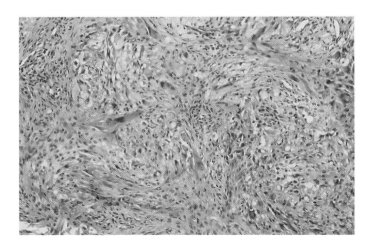

Fig. 48.11 Epithelioid sarcoma. In this area, pleomorphic spindle-shaped cells in a fascicular pattern merge with less well-defined cells.

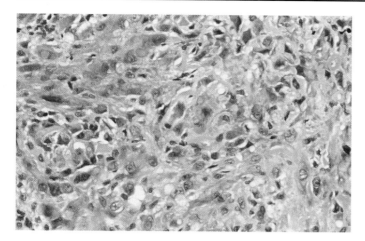

Fig. 48.12 Epithelioid sarcoma. An area of pleomorphic epithelioid cells.

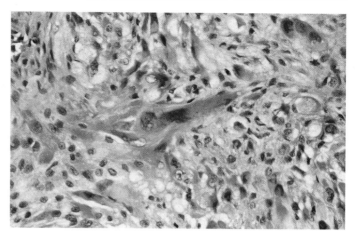

Fig. 48.15 Epithelioid sarcoma. A grossly pleomorphic spindle cell dominates the center of the field surrounded by scattered, ill-defined, pale epithelioid cells.

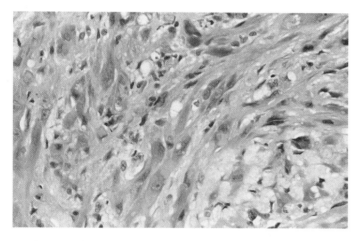

Fig. 48.13 Epithelioid sarcoma. Higher power view of spindle cells with abnormally large, vesicular nuclei.

BEHAVIOR AND MANAGEMENT

Of the 202 patients with epithelioid sarcoma reported by Chase & Enzinger,[35] 77% developed recurrences and 32% of these died. Although epithelioid sarcoma is therefore a highly malignant tumor, many variables, such as the primary site, affect the prognosis.

Early radical excision is the first essential. Enzinger & Weiss[17] also recommend that radiotherapy should be combined with surgery and prolonged multiagent chemotherapy.

REFERENCES

1. Abrikossoff A 1926 Ueber Myome, ausgehend von der quergestreifen willkürlicher Muskulatur. Virchows Arch [A] 260: 215–233
2. Fisher ER, Wechsler H 1962 Granular cell myoblastoma – a misnomer. Electron microscopic and histochemical evidence concerning its Schwann cell derivation and nature (granular cell schwannoma). Cancer 15: 936–954
3. Rode J, Dhillon AP, Papadaki L 1982 Immunohistochemical staining of granular cell tumour for neurone specific enolase: evidence in support of a neural origin. Diagnost Histopathol 5: 205–211
4. Armin A, Connelly EM, Rowden G 1983 An immunoperoxidase investigation of S-100 protein in granular cell myoblastomas: evidence for Schwann cell derivation. Am J Clin Pathol 79: 37–44
5. Thompson SH 1984 Myoglobin content of granular cell tumor of the tongue. Oral Surg Oral Med Oral Pathol 57: 74–76
6. Stewart CM, Watson RE, Eversole LR, Fischlswieger W, Leider AS 1988 Oral granular cell tumors: a clinicopathologic and immunocytochemical study. Oral Surg Oral Med Oral Pathol 65: 427–435
7. Baden E, Divaris M, Quillard J 1990 A light microscopic and immunohistochemical study of a multiple granular cell tumor and review of the literature. J Oral Maxillofac Surg 48: 1093–1099
8. Mentzel T, Wadden C, Fletcher CDM 1994 Granular cell change in smooth muscle tumour of skin and soft tissue. Histopathology 24: 223–231
9. Ogus HD, Bennett MH 1978–1979 Carcinoma of the dorsum of the tongue: a rarity or misdiagnosis. Br J Oral Surg 16: 115–124
10. Garlick JA, Dayan D, Buchner A 1992 A desmoplastic granular cell tumour of the oral cavity: report of a case. Br J Oral Maxillofac Surg 30: 119–121
11. Zuker RM, Buenchea R 1993 Congenital epulis: review of the literature and report of a case. J Oral Maxillofac Surg 51: 1040–1043
12. McMahon MG, Mintz S 1994 In utero diagnosis of a congenital gingival granular cell tumor and immediate postnatal surgical management. J Oral Maxillofac Surg 1994; 52: 496–498
13. Rohrer MD, Young ASK 1982 Congenital epulis (gingival granular cell tumor): ultrastructural evidence of origin from pericytes. Oral Surg Oral Med Oral Pathol 52: 56–63

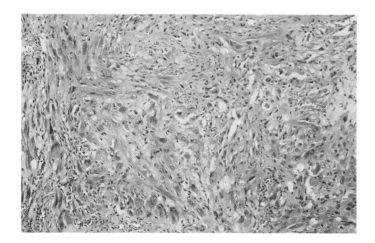

Fig. 48.14 Epithelioid sarcoma. An area predominantly of ill-defined streams of fibroblast-like cells intermingled with some epithelioid cells.

14. Zarbo RJ, Lloyd RV, Beals TF, McClatchey KD 1983 Congenital gingival granular cell tumor with smooth muscle cytodifferentiation. Oral Surg Oral Med Oral Pathol 56: 512–520

15. Damm DD, Cibull ML, Geissler RH, Neville BW, Bowden M, Lehmann JE 1993 Investigation into the histogenesis of congenital epulis of the newborn. Oral Surg Oral Med Oral Pathol 76: 202–212

16. Zarbo RJ, Lloyd RV, Beaks TF, McClatchey KD 1983 Congenital granular cell tumor with smooth muscle cytodifferentiation. Oral Surg Oral Med Oral Pathol 56: 512–520

17. Enzinger FM, Weiss SW 1995 Soft tissue tumors, 3rd edn. CV Mosby, St Louis

18. Carson HJ, Tojo DP, Ghosh L, Molnar ZV 1993 Primary alveolar soft part sarcoma of the tongue of an elderly man. A case report and review of the literature. Oral Surg Oral Med Oral Pathol 76: 62–67

19. Marker P, Jensen ML, Siemssen SJ 1995 Alveolar soft part sarcoma of the oral cavity: report of a case and review of the literature. J Oral Maxillofac Surg 53: 1203–1208

20. Porter KM, Porter SR, Scully C 1988 Lingual metastasis of alveolar soft part sarcoma. Oral Surg Oral Med Oral Pathol 65: 742–744

21. Sciot R, Dal Cin P, De Vas R, van Damme B 1993 Alveolar soft part sarcoma: evidence of its myogenic origin and the involvement of 17q25. Histopathology 23: 439–444

22. Daly JM, Gutenberg SA 1988 Benign mesenchymoma of the palate. Report of a case. J Oral Maxillofac Surg 46: 890–892

23. Micheau CR, Gerard-Merchant R, Cachin Y 1968 Les tueurs rares de la langue. Etude anatomo-pathologique (à propos de 178 cas). Arch Anat Pathol 16: 119–128

24. Takenoshita Y, Mihashi T, Horinouchi Y, Oka M 1991 Benign mesenchymoma of the tongue. Report of a case, with review of the literature. J Cranio-Maxillo-Fac Surg 19: 161–165

25. Couwenhoven R, Mostofi R, Levin S, Goldman S 1985 Intraoral benign mesenchymoma. Oral Surg Oral Med Oral Pathol 59: 619–622

26. Stout AP 1948 Mesenchymoma, the mixed tumor of mesenchymal derivatives. Ann Surg 127: 278–290

27. Shmookler BM, Enzinger FM, Brannon RB 1982 Orofacial synovial sarcoma. A clinicopathologic study of 11 new cases and review of the literature. Cancer 50: 269–276

28. Massarelli G, Tanda F, Salis B 1978 Synovial sarcoma of the soft palate: report of a case. Hum Pathol 9: 431–435

29. Holtz F, Magielski JE 1985 Synovial sarcomas of the tongue base: the seventh reported case. Arch Otolaryngol 24: 481–485

30. Novotny GM, Fort TX 1971 Synovial sarcoma of the tongue. Arch Otolaryngol 1971; 94: 77–80

31. Nunez-Alonso C, Gashi EN, Christ ML 1979 Maxillofacial synovial sarcoma: light and electron microscopic study of two cases. Am J Surg Pathol 3: 23–30

32. DelBalso AM, Pyatt RS, Busch RF, Hirokawa R, Fink CS 1982 Synovial cell sarcoma of the temporomandibular joint. Arch Otolaryngol 108: 520–522

33. Carillo R, El-Naggar AK, Rodriguez-Peralto JL, Batsakis JG 1992 Synovial sarcoma of the tongue: case report and review of the literature. J Oral Maxillofac Surg 50: 904–906

34. Karr RA, Best CG, Toth BB 1991 Synovial sarcoma metastatic to the mandible: report of two cases. J Oral Maxillofac Surg 49: 1341–1346

35. Chase DR, Enzinger FM 1985 Epithelioid sarcoma. Diagnosis, prognostic indicators, and treatment. Am J Surg Pathol 9: 241–263

36. Jameson CF, Simpson MT, Towers JF 1990 Primary epithelioid sarcoma of the palate. J Oral Maxillofac Surg 19: 240–242

37. Fisher C 1988 Epithelioid sarcoma: the spectrum of ultrastructural differentiation in seven immunohistochemically defined cases. Hum Pathol 19: 265–275

Tumors and tumor-like lesions of lymphoid tissue

Lymphomas, midline granuloma syndromes, and granulocytic sarcoma

49

Hodgkin's disease and non-Hodgkin lymphomas

Lymphomas are solid tumors of any type of lymphocyte; they are all malignant. They comprise Hodgkin's disease and non-Hodgkin lymphoma, but in the following account the latter are referred to simply as lymphomas. Leukemias, by contrast, typically do not form solid tumors, but affect the bone marrow and blood. However, lymphocytic lymphomas may have features of both diseases. Myeloma and Langerhans cell histiocytosis also arise from lymphoreticular cells, but particularly affect bones; these are discussed in Chapters 29 and 30.

HODGKIN'S DISEASE

Hodgkin's disease frequently involves the cervical lymph nodes (where it may be mistaken for a submandibular salivary gland tumor), but only exceptionally rarely affects the oral cavity. Males are predominantly affected overall, but there is equal male and female representation in nodular sclerotic disease. The peak incidence is in the third and fourth decades, but almost any age can be affected after early infancy. The nodular sclerosis type may be associated with the bizarre symptom of alcohol-induced pain in lymph nodes.

Hodgkin's disease is associated with depressed immune function which is aggravated by treatment, and abnormal susceptibility to infection.

CLINICAL FEATURES

Oral lesions due to Hodgkin's disease are exceptionally uncommon. They form nondescript soft tissue swellings and are not clinically distinguishable from non-Hodgkin lymphomas. Jaw involvement is even more infrequent. Cohen et al[1] reported a case and, from a review of the literature, quoted a frequency of jaw involvement in Hodgkin's disease of less than 2 in 2000 cases. They concluded that the prognosis for Hodgkin's disease affecting the jaw was very poor.

Hodgkin's disease may be associated with HIV infection, and may also then affect the oral cavity. Microscopically, it does not differ from the disease in HIV-negative persons, but the prognosis is far poorer.

MICROSCOPY

The cellular picture varies widely, as indicated in the classification (Tables 49.1 and 49.2), and there is growing evidence that Hodgkin's disease comprises more than one neoplastic entity. Most types appear to start in the T-cell region of lymph nodes, but lymphocyte-predominant Hodgkin's disease appears to be of B-cell origin.

Hodgkin's cells are histiocyte-like, with large eosinophilic nucleoli, or have paired (mirror-image) nuclei (Reed–Sternberg

Table 49.1 Ann Arbor classification of Hodgkin's disease*

Stage I	Involvement of a single lymph node region or a single extralymphatic organ or site
Stage II	Involvement of two or more lymph node regions on the same side of the diaphragm, or localized involvement of extralymphatic organ or site and of one or more lymph node regions on the same side of the diaphragm
Stage III	Involvement of nodes on both sides of the diaphragm. there may also be: III_S splenic involvement III_E localized involvement of extralymphatic organ or site III_{ES} involvement of both of the above
Stage IV	Diffuse or disseminated involvement of one or more extralymphatic organs or tissues, with or without associated lymph node involvement

*Each stage is further qualified with the suffix A if systemic symptoms are absent, or B if there are fever, night sweats, or more than 10% loss of weight in the previous 6 months.

Table 49.2 Rye classification of Hodgkin's lymphoma

Nodular sclerosis
Lymphocyte predominant
Mixed cellularity
Lymphocyte depleted

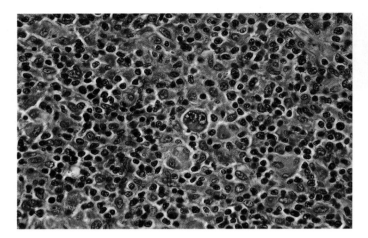

Fig. 49.1 Hodgkin's lymphoma. Classical binucleate Reed–Sternberg cell, showing prominent eosinophilic nucleoli.

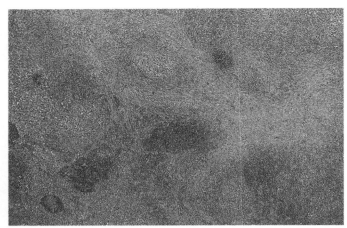

Fig. 49.2 Hodgkin's lymphoma, nodular sclerosing variant. Cellular nodules are separated by bands of fibrous tissue extending into and dividing the node.

giant cells); diagnosis depends largely on recognizing these cells (Fig. 49.1). However, they are frequently difficult to find and, as with non-Hodgkin's lymphoma, any superimposed inflammation adds to the difficulties.

Hodgkin's disease, particularly of the lymphocyte-depleted reticular type, may sometimes be difficult to distinguish from non-Hodgkin's lymphomas by microscopy. However, the distinction is important as the chance of permanent cure of some types of Hodgkin's disease is high. The overall 5-year survival rate may be as high as 80%, but the considerable improvement in the prognosis of Hodgkin's disease has resulted from precise staging (Table 49.1). Before accurate staging methods had been devised, relapse was frequently the result of failure to identify and treat occult deposits.

Factors which adversely affect prognosis are, therefore:

- advanced stage
- advanced age
- systemic symptoms (fever, night sweats, and weight loss)
- abnormal hematological findings
- Aggressive histological subtype (nodular sclerotic variant with lymphocyte depletion and, particularly, lymphocyte-depleted types).

NODULAR SCLEROSIS HODGKIN'S DISEASE

The normal nodal architecture is replaced by nodules of Hodgkin's tissue separated by bands of fibrous tissue (Fig. 49.2).

The nodules consist of a mixture of cells that are seen in other subtypes of the disease, but lacunar cells are a characteristic finding. These have complex often multilobed nuclei, which are surrounded by a clear space left by dissolution of the lipid-rich cytoplasm during processing. The large nucleus contains the prominent eosinophilic nucleolus typical of the Hodgkin's cell. By contrast, classical Reed–Sternberg cells are few.

The amount of collagen can vary widely, and in extreme cases almost the whole node is fibrotic. The cellular picture also varies from subtypes in which lymphocytes predominate, but lacunar and Reed–Sternberg cells are scanty (NS I), to those in which lymphocytes are scanty and Hodgkin's cells are numerous (NS II). The latter is aggressive and has a strong tendency to involve the mediastinum. However, a worse prognosis for NS II is disputed.

LYMPHOCYTE-PREDOMINANT HODGKIN'S DISEASE

Lymphocytes, sometimes mixed with bland histiocytes, are abundant, but Hodgkin's and Reed–Sternberg cells are scanty. The pattern is usually nodular without fibrosis. Also characteristic is the presence of so-called popcorn cells, which are a Reed–Sternberg cell variant with a multilobed nucleus, also seen in lymphocyte-predominant nodular-sclerosis Hodgkin's disease.

Lymphocyte-predominant Hodgkin's disease typically gives rise to localized, asymptomatic lymphadenopathy in the neck or inguinal region. The prognosis is good with appropriate treatment.

MIXED CELLULARITY HODGKIN'S DISEASE

Mixed cellularity Hodgkin's disease is the second most common type, but accounts for less than 20% of cases.

Histologically, lymphocytes are mixed with histiocytes, plasma

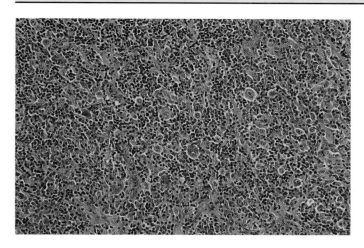

Fig. 49.3 Hodgkin's lymphoma, mixed cellularity variant. There is a diversity of cell types, including typical (binucleate) and mononuclear Reed–Sternberg cells, histocytes, lymphocytes, and plasma cells.

cells, eosinophils, Hodgkin's cells, and Reed–Sternberg cells (Fig. 49.3). The last are relatively numerous.

Mixed cellularity Hodgkin's disease is relatively aggressive, and in more than 50% of cases is in an advanced stage at presentation. Over a third of patients have systemic symptoms and the overall survival rate is poor.

LYMPHOCYTE-DEPLETED HODGKIN'S DISEASE

Lymphocyte-depleted Hodgkin's disease accounts for less than 2% of cases. There are two subtypes:

- *Lymphocyte-depleted, reticular type Hodgkin's disease.* Lymphocytes are scanty but pleomorphic Reed–Sternberg cells are numerous and frequently atypical.
- *Lymphocyte-depleted, diffuse-fibrosis type Hodgkin's disease.* Scattered Reed–Sternberg cells, often bizarre in character, are mixed with scanty lymphocytes, plasma cells, and eosinophils in a stroma of amorphous eosinophilic material. The fibrous tissue is not collagenous but argyrophil.

Lymphocyte-depleted, diffuse-fibrosis type Hodgkin's disease. carries the worst prognosis, with a high proportion of patients having systemic symptoms, together with hepatic and bone marrow involvement, often without significant lymphadenopathy.

BEHAVIOR AND MANAGEMENT

Precise histological diagnosis and staging are the prerequisites. In general, patients with stage IA or IIA disease are treated with external megavoltage radiotherapy to all affected nodes. Patients with stage IB or IIB disease are treated with combination chemotherapy, such as nitrogen mustard, vincristine (Oncovin), prednisolone, and procarbazine (MOPP). Stage IIIA disease may be treated by radiotherapy, but now is more frequently treated with chemotherapy, as are stages IIIB, IVA, and IVB.

NON-HODGKIN LYMPHOMAS

The aetiology of lymphomas is unknown, but they are more frequent in the following:

- Rheumatoid arthritis, Sjögren's syndrome and benign lymphoepithelial lesion.
- After immunosuppressive treatment, particularly for organ transplantation, and cytotoxic chemotherapy.
- Acquired immune deficiency syndrome and some other immunodeficiency states.
- After irradiation.

Burkitt's lymphoma, some T-cell lymphomas, and many lymphomas in patients with AIDS are associated with the Epstein–Barr virus (EBV). T-cell lymphomas may be EBV associated, but others are seropositive for the human T-cell lymphotropic virus (HTLV).

Exposure to asbestos has been reported to be associated with a raised incidence of oral lymphomas, but this has not been widely confirmed.

Oropharyngeal lymphomas are uncommon but most frequently arise in Waldeyer's ring which, after the gastrointestinal tract, is the second most common site of extranodal lymphomas. The tonsil and soft palate are the sites for about 80% of them. Some are low-grade B-cell lymphomas, but they are heterogeneous. Only a minority can be confirmed as mucosa-associated lymphoid tissue (MALT) lymphomas, which in their early stages are of very low grade. Wright[2] has reviewed the difficulties involved in categorizing these tumors. In salivary glands, by contrast, a high proportion of lymphomas arising in lymphoepithelial lesions or Sjögren's syndrome appear to be of MALT type, as discussed in Chapter 53.

Oral HIV-associated lymphomas are more frequent, particularly in drug abusers, than in HIV-negative persons, but are still uncommon. Overall, they account for 2% of oral neoplasms in patients with AIDS. They are more frequently extranodal, are usually immunoblastic, and respond so poorly to treatment that survival is likely to be only of the order of months. Typical appearances are rapidly growing masses, which sometimes ulcerate, in such sites as the gingivae or fauces.[3] Herndier et al[4] have described the clinical and microscopic features of AIDS-associated lymphomas, and have discussed in detail the phenotypes and other aspects of the molecular biology. Lozada-Nur et al[5] have reported primary intraoral lymphomas in seven patients with AIDS. One was on the mandibular gingiva, and the remainder were on the palate. In one patient the lymphoma was the AIDS-defining illness; all other patients had previously had *Pneumocystis carinii* pneumonia, and the length of time between the diagnosis of HIV infection ranged from 7 months to 10 years. All the lymphomas were of B-cell lineage, and six were of the high-grade, diffuse large-cell type. None expressed CD3 or CD30 antigens. All were positive for EBV-encoded RNA. Despite multidrug chemotherapy with or without radiotherapy, none of the patients survived for more than 8 months.

Salivary glands, particularly the parotids, which have a lymphoid component, can occasionally also be the site of origin (see Ch. 53).

Wolvius et al[6] have described 34 oral lymphomas, of which 12 originated in bone (see below).

CLINICAL FEATURES

Lymphomas most frequently affect persons of middle age or over. The age range of the cases presented by Wolvius et al[6] was 3–88 years, with a mean of 59 years. Oral lymphomas typically form nondescript, diffuse, usually soft, painless swellings, which may become ulcerated by trauma. Slootweg et al[7] point out that oral lymphomas, apart from those arising in Waldeyer's ring, are notorious for mimicking inflammatory diseases of the periodontal tissues or jaws. Gingival masses due to HIV-associated lymphomas are well recognized. The regional lymph nodes are not usually involved at first, and diagnosis depends on the microscopic findings and related investigations.

Nasopharyngeal lymphoma is a rare cause of midfacial destructive disease, and can cause swelling and ulceration of the palate as the presenting feature, as discussed later.

MICROSCOPY: GENERAL ASPECTS

Approximately 85% of lymphomas are B-cell tumors. According to their stage of differentiation, they give rise to different histologic types of tumor which can be graded in terms of behavior as shown, for example, in the Working Formulation (Table 49.3). Non-Hodgkin lymphomas appear as solid sheets of lymphocytes, which may be predominantly small or large. They may be diffuse or have a follicular pattern. As can be seen from the Working Formulation, follicular lymphomas are generally low or intermediate grade and have a better prognosis. Invasion or destruction of adjacent tissues may be seen, and helps to confirm the malignant nature of these tumors. An additional problem in the mouth is that, if traumatized, superimposed inflammation

Table 49.3 Working Formulation classification for non-Hodgkin lymphomas

Behaviour		Histology
I	Low grade	Small lymphocytic Follicular, small cleaved cell Follicular, mixed small cleaved and large cell
II	Intermediate grade	Follicular, large cell Diffuse, small cleaved cell Diffuse, mixed small and large cell Diffuse, large cell
III	High grade	Large cell, immunoblastic Lymphoblastic Diffuse, small non-cleaved cell

can cause a lymphoma to appear reactive rather than neoplastic microscopically. In addition to the cytological features, which determine the grade of a tumor, a useful test is detection of a change from polyclonality (production of both λ and κ immunoglobulin light chains) of lymphoepithelial or reactive lesions to monoclonal production (light-chain restriction) usually of κ light chains, by the neoplastic cells. However, recognition of a lymphoproliferative lesion as a malignant lymphoma may be difficult, and grading, which largely determines treatment and prognosis, even more difficult.

Isaacson & Norton[8] have described and illustrated in detail the pathology of lymphomas of the upper aerodigestive tract. Nevertheless, identification of morphological differences between the cells requires considerable experience, and the Working Formulation takes no account of T-cell lymphomas. Thus the category of large-cell lymphoma, which includes both B- and T-cell lymphomas and anaplastic, DC30-positive tumors, is a heterogeneous group in terms of clinical presentation and behavior. This is therefore a difficult area of microscopy, and many classifications have been devised. As a consequence, precise categorization depends mainly on immunophenotyping. Recognition of specific gene rearrangements may also be informative. Thus, translocation of the *bcl-2* gene is found in over 80% of follicular lymphomas, but the expression of both *p53* and *bcl-2* in large B-cell lymphomas appears to confer a poor prognosis. The importance of *bcl-6* gene rearrangements in large B-cell lymphomas in determining behavior has not yet been widely confirmed. Increasingly, polymerase chain reaction (PCR) is being used for the diagnosis of lymphomas, particularly in small specimens, as reviewed by Chan & Greiner.[9]

In the series presented by Wolvius et al,[6] 12 of 34 oral lymphomas were of the diffuse centroblastic type (Kiel classification). Two cases from the palate were MALT lymphomas forming characteristic lymphoepithelial lesions. Histological grading showed four low-grade (12%), 19 intermediate-grade (56%), and 11 high-grade (32%) tumors. Of 33 patients staged according to the Ann Arbor protocol: 20 were in stage I; one was in stage II, with involvement of the submandibular nodes; one was in stage III, with involvement of paraaortic and inguinal lymph nodes; and 11 were in stage IV, with involvement of cervical, supraclavicular, abdominal, and inguinal lymph nodes.

The classification given in Table 49.3 does not distinguish between B-cell and T-cell tumors. This is done in the Kiel classification (Table 49.4), which includes several different types of lymphoid tumors that cannot be discussed here.

The main histological groups of lymphomas can be summarized as follows, although there are many subtypes:

- lymphocytic lymphomas
- follicle center cell lymphomas
- Immunoblastic lymphomas
- Burkitt-type lymphoma
- MALT lymphoma
- T-cell lymphomas

Table 49.4 Kiel Classification of lymphomas (modified)

B-cell lymphomas	T-cell lymphomas
Low grade	*Low grade*
Lymphocytic	Lymphocytic
Lymphoplasma/cytoid/plasmacytic	Small cerebriform cell (mycoses fungoides and Sézary's syndrome)
Centroblastic centrocyte follicular	Pleomorphic small cell
Centroblastic centrocytic diffuse	Angioimmunoblastic lymphadenopathy
Centrocytic	T-zone lymphoma
	Lymphoepitheloid lymphoma
High grade	*High grade*
Centroblastic	Immunoblastic
Immunoblastic	Pleomorphic medium and large cell (HTLV-1)
Lymphoblastic	
Anaplastic (CD30)	Anaplastic (CD30)
Burkitt's lymphoma	Lymphoblastic

LYMPHOCYTIC LYMPHOMAS

Adults are predominantly affected. The disease is indolent and many patients die from other causes. They frequently are abnormally susceptible to bacterial infections due to an associated hypogammaglobulinemia. However, in 5–10% of cases there is transformation to immunoblastic lymphoma, which is resistant to treatment. Many regard lymphocytic lymphoma and chronic lymphocytic leukemia as variants of the same disease.

In most cases, lymphocytic lymphoma is disseminated, with splenic, liver, and bone marrow involvement.

Microscopy

These are neoplasms of small, functionally immature lymphocytes. Over 90% are B-cell tumors. The nodal architecture is replaced by a dense infiltrate of small round lymphocytes with occasional larger cells (prolymphocytes) scattered among them or in small aggregates.

FOLLICLE CENTER CELL LYMPHOMAS

These are neoplasms of germinal center cells and, therefore, are B-cell tumors.

Microscopy

Germinal centers are reproduced to a varying degree, particularly in follicular types. However, follicle center cell lymphomas can also show a mixed pattern of follicular and diffuse lymphoma or be entirely diffuse, particularly in the case of centroblastic and centrocytic lymphomas.

Cytologically, there may be a mixture of centrocytes and centroblasts (centrocytic/centroblastic lymphoma). Alternatively, only a single cell type is represented. These are known as centro-

cytic or centroblastic lymphomas according to the cell type, and they have a diffuse pattern (Figs 49.4–49.7).

Centrocytic/centroblastic lymphomas

These are one of the most common types of non-Hodgkin's lymphomas. They are diseases of the elderly, with a peak incidence in the sixth and seventh decades, and are rare in children or young adults. The most common clinical picture is of painless, slowly progressive lymphadenopathy, which is usually widespread. Up to half the patients have systemic symptoms. Typically, response to treatment is initially good, but recurrence is the rule. The disease therefore has a prolonged course interrupted by therapeutic remissions, and cure is rare.

Microscopy

The picture is variable, but centrocytic/centroblastic lymphomas contain all the cells normally present in germinal centers, namely, centroblasts and centrocytes, which are the neoplastic cells, as

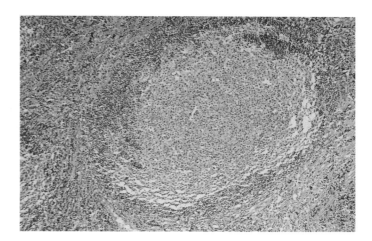

Fig. 49.4 Follicle center cell lymphoma. Low-power view showing the well-developed follicular pattern.

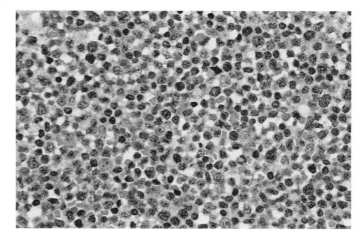

Fig. 49.5 Follicle center cell lymphoma. Higher power view showing the center of a follicle composed of mixed centrocytes and centroblasts.

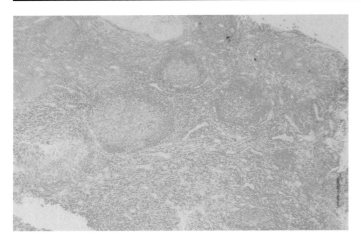

Fig. 49.6 Follicle center cell lymphoma. Low-power view of staining for bcl-2 protein, showing that the follicles are strongly positive.

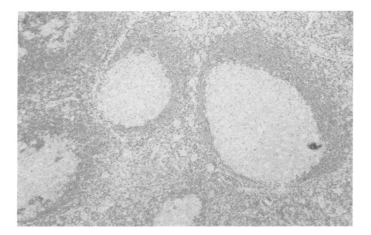

Fig. 49.7 Reactive lymph node showing, in contrast with Figure 49.6, an absence of bcl-2 expression in the follicles.

well as non-neoplastic T lymphocytes (mostly CD4+), and dendritic reticulum cells.

The lymph-node architecture is replaced by crowded follicles, which often extend through the capsule. Usually there is a predominance of centrocytes (small irregular lymphocytes, so-called, 'small cleaved cells'), while predominance of centroblasts (larger nucleated, noncleaved lymphoid cells) suggests a poorer prognosis. Other indications of high tumor grade and resistance to treatment are larger pleomorphic centroblasts and loss of follicular pattern.

Centrocytic (diffuse, small cleaved cell) lymphomas

Centrocytic lymphomas usually present with lymphadenopathy alone, but can, less frequently, have a leukemic blood picture.

Microscopy

The lymph-node architecture is replaced by a uniform, diffuse

infiltrate of small centrocytes, but there is sometimes a suggestion of a follicular pattern due to persistence of aggregates of dendritic reticulum cells. Benign reactive follicles may also become entrapped, as the neoplastic cells have a tendency selectively to replace the mantle zone.

The tumor cells are generally of uniform size, slightly larger than small lymphocytes, and have distinctive, irregular, heterochromatic nuclei. Although the neoplastic cells are morphologically identical to the centrocytes present in reactive follicles, immunophenotyping has shown that, unlike the latter, which express SIgM and are CD10+, but are negative for SIgD and CD5+, the neoplastic centrocytes express both SIgM and SIgD, and are CD5 but not CD10 positive.

Prognosis

The usual course is an initially good response to treatment followed by fatal recurrence of disseminated disease.

Centroblastic (diffuse large, noncleaved cell) lymphoma

Centroblastic lymphomas are high-grade tumors that affect adults. They represent about 5% of malignant lymphomas and usually cause regional lymphadenopathy. However, the tumor has frequently already disseminated to the bone marrow and spleen, when enlarged lymph nodes are noticed.

Microscopy

The normal nodal tissue is usually entirely replaced by a diffuse infiltrate of large blast cells, but a residual follicular pattern may persist. The neoplastic lymphocytes have round nuclei with 2–5 nucleoli, which typically lie next to the cell membrane. There is a narrow but distinct rim of cytoplasm. Immunophenotyping confirms the B-cell origin of these tumors, and immunocyto-chemistry shows light-chain restriction and, sometimes, production of considerable quantities of immunoglobulin (Fig. 49.8).

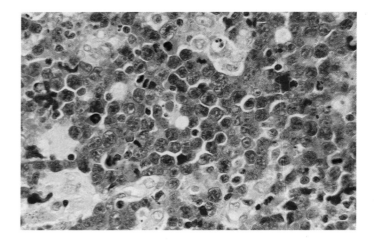

Fig. 49.8 High-grade B-cell lymphoma. High-power view showing cellular pleomorphism, with mitotic figures and blast cells with prominent nucleoli.

Prognosis

In the past, centroblastic lymphoma had a uniformly poor prognosis with rapid deterioration, but cure of a significant number of cases is possible with current chemotherapy.

IMMUNOBLASTIC (LARGE-CELL) LYMPHOMA

Immunoblastic lymphoma is the most common type of high-grade lymphoma. It may arise de novo or as a consequence of transformation of the other types of lymphoma already mentioned. It is most common in later adult life, but a wide age range can be affected. It usually causes nodal disease, but can also be extranodal.

Microscopy

There is uniform infiltration of the node or extranodal tissue with immunoblasts. They have large round nuclei with a central nucleolus, a prominent nuclear membrane, and sometimes show plasmacytic differentiation. Occasionally, there is gross pleomorphism, producing a picture resembling that of Hodgkin's disease. Immunophenotyping is then required to confirm the B-cell nature of the neoplasm.

Prognosis

In the past immunoblastic lymphoma had a worse prognosis than any other type of B-cell lymphoma and the outcome was uniformly fatal. However, a cure rate of up to 40% may now be possible with current chemotherapy.

BURKITT'S (SMALL NONCLEAVED CELL) LYMPHOMA

This type of lymphoma, which is endemic in East Africa, has its onset in childhood. It was the first type of lymphoma where association with EBV was demonstrated, and the EBV virome can be shown to be incorporated within the neoplastic lymphocytes.

Clinical features

Endemic Burkitt's lymphoma is peculiar in its onset at an average age of 7 years, its predominantly extranodal distribution, and with jaw involvement as the single most common initial site. Spread to the surrounding oral soft tissues and parotid glands, and involvement of nonlymphoid abdominal viscera are common. This tumor is one of the most rapidly growing, with a cell-doubling time of less than 24 hours.

Over 95% of cases respond completely to single-dose chemotherapy and, although there is a high relapse rate, especially in those with widespread disease, the overall survival rate is approximately 50%. Also unlike other lymphomas, there is little or no response to radiotherapy.

Microscopy

Burkitt's lymphoma presents a monomorphic picture of medium-size blast cells with round nuclei and 2–3 nucleoli, which are usually apposed to the nuclear membrane, but scanty cytoplasm. There is a high rate of mitotic activity, and scattered macrophages, which characteristically give the otherwise dark sheets of cells a 'starry sky' appearance, can sometimes be seen to have ingested dead tumor cells (Figs 49.9–49.11).

A histologically similar tumor is occasionally encountered in children and adults in the West, but differs in that gut-associated lymphoid tissue is predominantly affected and it is rarely associated with the EBV genome or high EBV antibody titers. However, jaw involvement is far more frequent than with other lymphomas.

Lymphoma resembling Burkitt's lymphoma microscopically can also be a complication of immunosuppressive treatment and of AIDS, and in about 50% of the latter is associated with EBV.

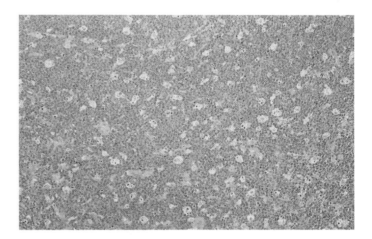

Fig. 49.9 Burkitt's lymphoma. Low-power view showing the uniform cellular picture and starry sky appearance due to scattered macrophages.

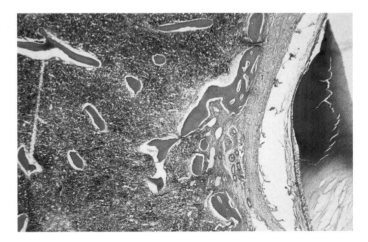

Fig. 49.10 Burkitt's lymphoma from the jaw of a young child, showing the typical pattern of small dark cells invading alveolar bone, with a developing tooth on the right.

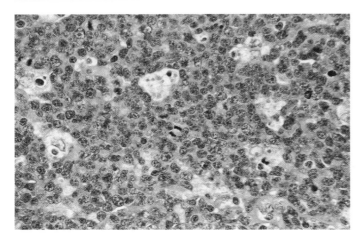

Fig. 49.11 Burkitt's lymphoma. High-power view, showing the monomorphic lymphoblasts and scattered histiocytes.

Burkitt's lymphoma of the jaw

As mentioned earlier, jaw involvement is typical of endemic African Burkitt's lymphoma. Nonendemic ('American') Burkitt's lymphoma also affects the jaws far more frequently than the more common lymphomas. Sariban et al[10] found that 16 of 100 patients with this disease had jaw involvement at presentation and two more at relapse. Single-quadrant mandibular involvement was most common. Fourteen patients presented with dental symptoms. Toothache and perioral numbness were the most frequent symptoms in adults. Toothache, loose teeth, or intra- or perioral swelling were the most common complaints in children. Three patients, all children, had disease limited to the jaw.

Six of the 18 patients (four children and two adults) were alive, off chemotherapy, and free from disease 2–15 years after diagnosis (mean period of follow-up 7 years). Of the 12 patients who died, nine had widespread disease. After an initial response to chemotherapy, resistance developed. However, three patients died from the toxic effects of chemotherapy, with no evidence of tumor recurrence at autopsy.

Wang et al,[11] using more recent data from the American Burkitt's Lymphoma Registry, found jaw involvement in only 7% and cervical lymphadenopathy in 16% of cases. They summarized the findings of previous series and presented seven new cases of head and neck disease. Of these, four had jaw, one had sinus, and two had oral involvement.

MALT LYMPHOMA

Mucosa-associated lymphoid tissue (MALT) lymphomas are low-grade tumours that particularly arise in the stomach, small intestine, salivary glands, thyroid, and lung, but infrequently in the oral cavity.

MALT lymphomas have been of particular interest because, in those arising in the stomach, *Helicobacter pylori* appears to provide a strong antigenic stimulus and eradication of this bacterium may cause regression of the tumor. MALT lymphomas

can also be exceedingly indolent and can spread to other mucosal sites ('homing').

Microscopy

Wright[2] summarized the features of MALT lymphomas as follows:

1. They are composed predominantly of centrocyte-like cells the morphology of which ranges from lymphocyte-like to monocyte-like appearances (Figs 49.12–49.15).
2. Some of these tumors show plasmacytic differentiation and the plasmacytoid cells tend to show microanatomical separation from the centrocyte-like cells (Fig. 49.16).
3. Small clusters of centrocyte-like cells infiltrate and destroy epithelium, forming lymphoepithelial lesions.
4. Tumor cells infiltrate pre-existing reactive lymphoid follicles (follicular colonization). This may give the tumor a nodular appearance.

Monocytoid B-cell lymphomas, in which the malignant lymphocytes have rather bland-looking nuclei and relatively abundant clear cytoplasm, were thought to be a distinct entity and to arise particularly frequently in Sjögren's syndrome. However, monocytoid B cells can also be seen in MALT lymphomas. MALT and monocytoid B-cell lymphomas, if distinct entities, are therefore closely related and distinct from other low-grade B-cell lymphomas in their behavior.

Although MALT lymphomas can be indolent, they tend to progress to high-grade tumors and are then difficult to recognize as being of MALT origin, unless residual areas of low-grade tumor can be found.

General aspects of management

Prognosis depends both on the tumor-cell phenotype and also on the tumor stage. Staging investigation to determine the extent of spread of the tumor includes physical examination, blood picture

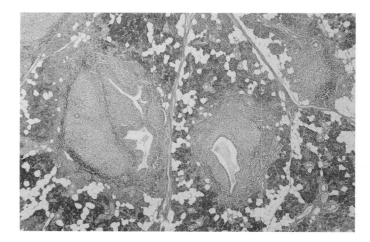

Fig. 49.12 MALT lymphoma. Low-power view of focal lymphoepithelial lesions in parotid gland. Proliferation areas of pale centrocyte-like cells are conspicuous.

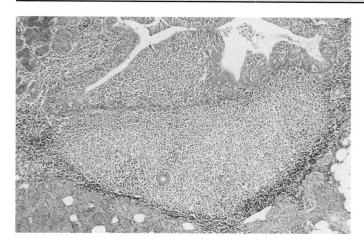

Fig. 49.13 MALT lymphoma. Higher power view showing pale centrocyte-like cells infiltrating the duct epithelium.

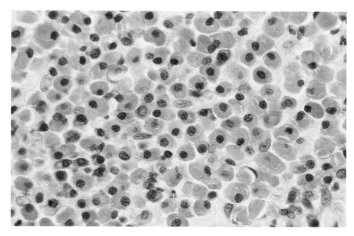

Fig. 49.16 MALT lymphoma. High-power view showing an area of plasmacytoid cells (an uncommon feature).

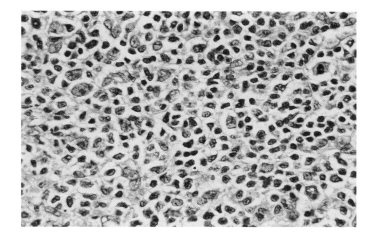

Fig. 49.14 MALT lymphoma. High-power view showing an area of cells with centrocyte-like morphology.

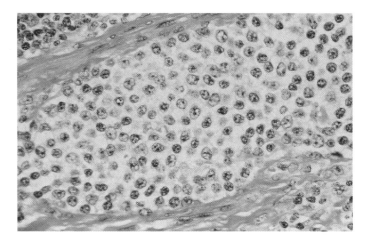

Fig. 49.15 MALT lymphoma. High-power view showing an area of monocytoid cells.

and ESR, chest radiographs, bipedal lymphogram, bone marrow biopsy, and computed tomography scanning or magnetic resonance imaging to detect affected nodes in the abdomen.

The few cases with disease localized to a single node or extranodal site (stage I) and those with limited spread (stage II) are treated by irradiation. Early stage MALT lymphomas (see below), in particular, are likely to respond to local treatment. However, the majority of patients with oral or perioral lymphomas have disseminated disease (stage III or IV), and treatment is by radiotherapy, combination chemotherapy, or both. Oral complications of such treatment (e.g. ulceration and infection) are common. The overall 5-year survival rate for non-Hodgkin lymphomas is about 30%. Of the 34 oral cases presented by Wolvius et al,[6] the mean recurrence-free interval was 31 months and the mean survival time was 38 months.

PRIMARY LYMPHOMA OF BONE

Involvement of the jaws is typical of African Burkitt's lymphoma but, rarely, other primary lymphomas can arise in bone. Pileri et al[12] have reported in detail 17 cases affecting the mandible. Pain at the site and swelling are typical, but there are no distinctive clinical features. Radiographically the tumor forms a poorly demarcated area of bone destruction. Diagnosis depends entirely on the microscopic findings and exclusion of disseminated lymphoma.

Microscopy

Parker & Jackson[13] established primary lymphoma of bone as an entity, but termed it 'primary reticulum cell sarcoma of bone,' as the lymphocytes resembled histiocytes. This term persisted for many years, but most primary lymphomas of bone are intermediate grade, diffuse, large-cell lymphomas. The lymphocyte nuclei are larger, with fine nuclear chromatin and more abundant cytoplasm than those of histiocytes. Of 11 cases evaluated by

Pettit et al,[14] all were large-cell lymphomas. Of these, nine were of large cleaved cell type and the other two were large cell, but not otherwise specified. The frequency of multilobated cells was, therefore, high. Fine reticulin fibers surround single or small groups of these lymphocytes.

Diagnosis, and particularly differentiation from Ewing's sarcoma, depends on immunostaining or gene product analysis, which will indicate whether these large cells are B or T lymphocytes. Differentiation from Ewing's sarcoma is particularly important because of its far worse prognosis.

Behavior and management

Disseminated lymphoma should first be excluded. In the case of a true primary lymphoma of bone, excision should be followed by multiagent chemotherapy. Fechner & Mills[15] quote 5- and 10-year survival rates respectively, for primary skeletal lymphoma, of 58% and 53%, but the prognosis deteriorates once other bones become involved. Few data on the prognosis after modern treatment of these uncommon tumors in the jaws are available, but they probably have a better prognosis than most soft-tissue non-Hodgkin lymphomas.

T-CELL LYMPHOMAS

As mentioned earlier, T-cell lymphomas are uncommon, particularly in the oropharyngeal region. By contrast, they comprise the majority of extranodal nasopharyngeal lymphomas. These can give rise to the *midline granuloma syndrome*, where they can be confused with Wegener's granulomatosis, as discussed below.

HTLV-related T-cell lymphomas are more frequently seen in certain endemic areas such as parts of Japan. They appear to carry a poorer prognosis, as reported by Kurihara et al,[16] who found that among 11 orofacial lymphomas in Japan, four were HTLV-related and were T-cell neoplasms, while the remaining HTLV-unrelated neoplasms were mostly of B-cell origin and carried a better prognosis.

Sirois et al[17] reported eight cases of cutaneous T-cell lymphoma that involved the oral cavity, but could find reports of only 22 earlier examples in the English-language literature and 30 worldwide. All but one of their eight cases had active skin disease at the time of oral involvement, despite topical or systemic chemotherapy. Five patients had typical mycosis fungoides (all but one of them in the tumor phase), one had erythroderma without blood involvement, and one developed a facial tumor before typical plaques of mycosis fungoides appeared elsewhere.

Immunophenotyping showed an aberrant T-helper-cell phenotype in three cases and a T-suppressor-cell phenotype in two. The oral lesions comprised multiple or solitary ulcerated plaques, multiple papules or nodules, multiple erosions, or solitary ulcerated tumors. Gingival lesions were most common (five cases), while the palate and tongue were each involved with solitary ulcerated tumors.

Rosenberg et al[18] have reported two cases of CD30-positive T-cell lymphomas of the oral mucosa, which presented as palatal and gingival ulcers. One patient had previously undergone cytotoxic treatment for chronic lymphatic leukemia.

Isaacson & Norton[8] discuss extranodal lymphomas of the upper aerodigestive tract, but limit their description of those arising from Waldeyer's ring to tonsillar tumors. However, they note that, what appears to be a distinct group of high-grade lymphomas of T-cell or possibly natural killer cell (NKC) phenotype, has a predilection for the upper aerodigestive tract, including the mouth.

High-grade T-cell lymphomas have highly variable histology. This is abundantly illustrated by the fact that nasopharyngeal T-cell lymphomas were not recognized as lymphomas until relatively recently.

The neoplastic cells vary widely in size, and typically have complex pleomorphic nuclei with a variable amount of pale-staining cytoplasm. Furthermore, necrosis is often significant, so that inflammatory cells can obscure the neoplastic infiltrate (Figs 49.17–49.19).

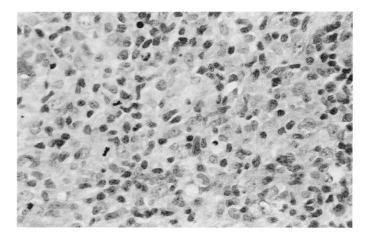

Fig. 49.17 T-cell lymphoma. Higher power view, showing the typical pleomorphic picture of lymphocytes, many with irregular nuclear outlines.

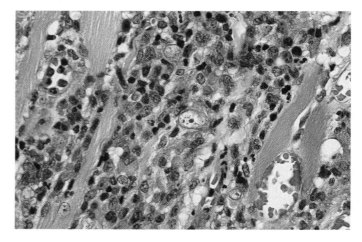

Fig. 49.18 T-cell lymphoma. Higher power view, showing a high-grade tumor composed of pleomorphic and immunoblast-like cells, invading tongue muscle.

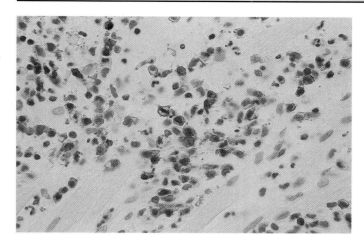

Fig. 49.19 T-cell lymphoma. Immunocytochemistry showing positive staining with CD-3 T-lymphocyte surface marker.

Isaacson & Norton[8] state that only a third of cases of T-cell lymphomas of the upper aerodigestive tract are CD3 positive in cryostat sections, but that more are positive with polyclonal antisera in paraffin sections, when the CD3 antigen is frequently cytoplasmic. They also state that up to 75% of these tumors express NKC antigens, particularly CD56, and that there is a high rate of expression of the lymphocyte activation markers HLA-DR, CD25, and CD30.

Management

The first requirement is accurate microscopic diagnosis followed by staging. In general, radiotherapy alone is satisfactory for nonextensive stage I, low or intermediate grade disease. Chemotherapy, such as the CHOP (cyclophosphamide, doxorubicin, vincristine and prednisolone) regimen, is used for widespread stage I or II disease. Whether combined modality treatment is beneficial for disseminated disease is uncertain. Overall, prolonged remissions can be obtained for low-grade tumors, but the possibility of cure is doubtful unless disease is localized to one or two nodes, which are treated surgically or by radiotherapy. The early mortality from high-grade lymphomas is high, but aggressive chemotherapy can bring about prolonged remission and, paradoxically, cure in some cases. Supportive treatment, including transfusions as necessary and aggressive treatment of infections, is important.

Nasopharyngeal T-cell lymphoma and midline granuloma syndromes (lethal midline granuloma, midfacial destructive disease, etc.)

Midline granulomas are granulomas mainly in the sense of the clinical appearance of granulomatous destruction of tissues, particularly of the nasal cavity, but sometimes extending into the mouth. Proliferation, ulceration, and crusting of the nasal or paranasal tissues typically leads to destruction (occasionally gross) of the midfacial tissues. Later, other organs are involved, and the outcome is typically fatal. Wegener's granulomatosis was the first disease to be recognized as a cause of these syndromes, and it is discussed here as it is usually clinically indistinguishable from a nasopharyngeal T-cell lymphoma in its early stages.

Specific infections, such as tuberculosis, leprosy, or the deep mycoses, have produced a somewhat similar clinical picture, particularly in the past, but only the idiopathic types are discussed here. These comprise two main diseases, namely:

- peripheral T-cell (rarely B-cell) angiocentric lymphomas
- Wegener's granulomatosis (a form of necrotizing vasculitis).

NASOPHARYNGEAL T-CELL LYMPHOMAS

Some of these nasopharyngeal lymphomas can cause midfacial destruction. The cellular picture is pleomorphic, and a variety of terms had been given to these lesions until the introduction of T-cell markers confirmed their nature. Confusion has arisen particularly because of the tendency for the tumor cells sometimes to surround or destroy blood vessels and so to mimic closely true vasculitis.

As mentioned earlier, these tumors, by their involvement of the nasal passages, are not reliably distinguishable clinically in their earlier stages from Wegener's granulomatosis. The age and sex distribution seems also to be similar.

Early features are nasal obstruction and serosanguinous discharge from or crusting of the nostrils. In neglected cases, massive destruction of the center of the face and secondary infection may follow.

Oral lesions, unlike those of Wegener's granulomatosis, typically consist of boggy palatal swelling and ulceration. The latter may consist of no more than a small central crater or result from extensive palatal necrosis. Bone destruction can lead to loosening of upper teeth. Involvement of regional lymph nodes is unusual until the tumor disseminates.

MICROSCOPY

The cellular picture is pleomorphic, with many large or immunoblast-like cells and relatively few small lymphocytes. A striking feature is the angiocentric distribution of the tumor cells and angiodestruction, which mimics vasculitis. Epithelium may also be invaded, and extensive areas of necrosis may be seen. Unlike Wegener's granulomatosis, giant cells are absent, and granulocytes are few unless infection is superimposed. However, in biopsies from the mouth the picture is frequently obscured by necrosis, superimposed inflammation and, consequently, a mixed cell population (Figs 49.20–49.22).

In the past some of the cases were categorized as 'lymphomatoid

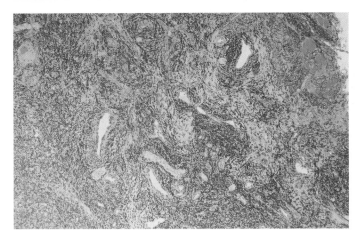

Fig. 49.20 Angiocentric T-cell lymphoma. Low-power view, showing conspicuously dense perivascular distribution of lymphocytes.

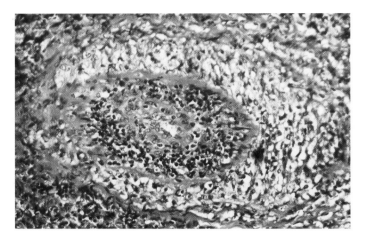

Fig. 49.21 Angiocentric T-cell lymphoma. Higher power view, showing infiltration of a small vessel wall.

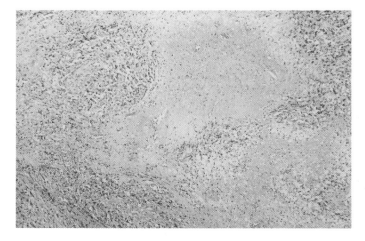

Fig. 49.22 T-cell lymphoma. Low-power view, showing large areas of necrosis typical of a nasopharyngeal lymphoma.

granulomatosis,' but it is widely accepted now that this is a T-cell lymphoma.

Rare cases of B-cell lymphomas causing midline granuloma syndrome have been reported by Hirota et al[19] and Maxymiw et al.[20] In both cases there was palatal necrosis and ulceration. In the case reported by Maxymiw et al,[20] there were also angiocentric and angiodestructive changes suggestive of a T-cell lymphoma.

BEHAVIOR AND MANAGEMENT

Adequate biopsy is essential. In the case of palatal involvement the biopsy should extend deeply, and be repeated if necessary, to obtain material uncontaminated by superimposed inflammation or necrosis.

Some of these tumors have a slow and remittent course, but eventually disseminate. The main principles of treatment are radiotherapy, usually with combination chemotherapy.

WEGENER'S GRANULOMATOSIS

In fully developed form, Wegener's granulomatosis comprises the triad of granulomatous inflammation of the nasal region, and pulmonary and lung involvement.

Wegener's granulomatosis is regarded as being immunologically mediated. It is frequently classified with the connective tissue diseases, but with questionable justification, as there are no immunological abnormalities linking Wegener's granulomatosis with these disorders. Neutrophil anticytoplasmic antibodies have been detected and may be useful in diagnosis, but are not specific to Wegener's granulomatosis.

INCIDENCE

Men appear to be more frequently affected and the peak age of incidence is between 40 and 55 years. The disease has, rarely, also been seen in children.

CLINICAL FEATURES

Early features of Wegener's granulomatosis typically consist of granulomatous inflammation of the nasal cavity and variable degrees of destruction. Later, destruction of the nasal septum can lead to a saddle nose deformity.

Oral lesions

Wegener's granulomatosis can give rise to a distinctive proliferative gingivitis with a granular surface and deep red in color, that has been described as 'strawberry gums.' This can form the earliest clinical manifestation of the disease. A few or many teeth may be involved. This form of gingivitis, after confirmation by biopsy, can allow treatment to be started at an unusually early stage. Mucosal ulcers may develop in the later stages and may dominate the picture. Unlike the palatal ulceration that may result from a nasopharyngeal lymphoma, the ulcers of Wegener's granulomatosis can be large, shallow, and widely distributed. Cervical lymphadenopathy may be present.

MICROSCOPY

There is widespread inflammation, with a mixed cellular picture and, frequently, numerous eosinophils. An essential feature is necrotizing vasculitis of small arteries, associated with giant cells. The giant cells are not necessarily directly involved in the vasculitis, and may just as frequently be found in the adjacent tissues. They are typically compact, with four or five nuclei and an irregular outline, but may resemble Langhans giant cells. Granulomas, although characteristic of this disease, are inconspicuous, usually difficult to find, and are rarely seen in oral biopsies, as are foci of necrosis and microabscesses[21] (Figs 49.23 and 49.24).

Biopsies of gingival lesions typically show only the giant cells, and are unlikely to show vasculitis because no arteries of sufficient size are likely to be included. In addition, gingival tissues show superficial proliferation, throwing the epithelium up into folds, which produce the granulomatous appearance seen clinically.[22]

BEHAVIOR AND MANAGEMENT

Early recognition of Wegener's granulomatosis is essential, as it can be considerably more rapidly fatal than a peripheral T-cell lymphoma. A few cases can be recognized early by the gingival lesions that precede systemic disease. Later manifestations are typically pulmonary cavitation and renal disease, which is the main cause of death. Joint pains are common and rashes are sometimes a feature. The diagnosis must be established by biopsy at the earliest possible moment, and detection of antineutrophil cytoplasmic antibodies (ANCAs) is helpful. The latter show fine granular cytoplasmic fluorescence and are present in approximately 85% of cases. The value of antineutrophil cytoplasmic antibodies in diagnosis has been reviewed by Burrows & Lockwood.[23] They have reported that staining for classical antineutrophil cytoplasmic antibodies (cANCAs) is more strongly positive in Wegener's granulomatosis than in polyarteritis nodosa, microscopic polyarteritis, or Churg–Strauss syndrome. Staining for perinuclear (pANCAs) is positive in all of these apart from classical polyarteritis nodosa where it is weak. Although antineutrophil cytoplasmic antibodies are not specific to Wegener's granulomatosis, the clinical picture produced by other forms of vasculitis is quite different. By contrast, they are highly informative for distinguishing Wegener's granulomatosis from nasopharyngeal lymphoma when it presents a similar clinical picture and, frequently, arteritis-like changes histologically, as discussed earlier.

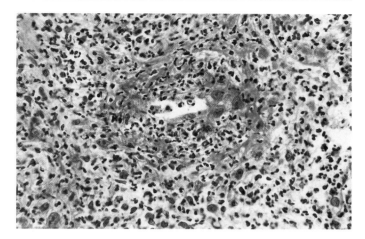

Fig. 49.23 Wegener's granulomatosis. High-power view, showing a similar pattern of angiodestruction to that of a T-cell lymphoma, but the cells are polymorphonuclear leucocytes.

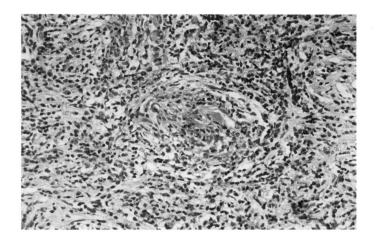

Fig. 49.24 Wegener's granulomatosis. Lower power view, showing complete vessel destruction and many eosinophils (a typical feature of this disease).

Examination of the nasopharynx, chest radiographs, renal function tests and, if appropriate, lung biopsy should also be carried out. Hematuria is likely to indicate glomerulonephritis and a poor prognosis.

Early treatment with cytotoxic drugs, such as cyclophosphamide or azathioprine, may be successful. Arrest of the disease with cotrimoxazole has been reported on several occasions, but remains a controversial treatment.[24]

Common features and important differences between Wegener's granulomatosis and nasopharyngeal T-cell lymphomas are summarized in Table 49.5. While a typical site for angiocentric peripheral T-cell lymphomas is in the nasopharynx, Khan et al[25] have reported bilateral salivary gland involvement with extensive destruction, which they considered was probably of the same nature. Genotypic analysis was inconclusive, but peripheral T-cell lymphomas can show genotypic heterogeneity.

Table 49.5 Midline granuloma syndromes

Wegener's granulomatosis	Nasopharyngeal T-cell lymphoma
Nasopharyngeal lesions Ulceration, discharge, granulation and crusting Destruction of the nasal septum	*Nasopharyngeal lesions* Ulceration, discharge, granulation and crusting Can ultimately cause severe midfacial destruction
Oral lesions Proliferative gingivitis (strawberry gums) Mucosal ulceration, sometimes widespread	*Oral lesions* Extension into the mouth is most likely to be via the palate, which appears ulcerated as a result of perforation
Microscopy Necrotizing arteritis with giant cells	*Microscopy* Pleomorphic cellular picture, but typically with angiocentric and angiodestructive infiltrations mimicking arteritis Identification of T-cells by immunocytochemistry is required
Immunological findings Antineutrophil cytoplasmic antibodies (ANCAs) present	
Spread Mainly to the lungs and kidneys	*Spread* Late-stage nasopharyngeal lymphoma disseminates in a generally similar way to other lymphomas
Treatment Cyclophosphamide and/or azathioprine may be effective if given early	*Treatment* Radiotherapy, usually supplemented with combination chemotherapy

* Either may be the presenting sign.

Systemic mastocytosis

Systemic mastocytosis is a systemic disease characterized by mast cell proliferation and infiltration of the tissues, causing heterogeneous manifestations. The cutaneous form of the disease is known as *urticaria pigmentosa*, in which there may be single or multiple aggregations of mast cells. These give rise to lightly pigmented plaques or swellings, which swell when scratched, due to release of mast cell proteases. Systemic mastocytosis affects approximately 10% of patients with urticaria pigmentosa, or may develop de novo. Tissues that may be infiltrated include bone, lymph nodes, liver, and spleen. Rarely, large numbers of mast cells may spill over into the blood to cause mast cell leukemia. Systemic mastocytosis typically affects those in the sixth or seventh decades.

Fechner & Mills[15] state that 45–70% of patients with systemic mastocytosis have radiographically detectable osseous lesions. However, Medina et al[26] have reported what is believed to be the first reported case of systemic mastocytosis involving the mandible. In this patient, a 29-year-old female, the diagnosis of systemic mastocytosis had been made 20 years earlier as a result of skin lesions and bone marrow infiltration. Radiographs showed a 1.5 cm × 2.0 cm area of radiolucency around a molar root. This was found to be a smooth-walled bony cavity containing friable material that was readily enucleated. Microscopy showed sheets of mast cells that showed metachromatic staining of the granules with toluidine blue. They were also Giemsa, chloroacetate esterase, leucocyte common antigen, and neuron-specific enolase positive, but were chromogranin and S-100 negative. Electron microscopy confirmed most of the population to be typical mast cells, but approximately 20% of them were T (tryptase positive, chymase negative) mast cells.

MANAGEMENT

Systemic symptoms such as malaise, fever, headache, or joint pains are frequently present, but are of little value in suggesting so uncommon a disease. However, the majority of patients with systemic mastocytosis have urticaria pigmentosa, and may have experienced acute exacerbations of their disease due to release of mast cell mediators. These anaphylactoid reactions include urticaria, flushing, bronchoconstriction, acute hypotension, vomiting, and diarrhea. The hypotension causes tachycardia and can lead to fatal circulatory collapse. Factors that can trigger such reactions include drugs (such as penicillin, aspirin, morphine, sulfonamides, procaine-containing local anesthetics, and several intravenous general anesthetic agents), foods, (particularly peanuts or chocolate), exposure to extremes of temperature, and emotional stress.

Even in the absence of signs or symptoms of mastocytosis, biopsy of a jaw lesion showing tumor-like aggregations of mast cells should provide the diagnosis. However, operative procedures can sometimes lead to prolonged bleeding due to defective hemostasis possibly caused by mast cell heparin release. Prolonged follow-up is required because of the possibility of progressive hematological disease in a minority.

Granulocytic sarcoma (chloroma)

Granulocytic sarcomas are solid tumors of immature granulocytes. They are usually associated with acute, but occasionally with chronic, myelogenous leukemia or other myeloproliferative disease such as polycythemia vera or myeloid metaplasia. Granulocytic sarcoma usually forms during a blastic crisis, but can precede leukemic changes in the blood or even the bone marrow. Most oral granulocytic sarcomas have been in the jaws, and the first such case reported appears to be the one described by Brooks et al[27] – a granulocytic sarcoma of the maxilla in a child. Ficarra et al[28] have reported a submucosal, soft tissue granulocytic sarcoma in an aleukemic patient and reviewed seven earlier cases. In addition to these, Timmis et al[29] reported a granulocytic sarcoma of the retromolar soft tissue of the mandible in another aleukemic patient, and Dreizen et al[30] reported eight cases involving the head and neck. Of these, one was in the gingivopalatal mucosa and another was in the cheek. Of eight patients where the sex was recorded, all but two were females. Eisenberg et al[31] have reported another case in an aleukemic male, and reviewed the condition in detail.

CLINICAL FEATURES

Granulocytic sarcoma of the soft tissues typically causes a swelling with intact surface and minimal symptoms. The tumor in the case reported by Eisenberg et al[31] was unusual in that it appeared as multiple erythematous nodules on the free and attached gingiva, and submandibular lymphadenopathy. Tumors of the jaws may sometimes be, but are not invariably, painful. Radiographically, intraosseous lesions show an ill-defined area of radiolucency.

MICROSCOPY

The soft tissue mass may sometimes have the greenish tinge, which justifies the term *chloroma*, due to the presence of myeloperoxidase, but the color fades on exposure to air.

Hematoxylin and eosin staining shows a densely cellular tumor consisting of large round to oval cells. The cytoplasm is scanty and eosinophilic, and not obviously granulocytic. The nuclei are vesicular with prominent nucleoli, and mitotic figures may be abundant. Stroma is scanty and the tumor is poorly circumscribed. The appearances mimic those of a large-cell lymphoma or metastatic carcinoma, for either of which granulocytic sarcoma has sometimes been mistaken. However, large areas or the whole section may appear reddish, and this is highly suggestive. Naphthol–ASD–chloracetate staining clearly demonstrates cytoplasmic granules, and confirms the diagnosis. Eisenberg et al[31] have described other techniques, including Wright–Giemsa stain, which shows the delicate nuclear chromatin pattern and nucleoli, and cytoplasmic granules. However, the diagnosis is otherwise difficult in the absence of overt leukemia and if eosinophilic myelocytes are not seen.

BEHAVIOR AND MANAGEMENT

The prognosis is that of myelogenous leukemia, although the individual tumors readily respond to radiation or combination chemotherapy. Although the prognosis of adult myelogenous leukemia is improving, reported cases of granulocytic sarcoma have survived more or less briefly. The patient reported by Timmis et al[29] died only 13 days after the oral biopsy, and was found to have multicentric granulocytic sarcomas of the skeleton, but showed no leukemic cells in the blood or bone marrow. The patient reported by Eisenberg et al[31] received successful bone-marrow transplantation after initial chemotherapy had failed.

Follicular dendritic cell tumor

This rare tumor affects lymph nodes, but two examples have been reported in the oral cavity by Chan et al.[32] It is mentioned here largely to draw attention to a tumor which, as those authors suggested, may be mistaken for various sarcomas or some lymphomas.

Typical features are spindle cells in sheets, whorls, or storiform configurations, or having a syncytial-like appearance. These merged cell masses may appear fibrillary due to interdigitating cell processes, which can be visualized by electron microscopy. Multinucleate cells may be conspicuous and lymphocytes scattered throughout. In the tumors reported by Chan et al,[32] there were areas interspersed by narrow pseudovascular spaces, with plump tumor cells protruding into the lumina. Most of the nuclei have a delicate chromatin pattern and a single nucleolus. Immunoreactivity with at least two of the markers CD21, CD35, R4/23, and Ki-M4 provides valuable support for the diagnosis. Follicular dendritic cell tumors appear to be indolent, and any that have recurred after excision appear to have responded to re-excision.

REFERENCES

1. Cohen MA, Bender S, Struthers PJ 1984 Hodgkin's disease of the jaws. Review of the literature and report of a case. Oral Surg 57: 413–417
2. Wright DH 1994 Lymphomas of Waldeyer's ring. Histopathology 24: 97–99
3. Epstein JB, Scully C 1992 Neoplastic disease in the head and neck of patients with AIDS. Int J Oral Maxillofac Surg 21: 219–226
4. Herdier BG, Kaplan LD, McGrath MS 1994 Pathogenesis of AIDS lymphomas. AIDS 8: 1025–1049
5. Lozada-Nur F, de Sanz S, Silverman S et al 1996 Intraoral non-Hodgkin's lymphoma in seven patients with acquired immunodeficiency syndrome. Oral Surg Oral Med Oral Pathol Oral Radiol Endod 82: 173–178
6. Wolvius EB, van der Valk P, van der Wal JE et al 1994 Primary extranodal non-Hodgkin lymphoma of the oral cavity. An analysis of 34 cases. Oral Oncol Eur J Cancer B: Oral Oncol 30: 121–125
7. Slootweg PJ, Wittkampf ARM, Kulin PM, de Wilde PCM, van Unnik JAM. Extranodal non-Hodgkin's lymphoma of the oral tissue. J Max-Fac Surg 13: 85–92
8. Issacson PG, Norton A 1994 Extranodal lymphomas. Churchill Livingstone, Edinburgh
9. Chan WC, Greiner TC 1994 Diagnosis of lymphomas by the polymerase chain reaction. Am J Clin Pathol 101: 273–274
10. Sariban E, Donahue A, Magrath IT 1984 Jaw involvement in American Burkitt's lymphoma. Cancer 53: 1777–1782
11. Wang MB, Strasnick B, Zimmerman MC 1992 Extranodal Burkitt's lymphoma of the head and neck. Arch Otolaryngol Head Neck Surg 118: 193–199
12. Pileri SA, Montanari M, Falini B et al 1990 Malignant lymphoma involving the mandible. Clinical morphologic and immunohistochemical study of 17 cases. Am J Surg Pathol 14: 652–659
13. Parker F, Jackson H 1939 Primary reticulum cell sarcoma of bone. Surg Gynaecol Obstet 68: 45–53
14. Pettit CK, Zukerberg LR, Gray MH et al 1990 Primary lymphoma of bone. A B-cell neoplasm with a high frequency of multilobated cells. Am J Surg Pathol 14: 329–334
15. Fechner RE, Mills SE 1992 Tumors of the bones and joints. Atlas of tumor pathology. Armed Forces Institute of Pathology, Washington, DC, third series, fascicle 8
16. Kurihara K, Kohno H, Miyamoto N, Chikamori Y, Kondo T 1990 Pathologic characteristics of human T-cell lymphotropic virus (HTLV)-related extranodal orofacial lymphomas. Oral Surg Oral Med Oral Pathol 70: 199–205
17. Sirois DA, Miller AS, Harwick RD, Vonerheld EC 1993 Oral manifestations of cutaneous T-cell lymphoma. A report of eight cases. Oral Surg Oral Med Oral Pathol 75: 700–705
18. Rosenberg A, Biesma DH, Sie-Go DMD, Slootweg PJ 1996 Primary CD30-positive T-cell non-Hodgkin's lymphoma of the oral mucosa. Report of two cases. Intl J Oral Maxillofac Surg 25: 57–59
19. Hirota J, Osaki T, Yoneda K et al 1992 Midline malignant B-cell lymphoma with leukaemic transformation. Cancer 70: 2958–2962

20. Maxymiw WG, Patterson BJ, Wood RE, Meharchand JM, Munro AJ, G'orska-Flipot I 1992 B-cell lymphoma presenting as a midfacial necrotizing lesion. Oral Surg Oral Med Oral Pathol 74: 343–347

21. Devaney KO, Travis WD, Hoffman G, Leavitt R, Lebovics R, Fauci AS 1990 Interpretation of head and neck biopsies in Wegener's granulomatosis. A pathologic study of 126 biopsies in 70 patients. Am J Surg Pathol 14: 555–564

22. Cawson RA 1965 Gingival changes in Wegener's granulomatosis. Br Dent J 118: 30–33

23. Burrows NP, Lockwood NW 1995 Antineutrophil cytoplasmic antibodies and their relevance to the dermatologist. Br J Dermatol 132: 173–181

24. Hoffman GS, Kerr GS, Leavitt RY et al 1992 Wegener granulomatosis: an analysis of 158 patients. Ann Intern Med 116: 488–498

25. Khan SM, Bailey IS, Addis BJ 1991 Angiocentric immunoproliferative lesion presenting as bilateral salivary gland swellings: a case report with genotypic analysis. Histopathology 19: 96–98

26. Medina R, Faecher RS, Stafford DS, Zander DS, Baughman RA 1994 Systemic mastocytosis involving the mandible. Oral Surg Oral Med Oral Pathol 78: 28–35

27. Brooks HW, Evans AE, Glass RM, Pang EM 1974 Granulocytic sarcoma of the head and neck in childhood. The initial manifestation of myeloid leukaemia in three patients. Arch Otolaryngol 100: 306–308

28. Ficarra G, Silverman S, Quivey JM, Hansen LS, Gianotti K 1987 Granulocytic sarcoma (chloroma) of the oral cavity: a case with a leukaemic presentation. Oral Surg Oral Med Oral Pathol 63: 709–714

29. Timmis DP, Schwartz JG, Nishioka G, Tio F 1986 Granulocytic sarcoma of the mandible. J Oral Maxillofac Surg 44: 814–818

30. Dreizen S, McCredie KB, Keating MJ 1987 Mucocutaneous granulocytic sarcomas of the head and neck. Oral Pathol Med 16: 57–60

31. Eisenberg E, Peters ES, Krutchkoff DJ 1991 Granulocytic sarcoma (chloroma) of the gingiva; report of a case. J Oral Maxillofac Surg 49: 1346–1350

32. Cahn JKC, Tsang WYW, Tang SK, Lee AWM 1994 Follicular dendritic cell tumors of the oral cavity. Am J Surg Pathol 18: 148–157

Non-neoplastic lymphoproliferative diseases 50

A variety of conditions may simulate lymphomas clinically, histologically, or both, and may occasionally have to be considered in the differential diagnosis. Most of them affect lymph nodes, but some can affect the oral tissues.

Sinus histiocytosis

Sinus histiocytosis is typically seen in nodes draining carcinomas. It is a rare cause of cervical lymphadenopathy, but the swelling may be mistaken for a metastasis.

MICROSCOPY

There are prominent distended lymphoid sinusoids. The sinuses are filled with histiocytes and the endothelial cells are often grossly enlarged.

MANAGEMENT

The condition is benign and requires no treatment.

SINUS HISTIOCYTOSIS WITH MASSIVE LYMPHADENOPATHY (ROSAI–DORFMAN DISEASE)

This disease is also rare, but particularly affects blacks. As the name implies, lymphadenopathy can be gross. It can occasionally be extranodal, and salivary glands and other sites may be involved. Fever and neutrophil leucocytosis may be associated, but most cases resolve spontaneously.

MICROSCOPY

The lymph node sinuses are filled with very large histiocytes, some of which have engulfed lymphocytes, and there is a reactive plasmacytosis.

Benign lymphoid hyperplasia of the palate

This rare lymphoproliferative lesion is similar to the so-called pseudolymphoma of other sites. Wright & Dunsworth[1] appear to have been the first to recognize its distinctive features and of the ability of previously reported lesions to persist for 4–12 years without lymphomatous change. Seven more examples were reported by Bradley et al,[2] another by Kabani et al,[3] and two more by Napier & Newlands.[4]

Clinically, there is typically a firm painless swelling to one side of the soft palate.

MICROSCOPY

Multiple germinal centers are present and may have a rim of well-differentiated B lymphocytes together with a mixed, mainly mononuclear infiltrate with many plasmacytoid lymphocytes. Immunohistochemistry carried out by Napier & Newlands[4] confirmed that the lesion was reactive rather than neoplastic by virtue of polyclonal light chain restriction in the germinal centers, mature and immature B-cells in the mantle zone with both B and T lymphocytes in the extramantle zone.

MANAGEMENT

If lymphoma can be excluded, prolonged follow-up is required to exclude the possibility of lymphomatous change or to treat it early if it should happen. However, follow-up has in some cases been as long as 10 years, and as far as is known lymphomatous change has not been seen.

Palatal infiltration in Sjögren's syndrome

Very occasionally, palatal swelling due to lymphoplasmacytic infiltration is a manifestation of Sjögren's syndrome. Cooper[5] described it in a 69-year-old woman with advanced disease, and reviewed earlier reports. Histologically, the changes are essentially the same as those seen in the salivary glands.

Langerhans cell histiocytosis

Cervical lymph nodes can be enlarged, sometimes massively, either in isolation or, more frequently, in association with multisystem disease (see Ch. 30).

Giant (angiofollicular) lymph node hyperplasia (Castleman's disease)

This rare condition usually affects the thorax, but in 15–20% of cases causes a cervical mass resembling a lymphoma.[6] Its cause is unknown, but it can be a complication of HIV infection.

MICROSCOPY

The salient features are gross hyperplasia of lymphoid follicles, in which lymphocytes form tight concentric layers around blood vessels, with swollen endothelial cells, which frequently proliferate. The interfollicular tissue is highly vascular (Figs 50.1 and 50.2). Several variants of this picture have been described, and in the rare plasma-cell type there may be monoclonal immunoglobulin production.

MANAGEMENT

Although the condition is benign, the mass may be so large that resection may be justified. This does not merely confirm the diagnosis, but is usually curative. Otherwise, a short course of high-dose corticosteroids or a single other immunosuppressive drug is effective. Combination cytotoxic chemotherapy should be avoided. The condition is not radiosensitive.

Lymphomatous change is a rare but recognized complication, and malignant blood vessel tumours, particularly Kaposi's sarcoma in patients with the acquired immune deficiency syndrome, are another.[7]

Infectious mononucleosis

The enlarged lymph nodes of infectious mononucleosis are rarely biopsied unless the presentation is atypical or lymphadenopathy

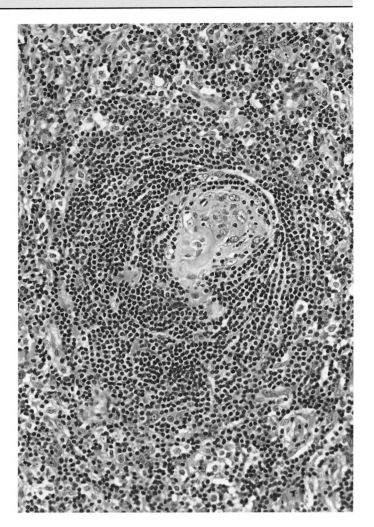

Fig. 50.1 Angiofollicular lymphoid hyperplasia, hyaline vascular type. Concentrically packed lymphocytes surround a vessel with thickened endothelium.

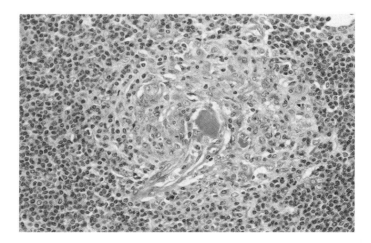

Fig. 50.2 Angiofollicular lymphoid hyperplasia, hyaline vascular type. At higher power, hyaline change at the center of the pseudofollicle is more conspicuous.

is persistent. Involvement of the lingual tonsils at the base of the tongue has been described clinically by Har-el & Jephson.[8] Exceptionally rarely, the lymphoid tissue of the foliate papillae has also been involved, as has been illustrated with the histologic changes by Cawson et al.[9] The variety of histologic changes in the lymph nodes or tonsils of 10 patients has been described by Childs et al.[10] Two of these patients had asymptomatic lymphadenopathy, no peripheral blood lymphocytosis, and negative serology by Monospot testing.

MICROSCOPY

The appearances are varied, possibly according to the stage of the disease when the biopsy was taken,[11] and have been described in detail by Stansfeld.[12] However, the follicles are soon overrun by proliferating lymphoid cells. The initial lymphocytic transformation and proliferation take place in the paracortex. Scattered immunoblasts appear in the T-zones, which expand rapidly until the follicles may disappear almost entirely and actively dividing immunoblasts replace the small lymphocytes. The blast cells are mainly mononuclear, but binucleate and atypical cells can closely resemble Reed–Sternberg cells (Fig. 50.3).

Several features that help to differentiate these changes from lymphomas have been described by Stansfeld.[12] First, the immunoblasts are typically in clumps interspersed by other cells, rather than uninterrupted sheets. Second, the immunoblasts vary in the strength of the cytoplasmic basophilia. Many show an intensity of basophilic and pyroninophilic cytoplasmic staining that would be unusual in malignant cells. Third, the large pyroninophilic immunoblasts are present not merely in the pulp, but also stuff the sinuses, which become dilated as a consequence. At this stage many of the immunoblasts show features of plasmacytoid differentiation.

These changes may be easier to describe than recognize, but diagnosis is usually helped by the clinical and serological changes.

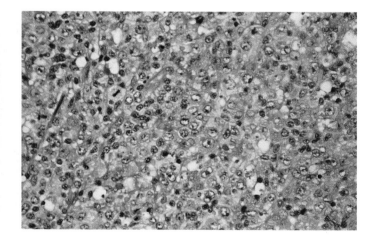

Fig. 50.3 Infectious mononucleosis. The lymphoma-like appearances in this lymph node are enhanced by large, Reed–Sternberg-like cells.

Phenytoin and other drug-associated lymphadenopathies

Of the many possible side-effects of phenytoin, a rare effect is lymphadenopathy, which can develop within a few weeks or months, but more frequently after long-term treatment. Lymphadenopathy caused by phenytoin (unlike that caused by many other drugs) is not generally associated with serum-sickness-like symptoms of fever, rashes, and joint pain. The importance of phenytoin-associated lymphadenopathy is that the microscopic changes can closely mimic Hodgkin's disease.

Cervical lymph nodes are frequently first affected, but lymphadenopathy usually becomes widespread.

MICROSCOPY

The appearances are varied, but the nodal architecture can be completely obliterated by a pleomorphic picture with proliferation of large immunoblast-like cells, which may be binucleate or multinucleate and closely resemble Reed–Sternberg calls. Although Stansfeld[12] considers that these changes have in the past been mistaken for malignant lymphoma, he accepts that there is also a small risk of lymphoma if the condition is allowed to progress.

The diagnosis is likely to be suggested by a history of treatment with phenytoin, or by the finding of associated gingival hyperplasia. If the latter is absent and the patient fails to disclose the necessary information about drug treatment (epilepsy is frequently not admitted by sufferers) so that lymph node biopsy is carried out, a specialist opinion may be needed, and Stansfeld[12] admits that at times the differential diagnosis from Hodgkin's disease may sometimes be extraordinarily difficult.

BEHAVIOR AND MANAGEMENT

Substitution of phenytoin with another anticonvulsant such as carbamazepine should allow the lymphadenopathy to subside and confirm the diagnosis.

Other drugs that can cause lymphadenopathy include penicillin (rarely), phenylbutazone (virtually obsolete), and some other nonsteroidal anti-inflammatory drugs and some antimalarials. As mentioned earlier, lymphadenopathy with these drugs is typically associated with serum-sickness-like features.

REFERENCES

1. Wright JM, Dunsworth AR 1983 Follicular hyperplasia of the hard palate: a benign lymphoproliferative process. Oral Surg 55: 162–168
2. Bradley G, Main JHP, Birt BD, From L 1987 Benign lymphoid hyperplasia of the palate. J Oral Pathol 16: 18–26
3. Kabani S, Cataldo E, Folkerth R et al 1988 Atypical lymphohistiocytic infiltrate (pseudolymphoma) of the oral cavity. Oral Surg Oral Med Oral Pathol 66: 587–592
4. Napier SS, Newlands C 1990 Benign lymphoid hyperplasia of the palate: report of two cases and immunohistochemical profile. J Oral Pathol Med 19: 221–225
5. Cooper JC 1976 Oral swelling in Sjögren's syndrome. Br J Oral Surg 14: 128–136
6. Wolf M, Kessler A, Horovitz A 1991 Benign angiofollicular lymph node hyperplasia

(Castleman's disease) presenting as a solitary cervical mass. J Oral Maxillofac Surg 49: 1129–1131

7. Gerald Q, Kostianovsky M, Rosai J 1990 Development of vascular neoplasia in Castleman's disease. Am J Surg Pathol 14: 603–614

8. Hare-El G, Jephson JS 1990 Infectious mononucleosis complicated by lingual tonsillitis. J Laryngol Otol 104: 651–653

9. Cawson RA, Binnie WH, Eveson JW 1994 Color atlas of oral disease, 2nd edn. Mosby Wolfe, London, p 18.18–18.19

10. Childs CC, Parham DM, Berard CW 1987 Infectious mononucleosis. The spectrum of morphologic changes simulating lymphoma in lymph nodes and tonsils. Am J Surg Pathol 11: 122–132

11. Gowing NFC Infectious mononucleosis: histopathologic aspects. In: Sommers SC (ed) Pathology Annual. Appleton-Century-Crofts, New York p 1–20

12. Stansfeld AG 1992 In: Lymph node biopsy and interpretation, 2nd edn (Stansfeld AG, d'Ardenne AJ, eds). Churchill Livingstone, London, p 102–105

Salivary gland tumors

Benign salivary gland tumors and general aspects

51

Thackray & Sobin's 1972 classification[1] of salivary gland tumors, shown in Table 51.1, is still widely used, although it is now accepted that mucoepidermoid and acinic cell 'tumors' are carcinomas. Since this classification was constructed, many more tumors have been recognized.

To take these changes into account, in 1991 another classification was proposed by the World Health Organization (WHO) Collaborating Center for Salivary Gland Tumors.[2] This classification is shown in modified form, as used in this text, in Table 51.2. This classification has discarded the category of 'monomorphic' adenomas as a single group distinguishable in their behavior from pleomorphic adenomas.

INCIDENCE

The peak incidence for benign tumors is in the sixth decade and, for malignant tumors, the seventh. Thus in the third decade, nearly 95% of tumors are benign, but by the seventh decade and after, 30% of tumors are malignant. Overall, women are only slightly more frequently affected until the eighth and ninth decades, after which age women are almost twice as frequently affected as men. This, however, must be related to a female predominance of 2 : 1 at these ages in the general population. For some tumors there is a female, but in others, a male preponderance, as discussed later.

Overall, more than 70% of salivary gland tumors are in the parotid, 11% are in the submandibular glands, and the remainder may be distributed as shown in Table 51.3, but there may be some variation from country to country. In purely relative terms, malignant tumors are more frequent in the minor salivary glands: thus only 16% of parotid, but 78% of sublingual and 46% of minor gland, tumors are malignant.

As to the sites of minor gland tumors (approximately 14% of all salivary gland tumors), 54% are in the palate, 20% in the lips, and 10% in the buccal mucosa.

Table 51.1 Classification of salivary gland tumors (after Thackray & Sobin[1])

Epithelial tumors
A. Adenomas
   1. Pleomorphic adenoma (mixed tumor)
   2. Monomorphic adenoma
      (a) Adenolymphoma (Warthin's tumor)
      (b) Oxyphilic adenoma (oncocytoma)
      (c) Other monomorphic adenomas
B. Mucoepidermoid tumor
C. Acinic cell tumor
D. Carcinomas
   1. Adenoid cystic carcinoma
   2. Adenocarcinoma
   3. Squamous cell carcinoma
   4. Undifferentiated carcinomas
   5. Carcinoma in pleomorphic adenoma

Nonepithelial tumors
Hemangioma
Lymphangioma
Neurofibroma
Lipoma
Others, including malignant variants of the above
Lymphoma

CLINICAL FEATURES

Salivary gland tumors cause swellings and are sometimes painful. A painful salivary gland swelling strongly suggests malignancy, but nonmalignant parotid swellings, such as infections, some Warthin's tumors, and a few cases of Sjögren's syndrome, can also be painful. There are no reliable clinical indicators of malignancy. However, rapid growth, pain, lymphadenopathy and, in the case of the parotid gland, facial palsy are strongly suggestive and are likely to indicate a poor prognosis. Beyond that there are no clinical features peculiar to specific salivary gland tumors and, as yet, no imaging techniques will reliably distinguish benign from malignant tumors. Frequently also, neoplasms cannot be distinguished from non-neoplastic disease until the microscopic findings are available.

Within the mouth, salivary gland tumors may be firm or rubbery, and may feel lobulated. If benign, they are mobile on deeper tissues, and the overlying mucosa is normal, unless traumatized, but sometimes appears bluish. Growth of some adenomas can be exceedingly slow.

Table 51.2 WHO (1991) Histopathological classification of salivary gland tumors (modified)

I Adenomas
Pleomorphic adenoma
Myoepithelioma
Warthin's tumor (adenolymphoma)
Oncocytoma
Duct adenomas
   Basal cell adenoma and membranous variant
   Canalicular adenoma
Sebaceous adenoma and sebaceous lymphadenoma
Duct papillomas
   Inverted duct papilloma
   Intraduct papilloma
   Sialadenoma papilliferum
Papillary cystadenoma

II Carcinomas
Mucoepidermoid carcinoma
Acinic cell carcinoma
Adenoid cystic carcinoma
   Cribriform/tubular
   Solid
Adenocarcinoma (not otherwise specified)
   Papillary cystadenocarcinoma
   Mucinous adenocarcinoma
Carcinoma in pleomorphic adenoma
   Intracapsular (noninvasive)
   Invasive
   Carcinosarcoma
Metastasizing pleomorphic adenoma
Polymorphous low-grade (terminal duct) adenocarcinoma
Epithelial–myoepithelial duct carcinoma
Salivary duct carcinoma
Basal cell (basaloid) carcinoma
Sebaceous carcinoma
   Sebaceous carcinoma with lymphoid stroma
Oncocytic carcinoma
Squamous cell carcinoma
Adenosquamous carcinoma
Undifferentiated carcinoma
   Small cell and neuroendocrine carcinomas
Undifferentiated carcinoma with lymphoid stroma
Other carcinomas

III Mesenchymal tumors
Angiomas
Lipomas
Neural tumors
Other benign mesenchymal tumors and hamartomas
Sarcomas

IV Malignant lymphomas

V Secondary tumors

VI Unclassified tumors

VII Tumor-like disorders
Sialosis (sialadenosis)
Oncocytosis
Necrotizing sialometaplasia (salivary gland infarction)
Benign lymphoepithelial lesion
Salivary gland cysts
HIV-related cysts and other disorders
Kuttner tumor (chronic submandibular sialadenitis)

Table 51.3 Distribution of tumors in minor and major salivary glands*

Frequency at site (%) Tumor	Palate	Lips	Buccal mucosa	Total minor glands	Total major glands
Adenomas					
Pleomorphic	47	44	37	43	63
Other	6	30	13	11	7
Carcinomas					
Mucoepidermoid	9	–	8	9	2
Acinic cell	1	4	–	2	2
Adenoid cystic	12	9	13	13	4
Adenocarcinomas	12	9	18	12	3
Squamous cell	1	–	3	1	1
Undifferentiated	1	3	3	2	2
Carcinoma in pleomorphic adenoma	8	3	5	7	4

* Percentages are rounded up to whole figures. A few tumors in the tongue, pharynx, tonsil, retromolar fossa, alveolar ridge, maxillary tuberosity, and ethmoid have been omitted, as there was often only a single tumor in each of these sites.

Pleomorphic adenoma

Pleomorphic adenomas account for 63% of parotid, 60% of submandibular, and 43% of minor gland tumors. By contrast, they are rarely seen in the sublingual gland. Almost any age can be affected, but the peak incidence is in the fourth and fifth decades. There is a slight female preponderance.

CLINICAL FEATURES

Pleomorphic adenomas of the parotid gland have no distinctive features, but are slow-growing, painless, do not cause facial palsy and, if neglected, can reach an enormous size. At operation they vary in texture according mainly to their mucinous or collagenous content. Intraoral pleomorphic adenomas can sometimes be felt to be lobulated and may have a submucosal bluish tint.

MICROSCOPY

The main components are duct cells, often producing a multiplicity of duct-like structures, and sheets of epithelial or myoepithelial cells. The latter are not reliably identifiable by light microscopy as they may be small, dark and nondescript, spindle-shaped or resemble plasma cells. Squamous metaplasia of epithelial cells is common. The result is a mixed and variable picture of epithelial and myoepithelial cells together with mucoid or myxomatous tissue, which may form the bulk of the tumor. Cartilage or, less frequently, true bone may form. According to Seifert et al,[3] myxoid material forms 80% of the bulk of 55% of pleomorphic adenomas. These can thus readily burst at operation. At the other extreme, cartilage can rarely form the predominant component, causing the tumor to be hard and glistening when cut across. Another uncommon variant is a predominantly fatty tumor. Fat is a normal finding in parotid glands, but an occasional pleomorphic adenoma may at first appear lipomatous.[4] Electron microscopy studies have shown transition of myoepithelial cells to adipocytes. There is no proven correlation between these varied appearances and clinical behavior, but Seifert et al[3] state that recurrence may be more common with stroma-rich (mucoid) variants and carcinomatous change is most frequent in highly cellular tumors (Figs 51.1–51.4).

The mixed and varied microscopic pictures are well known, but widespread misapprehensions persist about the capsule and have led to frequent attempts to enucleate parotid gland tumors. Encapsulation may appear complete in the plane of section, but the tumor, despite being benign, can bulge through or infiltrate the capsule. Focal infiltration of the capsule is common and sub-capsular clefts can provide false planes of cleavage. Whole-organ

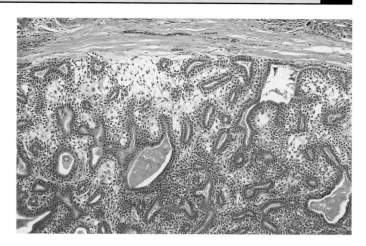

Fig. 51.3 Pleomorphic adenoma. Multiple duct-like structures with bilayered linings dominate the scanty mucoid stroma. The capsule is intact in this area.

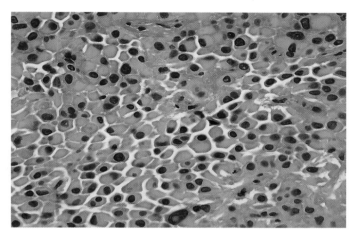

Fig. 51.4 Pleomorphic adenoma. Hyaline (plasmacytoid) myoepithelial cells.

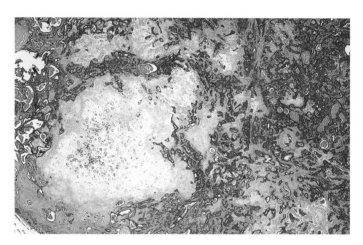

Fig. 51.1 Pleomorphic adenoma. A typical area of cartilage is surrounded by many duct-like structures.

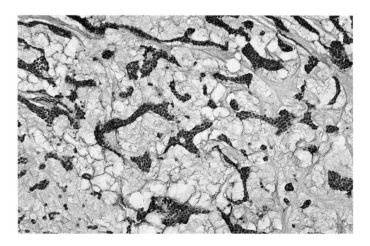

Fig. 51.2 Pleomorphic adenoma. Strands of myoepithelial cells are surrounded by mucoid stroma

sectioning of excised parotid pleomorphic adenomas by Lam et al[5] showed that in *all* cases the capsule was infiltrated by tumor, and that in a third of cases the capsule was incomplete, with tumor in direct contact with salivary tissue (Figs 51.5 and 51.6). Apparently isolated islands of tumor can also occasionally form outgrowths of the main mass and be joined to it only by a slender isthmus.

The main sources of diagnostic difficulties include extensive oncocytic change mimicking an oncocytoma. Alternatively, the myoepithelial cells may become clear, although confusion with any of the recognized clear cell tumors is unlikely, unless the specimen is inadequate. However, clear cell carcinomas occasionally develop in pleomorphic adenoma.

Also suggesting malignancy are areas of necrosis. Allen et al[6] noted necrosis in five pleomorphic adenomas, of which three had undergone sudden swelling and become painful. They concluded that these tumors were benign, but the periods of follow-up ranged from only 3 months to 3 years. More difficult is the presence of epithelial dysplasia. Atypia is frequently intracapsular,

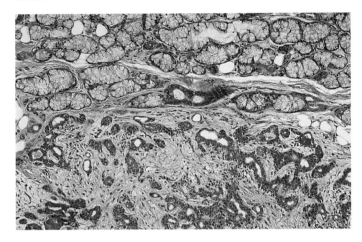

Fig. 51.5 Pleomorphic adenoma. Tumor, without any capsule, abuts onto normal salivary tissue in this area. This is a feature of most pleomorphic adenomas, but several sections may have to be examined.

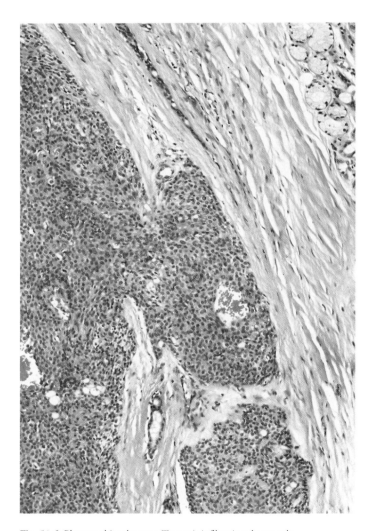

Fig. 51.6 Pleomorphic adenoma. Tumor is infiltrating the capsule.

but careful searching is necessary to exclude invasion. Also important is extensive fibrotic change (scarring), which is typically seen in neglected, long-standing tumors. Malignant change is particularly frequent in scarred areas, but only slender strands of carcinoma cells may be found after a thorough search.

BEHAVIOR AND MANAGEMENT

Pleomorphic adenomas, although capable of malignant change, are benign, but expand and grow in localized areas of proliferation to form irregular nodular masses. However, it is the surgical difficulties of managing parotid gland tumors that has led them to be regarded as 'semi-malignant' in the past. Management problems include the following:

- The risk of damage to the facial nerve is great, particularly when removing irregularly shaped tumors.
- Biopsy of parotid gland tumors is not feasible because of their ability to seed in the line of incision to produce multiple recurrences.
- The capsule is often incomplete and its integrity cannot be assumed if there is an unwise attempt at enucleation.
- Mucinous tumors can readily burst to produce multiple seedlings if enucleation is attempted.
- Removal of recurrences, which are typically multifocal, becomes more difficult with each attempt, and the end result can be innumerable nodules of tumor, spreading along the neck far beyond the original site.
- Treatment of recurrences increases the risk of having to resect the facial nerve. Alternatively, recurrences may prove to be unmanageable.
- The chances of malignant change are greater in recurrences, increase with each subsequent recurrence, and may be increased further if radiotherapy is used.

In short, the ability of seeded tumor cells to proliferate outside the original margins, and particularly in the incision scar, after incisional biopsy or incomplete excision is well established. Malignant change is also more frequent in scarred areas. Recurrences may not become apparent for 10 or even 20 years and this can give a false sense of the completeness of excision and encourage a dangerously conservative treatment policy. High reported cure rates after enucleation are based on inadequate duration of follow-up.

These considerations make it clear that incisional biopsy of parotid gland tumors should not be carried out in any circumstances. Currently, fine-needle aspiration cytology is acceptable and useful, although doubts have been expressed about its safety.[7] So-called 'enucleation' is also contraindicated, and it is essential to remove pleomorphic adenomas completely by total or subtotal parotidectomy at the first operation.

There is no case for irradiation as a supplement to surgery. There is no evidence of its benefit and it may increase the chances of or accelerate malignant change.[8] If re-operation is necessary post-irradiation scarring and ischemia greatly increase the difficulties.

Areas of epithelial atypia in the tumor without evidence of invasion (also sometimes termed 'intracapsular carcinoma' or 'carcinoma in situ') inevitably causes concern. If it is possible to be confident that this change is confined within the substance of the tumor, then it can be treated like other pleomorphic adenomas by parotidectomy or wide excision of other glands. However, follow-up must be rigorous.

Myoepithelioma

Myoepithelial tumors are rare and can be regarded as a variant of pleomorphic adenoma. The term 'myoepithelioma' is frequently used for tumors where myoepithelial cells predominate but some elements of a pleomorphic adenoma are present. 'Pure' myoepitheliomas are rare. Ellis & Gnepp[9] found 50 reports of these tumors. Almost any age could be affected, but the average was 40 years. Forty-eight per cent of these tumors were in the parotid glands and 52% were in minor glands.

MICROSCOPY

Spindle-cell myoepitheliomas, the most common type, are highly cellular and consist of elongated, slender spindle cells forming interlacing streams with little stroma. They therefore resemble mesenchymal tumors such as neurofibroma. Occasionally, immunocytochemistry is required to detect the typical double staining of myoepithelial cells with high-molecular-weight keratin markers as well as mesenchymal markers, particularly S-100 protein, vimentin, and smooth-muscle-specific actin.

Aggressive behavior may not be entirely predictable from the microscopic appearances, but mitotic activity and cellular pleomorphism are highly suspicious.

Myoepitheliomas are usually benign and should be treated accordingly, but all grades can be seen between spindle cell myoepitheliomas and myoepithelial carcinomas. The latter show mitotic activity and cellular pleomorphism, giving them a sarcomatoid appearance.

Plasmacytoid myoepitheliomas consist of elliptical or rounded cells, with hyaline, basophilic cytoplasm, and eccentrically placed nuclei. They typically have a loose, abundant, myxoid stroma. Although a solitary plasmacytoma can very occasionally form in a parotid gland there should be little chance of mistaking it for a plasmacytoid myoepithelioma (Figs 51.7 and 51.8).

Doubts are being expressed about both the nature and behavior of plasmacytoid myoepitheliomas. Franquemont & Mills[10] found that staining for desmin and muscle-specific and smooth-muscle actins was negative, and suggested that these plasmacytoid cells should not be classified as myoepithelial.

Unlike the spindle-cell type, plasmacytoid myoepitheliomas were thought not to have any potential for aggressive behavior.

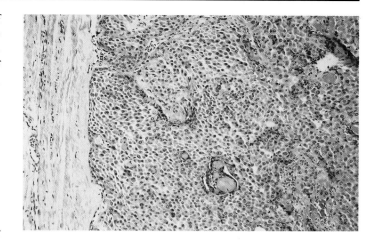

Fig. 51.7 Myoepithelioma, plasmacytoid type.

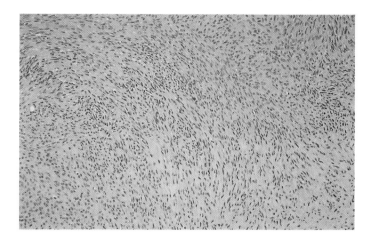

Fig. 51.8 Myoepithelioma, spindle-cell type.

Nevertheless, Di Palma & Guzzo,[11] in reporting 10 malignant myoepitheliomas, included two of plasmacytoid configuration.

BEHAVIOR AND MANAGEMENT

Myoepitheliomas should be removed by parotidectomy or wide excision in other sites.

Monomorphic adenomas

The 1992 WHO classification has abandoned this term for benign salivary gland tumors that have a less varied cellular picture than pleomorphic adenomas and lack their myxochondroid stroma. Instead, a variety of benign tumors has been categorized which, in contrast to pleomorphic adenoma are usually better circumscribed, have less tendency to recur and are generally less difficult to manage.

WARTHIN'S TUMOR (ADENOLYMPHOMA, CYSTADENOLYMPHOMA)

In the parotid glands, Warthin's tumor forms 14% of neoplasms. Strangely, there has in the past been a heavy preponderance of males with this tumor, and in the last edition of this text Lucas[12] noted that 85–90% of these tumors were in males. However, a male/female ratio of 10 : 1 has undoubtedly fallen to only 1.6 : 1, as shown by Eveson & Cawson[13] in an analysis of 278 of these tumors and in other recent series. The age range of those affected is 50–70 years.

Warthin's tumor affects the parotid glands, and the authenticity of those reported in other glands has been questioned by Eveson & Cawson[13] from a study of 278 of these tumors. However, van der Wal et al[14] were able to find 10 cases in other sites during a 20-year period.

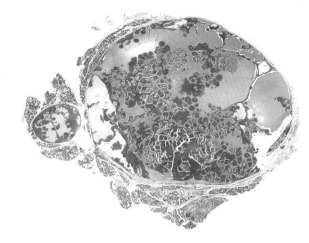

Fig. 51.9 Warthin's tumor. Whole mount showing the papillary cystic configuration in two separate tumors.

CLINICAL FEATURES

Warthin's tumors usually cause soft painless swellings, but sometimes there can be pain or rapid expansion, probably as a result of the partly cystic nature of most of them. Occasionally, the tumor is bilateral or multifocal in a single gland. Lam et al,[15] by step-serial whole-organ sectioning of 26 parotid glands, found multiple Warthin's tumors in 13 cases, thus confirming the findings of earlier studies that lacked histological confirmation. The greatest number of Warthin's tumors in a single gland was four, and bilateral tumors were present in three of 24 patients.

MICROSCOPY

Warthin's tumors have a thin capsule and consist of tall, columnar, finely granular, eosinophilic epithelial cells surrounding lymphoid tissue, which frequently forms germinal follicles. The epithelium typically forms papillary projections into cystic spaces. As noted by Warthin,[16] ciliated epithelium is occasionally identifiable. The amounts of epithelial and lymphoid stroma are highly variable and either may predominate (Figs 51.9–51.11).

Occasionally, part of the tumor can undergo apparently spontaneous necrosis (infarction), and epithelioid granulomas resembling those of tuberculosis can form. These were found in 20 of 278 Warthin's tumors by Eveson & Cawson.[17] Taxy[18] has also described squamous and mucinous metaplasia in foci of necrosis giving rise to appearances resembling squamous or mucoepidermoid carcinoma. Warthin's tumor can also occasionally be concurrent with other salivary gland tumors, rarely show lymphomatous change, or even more rarely have carcinoma developing in it (Fig. 51.12).

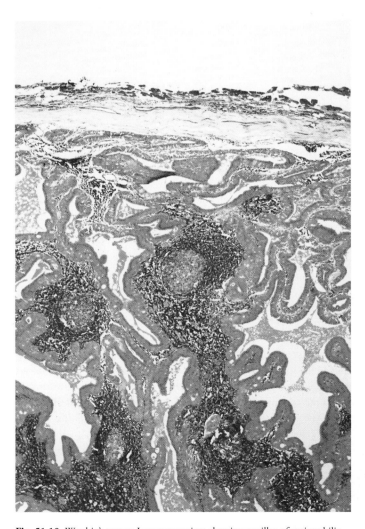

Fig. 51.10 Warthin's tumor. Low-power view, showing papillae of eosinophilic epithelium that lack a lymphoid tissue core in some parts.

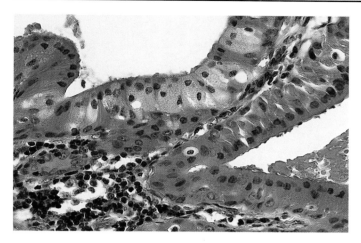

Fig. 51.11 Warthin's tumor. Higher power view, showing the tall columnar epithelial cells with peripheral nuclei and a basal layer of small cells.

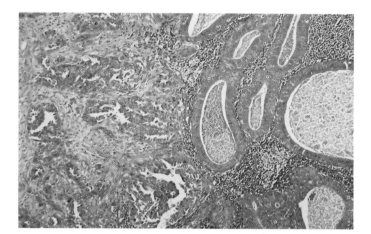

Fig. 51.12 Carcinoma in Warthin's tumor.

HISTOGENESIS

The clinicopathologic features of Warthin's tumor have aroused considerable speculation, as reviewed by Gallo.[19] The lymphoid stroma has similar proportions of T and B lymphocytes as does a normal lymph node, and it seems likely that Warthin's tumors arise in heterotopic salivary gland tissue in intraparotid lymph nodes. However, in reviewing 140 Warthin's tumors, Gallo[19] found that 32% of patients had autoimmune disease, as compared with 4.4% of 380 patients with pleomorphic adenomas. Gallo[19] also found that nine consecutive patients with Warthin's tumor had higher levels of VCA and EA antibodies to Epstein–Barr virus than did patients with pleomorphic adenomas or healthy controls, and postulated a role for this virus in the pathogenesis.

BEHAVIOR AND MANAGEMENT

Warthin's tumor is completely benign. Lam et al[15] suggest that

superficial parotidectomy is appropriate because most parotid lymph nodes lie in the superficial lobe. Excision is curative. Recurrence may result from incomplete removal of the tumor or from it being multifocal. Carcinomatous or lymphomatous change has been reported,[20] but is extraordinarily uncommon.

ONCOCYTOMA (OXYPHILIC ADENOMA)

Oncocytomas form 0.5% of epithelial salivary gland tumors. They particularly affect those in the seventh or eight decades and are more frequent in women. The parotid glands are the usual site.

MICROSCOPY

Oncocytomas consist of distinctive, uniform, plump, polygonal cells with abundant, granular eosinophilic cytoplasm, separated by fine fibrous septa. Occasionally, transition of oncocytes to clear cells can be seen, as discussed below. Oncocytomas consisting entirely of clear cells are a recognized entity, but are exceedingly rare (Figs 51.13–51.16).

The main consideration in differential diagnosis is to distinguish oncocytomas from oncocytic change in other tumors and the even more uncommon oncocytic carcinomas.

Oncocytomas are benign, and Brandwein & Huvos[21] suggest that even perineural invasion is compatible with benign behavior.

BEHAVIOR AND MANAGEMENT

Excision is normally curative. Reported recurrences may be due to incomplete removal or to unrecognized oncocytic change in a carcinoma.

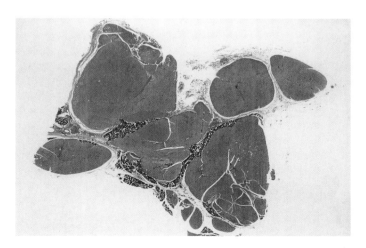

Fig. 51.13 Oncocytoma. A whole mount shows the uniformly eosinophilic appearance of the tumor.

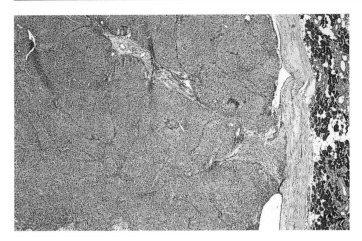

Fig. 51.14 Oncocytoma. The tumor cells have a suggestion of a thecal configuration.

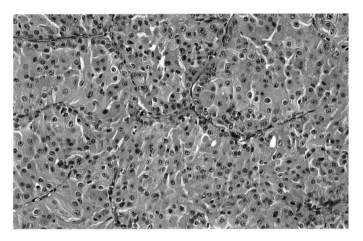

Fig. 51.15 Oncocytoma. Higher power view shows the polygonal, uniformly eosinophilic cells separated by fine fibrous septa.

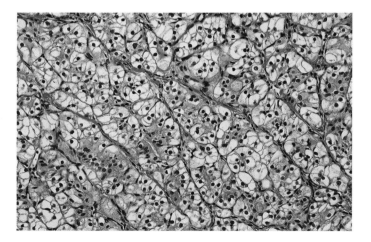

Fig. 51.16 Oncocytoma. Clear-cell variant showing a resemblance to a renal cell carcinoma.

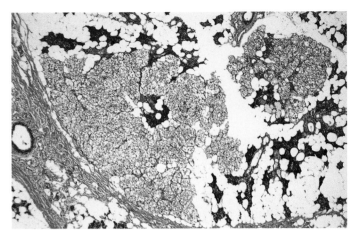

Fig. 51.17 Multinodular oncocytic hyperplasia. Low power view, showing extensive clear-cell change.

MULTIFOCAL NODULAR ONCOCYTIC HYPERPLASIA

Foci of oncocytic cells resembling oncocytomas may be seen, but they are small (up to 1 cm across), multiple, and interspersed with normal salivary tissue. It is possible that oncocytomas arise by confluence of these foci. Clear cells are most frequently seen in these foci which may thus mimic a clear-cell tumor infiltrating the gland (Fig. 51.17).

ONCOCYTOSIS

Oncocytic change, which is occasionally extensive, can be seen as an age change in normal duct tissue and in other tumors such as pleomorphic adenomas or, more important, in adenocarcinomas. As oncocytomas are benign, it is necessary to differentiate them from oncocytic change in other tumors that are far more difficult to manage. Palmer et al[22] have shown that a significant number of oncocytomas may have been categorized incorrectly. In a reassessment of 26 tumors previously classified as oncocytomas, they found that nine of them were pleomorphic adenomas with oncocytic change (Fig. 51.18).

DUCT ADENOMAS

Seventy-five per cent of duct adenomas are found in the parotid glands, 22% are in the minor glands, where the lip is a site of predilection, but very few are found in other glands. Duct adenomas constitute about 20% of all adenomas. They comprise basal cell (tubular, trabecular, and membranous types) and canalicular types, which form slow-growing, well-circumscribed swellings.

Tubular adenomas

These consist of tubules, containing eosinophilic secretions. The tubules have a lining of small dark epithelial cells and an outer

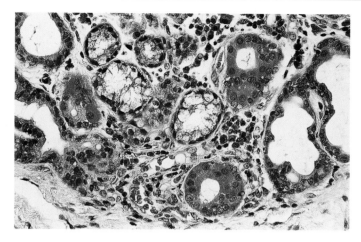

Fig. 51.18 Oncocytosis. An early stage of oncocytosis, which is seen in some of the duct cells.

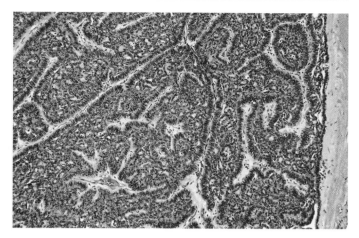

Fig. 51.19 Basal cell adenoma, trabecular type.

layer of myoepithelial cells, which may also form strands extending between the tubules, or may be few and inconspicuous. The stroma is usually scanty and unremarkable, but a rare variant shows myoepithelial stromal proliferation.

Trabecular adenomas

These consist of a monotonous pattern of cords, which are uniform in width, and composed of darkly staining cells in a sparse, featureless stroma. Rarely, a trabecular adenoma shows oncocytic change and may mimic an oncocytoma (Figs 51.19 and 51.20).

Membranous basal cell adenomas

These adenomas are rare. They have a thick, eosinophilic, periodic acid/Schiff (PAS)-positive hyaline layer surrounding the epithelium, which may contain lumens and hyaline material (Fig. 51.21). They are usually multilobular and may be incompletely encapsulated. They can also contain foci of normal salivary tissue, which add to the impression of invasiveness and enhance their similarities to an adenoid cystic carcinoma.

Membranous basal cell adenomas most frequently affect the parotid glands and then may be associated with multiple similar (turban) tumors of the scalp. They are sometimes, therefore, termed *dermal analog tumors of the parotid*. They may rarely undergo malignant change.

Canalicular adenomas

These were brought to prominence by Nelson & Jacoway,[23] who reported 29 cases and noted that several of them had been mistaken for adenoid cystic or other carcinomas. Twenty-three of the 29 cases involved the upper lip.

Unlike tubular adenomas, the canalicular type lacks myoepithelial cells surrounding the duct-like structures or cords of columnar or

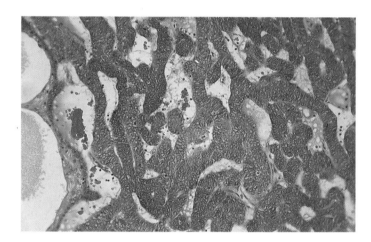

Fig. 51.20 Basal cell adenoma. This is a trabecular type, but was an intraosseous tumor.

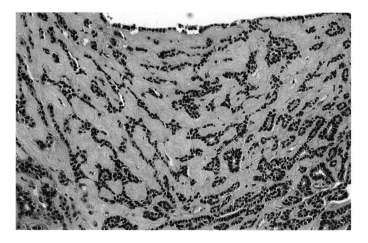

Fig. 51.21 Basal cell adenoma, membranous type.

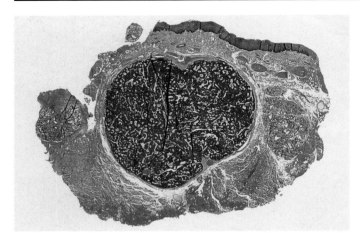

Fig. 51.22 Canalicular adenoma of the lip.

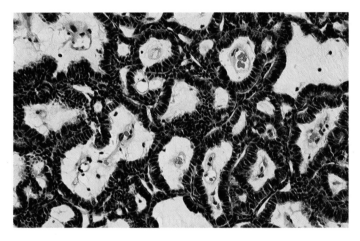

Fig. 51.23 Canalicular adenoma. Extensive stromal degeneration has left only outlines of blood vessels persisting.

cuboidal epithelial cells. Cyst formation may be prominent, while degeneration of the stroma may leave it virtually structureless, and often only ghosts of blood vessels remain (Figs 51.22 and 51.23).

Ferreiro,[24] from an immunohistochemical analysis of six canalicular adenomas, showed immunoreactivity for keratins AE1/AE3, but only one was weakly positive for EMA. All were vimentin and S-100 positive, but CEA and actin negative. These findings contrasted with five cases of polymorphous low-grade adenocarcinoma, all of which were positive for S-100 protein, and six cases of adenoid cystic carcinoma, which were all positive for CEA and S-100 protein.

BEHAVIOR AND MANAGEMENT

Excision is normally curative. As already mentioned, the chief risk with duct adenomas is that of confusing some of them with adenoid cystic carcinomas or basal cell adenocarcinomas. A thorough search of many fields may occasionally be necessary to confirm absence of invasion. If the biopsy is small it may be impossible to make the necessary distinction.

CLEAR CELL ADENOMA

In the past, benign clear cell tumors have been described, but their existence is highly questionable. Most clear cell tumors are malignant, despite a cytologically benign appearance.

PAPILLARY CYSTADENOMA

Papillary cystadenomas are uncommon, and in the past have been misdiagnosed. Ellis & Auclair[25] have described and illustrated the varied appearances of these tumors. They noted that only 25% showed a distinct fibrous capsule, and in some cases there were irregular margins, which might suggest infiltrative behaviour. The size and number of cysts were also variable, but when large invariably showed papillary growth into the lumen. Other cases showed duct-like structures, which Ellis & Auclair[25] believed could develop into cysts. The epithelium may be cuboidal or columnar, and in the latter case could be oncocytic and resemble a Warthin's tumor lacking lymphoid stroma (Fig. 51.24).

However, these workers noted that differences between cyst adenomas and low-grade papillary cystic adenocarcinomas could be subtle unless invasion of surrounding structures was seen. Moreover, as reported by Mills et al,[26] the latter could take between 10 and 20 years to recur, and could readily be thought to be benign (Figs 51.25 and 51.26).

Ellis & Auclair,[25] from the data available to them, considered that papillary cystadenomas were unlikely to recur after conservative but complete surgical excision.

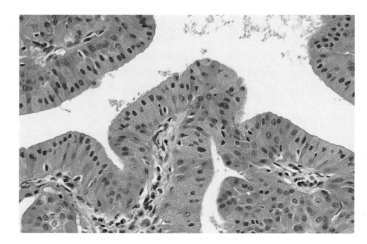

Fig. 51.24 'Papillary cystadenoma.' At high power the tumor can be seen to be a stroma-poor Warthin's tumor resembling areas of the tumor shown in Figure 51.10.

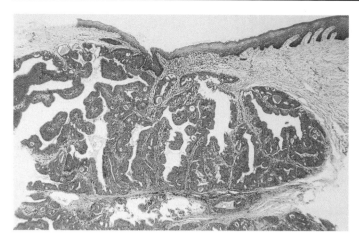

Fig. 51.25 'Papillary cystadenoma.' Low-power view, showing a much folded epithelium lining microcysts.

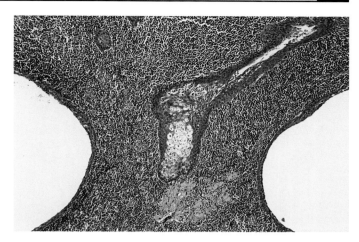

Fig. 51.27 Sebaceous lymphadenoma. Sebaceous tissue and cysts are set in a dense lymphoid stroma.

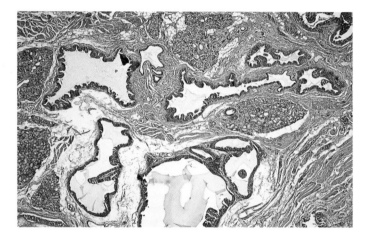

Fig. 51.26 Papillary cystadenoma. Another cytologically benign tumor that, nevertheless, appears to be infiltrating the gland and may ultimately prove to be malignant.

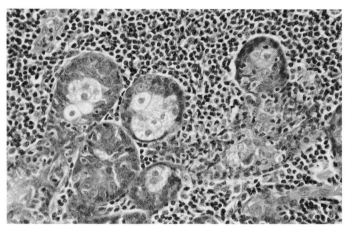

Fig. 51.28 Sebaceous lymphadenoma. Higher power view, showing sebaceous lobules and lymphoid stroma.

SEBACEOUS LYMPHADENOMA AND SEBACEOUS ADENOMA

Both of these tumors are rare. The sebaceous lymphadenoma resembles a Warthin's tumor, but with sebaceous cells forming solid masses and sebaceous cysts in place of the oncocytic cells. The pure sebaceous adenoma is particularly rare, but consists of solid masses of sebaceous tissue in a fibrous stroma (Figs 51.27 and 51.28).

Sebaceous elements can, rarely, also be seen in pleomorphic adenomas.

DUCT PAPILLOMAS

SIALADENOMA PAPILLIFERUM

Most of these rare tumors are in the minor glands, usually in the region of the junction of hard and soft palates. Unlike other salivary gland tumors, they form painless exophytic growths. They resemble papillomas of the oral mucosa, but grow from the orifice of a minor gland. The mean age of incidence is 59 years, but almost any age can be affected.

Microscopy

The superficial part closely resembles a squamous cell papilloma and consists of stratified squamous epithelium thrown up into papillae with a fibrovascular core. More deeply this epithelium merges with proliferating, dilated duct-like structures and, frequently, microcysts with papillary projections in their lumens (Figs 51.29 and 51.30)

Behavior and management

Local excision appears to be curative.

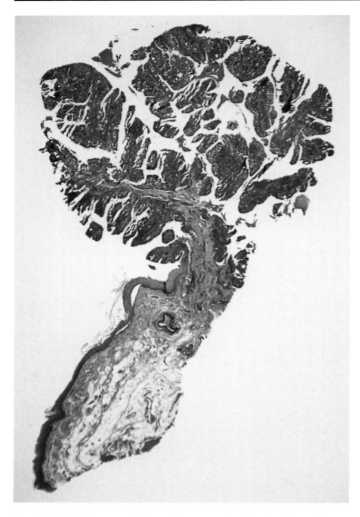

Fig. 51.29 Sialadenoma papilliferum. Low-power view, showing the papillary extraglandular component.

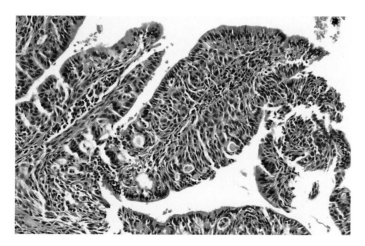

Fig. 51.30 Sialadenoma papilliferum. Irregular papillary processes are covered by pseudostratified columnar epithelium and have a core of vascular connective tissue.

INVERTED DUCT PAPILLOMA

Clark et al[27] found only five reports of inverted duct papillomas of salivary glands, but Hegarty et al[28] concluded that 17 had been described by then, and added another. Clinically, the latter found patients to have been aged between 32 and 66 years. In these patients the tumors formed smooth discrete masses 1–1.5 cm in diameter in various sites within the oral cavity, but in the lower lip in 11 of 18 cases. There were no distinctive features to suggest the diagnosis, apart from a mucosal punctum at the tip of the swelling.

Microscopy

An inverted duct papilloma typically forms just within the orifice of a duct of a gland, or its epithelium may be continuous with that of the surface mucosa. It consists of thick papillae covered by basaloid or squamous cells, and may contain a few goblet or columnar cells. The papillary overgrowth fills and dilates the duct lumen, and also bulges into, but does not infiltrate, the lamina propria. Microcysts lined by squamous or columnar epithelium occasionally form. These features have been unusually clearly illustrated by Hegarty et al[28] in their report of this tumor in the lip of a 50-year-old male (Figs 51.31 and 51.32).

Behavior and management

Excision appears to be curative and there is no evidence of a similar propensity for recurrence to that of inverted papillomas of the nasal cavity.

INTRADUCT PAPILLOMA

Intraduct papilloma is the most uncommon of all duct papillomas. It differs from the inverted duct papilloma in that its origin is more deeply in the salivary gland duct.

Microscopy

Intraduct papillomas consist of fibrovascular papillae covered by columnar or cuboidal epithelium, which forms a mass that distends the duct lumen to form a cyst-like cavity. Unlike inverted duct papillomas, the tumor does not extend into the duct wall, but obstruction by the tumor can give rise to secondary duct dilatation proximally.

Behavior and management

Excision is curative.

ADENOMATOID HYPERPLASIA OF MINOR SALIVARY GLANDS

Benign non-neoplastic enlargement of minor oral salivary glands

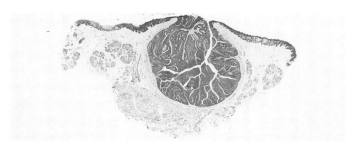

Fig. 51.31 Inverted duct papilloma. The origin from the duct close to its orifice and invagination of the lamina propria.

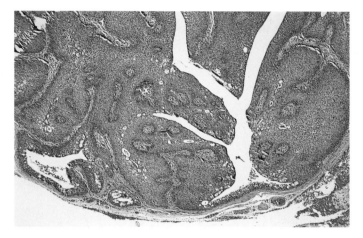

Fig. 51.32 Inverted duct papilloma. Higher power view, showing the basaloid epithelium and many goblet cells.

is an uncommon but recognized entity. Its distinction from a salivary gland tumor is important. Giansanti & Waldron[29] appear to have been the first (1971) to describe the histologic features in two cases, while the largest series (40 lesions) is that reported by Buchner et al.[30] Barrett & Speight[31] have added 20 new cases, and reviewed the condition.

CLINICAL FEATURES

Adenomatoid hyperplasia of minor salivary glands usually gives rise to a painless, tumor-like swelling of the palate, as observed in 19 of the 20 cases reported by Barrett & Speight.[31] Twelve of the 19 tumors affected the hard palate, eight affected the junction of the hard and soft palate, and two were in the soft palate. Uncommon complaints are an increase in the size of the lesion, or dysphagia. The age range of those affected is wide, with a mean age ranging from 39 to 50 years in the different series. There is a slight male preponderance. The cause is unknown, but Buchner et al[30] suggested that it was sometimes a reaction to chronic trauma, while Barrett & Speight[31] noted that 14 of their patients were tobacco smokers, wore dentures, or both.

MICROSCOPY

The glandular tissue is hyperplastic. It is morphologically otherwise normal, but some isolated lobules may appear hypertrophic and the acini may be filled with excessive mucus, which pushes the nucleus to the basal aspect of the cells. Duct dilatation may be noted, particularly superficially, deep to the mucosa, and mucous spillage is sometimes seen.

Inflammation, when present, tends to be focal and limited to a few lobules.

BEHAVIOR AND MANAGEMENT

Adenomatoid hyperplasia of minor salivary glands is benign. Once the diagnosis has been confirmed by microscopy, the lesion can be excised. Complete excision is curative.

SCLEROSING POLYCYSTIC ADENOSIS OF MAJOR SALIVARY GLANDS

Smith et al[32] have described nine cases of this slow-growing non-neoplastic lesion. Patients ranged in age from 12 to 63 years, and there was no gender preponderance. The parotid glands were involved in all but one case.

MICROSCOPY

The masses are circumscribed, but lack encapsulation and consist of sclerotic, hyalinized connective tissue with appearances reminiscent of fibrocystic breast disease. Hyperplastic ductal and acinar elements are distributed in the fibrous tissue and frequently are associated with ductal ectasia. The lining of these dilated ducts frequently shows apocrine-like metaplasia and hyperplasia, sometimes with formation of transluminal bridges, giving a cribriform appearance, or surrounding eosinophilic globules. Foci of the acinar components may contain large, strongly eosinophilic, PAS-positive cytoplasmic granules. A lymphocytic infiltrate of variable intensity accompanies the epithelial proliferation (Figs 51.33 and 51.34).

BEHAVIOR AND MANAGEMENT

As Smith et al[32] point out, several of these lesions had been mistaken for mucoepidermoid or other carcinomas or pleomorphic adenomas, and it is important that this distinction should be made.

All the cases reported by Smith et al[32] had been treated by local or, in one case, wide excision, or superficial lobectomy. Of the cases where data were available, one recurred after 56 months but the patient was disease-free 30 months later after total parotidectomy and radiotherapy. Another had multiple recurrences over a period of 9 years. The three remaining patients on whom

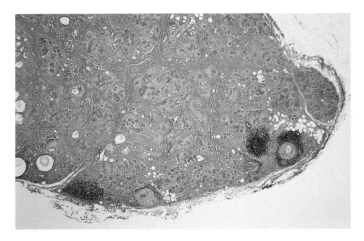

Fig. 51.33 Sclerosing polycystic adenosis. Low-power view, showing the fibrous nature of the mass with foci of hyperplastic glandular tissue and a few small cysts.

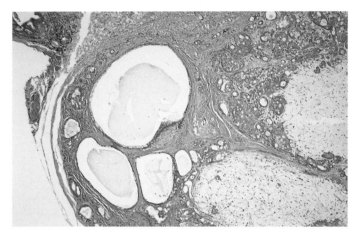

Fig. 51.34 Sclerosing polycystic adenosis. Cysts have epithelial linings that contain mucous cells.

information was available remained disease-free for periods of 7–27 months.

NECROTIZING SIALOMETAPLASIA

This tumor-like lesion is seen virtually exclusively in the minor glands of the palate. It is of unknown cause, although it is thought to result in part from cigarette smoking. It is far more frequent in the USA than in Britain.

Middle-aged males are predominantly affected. Typically, the patient develops a relatively painless ulcerated swelling on the hard palate midway between the midline and gingival margin often in the first molar region. The base of the ulcer is often on the underlying bone, and the margins are irregular and heaped up or everted. The ulcer, which may be 15–20 mm in diameter,

clinically resembles a squamous cell carcinoma for which it has, in the past, also been mistaken on microscopy.

MICROSCOPY

Chronic inflammation of minor salivary tissue leads to necrosis of acini. The duct tissue, which undergoes squamous metaplasia, proliferates, giving a pseudo-epitheliomatous appearance. (Figs 51.35 and 51.36).

BEHAVIOR AND MANAGEMENT

These lesions may be excised for diagnostic purposes, but usually heal spontaneously within 8–10 weeks. An acrylic cover plate is sometimes needed to protect the healing area, particularly at meal times.

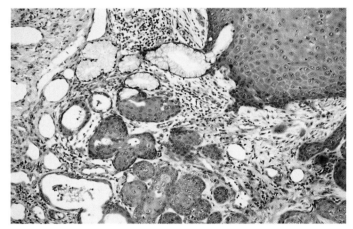

Fig. 51.35 Necrotizing sialometaplasia. Low-power view, showing extensive inflammatory infiltrate, and metaplasia of duct epithelium, giving a pseudoepitheliomatous appearance.

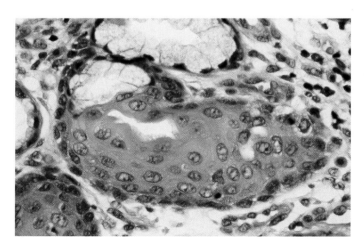

Fig. 51.36 Necrotizing sialometaplasia. Higher power view, showing the islands of metaplastic epithelium and some mucous cells.

REFERENCES

1. Thackray AC, Sobin LH 1972 Histological typing of salivary gland tumours. World Health Organization, Geneva
2. Seifert G in collaboration with pathologists in 6 countries 1991 Histological typing of salivary gland tumors. Springer-Verlag, Berlin
3. Seifert G, Miehlke A, Haubrich J, Chilla R 1986 Diseases of the salivary glands. Georg Thieme Verlag, Stuttgart
4. Ng WK, Ma L 1995 Pleomorphic adenoma with extensive lipometaplasia. Histopathology 27: 285–288
5. Lam KH, Wei WI, Ho HC, Ho CM 1990 Whole organ sectioning of mixed parotid tumours. Am J Surg 160: 377–381
6. Allen CM, Damm D, Neville B, Rodu B, Page D, Weathers DR 1994 Necrosis in benign salivary gland tumours. Not necessarily a sign of malignant transformation. Oral Surg Oral Med Oral Pathol 78: 455–461
7. Hix WR, Aaron BL 1990 Needle aspiration of lung cancer. Risk of tumor implantation is not negligible [editorial]. Chest 97: 516–517
8. Watkin GT, Hobsley M 1986 Should radiotherapy be used routinely in the management of benign parotid tumours. Br J Surg 73: 601–603
9. Ellis GL, Gnepp DR 1988 Unusual salivary gland tumours. In: Woolf DR (ed) Pathology of the head and neck. Churchill Livingstone, New York
10. Franquemont DW, Mills SE 1993 Plasmacytoid monomorphic adenoma of salivary glands. Absence of myogenous differentiation and comparison with spindle cell myoepithelioma. Am J Surg Pathol 17: 136–153
11. Di Palma S, Guzzo M 1993 Malignant myoepithelioma of salivary glands: clinicopathological features of ten cases. Virc Arch A Pathol Anat 423: 389–396
12. Lucas RB 1984 Pathology of tumours of the oral tissues, 4th edn. Churchill Livingstone, Edinburgh
13. Eveson JW, Cawson RA 1986 Warthin's tumor (cystadenolymphoma) of salivary glands. A clinicopathologic investigation of 278 cases. Oral Surg Oral Med Oral Pathol 61: 256–262
14. Van der Wal JE, Davids JJ, van der Waal I 1993 Extraparotid Warthin's tumours – report of 10 cases. Br J Oral Maxillofac Surg 31: 43–44
15. Lam KH, Ho HC, Wei WI 1994 Multifocal nature of adenolymphoma of the parotid. Br J Surg 81: 1612–1614
16. Warthin AS 1929 Papillary cystadenoma lymphomatosum. J Cancer Res 13: 116–125
17. Eveson JW, Cawson RA 1989 Infarcted ('infected') adenolymphomas. A clinicopathological study of 20 cases. Clin Otolaryngol 14: 205–210
18. Taxy JB 1992 Necrotizing squamous/mucinous metaplasia in oncocytic salivary gland tumors. A potential diagnostic problem. Am J Clin Pathol 97: 40–45
19. Gallo O 1995 New insights into the pathogenesis of Warthin's tumour. Oral Oncol, Eur J Cancer B: Oral Oncol 31: 211–215
20. Bengoechea O, Sanchez F, Larrinaga B, Martinez–Penueal JM 1989 Oncocytic adenocarcinoma arising in a Warthin's tumour. Pathol Res Pract 185: 907–911
21. Brandwein MS, Huvos AG 1991 Oncocytic tumors of major salivary glands. A study of 68 cases with follow-up of 44 patients. Am J Surg Pathol 15: 514–528
22. Palmer TJ, Gleeson MJ, Eveson JW, Cawson RA 1990 Oncocytic adenomas and oncocytic hyperplasia of salivary glands: a clinicopathological study of 26 cases. Histopathology 16: 487–493
23. Nelson JF, Jacoway JR 1973 Monomorphic adenoma (canalicular type). Report of 29 cases. Cancer 31: 1151–1153
24. Ferreiro JA 1994 Immunohistochemical analysis of salivary gland canalicular adenoma. Oral Surg Oral Med Oral Pathol 78: 761–765
25. Ellis GL, Auclair PL 1996 Tumors of the salivary glands. Atlas of tumor pathology. Armed Forces Institute of Pathology, Washington, DC, 3rd series, fascicle 17
26. Mills, SE, Garland TA, Allen MS 1984 Low-grade papillary adenocarcinoma of palatal salivary gland origin. Am J Surg Pathol 8: 367–374
27. Clark DB, Priddy RW, Swanson AE 1990 Oral inverted duct papilloma. Oral Surg Oral Med Oral Pathol 69: 487–490
28. Hegarty DJ, Hopper C, Speight PM 1994 Inverted ductal papilloma of minor salivary glands. J Oral Pathol Med 23: 334–336
29. Giansanti JS, Waldron CA 1971 Intraoral mucinous minor salivary gland lesions presenting clinically as tumors. Oral Surg Oral Med Oral Pathol 32: 918–922
30. Buchner A, Merrell PW, Capenter WM, Leider AS 1991 Adenomatous hyperplasia of minor salivary glands. Oral Surg Oral Med Oral Pathol 71: 583–587
31. Barrett AW, Speight PM 1995 Adenomatoid hyperplasia of oral minor salivary glands. Oral Surg Oral Med Oral Pathol Oral Radiol Endod 79: 482–487
32. Smith BC, Ellis GL, Slater LJ, Foss RD 1996 Sclerosing polycystic adenosis. A clinicopathologic analysis of nine cases. Am J Surg Pathol 20: 161–170

Carcinomas of salivary glands

52

The relative frequency of malignant compared with benign salivary gland tumors and the site to site variation in Table 51.3. Approximately 25% of salivary gland tumors in adults are malignant and the lowest *relative* frequency of malignant salivary gland tumors compared with benign tumors is in the parotid (15%) and the highest is in the sublingual glands (86%), although the overall numbers there are minute. Of the moderate numbers of salivary gland tumors in the minor glands, 46% are likely to be malignant.

CLINICAL FEATURES

Malignant salivary gland tumors usually grow more rapidly and may cause pain, particularly in the later stages. Typical features include fixation, ulceration, and involvement of regional lymph nodes. In the parotid gland, facial palsy is a highly significant sign and frequently implies a poor prognosis. Seifert et al[1] found that well-differentiated mucoepidermoid and acinic cell carcinomas never caused facial palsy, but the latter was present in 40–67% of the more malignant tumors and, in particular, in squamous cell, undifferentiated, and solid adenoid cystic carcinomas.

BEHAVIOR AND MANAGEMENT

Overall, only a minority of malignant salivary gland tumors betray their nature clinically. Few are recognized until after histology has been carried out. Therefore, there is usually pre-operative uncertainty about the best management of each individual patient, because of the impossibility of predicting behavior preoperatively and the absence of any guide that a conventional biopsy might provide. Preoperative fine-needle aspiration cytology followed by frozen-section confirmation during operation may, therefore, be valuable in suggesting a need for more radical procedures, and sometimes sacrifice of the facial nerve and neck dissection is indicated.

Mucoepidermoid carcinoma

Mucoepidermoid carcinomas formed 4.8% of all salivary gland tumors in the series reported by Seifert et al,[1] but only 2.8% of those in the series of the British Salivary Gland Tumour Panel. This represents 19.5% and 12%, respectively, of malignant epithelial tumors in these two series. Moreover, the relative frequency of mucoepidermoid carcinomas appears to be considerably greater in the USA; in the series reported by Foote & Frazell[2] for example, they formed 11% of all salivary gland tumors and 33% of the malignant tumors. In terms of individual glands, mucoepidermoid carcinomas form 1.5% of parotid gland tumors and approximately 10% of tumors of the minor glands, but are virtually never found in the sublingual glands.

The gender distribution is almost equal, with a peak incidence in the fifth decade, but any age can be affected.

CLINICAL FEATURES

Mucoepidermoid carcinomas are usually indistinguishable from benign tumors clinically, and Seifert et al[1] recorded that only 20% of high-grade mucoepidermoid carcinomas caused facial palsy and other clinical signs suggestive of malignancy.

Mucoepidermoid carcinoma is one of the most common types of postirradiation salivary gland tumors, and in a review of previous reports (including those relating to the survivors of the atomic bombing of Hiroshima and Nagasaki[3]) Watkin & Hobsley[4] noted that of the 70 malignant salivary gland tumors that resulted, 33 (47%) were mucoepidermoid carcinomas, which formed the single largest group.

Mucoepidermoid carcinoma is also the most frequent type of intraosseous salivary gland tumor, as discussed later.

MICROSCOPY

Mucoepidermoid carcinomas consist mainly of two distinct but contiguous cell types. These are epidermoid (squamous) cells and large, pale, faintly granular mucous cells. Microcyst formation is common, and mucoepidermoid carcinomas can occasionally consist of a large monolocular cyst with the tumor forming only a mural thickening. Careful assessment of the nature of the lining of salivary gland cysts is, therefore, essential (Figs 52.1–52.4).

In higher grade tumors the epidermoid element proliferates at the expense of mucous cells, so that the tumor tends to resemble a squamous cell carcinoma. However, small foci of mucin staining should be positive (Figs 52.5–52.7).

Adverse microscopic features include a small intracystic component, high mitotic activity, neural invasion, necrosis, and anaplasia. Occasionally, there is gross pleomorphism and nuclear hyperchromatism. However, even cytologically benign-looking tumors can be invasive and sometimes metastasize.

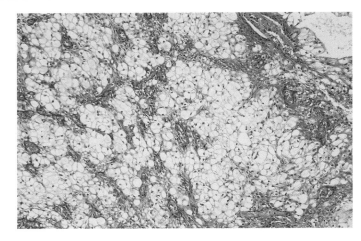

Fig. 52.3 Mucoepidermoid carcinoma. Clear cell change. Large areas of mucous cells have undergone hydropic change and are separated by strands of epidermoid cells.

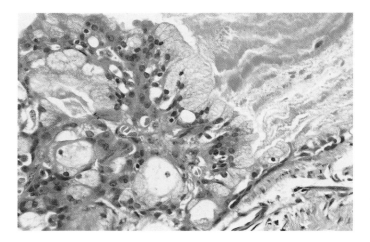

Fig. 52.1 Mucoepidermoid carcinoma. Low-power view, showing a typical cystic area of tumor with prominent mucous cells.

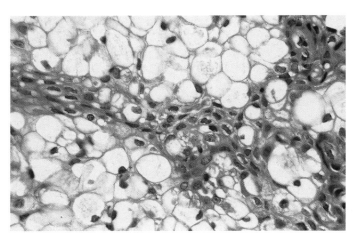

Fig. 52.4 Mucoepidermoid carcinoma with clear cell change. Higher power view, showing the water-clear cytoplasm of the mucous cells and the epidermoid cells.

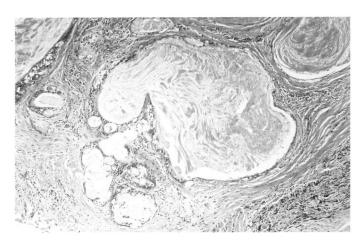

Fig. 52.2 Mucoepidermoid carcinoma. Higher power view, showing distended mucous cells backed by epidermoid cells in a typical, cytologically bland tumor.

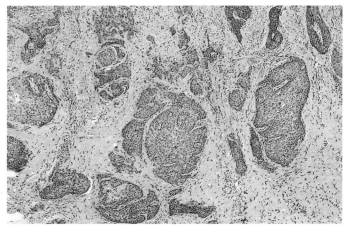

Fig. 52.5 Mucoepidermoid carcinoma. At low power the appearance of this higher grade tumor is essentially that of an epidermoid tumor.

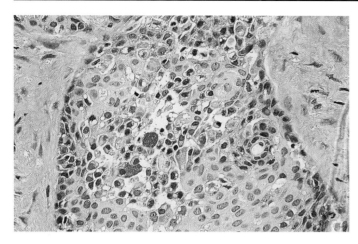

Fig. 52.6 Mucoepidermoid carcinoma. Mucin stain confirms the presence of a few mucous cells in a predominantly epidermoid tumor.

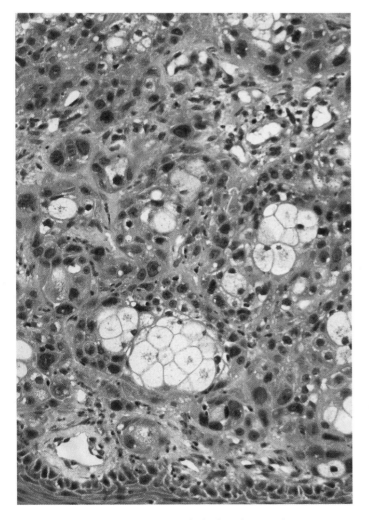

Fig. 52.7 Mucoepidermoid carcinoma. This high-grade tumor shows gross nuclear pleomorphism and hyperchromatism, and relatively few mucous cells.

BEHAVIOR AND MANAGEMENT

Spread through a gland is more diffuse than that of pleomorphic adenomas and may be aided by extravasation of mucus, carrying tumor cells with it. Even in the absence of microscopic evidence of invasion, all mucoepidermoid carcinomas should be regarded as malignant and excised completely. In a survey of 143 intraoral mucoepidermoid carcinomas, Auclair et al[5] found that a short history, production of symptoms, and location in the tongue or floor of the mouth, in association with microscopic criteria of malignancy, indicated a poor prognosis. Six out of 10 of their patients with high scores on these points died from their disease. Higher grade tumors should probably be treated like squamous cell carcinomas, but their response to radiotherapy is less predictable. Radiotherapy should only be used to supplement excision.

In a retrospective analysis of 749 reported cases, Hickman et al[6] found an estimated 5-year survival rate for mucoepidermoid carcinomas of 70.7% and a 10-year survival rate of 50%. Therefore, prognosis of these tumors appears to confirm that, overall, they are a relatively low-grade malignancy.

Acinic cell carcinoma

Over 85% of acinic cell carcinomas are found in the parotid glands, where they form about 3% of all tumors. Most of the remainder are found in the minor glands, but only rarely do they form in the sublingual or submandibular glands. Almost any age can be affected, but the peak incidence is in the seventh decade; there is a female preponderance of almost 2 : 1.

Seifert et al[1] noted that 17% of poorly differentiated acinic cell carcinomas caused facial palsy.

MICROSCOPY

Acinic cell carcinomas are infiltrative, but usually appear well circumscribed. The appearances are highly variable, but typically there is an almost uniform picture of large, granular basophilic cells closely resembling normal serous cells arranged in sheets or acinar configurations. There are usually many clear round spaces, which are thought to result from entrapped secretion. Frequently these spaces may be so numerous as to give the tumor a microcystic or lacy pattern. Occasionally, microcysts coalesce to form larger cystic cavities, and the tumor can assume a papillary cystic pattern. Vacuolated cells may be seen in over 33% of tumors and may be distinctive for acinic cell carcinomas. Smaller, cuboidal intercalated duct cells as well as acinic cells may also be seen. These have amphophilic or weakly eosinophilic cytoplasm and central nuclei. Occasional clear cells and their transition from granular cells may also be seen. Clear cells are occasionally numerous, but are rarely predominant (Figs 52.8–52.13).

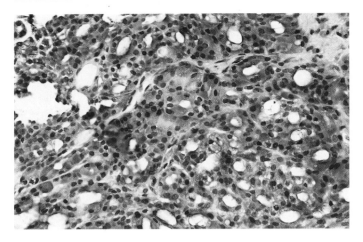

Fig. 52.8 Acinic cell carcinoma. Low-power view, showing a suggestion of acinar configuration of the basophilic cells.

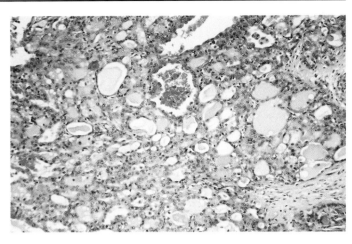

Fig. 52.11 Acinic cell carcinoma. This follicular pattern might be mistaken for a thyroid carcinoma.

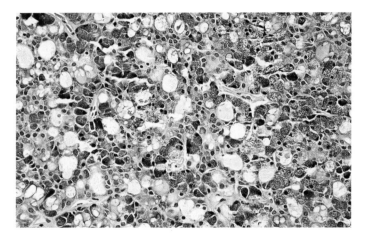

Fig. 52.9 Acinic cell carcinoma. At higher power, the tumor cells are seen to have a granular basophilic cytoplasm and the round clear areas that are typical of this tumor.

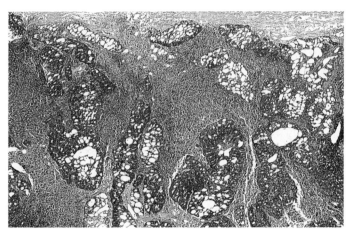

Fig. 52.12 Acinic cell carcinoma. This variant has a prominent lymphoid stroma. Some of the tumor processes show the lacy appearance that is also typical.

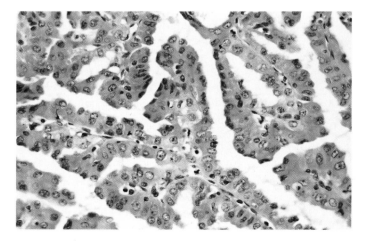

Fig. 52.10 Acinic cell carcinoma. A papillary cystic pattern is present in this area.

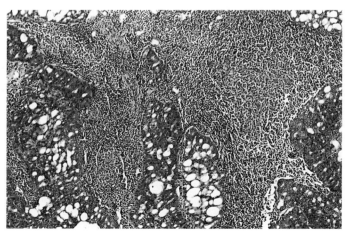

Fig. 52.13 Acinic cell carcinoma with lymphoid stroma. Another view, showing both granular cells and lacy areas.

Ellis & Gnepp[7] reported that, unexpectedly, acinic cell carcinomas frequently stain positively with mucicarmine and can mimic thyroid carcinomas, which may also contain intracellular mucin. This problem may have to be resolved by immunostaining for thyroglobulin or, if this fails, by investigation of the patient for a primary thyroid tumor.

Another variant has a dense lymphocytic stroma, which can extend with the tumor as it spreads into surrounding tissues.

Poorly differentiated acinic cell carcinomas, showing nuclear hyperchromatism and pleomorphism, are rarely seen.

BEHAVIOR AND MANAGEMENT

Despite the benign histologic appearance of most acinic cell carcinomas, their behavior is unpredictable. On the basis of only 101 reported cases suitable for analysis, Hickman et al[6] estimated the 5-year survival rate to be 82.2% and the 10-year survival rate to be 67.6%.

The findings of studies aimed at determining prognostic factors have been conflicting, but they confirm that recurrences may appear 20 years after the initial operation. Ellis & Corio,[8] in their analysis of 294 cases, found that no one tumor pattern or type was strongly indicative of a poor prognosis. However, they found that infiltrative growth, multinodularity, and stromal hyalinization were frequently seen in tumors that recurred or metastasized, and that an intercalated duct cell type of tumor was slightly more frequent among those that metastasized. The prognostic value of DNA cytometry appears to be limited,[9] but diploid tumors may show less tendency to metastasize, and tumors which show prominent necrosis, tubuloductal differentiation, and areas of loss of differentiation may be more aggressive.[10] Lewis et al[11] reported the findings in 90 patients with exceptionally long periods of follow-up. The primary treatment group of 63 patients had been followed for up to 45 years. The remainder (27 patients), who had been referred for recurrent disease, were followed up for a median period of 12 years. The authors calculated determinate survival probabilities of 90% at 5 years, 83% at 10 years, and 67% at 20 years. Forty-four per cent of the patients had local recurrences, 19% had metastases, and 25% died from their disease. Local recurrences first appeared up to 30 years after presentation, and death followed up to 38 years later. Clinical features associated with a poor prognosis were pain or fixation, signs of gross invasion, and treatment by local excision rather than parotidectomy. Microscopic features associated with a poor prognosis were a desmoplastic stromal reaction, atypia, or increased mitotic activity.

In view of the fact that even cytologically benign acinic cell carcinomas can occasionally metastasize, treatment (as with muco-epidermoid carcinomas) should be by parotidectomy, or wide excision of other glands. If the tumor is poorly differentiated, excision should be followed by radiotherapy.

Adenoid cystic carcinoma (cylindroma)

Adenoid cystic carcinomas form 30% of parotid, 30% of submandibular, and 40% of minor gland tumors, but only 1% of sublingual gland tumors. Unlike most other salivary gland tumors, 70% of adenoid cystic carcinomas are in the submandibular or minor salivary glands. An analysis by Hamper et al[12] of 96 cases showed that females accounted for 62.5% of cases, and that there were peak frequencies in the fourth and seventh decades.

CLINICAL FEATURES

The clinical features are similar to those of other salivary gland tumors, but facial palsy is particularly frequent, especially with the solid type. Pain from an unidentified source may also be due to a hidden adenoid cystic carcinoma.

MICROSCOPY

Small, darkly staining cells of uniform appearance comprise both duct-lining and myoepithelial-like cells. They are typically arranged in well-circumscribed, rounded groups surrounding more or less circular spaces to give a cribriform (Swiss cheese) pattern. Occasionally, there is a tubular configuration. Hyaline material often forms in the connective tissue surrounding the islands of tumor, and in their pseudolumens. This material may form in such large quantities as to spread the tumor cells into a lace-like pattern or into widely separated strands. At the opposite extreme there may be solid sheets of cells with a solid (basaloid) pattern and, sometimes, areas of necrosis. However, in all these variants it is often possible to find more typical cribriform areas (Figs 52.14–52.20).

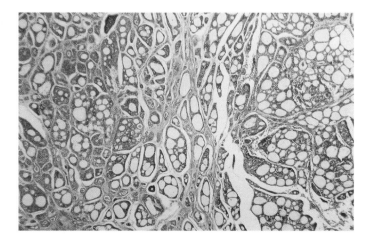

Fig. 52.14 Adenoid cystic carcinoma. Low-power view, showing the frequently seen cribriform pattern.

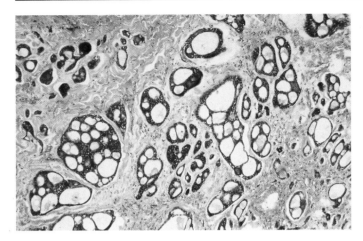

Fig. 52.15 Adenoid cystic carcinoma. Higher power view, showing the typical appearance of small, dark-staining cells in islands containing many microcysts.

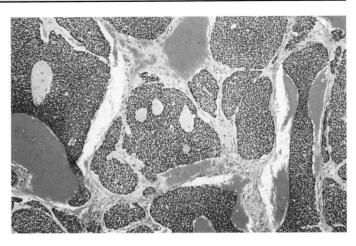

Fig. 52.18 Adenoid cystic carcinoma, solid type. Featureless sheets of small dark cells contain a few microcysts.

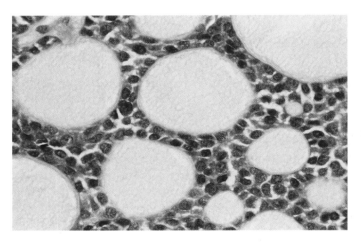

Fig. 52.16 Adenoid cystic carcinoma. Higher power view, showing the almost featureless tumor cells with scanty cytoplasm.

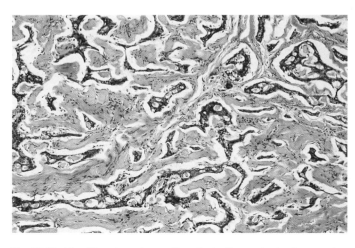

Fig. 52.17 Adenoid cystic carcinoma. Excessive hyaline production has spread the tumor cells out into slender strands.

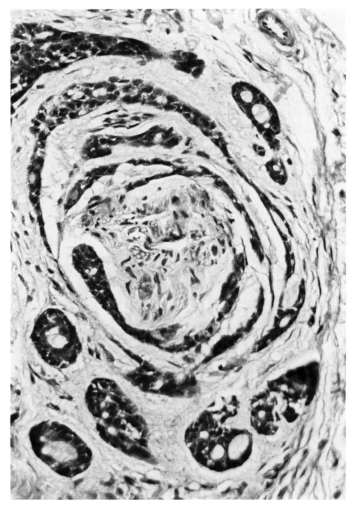

Fig. 52.19 Adenoid cystic carcinoma. Typical perineural invasion.

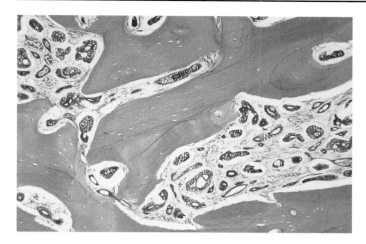

Fig. 52.20 Adenoid cystic carcinoma. Bone invasion.

In an immunohistochemical analysis of six cases by Ferreiro,[13] all were positive for CEA and S-100 protein. These findings contrasted with five cases of polymorphous low-grade adenocarcinoma, all of which were positive for S-100 protein but only one was positive for CEA.

BEHAVIOR AND MANAGEMENT

Behavior can be broadly related to the histologic configuration. In an analysis of 90 adenoid cystic carcinomas, Perzin et al[14] found that a solid configuration in more than 30% of the tumor area was associated with the worst prognosis, and the tubular type with the best. Santucci & Bondi,[15] on the basis of 25 tumors, further showed that the fewer the pseudolumens (gland-like spaces) per square millimeter of tumor, the lower were the chances of survival. Cleveland et al[16] confirmed that, for five solid-type maxillary adenoid cystic carcinomas, the mean survival time was only 2.5 years. Hamper et al,[12] using flow cytometry on 90 tumors, showed that a diploid histogram was associated with the longest survival times and that an atypical histogram was associated with the shortest. Van der Wal et al[17] noted that in 22 adenoid cystic carcinomas perineural invasion was more frequently associated with local recurrence, but correlation with distant metastasis was not statistically significant. With the aim of predicting the risk of metastases, Kim et al[18] have measured proliferating cell nuclear antigen (PCNA) activity by PC10 staining in 28 examples. The ratio of the number of positively staining cells compared with the total number of tumor cells was significantly higher in solid tumors. The index was also significantly higher for distantly metastasizing tumors (PC10 index, 21.5%) than for those without metastases (PC10 index, 11.1%). The PC10 index did not correlate with tumor size or with propensity for local recurrence.

Adenoid cystic carcinoma, although slow-growing, has a characteristically infiltrative pattern of growth. Perineural and intraneural invasion is typical of, but not unique to, this tumor. It can therefore spread along bony canals, sometimes far further than suggested by the radiographic area of bone destruction. Growth tends to be slow but inexorable, but metastatic spread is usually late. Metastases are more frequently to lungs and bone than to lymph nodes, but their growth may also be slow and allow survival for many more years.

Although, as already described, a variety of measures has been devised to predict the probable behavior of adenoid cystic carcinomas, there is no definitive protocol of management. For example, Blanck et al[19] reported 5- and 12-year survival rates of 73% and 39%, respectively, for 35 patients, even though only three of them underwent parotidectomy and 31 underwent local excision. The radical surgery of the Göttingen group[1] appeared to give no better results than those reported by Blanck et al.[19] Indeed, Seifert et al[1] admit that, despite recommending supraradical surgery even for small tumors, the method of treatment had very little influence on the outcome. Moreover, they could not confirm that radiotherapy prolonged survival. Doubts about the optimal treatment is reflected in the remarkable degree of spread of reported survival rates, which range from 0% at 10 years to 75% at up to 14 years. Hickman et al,[6] from reports of 1065 adenoid cystic carcinomas, estimated the 5-year survival rate to be 62.4% and the 10-year survival rate to be 38.9%. Seifert et al[1] give a 5-year recurrence or metastasis rate of 36% for the cribriform type and of 70% for the solid type with areas of necrosis. Their 8-year survival rate was 67% for the cribriform type and 32% for the solid type. Overall, they reported 5- and 12-year survival rates of 76% and 33% respectively.

Even though spread of this tumor is relentlessly infiltrative, the present consensus is that supra-radical surgery is not indicated, and mutilating surgery cannot be justified. The value of such surgery is unproven, and Seifert et al[1] suggest that it may even worsen the prognosis. As there may be even less room for maneuver in treating adenoid cystic carcinomas of intraoral glands, the prognosis may be worse than for the parotid gland. Quite frequently the postoperative history is one of limited local recurrences, each of which responds to local treatment, over the course of years. Adenoid cystic carcinomas should probably therefore be treated by radical resection (parotidectomy or its equivalent), with as wide a margin as is anatomically possible but compatible with reasonable rehabilitation. In the case of the parotid gland, sacrifice of branches of the facial nerve invaded by tumor may be unavoidable. Postoperative radiotherapy is usually also given, despite the lack of evidence that it prolongs survival.

Adenocarcinomas, not otherwise specified

Adenocarcinomas, not otherwise specified, show neoplastic duct or tubule formation microscopically, but no features indicating an origin from a pleomorphic adenoma.

Adenocarcinomas probably form less than 5% of salivary gland tumors. Approximately 48% of them are in the parotid, 10% in the submandibular, and 21% in minor salivary glands;

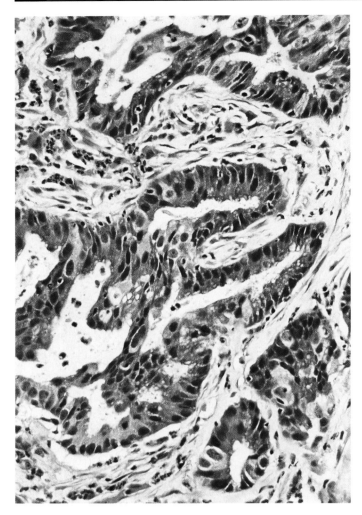

Fig. 52.21 Adenocarcinoma, not otherwise specified. Note the obvious glandular configuration.

fewer than 1% are in the sublingual glands. Males, usually in the seventh decade, appear to be affected almost twice as frequently as females.

MICROSCOPY

Adenocarcinomas consist of duct-like (tubular) structures. The cells may show significant atypia but the tubules are well formed, or the cytology may be relatively bland but the tubules are poorly formed. Invasion and destruction of surrounding tissues and, sometimes, perineural invasion may be seen (Fig 52.21).

BEHAVIOR AND MANAGEMENT

The behavior and prognosis of adenocarcinomas depend mainly on the degree of differentiation. Microscopically solid (undifferentiated) types tend to have the worst prognosis. Lymph-node metastasis and bloodstream spread are frequent with most types, although the rapidity with which this happens varies widely. Inevitably, the prognosis is also strongly affected by the extent of the primary tumor at operation. The overall 5-year survival rate is thought to be approximately 40%, but many previously reported adenocarcinomas would now be recategorized into other groups.

MUCINOUS ADENOCARCINOMA

This is a rare variant resembling its mucin-producing counterpart in the breast. Mucous cells and microcysts may cause it to simulate, to some degree, a mucoepidermoid carcinoma (Fig. 52.22).

BEHAVIOR AND MANAGEMENT

Adenocarcinomas progress rapidly. Treatment is by parotidectomy, if necessary with sacrifice of the facial nerve, or wide excision of other glands and, possibly, supplemented by radiotherapy.

PAPILLARY CYSTADENOCARCINOMA

Papillary cystadenocarcinoma typically affects the palate and is rare in other sites.

MICROSCOPY

Folds of epithelium project as papillary ingrowths into irregular cystic spaces. This epithelium appears cytologically benign, and such tumors, which may also shell out readily at operation, have been wrongly categorized in the past as papillary cystadenomas (Figs 52.23 and 52.24).

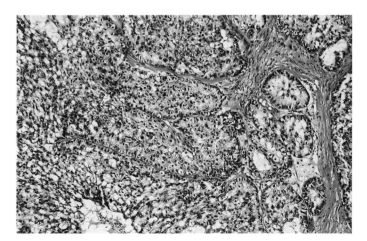

Fig. 52.22 Mucinous adenocarcinoma.

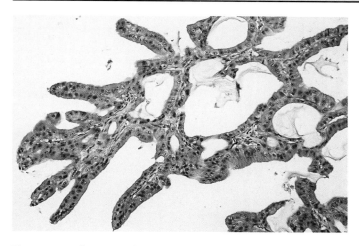

Fig. 52.23 Papillary cystic adenocarcinoma. Despite the cytologically bland appearance, extensive distant spread can develop, but typically only after a delay of 10 years or more.

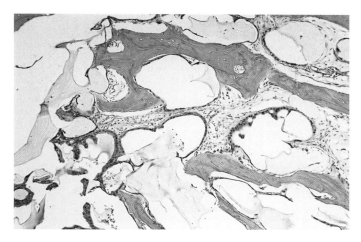

Fig. 52.24 Papillary cystic adenocarcinoma with mucin production. Bone has been invaded.

BEHAVIOR AND MANAGEMENT

Papillary cystadenocarcinomas can appear to respond to surgery but, despite wide excision and even radiotherapy, can metastasize and cause the death of patients only 15–30 years later.

Polymorphous low-grade adenocarcinoma (terminal duct carcinoma)

Polymorphous low-grade adenocarcinoma of minor salivary glands was first described by Evans & Batsakis in 1984.[20] Earlier, Batsakis et al[21] described a group of introral adenocarcinomas with a predominantly fascicular pattern as *terminal duct carcinomas,* but Evans & Batsakis[20] later concluded that these were variants of polymorphous low-grade adenocarcinomas.

INCIDENCE

Patients are usually aged between 50 and 75 years. Minor glands, particularly of the palate, are affected, and the tumor typically forms a firm painless swelling, which may later ulcerate. Vincent et al[22] evaluated 204 cases, including 15 of their own. Of 173 where the site was stated, 87 had arisen in the palate. The single next most frequent site (38 tumors) was the buccal mucosa. Only isolated examples of polymorphous low-grade adenocarcinoma of the parotid gland have been reported.[23,24]

Overall, Vincent et al[22] found women to be almost twice as frequently affected as men, and that the age at diagnosis was usually 40–70 years.

MICROSCOPY

Grossly, polymorphous low-grade adenocarcinomas appear circumscribed, but microscopically the surrounding tissue is infiltrated by slender strands of cells. In the bulk of the tumor, cytologically uniform, bland-looking cells of various shapes form a variety of configurations. The main microscopic pattern include the following:

- solid lobules surrounded by fibrous tissue
- cribriform areas containing hyaline stromal material
- duct-like structures
- fascicles of cells sometimes in a concentric (targetoid) arrangement
- papillary or papillary cystic structures.

The stroma is hyaline or mucinous, and fibrous and hyaline bands often separate different areas of the tumor. An unusual feature is the survival of relatively large areas of normal gland tissue or fat within the tumor. Perineural and intraneural invasion is a frequent finding (Figs 52.25–52.33)

Vincent et al[22] noted the frequency with which many cases of polymorphous low-grade adenocarcinomas had been misdiagnosed, most frequently as monomorphic adenomas or adenoid cystic carcinomas.

The immunohistochemical findings have been somewhat inconsistent. Gnepp et al[25] reported four cases which showed positive staining of more than 90% of the cells with epithelial membrane antigen and S-100 protein, while 75–95% stained with high-molecular-weight keratin. Variable numbers of cells stained positively, but with variable intensity, in all four tumors with muscle-specific antigen except in the cribriform areas, and with carcinoembryonic antigen. By contrast, EMA and CEA staining patterns in adenoid cystic carcinoma were similar and localized to ductal lumina. S-100 stained much less diffusely. Regezi et al[26] reported strong S-100 and weak actin staining of 14 polymorphous low-grade adenocarcinomas. By contrast, 14 of 15 adenoid cystic carcinomas stained positively for actin, but staining for glial fibrillary acidic protein and high- and low-molecular-weight keratins was similar for both kinds of tumor. Simpson et al[27] showed that staining of six polymorphous low-grade adenocarcinomas for keratin AE3 was weak or absent in four cases, but weakly

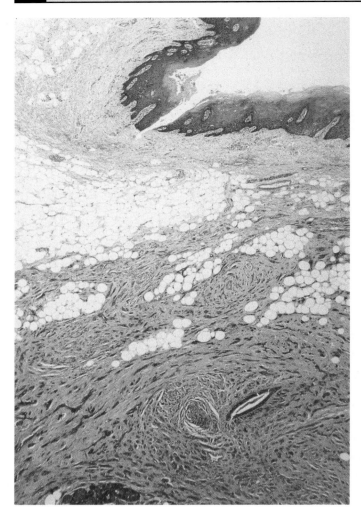

Fig. 52.25 Polymorphous low-grade adenocarcinoma. Low-power view, showing tumor deep to palatal epithelium and conspicuous involvement of normal fat.

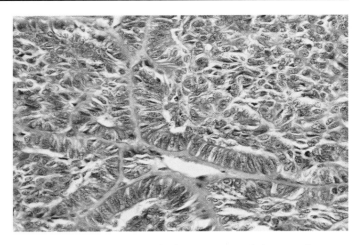

Fig. 52.27 Polymorphous low-grade adenocarcinoma. Lobular area with conspicuous palisaded peripheral cells.

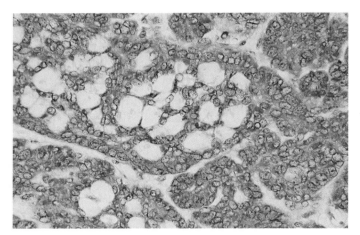

Fig. 52.28 Polymorphous low-grade adenocarcinoma. In this cribriform area the resemblance to adenoid cystic carcinoma is diminished by the 'washed-out' appearance of the tumor cells.

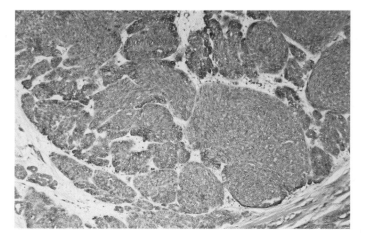

Fig. 52.26 Polymorphous low-grade adenocarcinoma. Lobular area, showing also the typical bland, 'washed-out' nuclei.

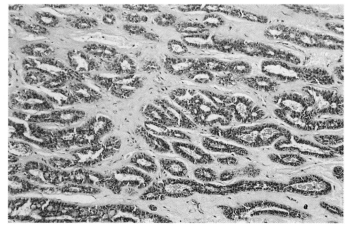

Fig. 52.29 Polymorphous low-grade adenocarcinoma. An area of duct-like structures.

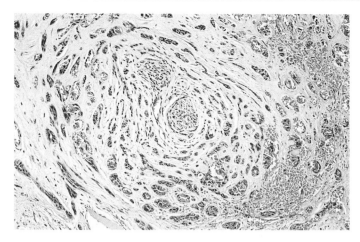

Fig. 52.30 Polymorphous low-grade adenocarcinoma. A targetoid area with encirclement of a nerve fiber.

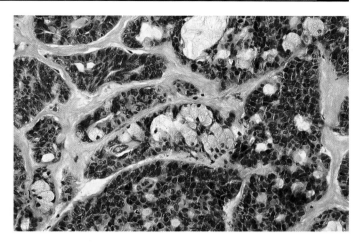

Fig. 52.33 Polymorphous low-grade adenocarcinoma. The prominent mucous cells cause this area to resemble a mucoepidermoid carcinoma.

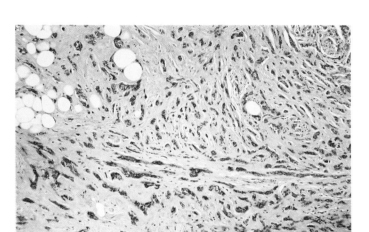

Fig. 52.31 Polymorphous low-grade adenocarcinoma. Indian filing of tumor cells and encirclement of fat lobules.

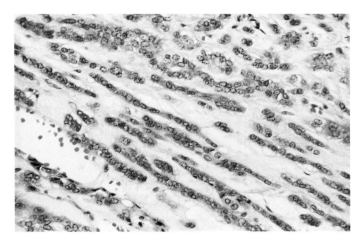

Fig. 52.32 Polymorphous low-grade adenocarcinoma. Strands of single cells in Indian file configuration, showing the typical washed-out nuclei.

positive in all six adenoid cystic carcinomas. Four of the latter stained weakly or negatively for S-100 protein, in contrast to five of the polymorphous low-grade adenocarcinomas, which stained more strongly with this antibody. As noted earlier, in five polymorphous low-grade adenocarcinomas Ferreiro[13] found all to be strongly positive for keratins AE1/AE3 and moderately or strongly positive for S-100 protein. Only one was weakly positive for CEA and one was weakly positive for actin. These findings contrasted with six adenoid cystic carcinomas, which showed similar staining for keratins AE1/AE3 and weakly positive in one case for actin, but all were moderately or weakly positive for CEA and S-100 protein.

Vincent et al[22] therefore concluded that the histologic features rather than special stains were more useful for differentiating polymorphous low-grade adenocarcinomas from other tumors.

BEHAVIOR AND MANAGEMENT

Because of their usual origin in minor salivary glands, polymorphous low-grade adenocarcinomas give rise to symptoms early. They are locally invasive, but only rarely metastasize.

Vincent et al[22] found a local recurrence rate of 17% for 116 cases within 1–19 years. Regional lymph node metastases were recorded in 9%. They suggested that polymorphous low-grade adenocarcinomas having a predominantly papillary configuration should be categorized as papillary cystadenocarcinomas, as the latter have a stronger tendency to metastasize (as described earlier).

Batsakis & El-Naggar,[28] using the term 'terminal duct carcinoma,' found from an analysis of reported cases that 6.6% of the papillary type metastasized and caused death of the patients in 13.3% of cases. By contrast, no reports of distant metastases were found for the nonpapillary type, although one of 80 patients died from the tumor.

Slootweg[24] re-examined 22 tumors categorized as polymorphous low-grade adenocarcinoma, papillary low-grade adenocarcinoma, papillary adenocarcinoma, or terminal duct carcinoma. He found that the highest rate of metastases was in those tumors that were entirely papillary-cystic or papillary-cystic with a lobular component. Moreover, he suggested that it was the presence rather than the extent of the papillary-cystic component that was important, and that metastases reproduced this configuration. However, in two entirely papillary-cystic tumors, metastases reproduced typical features of polymorphous low-grade adenocarcinoma.

Wide rather than local excision appears to be required, but each case should be assessed on its own merits. As the parotid gland is rarely affected, surgical difficulties should not be too great.

Salivary duct carcinoma

These tumors were termed 'duct carcinomas' because of their histologic resemblance to duct carcinomas of the breast. Nevertheless, this term may cause confusion with several other types of salivary gland carcinomas, which also arise from duct cells and, in particular, with 'terminal duct carcinoma' (low-grade polymorphous adenocarcinoma) and the 'intercalated duct carcinoma' (epithelial–myoepithelial carcinoma). Moreover, Seifert et al[1] use the term 'duct carcinoma' in this latter sense. The parotid glands are most frequently affected.[27,29–31] Analysis of 104 cases by Barnes et al[31] showed that 96% of salivary duct carcinomas arose in the major glands, were most frequent after the age of 50 years, and men were affected three times as frequently as women.

MICROSCOPY

Duct carcinomas consist of large pink or amphophilic cells with pleomorphic vesiculated nuclei and prominent nucleoli. Variable numbers of mitotic figures and both intraductal and infiltrating tumor proliferation may be seen. The intraductal component forms papillary, cribriform, or solid configurations. Solid areas may show ill-defined areas of necrosis or there may be comedo-like intraductal necrosis. Perineural, intraneural, or lymphatic spread may be seen (Figs 52.34–52.36).

Barnes et al[31] noted that in two of their cases there was residual pleomorphic adenoma, while Torteledo et al[32] reported 13 salivary duct carcinomas that had arisen in pleomorphic adenomas.

Delgado et al[30] found that most of the tumors also stained for one or more so-called breast-specific markers, but staining for estrogen receptors was consistently negative.

BEHAVIOR AND MANAGEMENT

Salivary duct carcinomas grow and spread rapidly. Variations in the microscopic appearances do not appear to correlate well with

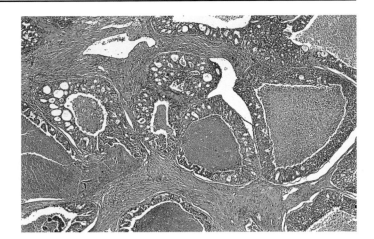

Fig. 52.34 Salivary duct carcinoma. Small duct-like spaces are surrounded by large eosinophilic cells.

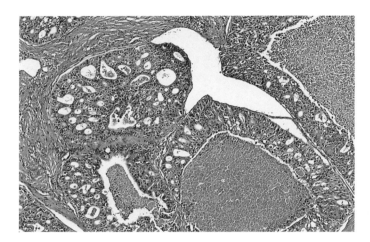

Fig. 52.35 Salivary duct carcinoma. Comedo-like necrosis is a typical finding and associated with a worse prognosis.

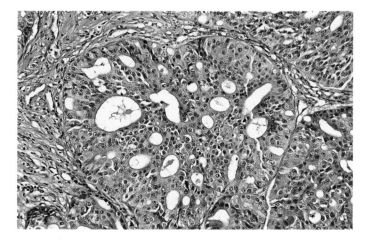

Fig. 52.36 Salivary duct carcinoma. Higher power view, showing large duct-like structures, surrounded by tumor cells with abundant eosinophilic cytoplasm with pleomorphic vesiculated nuclei and prominent nucleoli.

behavior, except that tumors showing necrosis have the worst prognosis. Intraductal salivary duct carcinoma is regarded as non-invasive, but Barnes et al[31] found that of four reported cases one developed infiltrative tumor a year later and another suffered two local recurrences.

Barnes et al,[31] by DNA image analysis of 13 salivary duct carcinomas, found no correlation of tumor ploidy with prognosis. In their analysis of 104 cases they found that a third of patients developed local recurrences, 59% had regional lymph node metastases, 46% developed systemic metastases, and 65% died from their disease, mostly within 4 years. The lungs are the most frequent site of metastases, closely followed by bones, but in many cases multiple sites are involved.

Complete excision followed by radiotherapy is usually advised. Barnes et al[31] also suggest that regional nodes should be treated by neck dissection or radiotherapy, even if not clinically involved. However, Ruiz et al[33] found that the outcome was unaffected by the aggressiveness of the treatment.

Clear cell tumors

Clear cell tumors, apart from the rare clear cell oncocytoma, should be regarded as at least potentially malignant and treated accordingly. The main types are as follows:

- clear cell oncocytoma
- clear cell mucoepidermoid and acinic cell carcinomas
- epithelial–myoepithelial (intercalated duct) carcinoma
- hyalinizing clear cell carcinoma
- metastatic renal cell carcinoma

Oncocytoma, and mucoepidermoid and acinic cell carcinomas have been described earlier, and the behavior of their clear cell variants does not differ from their more common conventional counterparts.

Clear cell carcinomas arising in pleomorphic adenomas have been reported.[34–36] None of the authors of the reports described these tumors as epithelial–myoepithelial carcinomas, although Cassidy & Connolly[36] considered that the tumor was of myoepithelial origin.

Ogawa et al[37] also reported three monophasic clear cell tumors of salivary glands, of which only one was S100 positive and showed focal staining for muscle-specific actin, and was considered to be a clear cell myoepithelioma. The others stained positively only for some epithelial markers, and it is doubtful how they should be categorized.

EPITHELIAL–MYOEPITHELIAL CARCINOMA

This tumor was originally described by Donath et al[38] and has been described in detail by Corio et al.[39] Approximately 40 cases have been reported. A similar example was shown as the last of a series of 'duct carcinomas' reported by Kleinsasser et al,[40] but salivary duct carcinomas are categorized as a separate group, as described earlier.

CLINICAL FEATURES

The mean age of patients appears to be about 60 years, and the peak incidence is in the seventh and eighth decades. Women have been affected in the ratio of 2 : 1. Over 80% of these tumors have been in the parotid glands and usually caused otherwise asymptomatic swellings. However, a minority have caused pain or facial weakness.

MICROSCOPY

Epithelial–myoepithelial carcinoma is typically multinodular and, although it appears circumscribed, encapsulation is incomplete. It consists of duct-like structures or larger spaces which sometimes contain eosinophilic periodic acid schiff (PAS) positive material. Alternatively, the cells may be predominantly in an organoid or thecal pattern with a well-defined basal membrane, which may be thickened and hyaline.

Small, dark cells line the duct-like spaces and are surrounded by large glass-clear cells, which usually predominate. The clear cells are considerably larger, of rounded polygonal shape, and usually contain glycogen (Figs 52.37 and 52.38).

The patterns and numbers of clear cells can vary between individual tumors or within a single example. In some areas there may only be solid sheets of clear cells. In others, there are cyst-like spaces into which there are papillary projections of tumor cells. Mitoses are rare, but there may be perineural infiltration or intravascular growth.

Electron microscopy and immunocytochemistry have confirmed that the dark cells are epithelial, but that the clear cells are myo-epithelial.[41] Positive staining for S100 protein, vimentin, myosin,

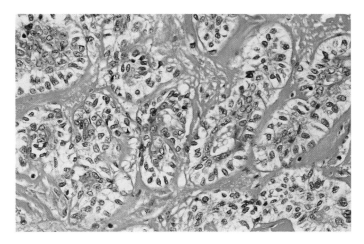

Fig. 52.37 Epithelial–myoepithelial carcinoma. A mantle of clear myoepithelial cells encloses the duct cells.

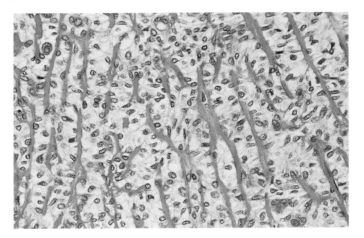

Fig. 52.38 Epithelial–myoepithelial carcinoma. In this tumor, clear myoepithelial cells dominate the picture, but retain a stranded configuration.

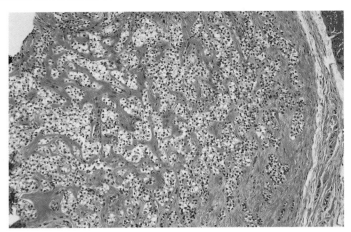

Fig. 52.39 Hyalinizing clear cell carcinoma. Cords of clear epithelial cells are surrounded by hyalinized bands of connective tissue.

and keratins may be useful in confirming the nature of the clear cells. Jones et al[42] reported that the outer layer of the myoepithelial cells reacts positively for α smooth-muscle actin. The small, dark cells are ductal epithelium with microvilli on some points on the luminal surface; they contain tonofilaments and are joined by desmosomes.

BEHAVIOR AND MANAGEMENT

Despite their relatively bland cytology, epithelial myoepithelial carcinomas have recurred significantly frequently, and some patients have died with metastases to lymph nodes, lung, or kidney. Seifert et al[1] suggest that the 5-year survival rate is 65%. Radical parotidectomy or en bloc resection of other glands is therefore indicated.

HYALINIZING CLEAR CELL CARCINOMA OF THE SALIVARY GLAND

Milchgrub et al[43] have presented 11 cases of yet another type of clear cell carcinoma in which the epithelium was surrounded by hyalinized bands with foci of myxohyaline stroma. Despite some microscopic resemblances to epithelial myoepithelial carcinoma, immunohistochemistry and electron microscopy failed to show myoepithelial cells. They noted four earlier examples which had been illustrated but not characterized as a distinct entity.

The patients comprised eight females and three males. Ages ranged from 34 to 78 years, with a mean of 55 years. Minor salivary glands were most frequently affected (nine cases). There was a single case in the parotid gland and another in the larynx.

MICROSCOPY

The tumor cells formed trabeculae, cords, or nests and infiltrated any residual acini or other soft tissues, such as the overlying oral mucosa. They were mostly round to polygonal, with clear, PAS-positive cytoplasm and central nuclei. The nuclear membranes frequently appeared indented with a suggestion of lobulation. Mitotic activity was noted in only two cases. In 10 of the 11 cases reported by Milchgrub et al,[43] there were polygonal cells with eosinophilic granular cytoplasm mingling with the clear cells, and appeared to represent a transition between the two types (Fig. 52.39).

The tumor cells were immunoreactive for low and high-molecular-weight keratins and epithelial membrane antigen. In two cases there was carcinoembryonic antigen reactivity. Immunoreactivity for S100 protein, smooth-muscle actin, and muscle-specific actin was consistently negative. Electron microscopy failed to show any cells with myoepithelial differentiation, zymogen, mucin, or dense core neurosecretory granules.

A distinctive feature was the stroma, which was desmoplastic in both the primary tumors and metastases. It sharply outlined the trabeculae and nests of tumor cells, and enhanced the streaming effect where the tumor cells were aligned in slender cords. In five cases the stroma was hyalinized and PAS-positive and, although resembling amyloid, was Congo red negative. In eight tumors there were also foci of loose myxoid stroma. Electron microscopy showed a prominent continuous layer of basal lamina surrounding most tumor cell nests.

Perinuclear invasion was seen in most cases, but vascular invasion was absent.

Eight of the 11 tumors reported by Milchgrub et al[43] had originally been reported as other types of carcinoma, such as poorly differentiated adenocarcinoma, epithelial myoepithelial carcinoma, mucoepidermoid carcinoma, acinic cell carcinoma, squamous cell carcinoma, carcinoma in pleomorphic adenoma, or calcifying epithelial odontogenic tumor.

BEHAVIOR AND MANAGEMENT

One of the patients reported by Milchgrub et al[43] presented with cervical nodal metastases, but no metastases developed in the remaining nine patients. Clinical follow-up, of duration 6 months to 11 years, showed no evidence of recurrent disease in any of the patients. Hyalinizing clear cell carcinoma therefore appears to be of low-grade malignancy and wide excision, possibly supplemented by radiotherapy, appears to be the treatment of choice.

METASTATIC RENAL CELL CARCINOMA (HYPERNEPHROMA)

When any feature suggests that a clear cell tumor of a salivary gland is a secondary deposit, the kidney is the only important source. Batsakis & McBurney[44] have claimed that renal cell carcinoma is the most frequent metastasis to the jaws and sinonasal regions. There have been several reports of metastases of renal cell carcinoma to the parotid gland and other oral sites such as the tongue.[45–47]

Metastases are frequently the first sign of a renal cell carcinoma. If renal symptoms are absent, microscopic hematuria alone may be found in 60% of patients, and about 50% have nonspecific systemic symptoms such as fever, fatigue, or loss of weight. Gross hematuria, pain in the loin, and a renal mass develop late, and present in only 10% of patients.

MICROSCOPY

Renal cell carcinoma consists of solid masses of clear cells with small eccentric nuclei in an organoid or trabecular arrangement. The blood vessels are typically dilated, form scattered sinusoids, and may leave foci of hemorrhage and deposits of hemosiderin. Granular cells may also be present, and in some cases predominate (see Figs 51.36 and 51.37).

Differentiation from epithelial–myoepithelial carcinomas microscopically can sometimes be very difficult. Ellis & Gnepp[7] suggest that a helpful distinguishing feature is that epithelial–myoepithelial carcinoma has small blood vessels running between the groups of tumor cells, but renal cell carcinomas have large sinusoids. In unblocked material, the presence of fat is typical of renal carcinomas, but is not invariably present.

If doubt remains, intravenous urography and, if necessary, a computed tomography (CT) or ultrasound scan should be carried out. Excision of a primary renal cell carcinoma and a metastasis has occasionally proved curative.

BEHAVIOR AND MANAGEMENT

In general, the appearance of a metastasis indicates a poor prognosis. All nine patients with renal cell carcinoma metastasizing to the tongue died within approximately 6 months. However, others have reported survival for many years.[48,49] Nephrectomy may occasionally also lead to regression of a metastasis.[50,51] According to Middleton,[52] nephrectomy in combination with excision of a

solitary metastasis gives the same survival rate as nephrectomy in patients without metastases.

The findings are therefore conflicting, but excision of a metastatic renal cell carcinoma in a salivary gland as well as nephrectomy may offer hope for the patient.

Basal cell adenocarcinoma

These tumors are predominantly found in the parotid or submandibular glands and the mean age affected is approximately 60 years. McCluggage et al[53] have reviewed in detail the literature on basal cell adenocarcinoma and considered the question of whether these tumors arise de novo or from a pre-existing basal cell adenoma.

MICROSCOPY

Multiple nodules of small dark cells with scanty cytoplasm are frequently surrounded by larger, eosinophilic or amphophilic cells, but the latter are rarely palisaded. A distinct perinodular, hyalinized basal membrane and hyaline intranodular droplets are frequently present.

Basal cell adenocarcinomas closely resemble basal cell adenomas, particularly the membranous variant, and diagnosis depends on finding cellular or nuclear pleomorphism, mitotic activity, foci of necrosis or, particularly, evidence of infiltration. This may be perineural or intravascular, even in cytologically benign-looking tumors. Some examples may have cribriform areas simulating an adenoid cystic carcinoma, while others show a more pleomorphic picture and frequent mitoses (Fig. 52.40).

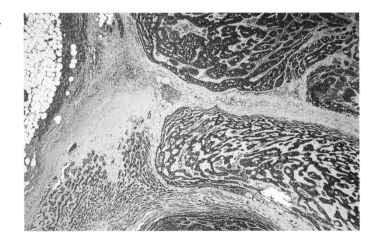

Fig. 52.40 Basal cell adenocarcinoma. Distinction from a basal cell adenoma can only be reliably made by recognition of invasive activity (below, left).

McCluggage et al,[53] by immunohistochemistry and electron microscopy, showed a dual population of ductal and myoepithelial cells, while flow cytometry showed DNA aneuploidy in one block.

BEHAVIOR AND MANAGEMENT

Most basal cell adenocarcinomas appear to be of low-grade malignancy. Recurrence or metastasis after wide excision is relatively uncommon, but occasionally metastases may appear more than a decade later. Total conservative parotidectomy (and its equivalent for other glands) therefore seems to be the minimal requirement. Microscopically high-grade tumors should be treated more radically.

Squamous cell (epidermoid) carcinoma

Squamous metaplasia in pleomorphic adenomas is common, but squamous cell carcinomas of salivary glands account for fewer than 3% of salivary gland tumors. They are a disease of the elderly. Men are more than twice as frequently affected as women at a mean age of 70 years (range 50–90 years). Nearly 70% of these tumors are in the parotid glands.

CLINICAL FEATURES

Squamous cell carcinomas of salivary glands do not seem to have any distinctive features, although they may be particularly firm on palpation and ulcerate readily. Facial palsy may also develop, and metastasis to regional nodes is rapid. In the mouth, squamous cell carcinomas of minor salivary glands may not be distinguishable from those arising from the mucosa.

MICROSCOPY

These tumors do not differ from squamous cell carcinomas from other tissues, and range from well-differentiated, keratinizing tumors to poorly differentiated examples without keratinization. However, it is essential to determine whether they are primary salivary gland tumors, metastases from elsewhere (with a correspondingly poor prognosis), or have spread from a mucosal or skin tumor. It may occasionally be difficult to distinguish them from high-grade mucoepidermoid carcinomas and to be certain that mucous cells are absent.

BEHAVIOR AND MANAGEMENT

Salivary gland squamous carcinomas are so uncommon that no reliable statement can be made about the response to treatment. Seifert et al[1] quote a 5-year survival rate of 40%. Treatment is by radical excision and radiotherapy.

Carcinoma of Stenson's duct

Carcinoma of Stenson's duct is even more uncommon than squamous cell carcinoma of the gland parenchyma. Its chief importance is that its usual presentation is a localized tender swelling. This may dilate the duct, produce a filling defect radiographically, and simulate an inflammatory lesion. Antimicrobial treatment can then delay diagnosis, with adverse effects on the patient's prognosis.

MICROSCOPY

These tumors range from well to poorly differentiated, but are otherwise typical squamous cell carcinomas and the duct may fill with keratin. The origin from the lining epithelium of Stenson's duct may be discernible, but its precise site of origin probably does not significantly affect either the management or the prognosis.

Mucoepidermoid carcinoma can also arise in Stenson's duct.

BEHAVIOR AND MANAGEMENT

Treatment is by radical excision and radiotherapy. Because of its superficial origin, symptoms and diagnosis should be earlier than in the case of intraglandular squamous cell carcinomas. However, so few cases have been reported, and the follow-up periods have been so short that it is not possible to gain any useful idea of the prognosis.

Adenosquamous carcinoma

Adenosquamous carcinoma is a rare neoplasm which, as the name implies, shows both adenoid and squamous differentiation. There have been reports of such tumors in many sites. Gerughty et al[54] described 10 cases, of which five were in the nasal or laryngeal areas and five were in the mouth. Ellis & Gnepp[7] reviewed 40 cases, and found that only minor oral glands were affected.

The main sites appear to be the floor of the mouth, posterior tongue and faucial area. Male patients outnumber females in the ratio of 2 : 1, and the peak age incidence has been in the sixth and seventh decades. Clinically, the tumor resembles squamous cell carcinoma of the mouth.

Reserve cells of the excretory duct epithelium may have the potential for both ductal and epidermoid differentiation. Alternatively, the appearances could be due to intermingling of two separate primary tumors.

MICROSCOPY

Adenosquamous carcinoma intermingles adenocarcinoma with squamous carcinoma but, unlike mucoepidermoid carcinoma, distinct and separate areas of both types of carcinoma are also seen.

Adenosquamous carcinoma should be distinguished from pseudoglandular areas in a squamous cell carcinoma. According to Ellis & Gnepp,[7] this latter appearance is seen only in carcinomas of the oral aspect of the lower lip and results from malignant acantholysis of the epidermoid cells to produce pseudolumens.

BEHAVIOR AND MANAGEMENT

Information from the few reported cases suggests that adenosquamous carcinoma is aggressive. All five oral cases reported by Gerughty et al[54] spread to regional lymph nodes, even though they were only 1 cm in size when biopsied. Three of the tumors also metastasized to the liver and lung.

Radical resection of glands appears to be necessary. Radiotherapy and prophylactic neck dissection should be considered, but their effect on survival is unknown.

Undifferentiated carcinomas

Undifferentiated carcinomas are rare and of similar frequency to squamous cell carcinomas. Sixty-three percent are in the parotid glands, while 22% are in the submandibular glands.

MICROSCOPY

A variety of appearances can be seen, but typically there are sheets of small cells that may be more or less spheroidal or spindle-shaped, have a basaloid appearance or can closely resemble an oat-cell carcinoma of the lung. The cells have large nuclei and the cytoplasm is scanty and poorly defined. Nuclear pleomorphism and mitotic activity may be prominent. The centers of cell masses may undergo necrosis. Neuroendocrine differentiation is sometimes detectable by means of such stains as Grimaleus in the first instance, but appears not to affect the prognosis. Large-cell undifferentiated carcinomas may also be seen occasionally.

BEHAVIOR AND MANAGEMENT

Metastasis from a distant site must be excluded as the prognosis is likely then to be hopeless. Even with primary salivary gland tumors, rapid spread of undifferentiated carcinomas, particularly to regional lymph nodes, is to be expected, while distant metastases are likely to be the chief cause of death. Despite the likelihood of earlier detection of undifferentiated salivary gland carcinomas from similar looking oat-cell carcinomas of the lung, their prognosis appears to be significantly worse.

Radical excision of the gland should be followed by radiotherapy. The 5-year survival rate is approximately 25%.[1]

Undifferentiated carcinoma with lymphoid stroma (lymphoepithelial carcinoma; malignant lymphoepithelial lesion)

Undifferentiated carcinoma with lymphoid stroma (UCLS) is common in some Eskimo races and Southern Chinese, but is very rare in those of European origin. Men are more frequently affected. Albeck et al[55] have reported familial clustering of these tumors as well as of nasopharyngeal carcinoma in Greenland natives, and suggest the possibility of transmission of a virulent strain of Epstein–Barr virus as a cause. There is little evidence that UCLS is preceded by benign lymphoepithelial lesion, and the earlier term 'lymphoepithelioma' is misleading.

MICROSCOPY

Ill-defined islands of poorly differentiated epithelium, which often appear syncytial, are buried in a dense stroma of lymphocytes. This appearance is identical to that of one type of nasopharyngeal carcinoma that is even more common in these racial groups, so that occasionally a salivary gland tumor is a metastasis from the nasopharynx. Better differentiated, low-grade tumors may also be seen (Fig. 52.41).

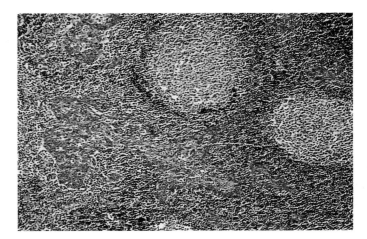

Fig. 52.41 Undifferentiated carcinoma with lymphoid stroma. Ill-defined islands of poorly differentiated epithelium appear syncytial and are buried in a dense lymphocytic stroma.

BEHAVIOR AND MANAGEMENT

The frequency of metastases is so high that, in addition to radical excision, there is some argument for neck dissection even in the absence of palpable nodes, unless the tumor is unusually well differentiated. Radiotherapy must be used if complete excision is not possible, but its value is uncertain.

Carcinoma in pleomorphic adenoma

Malignant change in a pleomorphic adenoma is more common in long-standing tumors (more than 10 years) or in multinodular recurrences. Thackray & Lucas[56] suggest that up to 25% of pleomorphic adenomas may undergo malignant change if left untreated for a decade or more, and that it is more frequent in recurrent and fibrotic tumors. As a consequence, carcinoma in pleomorphic adenoma is typically a tumor of older persons (mean age 63 years, range 25 to 83 years). The incidence is between 5% and 6% of epithelial tumors, but this may be an underestimate because of cases where the carcinoma has obliterated the adenomatous component.

CLINICAL FEATURES

Malignant change in pleomorphic adenoma is suggested by a sudden acceleration of growth or the onset of pain or facial palsy after years of gradual or episodic growth, or if seen in a recurrent tumor.

MICROSCOPY

Both pleomorphic adenoma and carcinoma can be seen contiguously. The malignant component may be small; alternatively, the original adenoma may be difficult to find. However, ghost-like areas of cartilage that tend to resist destruction are indicative of a pre-existent pleomorphic adenoma. In heavily scarred tumors only slender strands of malignant cells may be seen. The malignant component is most often an adenocarcinoma or undifferentiated carcinoma or, less frequently, other types of carcinoma.

As noted earlier, carcinoma in pleomorphic adenoma must be distinguished from atypia without invasive activity within the substance of a pleomorphic adenoma (Fig. 52.42).

BEHAVIOR AND MANAGEMENT

Recognition of carcinoma in pleomorphic adenoma is particularly important in that the prognosis appears to be poorer than for similar carcinomas arising de novo. Metastasis to lymph nodes

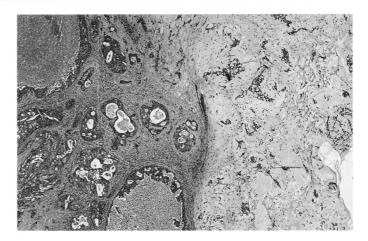

Fig. 52.42 Carcinoma in pleomorphic adenoma. A carcinoma with a cribriform configuration is juxtaposed with myxoid pleomorphic adenoma.

was reported in nearly 60% of cases by Seifert et al,[1] and later to distant sites. Treatment depends on the type of carcinoma and its extent, and should be by radical excision in the first instance.

On the basis of an analysis of 383 reported cases, the 5-year survival rate appears to be 55.7% and the 10-year rate 31%.[6]

Myoepithelial carcinoma (malignant myoepithelioma)

As described in Chapter 51, spindle-shaped myoepithelial cells can occasionally predominate in pleomorphic adenomas and, rarely, a pure spindle cell myoepithelioma may be seen. Malignant change involving these myoepithelial cells is exceedingly uncommon, but a case was reported by Dardick[57] and another by Singh & Cawson,[58] who also reviewed previous reports. Despite its distinctive appearances, myoepithelial carcinoma must be regarded as a variant of carcinoma in pleomorphic adenoma.

In the case reported by Singh & Cawson,[58] the malignant myoepithelial component had developed in and overgrown a pleomorphic adenoma to form a giant tumor (775 g) that extended down to the clavicle and had been present for 15 years. There was no pain or facial palsy.

MICROSCOPY

The most obvious feature is the pseudosarcomatous proliferation of the myoepithelial cells, which are predominantly spindle-shaped, with pleomorphic hyperchromatic nuclei and, sometimes, abnormal mitoses. The cell cytoplasm is fibrillar or vacuolated and there is strongly positive staining for actin, vimentin, and S100 protein. Interspersed among the spindle cells may be multinucleate giant cells and occasional plasmacytoid cells. Jie et al[59] have carried out quantitative analysis, using the IBAS II image system, of 12 myoepitheliomas and 10 myoepithelial carcinomas in order to help in the assessment of the aggressiveness of such tumors. They confirmed that myoepithelial carcinomas showed larger nuclei, which were frequently bizarre in shape and were significantly more frequently aneuploid.

Any residual pleomorphic adenoma shows the expected variety of appearances, including myxochondroid differentiation and calcification, but transition of some of the cells to pleomorphic, malignant, spindle-shaped myoepithelial cells may also be seen. Previously reported cases, such as those reported by Crissman et al[60] and Dardick,[57] showed generally similar features; the latter also described the ultrastructural changes. This patient showed no evidence of recurrence or metastases after 3 years.

BEHAVIOR AND MANAGEMENT

Too few cases have been reported to be certain that the prognosis of myoepithelial carcinoma is any more favorable than that of the more common type of carcinoma in pleomorphic adenoma. Radical parotidectomy with neck dissection, if necessary, therefore seems to be the most appropriate form of treatment.

Carcinosarcoma

Carcinosarcoma can be regarded as a rare variant of malignant change in pleomorphic adenoma in which both epithelial and stromal components are neoplastic. It probably comprises less than 0.2% of salivary gland tumors. Bleiweiss et al[61] and, more recently, Toynton et al[62] have each reported a case and reviewed earlier examples. Most patients have been in their sixth or seventh decade, and most were female. Carson et al[63] reported two cases with unusual stromal components, and summarized the findings in five other reports.

MICROSCOPY

The epithelial element is likely to consist of moderately well to poorly differentiated adenocarcinoma, which should be CAM 5.2 positive, but papillary cystic and epithelial–myoepithelial carcinoma may also be seen. The sarcomatous element is probably more frequently chondrosarcoma or osteosarcoma, and should stain positively for vimentin. Both elements may be S100 positive. In one of the cases presented by Carson et al,[63] residual pleomorphic adenoma was associated with epithelial–myoepithelial carcinoma and leiomyosarcoma.

BEHAVIOR AND MANAGEMENT

The sarcomatous element, as might be expected, appears to worsen the prognosis. Spread is frequently hematogenous, and

nodal involvement has been seen in only a minority of cases. Radical surgery is therefore indicated and local radiotherapy may be advisable because of the high risk of local recurrence. The scarcity of cases makes it impossible to assess the value of postoperative radio- or chemotherapy, and the outcome in reported cases has been almost uniformly poor.

Cytologically benign metastasizing mixed tumor

The term 'metastasing mixed tumor' is used for a particularly rare tumor, which resembles a cytologically benign pleomorphic adenoma, but is invasive and gives rise to metastases with equally benign cytological appearances. Such tumors have frequently not been distinguished from carcinoma in pleomorphic adenomas in reports. Males and females were equally frequently affected. Patients' ages ranged from 12 to 73 years (mean 35 years) and intervals between primary treatment and the appearance of metastases ranged from 2 to 52 years (mean interval 19.8 years).

MICROSCOPY

The appearances are those of a pleomorphic adenoma, with the exception that there may be clear signs of invasion and destruction of other tissues. Metastases retain the same benign appearances. Wenig et al[64] found neither histological variables nor flow cytometry to be successful for predicting metastasis. Qureshi et al[65] reported a case and in reviewing the literature found 23 other acceptable cases. Like others before them, they found no features predictive of potential for metastasis. Thus there appear to be no histological criteria for distinguishing a truly benign pleomorphic adenoma from one that will metastasize. Infiltration of the capsule, which, as mentioned earlier, is a frequent finding in pleomorphic adenomas, is not an indication for a potential to metastasize.

BEHAVIOR AND MANAGEMENT

The malignant nature of these tumors may sometimes only be confirmed by the appearance of metastases, which is most frequently to the lungs. Qureshi et al[65] also found that the most frequent site of metastases was the lungs (52%), but bony metastases developed in 48% of cases. In the 11 cases reported by Wenig et al,[64] all but one had at least one local recurrence before the appearance of metastases. The latter were sometimes found at the same time as the local recurrence, but one did not appear until 29 years later (this was 52 years after excision of the primary tumor). By contrast, histologically benign pleomorphic adenoma can occasionally metastasize without recurring locally. Qureshi et al[65] reported such a case and noted two others reported earlier.[66,67]

Despite the benign histological appearances of both the primary and metastatic tumors, Wenig et al[64] concluded that the mortality from the latter could be 22%. However, Qureshi et al[65] suggest that, as these tumors are slow growing, excision of metastases is worthwhile.

Since no features predictive of a potential for metastasis have as yet been found, this is another strong argument for radical excision of all pleomorphic adenomas.

Sebaceous carcinomas

Bailet et al[68] found that the parotid gland accounted for 29% of all sebaceous carcinomas of the head and neck region, and was second only to the eye. The mean age affected was 63 years.

MICROSCOPY

Sebaceous cells in sheets or nests show varying degrees of pleomorphism and nuclear atypia. Nevertheless, differentiation from sebaceous adenomas is sometimes difficult unless invasion is seen. There may also be a foreign body reaction to extravasated sebum.

Other difficulties in diagnosis may be caused by epidermoid carcinomas with foci of sebaceous differentiation, or by mucoepidermoid carcinomas. The latter, unlike sebaceous carcinomas, are mucin positive, but are negative for fat (Fig. 52.43).

BEHAVIOR AND MANAGEMENT

Of the 26 parotid gland sebaceous carcinomas reported by Bailet et al,[68] 18% died from their disease within 5 years. Radical excision possibly supplemented by radiotherapy appears to be the treatment of choice.

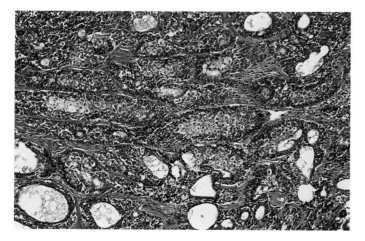

Fig. 52.43 Sebaceous carcinoma. Islands of sebaceous cells show large nuclei with prominent nucleoli.

SEBACEOUS CARCINOMA WITH LYMPHOID STROMA (SEBACEOUS LYMPHADENOCARCINOMA)

Sebaceous carcinoma with lymphoid stroma (sebaceous lymphadenocarcinoma) exceedingly uncommon. It consists of sebaceous cells, with varying degrees of loss of differentiation, often intermingled with benign sebaceous tissue in a dense lymphoid stroma. These tumors appear to be of lower grade malignancy than the 'pure' sebaceous carcinoma.

Oncocytic carcinoma (malignant oncocytoma)

This must be the most uncommon of all primary salivary gland tumors. Many of the earlier cases do not fulfil the two essential criteria of having oncocytes as the tumor cells and clear evidence of malignancy. Twenty-four cases fulfilling these criteria have been reviewed by Goode & Corio,[69] who attempted to define their characteristics. The majority showed gross pleomorphism, and all showed invasive activity or involvement of lymph nodes. Nevertheless, initial diagnoses of oncocytic adenoma had been made in several cases. However, even Goode & Corio,[69] although they recognize malignant change in an oncocytic adenoma as a category, do not distinguish it from adenocarcinoma with extensive oncocytic change. They also believe that cytologically benign oncocytomas can occasionally metastasize, as discussed earlier. Brandwein & Huvos[70] also emphasize that such features as pleomorphism, perineural, or vascular invasion can be compatible with benign behavior.

CLINICAL FEATURES

The parotid gland is chiefly affected, and only isolated cases have been reported in other glands. Most patients have been over 45 years and the mean age has been about 65 years. There seems to be no significant difference in sex distribution. The usual manifestation has been an asymptomatic swelling, but pain has been reported in a few cases.

MICROSCOPY

The tumor cells resemble those of a benign oncocytoma in that they are rounded or polygonal and have distinctly eosinophilic, granular cytoplasm, but differ in that there is noticeable pleomorphism, both nuclear and cellular, and significant numbers of mitoses. Also unlike benign oncocytoma, the cells may be in solid masses, cords, trabeculae, or papillae with small cysts, as well as in the expected alveolar arrangement. The oncocytic nature of these cells may be confirmed by staining with PTAH to confirm mitochondrial proliferation, or may be established unequivocally by electron microscopy.

The malignant nature of such tumors is indicated by gross pleomorphism evidence of invasion of surrounding tissues, by the appearance of metastases.

BEHAVIOR AND MANAGEMENT

True oncocytic carcinomas have a high incidence of recurrence after local excision, and this has been followed by metastasis. Of the 30 cases reviewed by Ellis & Gnepp,[7] 12 had cervical lymph node metastases and eight had distant metastases. Eight patients had died from their tumors.

Unfavorable prognostic features, Goode & Corio[69] suggest, are a large primary tumor and, microscopically, a predominantly cystic pattern, gross pleomorphism, or both.

Information is limited, but the reported behavior of cases of this rare tumor suggests that radical parotidectomy is probably the treatment of choice, and prophylactic neck dissection may have to be considered in view of the high reported incidence of nodal disease. Supplementary radiotherapy may also be considered, although its value is uncertain.

Epithelial salivary gland tumors in children

Only 3.5–5% of salivary gland tumors are in infants or children, but a major problem in their surgical management is the difficulty of avoiding damage to the developing facial nerve. The most common tumor type is the juvenile hemangioma, which is described later.

Epithelial salivary gland tumors in the young are considerably more frequently malignant than in adults. The parotid glands are most frequently affected, and Callender et al[71] reported that 21 of 29 epithelial salivary gland tumors in children were malignant. Shikani & Johns[72] found that pleomorphic adenomas formed 87% of the benign tumors, but the recurrence rate was between 20% and 40% after enucleation. Two of the recurrent tumors developed into highly aggressive carcinomas. Of the malignant tumors, mucoepidermoid carcinomas appear to be the most common type. Two of the 29 patients reported by Callender et al[71] died from their tumors.

In view of the high recurrence rate of pleomorphic adenomas and the high incidence of malignant tumors, radical parotidectomy seems to be necessary for epithelial salivary gland tumors in children. However, the chances of damaging the facial nerve are high, particularly in younger children, and even superficial parotidectomy of pleomorphic adenomas has a high chance of being followed by recurrence.

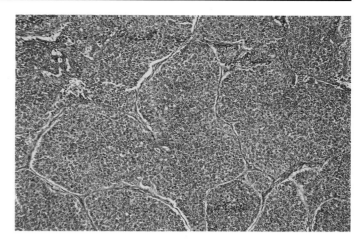

Fig. 52.44 Embryoma. Solid areas of small, dark epithelial cells are separated by fibrous strands and resemble a solid adenoid cystic carcinoma.

Embryoma (sialoblastoma)

Embryomas are congenital or neonatal salivary gland tumors and can be benign, but 25% may be malignant. Rarely, they are so large as to cause difficulties in delivery.

MICROSCOPY

Embryomas consist essentially of tissue resembling embryonic salivary gland epithelia in a loose mesenchymal stroma. The appearances vary, but typically consist of small dark cells with scanty cytoplasm forming duct-like structures, trabeculae or, occasionally, a cribriform pattern. They may therefore resemble a basal cell adenoma or adenoid cystic carcinoma. Like other embryonic epithelia, this tissue is able to grow infiltratively even when benign. Malignant embryomas may be recognized by greater atypia, but more objectively by invasion of such structures as nerves or blood vessels, and foci of necrosis (Fig. 52.44).

Treatment is clearly difficult and depends on the histological findings. In the case of malignant embryomas, interstitial irradiation may have to be considered, despite the patient's age.

Intraosseous salivary gland tumors

Rarely, salivary gland tumors form within the jaw from foci of ectopic tissue. The most common example of the latter is the enclavement of salivary gland tissue, known as the Stafne bone cavity, in the region of the angle of the mandible. Intraosseous salivary gland tumors arise most frequently near this site.

STAFNE'S IDIOPATHIC BONE CAVITY

Stafne's bone cavity has a cyst-like radiographic appearance. It is symptomless and only found by chance when it may be mistaken for cysts in the mandible.

The Stafne bone cavity is seen as a clearly demarcated round or oval radiolucency, nearly always below the inferior dental canal in the premolar, molar, or angle region of the mandible. It is a concave depression in the lingual aspect of the mandible and contains accessory lobes of the submandibular salivary gland. Very occasionally, a similar lesion is seen above the inferior dental canal and is found to contain accessory sublingual gland tissue. Even more rarely, similar enclaved islands of salivary tissue may be found in other parts of the mandible.

The diagnosis can be confirmed by sialography; no treatment is then necessary.

INTRAOSSEOUS SALIVARY GLAND TUMORS

RADIOGRAPHY

Intraosseous salivary gland tumors present a variety of appearances such as unilocular or multilocular cyst-like areas of radiolucency the nature of which is only recognizable after biopsy or excision. Malignant tumors are likely to show peripheral bone destruction and be less sharply circumscribed.

MICROSCOPY

Intraosseous salivary gland tumors do not differ microscopically from their soft-tissue counterparts. Most have been mucoepidermoid carcinomas, as reviewed by Waldron & Koh[73] and Brookstone & Huvos.[74] The latter found only seven benign tumors among 127 reported central salivary gland tumors.

An intraosseous salivary gland tumor might possibly be mistaken histologically for an odontogenic tumor, largely because of its location, but the chance of this happening should be small.

BEHAVIOR AND MANAGEMENT

If histology shows a malignant tumor, the possibility that it is a metastasis may be considered, but only because adenocarcinomas of other organs can occasionally resemble salivary gland tumors microscopically.

Treatment of intraosseous mucoepidermoid carcinomas or more malignant tumors should be by wide excision and, if necessary, grafting. Rare benign intraosseous tumors have been enucleated satisfactorily.

Metastatic tumors in salivary glands

Metastases to salivary glands are rare. The most frequent metastases are from skin tumors, particularly melanomas, and epidermoid carcinomas are usually in juxtaglandular nodes, as are many other metastases that appear as salivary gland tumors. Frequently, the possibility of a salivary gland tumor being a metastasis may be suspected, but metastatic renal cell carcinoma occasionally presents special problems, as noted earlier. Other metastases that could be mistaken for primary salivary gland carcinomas are adenocarcinomas from any of the many sites where they can originate, and thyroid carcinomas.

Illustrative of the range of tumors that can arise in the salivary glands is the report by Zachariades et al[75] of an extraskeletal Ewing's sarcoma that metastasized to the parotid gland in a 34-year-old female.

In the case of melanomas, as with other metastases, the prognosis is poor. The diagnosis is likely to be made only after parotidectomy, but Ball & Thomas[76] state that parotidectomy and elective neck dissection provide valuable locoregional palliation, although the long-term prognosis remains poor.

REFERENCES

1. Seifert G, Miehlke A, Haubrich J, Chilla R 1986 Diseases of the salivary glands. Georg Thieme Verlag, Stuttgart
2. Foote FW, Frazell EL 1954 Tumors of the major salivary glands. Atlas of tumor pathology. Armed Forces Institute of Pathology, Washington, DC, section IV, fascicle II
3. Takeichi N, Hirose F, Yamamoto H, Ezaki H, Fujikura T 1983 Salivary gland tumors in atomic bomb survivors, Hiroshima. Japan. II Pathologic study and supplementary epidemiologic observations. Cancer 52: 377–385
4. Watkin GT, Hobsley M 1986 Should radiotherapy be used routinely in the management of benign parotid tumours? Br J Surg 73: 601–603
5. Auclair PL, Goode RK, Ellis GL 1992 Mucoepidermoid carcinoma of intraoral glands. Evaluation and application of grading criteria in 143 cases. Cancer 69: 2021–2030
6. Hickman RE, Cawson RA, Duffy SW 1984 The prognosis of specific types of salivary gland tumors. Cancer 54: 1620–1624
7. Ellis GL, Gnepp DR 1988 Unusual salivary gland tumors. In: Gnepp DR (ed) Pathology of the head and neck. Churchill Livingstone, New York, p 627–631
8. Ellis GL, Corio RL 1983 Acinic cell adenocarcinoma. A clinicopathologic analysis of 294 cases. Cancer 52: 542–549
9. Hamper K, Mausch HE, Caselitz J et al 1990 Acinic cell carcinoma of the salivary glands: the prognostic relevance of DNA cytophotometry in a retrospective study of long duration (1965–1987). Oral Surg Oral Med Oral Pathol 69: 68–75
10. El-Naggar AK, Batsakis JG, Luna MA, McLemore D, Byers RM 1990 DNA flow cytometry of acinic cell carcinomas of major salivary glands. J Laryngol Otol 104: 410–416
11. Lewis JE, Olsen KD, Weiland LH 1991 Acinic cell carcinoma. Clinicopathol Rev Cancer 68: 172–179
12. Hamper K, Lazar F, Dietel M et al 1990 Prognostic factors for adenoid cystic carcinoma of the head and neck: a retrospective evaluation of 96 cases. J Oral Pathol Med 19: 101–107
13. Ferreiro JA 1994 Immunohistochemical analysis of salivary gland canalicular adenoma. Oral Surg Oral Med Oral Pathol 78: 761–765
14. Perzin KH, Gullane P, Clairmont AC 1978 Adenoid cystic carcinomas arising in salivary glands. A correlation of histologic features and clinical course. Cancer 48: 265–282
15. Santucci M, Bondi R 1989 New prognostic criterion in adenoid cystic carcinoma of salivary gland origin. Am J Clin Pathol 91: 132–136
16. Cleveland D, Abrams AM, Melrose RJ, Handlers JP 1990 Solid adenoid cystic carcinoma of the maxilla. Oral Surg Oral Med Oral Pathol 69: 470–478
17. Van der Wal JE, Snow GB, van der Waal I 1990 Intraoral adenoid cystic carcinoma. The presence of perineural spread in relation to site, size, local extension and metastatic spread in 22 cases. Cancer 66: 2031–2033

18. Kim K-H, Chung P-S, Rhee C-S, Kim W-H 1994 The manifestation of proliferating cell nuclear antigen in adenoid cystic carcinoma. Arch Otolaryngol Head Neck Surg 120: 1221–1225

19. Blanck C, Eneroth C-M, Jacobsson F, Jakobsson PA 1967 Adenoid cystic carcinoma of the parotid gland. Acta Radiol Ther Phys Biol 6: 177–196

20. Evans HL, Batsakis JG 1984 Polymorphous low grade adenocarcinoma of minor salivary glands. Cancer 53: 935–942

21. Batsakis JG, Pinkston GR, Luna MA, Byers RM, Tillery GW 1983 Adenocarcinomas of the oral cavity: a clinicopathologic study of terminal duct adenocarcinomas. J Laryngol Otol 97: 825–835

22. Vincent SD, Hammond HL, Finkelstein MW 1994 Clinical and therapeutic features of polymorphous low-grade adenocarcinoma. Oral Surg Oral Med Oral Pathol 77: 41–47

23. Ritland R, Lubensky I, LiVolsi VA 1993 Polymorphous low grade adenocarcinoma of the parotid salivary gland. Arch Pathol Lab Med 117: 1261–1263

24. Slootweg PJ 1993 Low-grade adenocarcinoma of the oral cavity: polymorphous or papillary? J Oral Pathol Med 22: 327–330

25. Gnepp DR, Chen JC, Warren C 1988 Polymorphous low grade adenocarcinoma of minor salivary gland. An immunohistochemical and clinicopathologic study. Am J Surg Pathol 12: 461–468

26. Regezi JA, Zarbo RJ, Stewart JCB, Courtney RM 1991 Polymorphous low grade adenocarcinoma of minor salivary gland. Oral Surg Oral Med Oral Pathol 71: 469–475

27. Simpson RHW, Clarke TJ, Sarsfield PTL, Babajews AV 1991 Salivary duct adenocarcinoma. Histopathology 18: 229–235

28. Batsakis JG, El-Naggar AK 1991 Terminal duct carcinomas of salivary tissues. Ann Otol Rhinol Laryngol 100: 251–253

29. Ruiz CC, Romero MP, Pérez MM 1993 Salivary duct carcinoma: a report of nine cases. J Oral Maxillofac Surg 51: 641–646

30. Delgado R, Vuitch F, Albores-Saavedra J 1993 Salivary duct carcinoma. Cancer 72: 1503–1512

31. Barnes L, Rao U, Krause J, Contis L, Schwartz A, Scalamonga P 1994 Salivary duct carcinoma. Part I. A clinicopathologic evaluation and DNA analysis of 13 cases with review of the literature. Oral Surg Oral Med Oral Pathol 78: 64–73

32. Tortoledo ME, Luna MA, Batsakis JG 1984 Carcinomas ex pleomorphic adenomas and malignant mixed tumours: histomorphologic indexes. Arch Otolaryngol 110: 172–176

33. Ruiz CC, Romero MP, Pérez MM 1993 Salivary duct carcinoma: a report of nine cases. J Oral Maxillofac Surg 51: 641–646

34. Litman CD, Alguacil-Garcia A 1987 Clear cell carcinoma arising in pleomorphic adenoma of the salivary gland. Am J Clin Pathol 88: 239–243

35. Klijanienko J, Michear C, Schwaab G, Marandas P, Friedman S 1989 Clear cell carcinoma arising in pleomorphic adenoma. J Laryngol Otol 103: 789–791

36. Cassidy M, Connolly CE 1994 Clear cell carcinoma arising in a pleomorphic adenoma of the submandibular gland. J Laryngol Otol 108: 529–532

37. Ogawa I, Nikai H, Takata T et al 1991 Clear cell tumors of minor salivary gland origin. An immunohistochemical and ultrastructural analysis. Oral Surg Oral Med Oral Pathol 72: 200–207

38. Donath K, Seifert G 1972 Zur Diagnose und Ultrastruktur des tubularen Speichelgangcarcinoms. Epithelial–myoepitheliales Schaltstrukcarcinom. Virch Arch (Pathol Anat) 356: 16–31

39. Corio RL, Sciubba JJ, Brannon RB, Batsakis JG 1982 Epithelial-myoepithelial carcinoma of intercalated duct origin. A clinicopathologic and ultrastructural assessment of sixteen cases. Oral Surg Oral Med Oral Pathol 53: 280–287

40. Kleinsasser O, Klein HJ, Hubner G 1968 Spiechelgangcarcinom. Ein den milchgangcarcinom analoge gruppe von speichdräsentumoren. Arch Klin Exp Ohren Nasen Kehlkopfheilkd 192: 100–105

41. Luna MA, Ordonez NG, Mackay B, Batsakis JG, Guillamondegui O 1985 Salivary epithelial–myoepithelial carcinomas of intercalated ducts: a clinical, electron microscopic, and immunocytochemical study. Oral Surg Oral Med Oral Pathol 59: 482–490

42. Jones H, Moshtael F, Simpson RHW 1992 Immunoreactivity of alpha smooth muscle actin in salivary gland tumours: a comparison with S100 protein. J Clin Pathol 45: 938–940

43. Milchgrub S, Gnepp DR, Vuitch F, Delgado F, Albores-Saavedra J 1994 Hyalinizing clear cell carcinoma of salivary gland. Am J Surg Pathol 18: 74–82

44. Batsakis JG, McBurney TA 1971 Metastatic neoplasms to the head and neck. Surg Gynaecol Obstet 133: 673–677

45. Sist TC, Marchetta FC, Milley PC 1982 Renal cell carcinoma presenting as a primary parotid gland tumour. Oral Surg Oral Med Oral Pathol 53: 499–502

46. Pisani P, Angeli G, Krengli M, Pia F 1990 Renal carcinoma metastasis to the parotid gland. J Laryngol Otol 104: 352–354

47. Okabe Y, Ohoka H, Nagayama I, Furukawa M 1992 View from beneath: pathology in focus. Renal cell metastasis to the tongue. J Laryngol Otol 106: 282–284

48. Tokich JJ, Harrison JH. Renal cell carcinoma: natural history and chemotherapeutic experience. J Urol 114: 371–374

49. Walter CW, Gillespie DR 1960 Metastatic hypernephroma of fifty years duration. Minnesota Med 43: 123–125

50. Holland JM 1973 Cancer of the kidney: natural history and staging. Cancer 32: 1030–1042

51. Garfield DH, Kennedy BJ 1972 Regression of metastatic renal cell carcinoma following nephrectomy. Cancer 30: 190–196

52. Middleton RG 1967 Surgery for metastatic renal cell carcinoma. J Urol 97: 973–977

53. McCluggage G, Sloan J, Cameron S, Hamilton P, Toner P 1995 Basal cell adenocarcinoma of the submandibular gland. Oral Surg Oral Med Oral Pathol 79: 342–350

54. Gerughty RM, Hennigar GR, Brown FM 1968 Adenosquamous carcinoma of the nasal, oral and laryngeal cavities. Cancer 22: 1140–1155

55. Albeck H, Bentzen J, Ockelmann HH, Nielsen NH, Bietlan P, Hansen HS 1993 Familial clusters of nasopharyngeal and salivary gland carcinomas in Greenland natives. Cancer 72: 196–200

56. Thackray AC, Lucas RB 1974 Tumors of the major salivary glands. Atlas of tumor pathology. Armed Forces Institute of Pathology, Washington, DC, second series, fascicle 10

57. Dardick I, van Nostrand AW 1985 Myoepithelial cells in salivary gland tumors – revisited. Head Neck Surg 7: 395–408

58. Singh R, Cawson RA 1988 Malignant myoepithelial carcinoma (myoepithelioma) arising in a pleomorphic adenoma of the parotid gland. Oral Surg Oral Med Oral Pathol 66: 65–70

59. Jie W, Qiguang W, Kaihua S, Chengrui B 1995 Quantitative multivariate analysis of myoepithelioma and myoepithelial carcinoma. Int J Oral Maxillofac Surg 24: 153–157

60. Crissman JD, Wirman JA, Harris A 1977 Malignant myoepithelioma of the parotid gland. Cancer 40: 3042–3049

61. Bleiweiss IJ, Huvos AG, Lara J, Strong EW 1992 Carcinosarcoma of the submandibular salivary gland. Cancer 69: 2031–2035

62. Toynton SC, Wilkins MJ, Cook HT, Stafford NDS 1994 True malignant mixed tumour of a minor salivary gland. J Laryngol Otol 108: 76–79

63. Carson HJ, Tojo DP, Chow JM, Hammadeh R, Raslan WF 1995 Carcinosarcoma of salivary glands with unusual stromal components. Report of two cases and review of the literature. Oral Surg Oral Med Oral Pathol Oral Radiol Endod 79: 738–746

64. Wenig BM, Hitchcock CL, Ellis GL, Gnepp DR 1992 Metastasizing mixed tumor of salivary glands. A clinicopathologic and flow cytometric analysis. Am J Surg Pathol 16: 845–858

65. Qureshi AA, Gitelis A, Templeton AA, Piasecki PA 1994 'Benign' metastasizing pleomorphic adenoma. A case report and review of the literature. Clin Orthopaed Rel Res 308: 192–198

66. Landolt U, Zobeli L, Pedio G 1990 Pleomorphic adenoma metastatic to the lung: diagnosis by fine needle aspiration cytology. Acta Cytol 34: 101–102

67. Girson M, Mendelsohn DB, Burns D, Mickey B 1992 Histologically benign pleomorphic adenoma of the calvaria. Am J Neuroradiol 12: 193–196

68. Bailet JW, Zimmerman MC, Arnstein DP, Wollman JS, Mickel RA 1992 Sebaceous carcinoma of the head and neck. Case report and literature review. Arch Otolaryngol Head Neck Surg 118: 1245–1249

69. Goode RK, Corio RL 1988 Oncocytic adenocarcinoma of salivary glands. Oral Surg Oral Med Oral Pathol 65: 61–66

70. Brandwein MS, Huvos AG 1991 Oncocytic tumors of the major salivary glands. Amer J Surg Pathol 15: 514–528

71. Callender DL, Frankenthaler RA, Luna MA, Lee SS, Goepfert H 1992 Salivary gland neoplasms in children. Arch Otolaryngol Head Neck Surg 118: 472–476

72. Shikhani AH, Johns ME 1988 Tumors of the major salivary glands in children. Head Neck Surg 10: 257–263

73. Waldron CA, Koh ML 1990 Central mucoepidermoid carcinoma of the jaws: report of four cases with analysis of the literature and discussion of the relationship to mucoepidermoid, sialodontogenic and glandular odontogenic cysts. J Oral Maxillofac Surg 48: 871–877

74. Brookstone MS, Huvos AG 1992 Central salivary gland tumors of the maxilla and mandible: a clinicopathologic study of 11 cases with an analysis of the literature. J Oral Maxillofac Surg 50: 229–236

75. Zachariades N, Koumoura F, Liapi-Avgeri G, Bouropoulo V 1994 Extraskeletal Ewing's sarcoma of the parotid region: a case report with detection of the tumour's immunophenotypical characteristics. Br J Oral Maxillofac Surg 32: 328–331

76. Ball ABS, Thomas JM 1990 Management of parotid metastases from cutaneous melanoma of the head and neck. J Laryngol Otol 104: 350–351

Nonepithelial tumors and tumor-like lesions of salivary glands

53

Almost any kind of mesenchymal tumor can develop in salivary glands, but overall they comprise fewer than 5% of salivary gland tumors. Lymphomas are the most common of them.

Sjögren's syndrome and salivary lymphoepithelial lesion

Sjögren's syndrome is characterized by dry eyes and dry mouth caused by a lymphoplasmacytic infiltrate replacing secretory cells. It is a connective tissue disease giving rise to a variety of auto-antibodies, of which SS-A and SS-B are of greatest diagnostic value. The traditional term *benign lymphoepithelial lesion* applies to the same histologic picture in patients in whom dry glands were apparently absent but, more probably, were unnoticed. However, the benign connotation is unjustified because of a risk of lymphomatous change in about 20% of cases.[1] This figure may be even higher after longer periods of follow-up. Another term, *myoepithelial sialadenitis*, which is favored by some, also seems inappropriate in that myoepithelial cells play no part in this lesion.

It is questionable whether *salivary lymphoepithelial lesion* is a separate entity from Sjögren's syndrome. The confusion has arisen because the parotid swelling of salivary lymphoepithelial lesion is clinically tumor-like and is treated surgically. The possibility of autoimmune disease is rarely considered, and it must be emphasized that remarkably few patients with proven xerostomia complain spontaneously of dry mouth. Postoperative investigation by Ostberg[2] showed that over 80% of patients with so-called benign lymphoepithelial lesion (salivary lymphoepithelial lesion) had symptoms or other abnormalities consistent with Sjögren's syndrome.

CLINICAL FEATURES

The diagnosis of salivary lymphoepithelial lesion is rarely made preoperatively and most cases are treated as tumors. However, it should be suspected in:

- women aged 50 years or over, with firm, smooth, diffuse parotid gland swellings that are not fixed superficially or deeply
- patients with bilateral parotid swellings, although unilateral swelling is more common
- patients with rheumatoid arthritis or any other connective tissue disease
- patients with dry mouth or eyes, although neither may be clinically obvious.

Pain is present in approximately 40% of patients.

MICROSCOPY

Both salivary lymphoepithelial lesion and Sjögren's syndrome are characterized by lymphoplasmacytic infiltration of salivary tissue. This is initially periductal, but it leads to progressive destruction of acini, which are replaced by the lymphoid infiltrate (Fig. 53.1). CD4 lymphocytes with production of proinflammatory cytokines such as interferon-γ can be detected in the focal infiltrates.

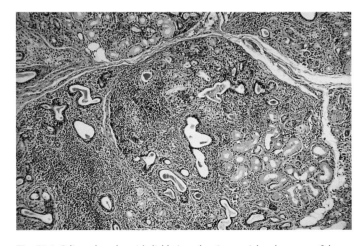

Fig. 53.1 Salivary lymphoepithelial lesion, showing partial replacement of the salivary gland by lymphoid tissue with dilated and proliferating ducts.

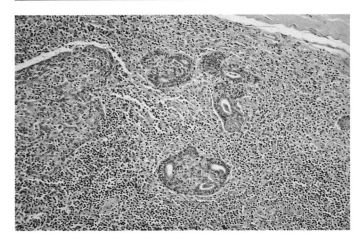

Fig. 53.2 Higher power view of a salivary lymphoepithelial lesion that is at a more advanced stage than the one shown in Figure 53.1. The gland has been totally replaced by lymphoid tissue, but islands of proliferating duct cells ('epimyoepithelial islands') can be seen.

Persistence and proliferation of duct epithelium gives rise to so-called 'epimyoepithelial islands,' which may contain hyaline material but lack myoepithelial cells (Fig. 53.2). This lympho-proliferation, unlike that of a lymphoma, is polyclonal and respects the lobular septa. Change to monoclonality, as discussed below, implies lymphomatous change.

SALIVARY LYMPHOEPITHELIAL LESIONS IN HIV INFECTION

Out of 15 salivary lymphoepithelial lesions, Smith et al[3] noted 12 typical examples in parotid gland resections from 11 males with generalized lymphadenopathy and at high risk of AIDS.

These lesions resemble salivary ('benign') lymphoepithelial lesions histologically in persons not infected with HIV except that cyst formation is common. They typically present as painless facial swellings in adult males, usually those aged of 20–40 years, who may also suffer from dry mouth or dry eyes.

MICROSCOPY

The parotid glands show typical features of salivary lymphoepithelial lesion with epimyoepithelial islands, but lymphoid follicles may be unusually prominent and may show changes suggestive of HIV-associated damage – namely, mantle zone effacement and follicle lysis. Also, microcysts lined by squamous or cuboidal epithelium are present and adjacent salivary tissue typically shows periductal and interstitial lymphocytic infiltrates. Sometimes the mass is almost entirely cystic, with no more than nodules of lymphoplasmacytic tissue forming mural thickenings.

Labouyrie et al[4] have demonstrated replication of HIV in these cystic lymphoepithelial lesions. Itescu et al[5] have shown that the lymphocytic infiltrate in HIV-associated salivary lesions,

unlike that of typical Sjögren's syndrome, consists of CD8 cells. Patients are typically also HLA DR5.[6] HIV-associated lympho-epithelial lesions can also undergo lymphomatous change.[7]

Tumor-like parotid gland swellings with changes typical of salivary lymphoepithelial lesion and, particularly with cyst formation, in an adult male below the age group at risk from Sjögren's syndrome is therefore strongly suggestive of HIV infection, especially also if autoantibodies typical of Sjögren's syndrome are absent. The main features in common with or differentiating them from Sjögren's include the following:

- The lesions are histologically the same as salivary ('benign') lymphoepithelial lesion, with epimyoepithelial islands, but typically show microcysts or are grossly cystic.
- Xerostomia is sometimes associated, but autoantibodies typical of Sjögren's syndrome are lacking.
- CD8 lymphocytes typically predominate in HIV-associated lesions, whereas in Sjögren's syndrome CD4 lymphocytes dominate the infiltrate.
- Also unlike Sjögren's syndrome, young adult males are predominantly affected.
- HIV-associated salivary lymphoepithelial lesions may also undergo lymphomatous change.

Lymphoma

Primary lymphomas of salivary glands are uncommon. They most frequently arise in intra- or periglandular lymphoid tissue, and are frequently a result of disseminated disease. Computed tomography (CT) scanning or other staging procedures are therefore essential.

Gleeson et al[8] analyzed the findings in 40 cases, and Wolvius et al[9] in 22 cases.

Occasionally, destruction of the nodal architecture makes it appear that the tumor has arisen in the gland parenchyma, but even in such cases the possibility that it is a secondary deposit needs to be excluded.

CLINICAL FEATURES

Lymphomas of salivary glands most frequently develop in the parotid glands, which have a significant content of lymphoid tissue. The submandibular gland accounts for 15–20% of cases, and the remainder are in the minor glands, particularly of the palate.

Lymphomas form firm swellings, usually grow rapidly, and have a history of little more than 6 months' duration. Pain and facial nerve palsy develop early in a minority. Fixation to deep or superficial structures and involvement of regional lymph nodes frequently develop later if the tumor is neglected. Most patients are aged between 50 and 70 years, and women are more frequently affected (in a ratio of 2 : 1), although in the series presented by Wolvius et al[9] there were 12 women and 10 men. In younger males especially, the possibility of HIV infection must be excluded. Exceptionally rarely, a lymphoma may develop in the lymphoid tissue of a Warthin's tumor.

MICROSCOPY

Most lymphomas of salivary glands are of the non-Hodgkin type. Most are B-cell lymphomas, including mucosa-associated lymphoid tissue (MALT) lymphomas, but almost any type of lymphoma may occasionally be found. The salivary tissue is replaced to a greater or lesser extent by sheets of lymphocytes, either diffusely or in a follicular pattern. The degree of maturation and differentiation is also variable, but are the same as in lymphomas in other sites. Signs of malignancy (namely, destruction of interlobular septa and capsule, and invasion of surrounding tissues) may be evident. Typing of lymphomas and sometimes even recognition of these tumors may be difficult.

Using current classifications, Wolvius et al[9] found that 15 of 22 salivary gland lymphomas were low grade and seven were high grade. In nine cases the growth pattern was follicular, and in 13 it was diffuse. All types of lymphoma in the Kiel classification were represented, except the lymphocytic type, and all the high-grade lymphomas were centroblastic, but the numbers of each were small.

MALT LYMPHOMA

MALT lymphomas can arise in salivary glands as a complication of Sjögren's syndrome or salivary lymphoepithelial lesions, and occasionally in the mouth. They are frequent in the stomach, small intestine, thyroid, and lung.

Although Shin et al[10] described a high frequency of monocytoid B-cell lymphomas in Sjögren's syndrome, monocytoid-like B cells can also be seen in MALT lymphomas. Shin & Sheibani[11] have emphasized the close microscopic similarities between these tumors. Harris[12] has confirmed the close relationship between MALT and monocytoid B-cell lymphomas, but noted that they were distinct from other low-grade B-cell lymphomas. Therefore, it is suggested that they should be grouped together as marginal zone B-cell lymphomas. Although these tumors are of very low grade and initially are curable with local treatment, if neglected they can evolve into high-grade lymphomas.

Microscopically, they consist predominantly of centrocyte-like cells, which range from lymphocyte-like to monocyte-like in appearance and have been described in Chapter 49.

Although they were the single most common type, only five of 22 salivary gland lymphomas analyzed by Wolvius et al[9] were of the MALT type.

LYMPHOMA IN SALIVARY LYMPHOEPITHELIAL LESION AND SJÖGREN'S SYNDROME

The incidence of lymphoma in salivary lymphoepithelial lesion or Sjögren's syndrome may be 20% or more.[13] Takahashi et al[14] found that of 32 salivary gland lymphomas the initial diagnosis had been 'myoepithelial sialadenitis' in nine cases. Lymphoma is typically a complication of long-standing disease and, therefore, is more likely to be seen in the elderly, particularly women. There is also a greater risk of lymphoma in patients with connective tissue disease, particularly rheumatoid arthritis (as mentioned earlier).

Lymphomatous change may be difficult to recognize among the lymphoproliferation characteristic of these diseases. Persistence of epimyoepithelial islands or of germinal centers does not preclude its presence. It is indicated by cytological features of malignancy, signs of invasion, and destruction of adjacent tissues. A more sensitive indicator is detection of expansion of a monoclonal B-cell population (Fig. 53.3). Schmid et al,[15] for example, considered areas of monotypic B-cell proliferation to represent lymphomatous

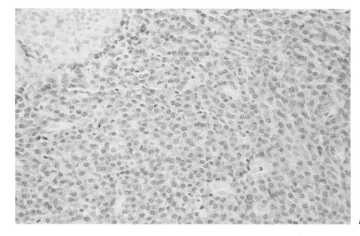

a

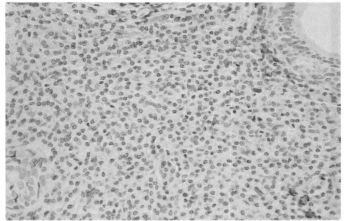

b

Fig. 53.3 An area of a lymphomatous change in a salivary lymphoepithelial lesion, showing a monoclonal population of B-cells stained by immunocytochemistry for κ (**a**) and λ (**b**) immunoglobulin light chains. The cells only express κ chains.

change in Sjögren's syndrome. Fishleder et al[16] and Freimark et al[17] also proposed that foci of monoclonality represented 'pre-lymphomatous change.' Even in histologically benign lesions, Falzon & Isaacson[18] have argued that a monoclonal B-cell population precludes the diagnosis of benign lymphoepithelial lesion. Moreover, immunoglobulin gene rearrangement in such a population may be identical to that in extrasalivary lymphomas in the same patient. Extensive areas of monoclonality are detectable by simple immunostaining, but a limited area may be masked by the general polyclonal infiltrate, and a more sensitive method is required.

Jordon et al[19] have pursued the detection of monoclonality in salivary lymphoepithelial lesions using the polymerase chain reaction (PCR) as well as immunohistochemistry and in situ hybridization, and reviewed previous work in this field. These methods in combination identified light-chain restriction in 77% (17 of 22) of cases. The single most sensitive method was by the PCR, which detected B-cell monoclonality in 68% of cases. Seven sequential biopsies were available from other sites, and six of them also showed B-cell monoclonality. Pablos et al[20] found, by PCR, clonal expansion of the heavy-chain immunoglobulin gene in the labial salivary glands of 13 patients with Sjögren's syndrome, but none developed a lymphoma within a mean period of follow-up of 4 years after biopsy. A B-cell lymphoma developed in another patient, but the clonal rearrangement of the tumor differed from the predominant rearrangement in the labial salivary glands at that time.

It may be noted that lip biopsies are frequently performed to confirm the diagnosis of Sjögren's syndrome, and they can be used for quantification of κ/λ ratios, and may therefore be valuable in the early detection of malignant lymphoproliferation. Thus Speight et al[21] have shown that lymphomatous change in Sjögren's syndrome can be predicted by in situ hybridization for κ and λ light chain mRNA in labial salivary glands. Of seven cases showing light-chain restriction, four developed low-grade MALT lymphomas, while a fifth died from disseminated lymphoma. Speight et al concluded that, when lymphoma develops in Sjögren's syndrome, lymphoma cells may disseminate to labial salivary glands before the onset of symptoms. Jordon et al[22] have also found, by in situ hybridization in 70 labial salivary gland biopsies, that 18.6% showed light-chain restriction. Subsequently, 30.7% of these patients were found to have extrasalivary lymphomas within a follow-up period of 18–156 months.

Although small areas of monoclonality can be identified by molecular techniques, they are so sensitive that the significance of positive findings is as yet controversial.

It would be surprising if light-chain restriction in 77% of salivary lymphoepithelial lesions, as reported by Jordon et al,[22] represented early lymphomatous change in every case. It may therefore be appropriate to suggest that detection of a small focus of monoclonality, if it does not indicate the presence or likelihood of lymphoma, should at least serve as a warning of the possibility and of the need to keep the patient under observation. In view of the age of most affected patients, lymphoma may not develop within the patient's lifetime, but expansion of a monoclonal B-cell population in salivary lymphoepithelial lesion must be regarded with some anxiety.

BEHAVIOR AND MANAGEMENT

Histologic typing and staging must be carried out as for a lymphoma in any other site. From the limited published data it appears that salivary gland lymphomas are usually stage I or II. Treatment is determined by the extent of disease as well as by the histologic subtype. Although the prognosis might be expected to be affected by the stage at presentation, this has not been confirmed in all reported series.[8]

Excision is likely to have been carried out in the first instance, but typing and staging determines the need for radiotherapy or chemotherapy or both.

Among 36 cases reported by Gleeson et al,[1] the median survival was only 49 months. Other reports have indicated considerably better survival rates, but overall the numbers are so small and the variables affecting prognosis so many, that generalizations are not useful.

HODGKIN'S DISEASE

Primary Hodgkin's disease of salivary glands is very rare. The figures are sometimes inflated by inclusion of disease of juxtaglandular cervical lymph nodes, but the gland parenchyma is rarely involved. However, a lymph node mass may occasionally be mistaken for a salivary gland tumor, particularly of the submandibular gland, but in many cases the disease has already disseminated. Unlike non-Hodgkin lymphomas, Hodgkin's disease has a peak in the third and fourth decades, and males predominate in the ratio of 4 : 1.

MICROSCOPY

Lymphocyte-predominant, nodular-sclerosing, and mixed types appear to be virtually equally frequent, but lymphocyte-depleted disease appears rare.

BEHAVIOR AND MANAGEMENT

Histological typing and staging investigation should be carried out. The findings should determine whether treatment is by radiotherapy or combination chemotherapy, and is by currently accepted protocols.

Hemangioma of the parotid gland

Juvenile hemangioma may be evident at birth, is usually seen before the age of 10 years, is more common in girls, and is exceedingly

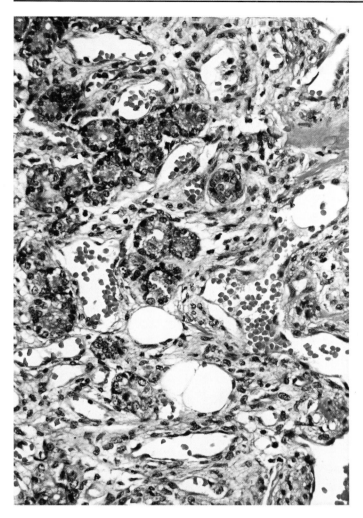

Fig. 53.4 Hemangioma of the parotid gland. Scattered acini persist among the proliferating blood vessels.

rare in adults. It gives rise to a soft, sometimes bluish, enlargement of the gland.

MICROSCOPY

The appearance is that of a hemangioma, usually of capillary type, in which isolated remnants of glandular tissue, particularly ducts, can be seen (Fig. 53.4). Rarely, these hemangiomas are partly or predominantly, cavernous or are mixed hemangiomas and lymphangiomas.

BEHAVIOR AND MANAGEMENT

Progress of these lesions is variable. Some may grow or even spread into adjacent tissue for a time, but spontaneous regression is also well recognized. However, the extent of the vascular proliferation may occasionally be so gross as to produce an arteriovenous shunt. This can rarely give rise to high-output circulatory failure.

If the tumor shows no signs of regressing, treatment should be delayed until the age of at least 5 years in order to lessen the risk of damaging the delicate, developing facial nerve. Excision, if it cannot be avoided, should be curative. Alternatives, such as injection of sclerosing agents or irradiation as primary treatment, or to reduce the bulk of the tumor preoperatively, are likely to cause complications outweighing possible benefits.

Other mesenchymal tumors of salivary glands

As mentioned earlier, mesenchymal tumors other than juvenile hemangiomas are rare in salivary glands. Lipomas and neural tumors are the most common types, but any other may occasionally be seen. These tumors do not differ from their counterparts in other sites.

Because of the rarity of mesenchymal tumors in salivary glands, it is not clear whether their behavior differs from that of histologically similar tumors elsewhere, and no practical comments can be made.

As mentioned earlier, a myoepithelioma may occasionally be mistaken microscopically for a mesenchymal tumor, but if necessary can be identified by immunohistochemistry.

PLASMACYTOMAS

Solitary plasmacytomas of salivary glands are rare. There is no evidence that they differ microscopically or in behavior from other solitary soft-tissue plasmacytomas. They can be readily distinguished from plasmacytoid myoepitheliomas, the cells of which lack typical cytological features of plasma cells and immunoglobulin formation and are only loosely aggregated in the stroma. The myoepithelial cells should also be identifiable with immunohistochemical markers (see Ch. 51).

SARCOMAS

Sarcomas form fewer than 1% of primary salivary gland tumors. Rhabdomyosarcomas and malignant fibrous histiocytomas are the most frequent types. Despite their superficial site, which enables early recognition, sarcomas of salivary glands appear to have a worse prognosis than their more deeply situated counterparts. The difficulties of surgery, particularly in the parotid region, may contribute to this poor prognosis.

JUXTAGLANDULAR TUMORS

Tumors of adjacent tissues occasionally involve or appear to involve salivary glands. An example is a lymphoma in the juxtaglandular lymph nodes, as discussed earlier.

Skin tumors can extend into the parotid gland in particular, but are likely to be recognized as such. Rarely, a jugulotympanic paraganglioma can mimic a parotid gland tumor. A mandibular or masseteric tumor can also involve the parotid region. All these possibilities are exceedingly rare, but should be borne in mind when a salivary gland tumor has unusual features.

REFERENCES

1. Gleeson MJ, Cawson RA, Bennett MH 1986 Benign lymphoepithelial lesion: a less than benign disease. Clin Otolaryngol 11: 47–51
2. Ostberg Y 1983 The clinical picture of benign lympho-epithelial lesion. Clin Otolaryngol 8: 381–390
3. Smith FB, Rajdeo H, Panesar N, Bhuta K, Stahl R 1988 Benign lympho-epithelial lesion of the parotid gland in intravenous drug users. Arch Pathol Lab Med 112: 743–745
4. Labouyrie E, Merlio JPH, Beylot-Barry M et al 1993 Human immunodeficiency virus type I replication within cystic lymphoepithelial lesion of the salivary gland. Am J Clin Pathol 100: 41–46
5. Itescu S, Brancato LJ, Buxbaum J et al 1990 A diffuse infiltrative CD8 lymphocytosis syndrome in human immunodeficiency virus (HIV) infection: a host immune response associated with HLA-DR5. Ann Intern Med 112: 3–10
6. Itescu S, Brancato LJ, Winchester R 1989 A sicca syndrome in HIV infection: association with HLA-DR5. Lancet ii: 466–468
7. Ioachim HL, Ryan JR, Blaugrund SM 1988 Salivary gland lymph nodes. The site of lymphadenopathies and lymphomas associated with human immunodeficiency virus infection. Arch Pathol Lab Med 112: 1224–1228
8. Gleeson MJ, Bennett MH, Cawson RA 1986 Lymphomas of salivary glands. Cancer 58: 699–704
9. Wolvius EB, van der Valk P, van der Wal JE et al 1996 Primary non-Hodgkin lymphoma of the salivary glands. An analysis of 22 cases. J Oral Pathol Med 25: 177–181
10. Shin SS, Sheibani K, Fishleder A et al 1991 Monocytoid B cell lymphoma in patients with Sjögren's syndrome: a clinicopathologic study of 13 patients. Hum Pathol 22: 422–430
11. Shin SS, Sheibani K 1993 Monocytoid B cell lymphoma. Am J Clin Pathol 99: 421–425
12. Harris NL 1993 Low-grade B-cell lymphoma of mucosa-associated lymphoid tissue and monocytoid B-cell lymphoma. Related entities that are distinct from other low-grade B-cell lymphomas. Arch Pathol Lab Med 117: 771–775
13. Gleeson MJ, Cawson RA, Bennett MH 1986 Benign lymphoepithelial lesion: a less than benign disease. Clin Otolaryngol 11: 47–51
14. Takahashi H, Cheng J, Fujita S et al 1992 Primary malignant lymphoma of salivary gland: a tumor of mucosa-associated lymphoid tissue. J Oral Pathol Med 21: 318–325
15. Schmid U, Helbron D, Lennert K 1982 Development of malignant lymphomas in myoepithelial sialadenitis (Sjögren's syndrome). Virch Arch A 395: 11–43
16. Fishleder A, Tubbs R, Hesse B, Levine H 1987 Uniform detection of immunoglobulin gene rearrangement in benign lymphoepithelial lesions. N Engl J Med 1118–1121
17. Freimark B, Fantozzi R, Bone R, Bordin G, Fox R 1989 Detection of clonally expanded salivary gland lymphocytes in Sjögren's syndrome. Arthritis Rheum 32: 859–869
18. Falzon M, Isaacson PG 1991 The natural history of benign lymphoepithelial lesion of the salivary gland in which there is a monoclonal population of B cells. A report of two cases. Am J Surg Pathol 15: 59–65
19. Jordan RCK, Odell EW, Speight PM 1996 B-cell monoclonality in salivary lymphoepithelial lesions. Oral Oncol, Eur J Cancer 32B: 38–44
20. Pablos JL, Carreira PE, Morillas L, Montalvo G, Ballestin C, Gomez-reino JJ 1994 Clonally expanded lymphocytes in the minor glands of Sjögren's syndrome patients without lymphoproliferative disease. Arthritis Rheum 37: 1441–1444
21. Speight PM, Jordan R, Colloby P, Nandha H, Pringle JH 1994 Early detection of lymphomas in Sjögren's syndrome by in situ hybridisation for κ and λ light chain mRNA in labial salivary glands. Eur J Cancer B: Oral Oncol 30: 244–247
22. Jordan RCK, Pringle JH, Speight PM 1995 High frequency of light chain restriction in labial salivary gland biopsies of Sjögren's syndrome detected by in situ hybridisation. J Pathol 177: 35–40

Choristomas and teratomas

Teratomas, choristomas, and related anomalies

54

Teratomas

Teratomas have been defined by Weaver et al[1] as tumors consisting of multiple tissues that, unlike hamartomas, are not indigenous to their site of origin. They are not merely malformations, but undergo progressive, often rapid, uncoordinated growth and invade adjacent tissues. Ovarian teratomas are well recognized, but very occasionally teratomas form in the oral cavity or nearby. Olivares-Pakzad et al[2] considered that the so-called 'hairy polyp' of the nasopharyngeal region was first reported by Brown-Kelly in 1918,[3] and, in addition to reporting another case, have reviewed the variants of these anomalies. They define teratomas as true neoplasms of presumed primordial germ-cell derivation and typically consisting of all three embryonic germ layers. These differentiate into somatic tissues that are nonindigenous to the site of origin. Hamartomas may similarly comprise all three germinal layers, but they are indigenous to the site of origin. Epignathi are complex proliferations that have been likened to a fetus in fetu, but are regarded by some as teratomas.

Sciubba & Younai[4] have presented a case of epipalatus (a teratoma arising from the palate) and reviewed 40 other teratomas arising from within the mouth or adjacent tissues such as the nasopharynx. In their case, the mass was approximately as large as the infant's head and caused death by obstructing the airway only minutes after birth. It was attached to the junction of the hard and soft palates by a stalk and was partially invested by epidermis with abundant cutaneous adnexae. Structures identified in this teratoma included epidermoid cysts, mature bone, and a joint in a fibrous capsule. The joint had a synovial space, while the bone had a normal epiphyseal growth plate and contained abundant hemopoietic marrow. Other elements were large areas of neuroglia, sympathetic ganglia, bronchial structures, salivary gland tissue, choroid plexus lining a cyst, hair follicles and sebaceous glands, and well-formed teeth, but no striated muscle.

In the example reported by Olivares-Pakzad et al,[2] a bilobed, polypoid mass extending from the hard palate protruded from the mouth of a 1-day-old boy. Associated anomalies were a mucosal band connecting the palate to the floor of the mouth. Other anomalies were a bifid tongue, cleft lower lip and soft palate, and a bifid-appearing mandible. The mass contained pilosebaceous units, mucous glands, and smooth muscle and had a core of myxoid fibroconnective tissue intermingled with reticulated mesenchyme and focal bundles of spindle cells with fibrillary or filamentous cytoplasm. There were also areas of anastomosing pseudovascular spaces with occasional multinucleate and clear cells. Immunohistochemistry showed the cells lining the cleft-like spaces to be positive for vimentin and epithelial membrane antigen, while electron microscopy indicated that they were meningothelial in type.

Hudson et al[5] reported what they believed to be the only case of a malignant teratoma of the mandible of a 14-year-old female. This tumor contained gastrointestinal epithelium showing malignant changes and multiple foci of embryonic cartilage.

BEHAVIOR AND MANAGEMENT

Large oral teratomas may be recognized in utero by ultrasonography, and radiographic demonstration of teeth in the mass is confirmatory. However, the size and location of oral teratomas may be such that affected infants may be stillborn or die soon after birth. These factors also make surgical resection very difficult, but if early respiratory obstruction can be overcome by immediate tracheostomy it has proved possible to remove large teratomas by multistage operations. Associated orofacial developmental defects have to be repaired at an appropriate time later.

Small oral teratomas may cause no difficulties in the immediate neonatal period, but they grow rapidly. El-Sayed,[6] for example, reported the uncomplicated delivery of an infant who had a mass behind the soft palate. This caused no trouble until 15 days later when it had grown so large as to cause respiratory embarrassment. This tumor contained fat, brain tissue, striated muscle, bone, hair follicles, and salivary gland tissue.

One to two per cent of ovarian teratomas may undergo malignant change, while foci of embryonal carcinoma may be found in testicular teratomas in patients over 5 years of age. Oral teratomas, which are mostly of the mature type and found at birth, are (with the exception mentioned earlier) benign, but threaten life because of their site.

Of 38 infants with teratomas reviewed by Sciubba & Younai,[4] where information was available, 16 were stillborn or died soon after.

Choristomas

A choristoma, as defined by Chou et al,[7] is a tumor-like growth of otherwise normal cells in an abnormal location. They reject the term *heterotopia* for this phenomenon as it does not reflect the tumor-like growth of the lesion. However, as discussed below, the term heterotopia is frequently used when choristomas are reported.

Chou et al[7] recognized the following categories of oral choristoma:

1. salivary gland choristoma
   (a) central
   (b) gingival
2. cartilaginous choristoma
3. osseous choristoma
4. lingual thyroid choristoma
5. glial choristoma
6. gastric mucosal choristoma.

CENTRAL SALIVARY GLAND CHORISTOMA

Chou et al[7] found only five reports that satisfied the criterion of salivary tissue completely enclosed in bone. These were usually in the body of the mandible and appeared radiographically as rounded areas of radiolucency with sclerotic margins which sometimes mimicked periapical granulomas. By contrast, Buchner et al[8] considered that 20 cases had been reported, and they presented four new ones. It is also surprising that if central salivary gland choristomas are as uncommon as Chou et al[7] suggest, central salivary gland tumors, which presumably arise from them, are so much more frequent. Waldron & Koh[9] alone found reports of 66 cases of intraosseous mucoepidermoid carcinomas. Other such reports are reviewed in Chapter 52.

GINGIVAL SALIVARY GLAND CHORISTOMA

Chou et al[7] found reports of four cases that appeared as solitary, asymptomatic tumor-like masses between 0.5 and 1.5 cm in diameter in the buccal or lingual gingiva.

Microscopically, both central and gingival salivary gland choristomas appear as encapsulated lobules of normal salivary gland acini of mixed type and ducts. Some chronic inflammatory cells may be present.

OSSEOUS CHORISTOMA

The first report of an osseous choristoma is credited to Monserrat in 1913,[10] who termed it *ostéome de la langue*. The term *osseous choristoma* was introduced by Krolls et al in 1972,[11] who noted that the term *osteomas of soft tissues* had persisted. Chou et al[7] were able to find reports of 39 examples, of which 85% were in the posterior dorsum of the tongue. Three others were in the middle third of the dorsum of the tongue, one in the lingual aspect of the anterior mandibular ridge, and one in the buccal mandibular vestibule.

Clinically, osseous choristomas form hard masses, which are sessile or pedunculated. They are covered by normal oral mucosa and are asymptomatic unless large enough to cause dysphagia or dysphonia.

Microscopically, osseous choristomas consist of well-circumscribed, lamellated bone surrounded by dense fibrous tissue. Osteocytes are present, but osteoblastic activity is minimal and any spaces are usually filled with fatty marrow.

Excision is normally curative, but Long & Koutnik[12] have reported an isolated example of recurrence of an osseous choristoma of the buccal soft tissues, 12 years after the original excision. From a review of the literature they concluded that this was the first recorded recurrence of an osseous choristoma, and Chou et al[7] concluded from their review that recurrence was unknown.

CARTILAGINOUS CHORISTOMA

The literature search by Chou et al[7] revealed 20 reported cases of cartilaginous choristomas. The tongue was involved in 17 cases, the buccal mucosa in two, and the soft palate in one. The ages of the patients ranged from 10 to 80 years.

These masses ranged in size from 1 to 13 cm in diameter and showed continued growth. The surface was sometimes inflamed, probably as a result of minor local trauma.

Microscopically, cartilaginous choristomas consist of hyaline cartilage, usually showing greater maturity centrally and surrounded by a dense fibrous perichondrium. The chondrocytes are normal and the hyaline matrix is well differentiated and mature. Thus there should be no difficulty in distinguishing these choristomas from extraskeletal chondrosarcomas (Fig. 54.1).

Excision of cartilaginous choristomas is required both because they can interfere with speech or swallowing and to confirm their nature. Recurrence is possible if the mass including the perichondrium is not removed entirely.

LINGUAL THYROID CHORISTOMA

Whether lingual thyroid tissue should be regarded as a choristoma may be questioned, because the normal thyroid gland primordium lies in the base of the tongue before descending into the neck. Small islands of thyroid tissue have been found in the tongue in up to 10% of autopsies.

The criteria of diagnosis of lingual thyroid choristoma used by Chou et al[7] were that it formed a tumor-like mass in the midline of the tongue between the foramen caecum and epiglottis, and that

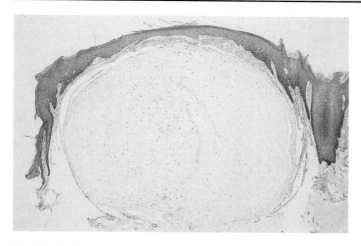

Fig. 54.1 Cartilaginous choristoma. This nodule of well-formed cartilage was present in the tongue.

its nature had been confirmed histologically or by radioactive iodine uptake.

Using these criteria, Chou et al[7] found 49 reports of lingual thyroid choristoma in patients ranging in age from 2.5 to 72 years. Females were affected in 80% of these cases. By contrast, Chou et al[7] noted that ectopic thyroid tissue was found in routine autopsies slightly more frequently in males. In 86% of the 49 cases there was no other functional thyroid tissue.

From a thyroid investigation center in Sri Lanka, Warnakulasuriya & Herath[13] found only eight lingual thyroids among 16 593 persons in a 25-year period.

Exceptionally rarely thyroid tissue can be present in some other site in the mouth than the tongue. Aguirre et al,[14] for example, have reported thyroid tissue in the left submandibular region.

Clinically, lingual thyroid choristomas form rounded swellings that are of variable size but are sometimes large enough to cause dysphagia, dysphonia, or even dyspnea. They are covered by normal mucosa and may appear bluish. Douglas & Barker[15] have reported an exceptional example where the entire substance of the tongue appeared to contain thyroid tissue.

Microscopically, lingual thyroid choristomas consist of mature or embryonic thyroid tissue, or a mixture of the two. Microfollicular fetal thyroid tissue is most frequently found and can be mistaken for carcinoma. However, carcinoma in lingual thyroid tissue is rare, so that Chou et al[7] found only three reports since 1965.

If the diagnosis is suspected it can be confirmed by scintiscanning so that biopsy, with its risk of significant bleeding, can be avoided. Magnetic resonance imaging supplemented by fine-needle aspiration cytology has considerable advantages if the facilities are available.

Management of lingual thyroid can be difficult if it is large enough to cause troublesome symptoms. Excision may be carried out if there is sufficient functional glandular tissue elsewhere but, as noted earlier, this is unusual. Treatment with iodine-131 is another option, but hypothyroidism is a well-recognized effect and has to be managed with thyroglobulin supplementation. Transplantation to another site is another possibility, but preliminary histological confirmation of the absence of carcinoma is essential.

Alderson & Lannigan[16] have reviewed the treatment options, and confirm that hypothyroidism is a common complication of excision but can sometimes be avoided by transplantation.

Although lingual thyroid can be the subject of any of the diseases such as hypothyroidism that can affect this gland, they are uncommon. Lingual thyroid cancer is also rare. Diaz-Arias et al[17] have reported a follicular carcinoma with clear cell change in a lingual thyroid, in which the diagnosis was confirmed for the first time immunohistochemically with thyroglobulin antibody and by electron microscopy.

LINGUAL SEBACEOUS CHORISTOMA

Sebaceous glands in the oral mucosa are present in up to 80% of persons, but do not normally become conspicuous until age advances. They are most frequently seen in the buccal and labial mucosae and appear as yellowish elevations of the surface beneath which a finely lobular pattern can be discerned. They are usually only a millimeter or two in diameter.

Intraoral sebaceous tissue may be regarded as choristomatous by virtue of being in an unusual site or because of the degree of hyperplasia. Chou et al[7] found reports of six lingual sebaceous choristomas that consisted of multiple lobules of sebaceous glandular tissue and ducts. They ranged from 2 to 20 mm in diameter.

Daley[18] has suggested that intraoral sebaceous hyperplasia should be defined as a lesion judged clinically to be a distinct abnormality that requires biopsy and which shows histologically one or more sebaceous glands, each with at least 15 lobules. Sebaceous glands in the oral cavity with fewer lobules are regarded by Daley[18] as within the range of normality.

GLIAL CHORISTOMA

Heterotopic brain tissue is rare, but most frequently appears in the region of the nose where it can cause respiratory obstruction. It is exceptionally rare in the oral cavity, so that Bychkov et al[19] considered that their case was the first fully authenticated example of glial heterotopia in the tongue. Chou et al[7] retrieved reports of 13 cases from the literature, and Garcia-Prats et al[20] were unable to find any more in a survey of the literature since 1900. Nevertheless, in addition to the one they presented, two others in the palate were reported by Al-Nafussi et al[21] and by Horie et al.[22] Two other cases of glial tumors of the oral cavity were reported by Morita et al.[23] Madjidi & Couly[24] also reported six cases in the face, including several impinging on or extending into the oral cavity. All of these, except one in a 10-year-old child with a mass in the cheek, were, as is typical of glial choristomas, seen in infants, usually within days or weeks of birth.

Lee et al[25] reported a particularly unusual glial choristoma in a 6-week-old infant. It extended into the oropharynx from the nasopharynx, and consisted of astrocytes, oligodendroglia, and cystic spaces lined by papillary structures resembling choroid plexus. Embedded in the mass was a pigmented neuroectodermal tumor.

Clinically, glial choristomas, although not true neoplasms, give rise to rapidly growing swellings consistent with the rapid growth of the brain in childhood. Lingual glial tumors typically form soft, smooth-surfaced polypoid masses. Respiratory distress is frequently the main symptom, or there may be difficulty in feeding. Gross facial asymmetry can result from glial tumors of the orbitozygomatic region.

MICROSCOPY

These masses consist of mature glial tissue, sometimes with differentiation to ependyma or choroid plexus. Neurones are frequently demonstrable. S100 protein, vimentin, and GFAP staining are positive. A variant, which should be termed *gliomatous teratoma*, shows scattered foci of squamous epithelium, striated muscle, and cartilage among the glia.

BEHAVIOR AND MANAGEMENT

Absence of communication with the brain should be confirmed by contrast computed tomography (CT) scanning. Complete excision is curative. Rarely, recurrence has followed incomplete resection.

GASTROINTESTINAL MUCOSAL CHORISTOMA (HETEROTOPIC ORAL GASTROINTESTINAL CYST)

Heterotopic gastric mucosa in the oral tissues usually gives rise to a cystic lesion. These rare cysts probably arise from displaced or residual embryonic rests as a result of an embryological anomaly leading to isolation of rests of gastic mucosa remaining after migration of the gastric anlage in the 3–4 mm embryo, from the neck in the region of the tongue. Fourteen cases of oral cysts with gastric or intestinal epithelial lining have been reviewed by Gorlin & Jirasak,[26] who added another.

Clinically, these cysts are seen in infants or young children, or occasionally later in life. In most cases, the cyst is in the anterior part of the tongue, but sometimes it is in the posterior part, the floor of the mouth, or the anterior neck, and may communicate with the surface. Males are affected three times as frequently as females.

Chou et al[7] found reports of 21 cases published since 1960, but numerous cases have been reported subsequently.[27–36]

MICROSCOPY

Gastric cystic choristomas are usually lined partly by gastric epithelium with chief and parietal cells, and partly by squamous epithelium. A muscularis mucosae is usually present. A lining partly or completely of intestinal epithelium containing Paneth, goblet and argentaffin cells is considerably more uncommon. The remainder of the lining usually consists of stratified squamous epithelium. In one of the two cases reported by Lipsett et al,[37] the cyst was lined by colonic epithelium, while the two cysts reported by Mir et al[32] were lined by squamous, gastric, intestinal, and respiratory epithelia. Bite & Cramer[29] reported a cyst of the upper lip lined by gastrointestinal and respiratory epithelium. The example reported by Khunamornpong et al[36] was unusual in that the tissue was on the anterior tongue and contained well-formed pancreatic tissue as well as gastrointestinal mucosa.

The most frequent site for oral gastrointestinal choristomas is the ventral surface of the tongue or floor of the mouth; less frequently, the anterior third or mid-dorsum of the tongue is involved. These lesions mostly arise in early infancy, but frequently remain untreated for many years.

Most oral gastrointestinal cysts form asymptomatic swellings but, unusually, the example reported by Burton et al[30] was noticed at birth as a bleeding ulcer. Peptic ulceration in a lingual lesion, as reported by Parikh et al,[28] is exceptional.

Excision is the treatment of choice and recurrence is very unusual.

REFERENCES

1. Weaver RG, Meyerhoff WL, Gates GA 1976 Teratomas of the head and neck. Surg Forum 27: 529–542
2. Olivares-Pakzad BA, Tazelaar HD, Dehner LP, Kasperbauer JL, Bite U 1995 Oropharyngeal hairy polyp with meningothelial elements. Oral Surg Oral Med Oral Pathol 79: 462–468
3. Brown-Kelly A 1918 Hairy or dermoid polyp of the pharynx and nasopharynx. J Laryngol Rhinol 33: 65–75
4. Sciubba JJ, Younai F 1991 Epipalatus: a rare introral teratoma. Oral Surg Oral Med Oral Pathol 71: 476–481
5. Hudson JW, Jaffrey B, Chase DC, Gray J 1983 Malignant teratoma of the mandible. J Oral Maxillofac Surg 41: 540–543
6. El-Sayed Y 1992 Teratoma of the head and neck. J Laryngol Otol 106: 836–838
7. Chou L, Hansen LS, Daniels TE 1991 Choristomas of the oral cavity: a review. Oral Surg Oral Med Oral Pathol 72: 584–593
8. Buchner A, Carpenter WM, Merrrell PW, Leider AS 1991 Anterior lingual salivary gland defect. Evaluation of twenty-four cases. Oral Surg Oral Med Oral Pathol 71: 131–136
9. Waldron CA, Koh ML 1990 Central mucoepidermoid carcinoma of the jaws: report of four cases with analysis of the literature and discussion of the relationship to mucoepidermormoid, sialodontogenic and glandular odontogenic cysts. J Oral Maxillofac Surg 48: 871–877
10. Monserrat M 1913 Ostéome de la langue. Bull Soc Anat 88: 282–283
11. Krolls SO, Jacoway JR, Alexander WN 1971 Osseous choristomas (osteomas) of intraoral soft tissue. Oral Surg Oral Med Oral Pathol 32: 588–595
12. Long DE, Koutnik AW 1991 Recurrent intraoral choristoma. Oral Surg Oral Med Oral Pathol 72: 337–379
13. Warnakulasuriya KA, Herath KB 1992 Investigating a lingual thyroid. Int J Oral Maxillofac Surg 21: 227–229
14. Aguirre A, de la Piedra M, Ruiz R, Portilla J 1991 Ectopic thyroid tissue in the submandibular region. Oral Surg Oral Med Oral Pathol 71: 73–76
15. Douglas PS, Barker AW 1994 Lingual thyroid: a review. Br J Oral Maxillofac Surg 32: 132–134
16. Alderson DJ, Lannigan FJ 1994 Lingual thyroid presenting after previous thyroglossal cyst excision. J Laryngol Otol 108: 341–343
17. Diaz-Arias AA, Biuckel JT, Loy TS, Croll GH, Puckett CL, Havey AD 1992 Follicular carcinoma with clear cell change arising in lingual thyroid. Oral Surg Oral Med Oral Pathol 74: 206–211
18. Daley TD 1993 Intraoral sebaceous hyperplasia. Diagnostic criteria. Oral Surg Oral Med Oral Pathol 75: 343–347
19. Bychkov V, Gatti WM, Fresco R 1988 Tumor of the tongue containing heterotopic brain tissue. Oral Surg Oral Med Oral Pathol 66: 71–73
20. Garcia-Prats MD, Rodriguez-Peralto JL, Carrillo R 1994 Glial choristoma of the tongue. Report of a case. J Oral Maxillofac Surg 52: 977–980
21. Al-Nafussi A, Hancock K, Sommerlad B, Carder PJ 1990 Heterotopic brain presenting as a cystic mass of the palate. Histopathology 17: 81–84

22. Horie N, Shimoyama T, Ozawa T, Ide F 1991 Heterotopic brain tissue in the palate: case report. J Oral Maxillofac Surg 49: 750–753
23. Morita N, Harada M, Sakamoto T 1993 Congenital tumors of heterotopic central nervous system tissue in the oral cavity: report of two cases. J Oral Maxillofac Surg 51: 1030–1033
24. Madjidi A, Couly G 1993 Heterotopic neuroglial tissue of the face. Oral Surg Oral Med Oral Pathol 76: 484–488
25. Lee SC, Henry MM, Gonzalez-Crussi F 1976 Simultaneous occurrence of melanotic neuroectodermal tumor and brain heterotopia in the oropharynx. Cancer 38: 249–253
26. Gorlin RJ, Jirasak JE 1970 Oral cysts containing gastric or intestinal mucosa – unusually embryological accident or heterotopia. J Oral Surg 28: 9–11
27. Awouters P, Reychler H 1991 Enteric duplication in the oral cavity. Int J Oral Maxillofac Surg 20: 12–14
28. Parikh DH, Ibrahim SK, Cook RC 1991 Peptic ulceration in a lingual sinus. J Pediatr Surg 26: 99–100
29. Bite U, Cramer HM 1992 Mixed heterotopic gastrointestinal and respiratory cyst of the lip. Plastic Reconstr Surg 90: 1068–1072
30. Burton DM, Kearns DB, Seid AB, Pransky SM, Billman G 1992 Tongue gastric choristoma: failure to localize by technetium-99 m pertechnetate scan. J Pediatr Otorhinolaryngol 24: 91–95
31. Martone CH, Wolf SM, Weskey RK 1992 Heterotopic gastrointestinal cyst of the oral cavity. J Oral Maxillofac Surg 50: 1340–1342
32. Mir R, Weitz, Evans J, Coren C 1992 Oral congenital cystic choristomas: a case report. Pediatr Pathol 12: 835–838
33. Lalwani AK, Lalwani RB, Bartlett PC 1993 Heterotopic gastric mucosal cyst of the tongue. Otolaryngol Head Neck Surg 108: 204–205
34. Surana R, Lsoty P, Fitzgerald RJ 1993 Heterotopic gastric cyst of the tongue in a newborn. Eur J Pediatr Surg 3: 110–111
35. Kinoshita Y, Honma Y, Otuka T, Shimura K 1994 Gastrointestinal mucosal cyst of the oral mucosa: report of a case and review of the literature. J Oral Maxillofac Surg 52: 1203–1205
36. Khunamornpong S, Yousukh A, Tnananuvat R 1996 Heterotopic gastrointestinal and pancreatic tissue of the tongue. A case report. Oral Surg Oral Med Oral Pathol Radiol Endod 81: 576–579
37. Lipsett J, Sparnon AL, Byard RW 1993 Embryogenesis of enterocystomas – enteric duplication cysts of the tongue. Oral Surg Oral Med Oral Pathol 75: 626–630

Metastatic tumors

55

Metastases in the jaws and soft tissues

Tumors can metastasize to the jaws, oral soft tissues, or salivary glands. Although the jaw is considerably less frequently involved than other bones, metastases are important because of the poor prognosis they carry.

Metastases to the jaws

Hirshberg et al[1] reviewed 390 well-documented reports of metastases to the jaws and found that in women (200 cases) the most common sites of primary tumors were breast (42%), adrenals (8.5%), genital organs (7.5%), and thyroid (6%). In men (184 cases), the most frequent sites of primary tumors were lungs (22.3%), prostate (12%) kidney (10.3%), bone (9.2%), and adrenals (9.2%).

CLINICAL FEATURES

Patients are usually middle-aged or elderly. Typical symptoms are pain, often severe, or swelling of the jaw. Paraesthesiae of the lip may be caused by involvement of a nerve trunk. The mandible is involved in over 80% of cases, particularly in the molar region. Although the maxilla was involved in only 13.6% (5.4% of metastases were in both jaws), in the cases reviewed by Hirshberg et al[1] localization there seemed to be related to the presence of teeth, which accounted for 93% of the maxillary cases. In the great majority (71%) the jaw deposit was recognized in the presence of a known primary neoplasm. However, in 37%, the jaw was the first recognized site of a metastasis and in 29.4% a deposit in the jaw formed the first sign of malignant disease.

RADIOGRAPHY

Typically, there is an area of radiolucency with a hazy outline (Fig. 55.1). It sometimes simulates an infected cyst, may be quite irregular and simulate osteomyelitis, or the entire mandible may have a moth-eaten appearance. Sclerotic areas may, rarely, be the

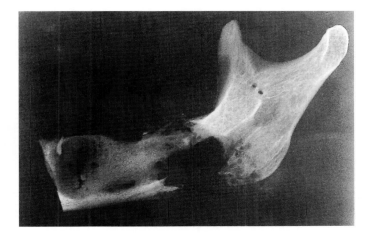

Fig. 55.1 Metastatic carcinoma. Radiography of the gross autopsy specimen shows a rounded but ill-defined area of radiolucency and pathological fracture of the mandible.

main feature, particularly prostatic cancer. Remarkably, Hirshberg et al[1] noted that in 5.4%, radiographs showed no pathological changes.

MICROSCOPY

Secondary deposits reproduce the histological pattern of the primary neoplasm and, as a result, there is a heavy preponderance of adenocarcinomas. Bone destruction by osteoclasts near the periphery of the deposit is the most common effect, but bone sclerosis can result particularly from metastases from the prostate. The latter are associated with raised prostate-specific antigen and acid phosphatase levels (Figs 55.2 and 55.3).

Examples of unusual metastases to the jaws include chordoma,[2] hepatocellular carcinoma,[3] mesothelioma,[4,5] malignant cystosarcoma phyllodes,[6] and neuroblastoma.[7] As noted in Chapter 47, Patton et al[8] in their analysis of 809 cases of metastases of malignant melanoma found that 15 had been in the oral soft tissues or jaws.

Some sarcomas, particularly Ewing's sarcoma, can metastasize to other bones, but the jaws are rarely involved.

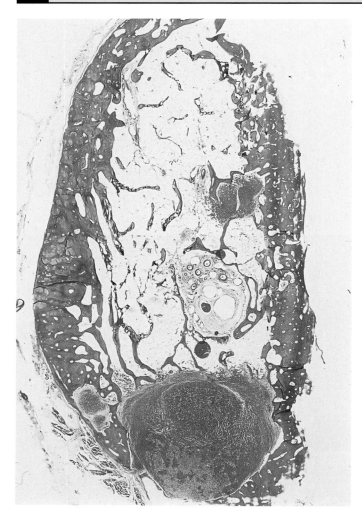

Fig. 55.2 Metastatic carcinoma below the inferior dental neurovascular bundle of the mandible.

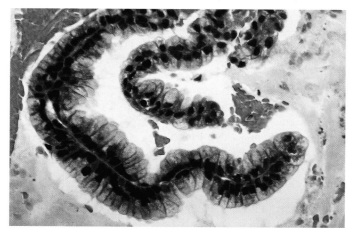

Fig. 55.3 Metastatic mucinous adenocarcinoma from the gut.

BEHAVIOR AND MANAGEMENT

Biopsy of the mass in the jaw will usually indicate whether it is a metastasis, and this may also be suggested by the history, especially of previous operations. General examination and radiographs of the rest of the skeleton may show other deposits. Blood examination is necessary to exclude anemia due to marrow replacement by metastases.

The primary tumor should be treated if this is still feasible, but bony metastases are a sign of bloodstream spread and only palliative treatment may be possible. Hirshberg et al[1] found that the mean time to death after recognition of metastases was only 7.3 months. However, they noted that most cases of jaw metastases had been reported before 1979. This poor prognosis may have changed as a result of improvements in treatment. Local irradiation may make the patient more comfortable and cause the tumor to regress for a time. Should the deposit fungate into the oral cavity or face, cryosurgery may help to control pain and hemorrhage, and reduce bulk.

Metastases to the oral soft tissues

Hatziotis et al[9] reported a granulosa cell carcinoma that had metastasized to the palatal gingiva, and found 48 cases of metastases to the oral soft tissues reported between 1945 and 1970. The primary tumors were most frequently carcinomas, but included a chondrosarcoma, chorionepithelioma, angiosarcoma, and retinoblastoma. Nineteen of these 48 deposits were in the gingiva or alveolar mucosa and 11 were in the tongue.

Hirshberg et al,[10] from an analysis of 157 reports of metastases to the oral soft tissues, found that men were more frequently affected (62%), and the most frequent primary sites in men were the lung (35.5%), kidney (16%), and skin (15%). In women, the most frequent primary sites were the breast (24%) and genital organs (17%). Thus, renal cell carcinoma, a relatively uncommon tumor, was overall the second most frequent source of oral soft tissue metastases in men.

Clinically, these metastases most frequently affected the gingiva or alveolar mucosa (55%) and tongue (27%), and generally resembled hyperplastic or reactive lesions, such as pyogenic granulomas, giant cell granulomas, or fibrous epulides. Ulceration was uncommon and noted in only 10% (Figs 55.4 and 55.5).

BEHAVIOR AND MANAGEMENT

While a destructive lesion in the jaws is likely to lead to consideration of the possibility of a malignant tumor as the cause, oral soft tissue metastases are far more deceptive in their clinical appearance. The need for histological confirmation of the nature of all oral soft tissue masses cannot be overemphasized, especially

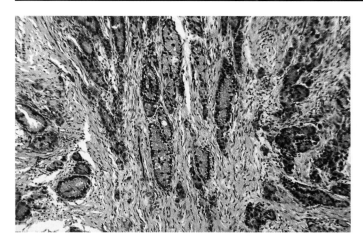

Fig. 55.4 Oral soft tissue metastasis from a gastric carcinoma.

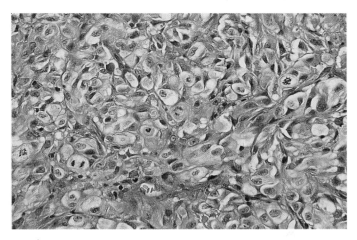

Fig. 55.5 Metastasis to the tongue. This illustrates some of the hazards of diagnosis by immunohistochemistry. The tumor was prostate-specific-antigen positive, but prostate biopsy showed no tumor and the metastasis proved to be a renal cell carcinoma, despite the paucity of clear cells.

as the oral metastasis preceded the diagnosis of the primary tumor in over 20% of the cases analyzed by Hirshberg et al.[10]

As with metastases to the jaws, those to the oral soft tissues are the result of bloodstream spread. In 10 cases of gingival metastases analyzed by Ellis et al,[11] survival after detection ranged from a mere 10 days to 29 months.

REFERENCES

1. Hirshberg A, Leibovich P, Buchner A 1994 Metastatic tumors to the jaw bones: analysis of 390 cases. J Oral Pathol Med 23: 337–341
2. Gorsky M, Silverman S, Greenspan D, Deluchi S, Merrell P 1983 Metastatic chordoma to the mandible. Oral Surg Oral Med Oral Pathol 55: 601–604
3. Barrera-Franco JL, Flores-Flores G, Mosquedo-Taylor A 1993 Mandibular metastasis as the first manifestation of hepatocellular carcinoma: report of a case and review of the literature. J Oral Maxillofac Surg 51: 318–321
4. Sproat CP, Brown AE, Lindley RP 1993 Oral metastasis in malignant pleural mesothelioma. Br J Oral Maxillofac Surg 31: 316–317
5. Kerpel SM, Freedman PD 1993 Metastatic mesothelioma of the oral cavity. Report of two cases. Oral Surg Oral Med Oral Pathol 76: 746–751
6. Yoshimura Y, Inoue Y, Mihara Y, Miura H 1991 Metastatic malignant cystosarcoma phyllodes. Report of a case presenting with an oral tumour and review of the literature. J Cranio Max Fac Surg 19: 227–231
7. Borle RM, Hazare VK, Bhowate RR, Borle SR 1991 Neuroblastoma metastatic to the mandible. J Oral Maxillofac Surg 49: 1124–1126
8. Patton LL, Brahim JS, Baker AR 1994 Metastatic malignant melanoma of the oral cavity. A retrospective study. Oral Surg Oral Med Oral Pathol 78: 51–56
9. Hatziotis JCh, Constaninou H, Papanayotou PH 1973 Metastatic tumors of the oral soft tissues. Oral Surg Oral Med Oral Pathol 36: 544–550
10. Hirshberg A, Leibovich P, Buchner A 1993 Metastases to the oral mucosa: analysis of 157 cases. J Oral Pathol Med 22: 385–390
11. Ellis GL, Jensen JL, Reingold IM, Barr RJ 1977 Malignant neoplasms metastatic to the gingivae. Oral Surg Oral Med Oral Pathol 44: 238–245

Index

Note: Page reference in *italics* refer to Figures; those in **bold** refer to Tables